the Elements

		IIIA	IVA	VA	VIA	VIIA	VIIIA or 0
							2 Helium **He** 4.00
		5 Boron **B** 10.81	6 Carbon **C** 12.01	7 Nitrogen **N** 14.01	8 Oxygen **O** 16.00	9 Fluorine **F** 19.00	10 Neon **Ne** 20.18
		13 Aluminum **Al** 26.98	14 Silicon **Si** 28.09	15 Phosphorus **P** 30.97	16 Sulfur **S** 32.06	17 Chlorine **Cl** 35.45	18 Argon **Ar** 39.95
IB	IIB						
29 Copper **Cu** 63.55	30 Zinc **Zn** 65.38	31 Gallium **Ga** 69.72	32 Germanium **Ge** 72.59	33 Arsenic **As** 74.92	34 Selenium **Se** 78.96	35 Bromine **Br** 79.90	36 Krypton **Kr** 83.80
47 Silver **Ag** 107.87	48 Cadmium **Cd** 112.41	49 Indium **In** 114.82	50 Tin **Sn** 118.69	51 Antimony **Sb** 121.75	52 Tellurium **Te** 127.60	53 Iodine **I** 126.90	54 Xenon **Xe** 131.30
79 Gold **Au** 196.97	80 Mercury **Hg** 200.59	81 Thallium **Tl** 204.37	82 Lead **Pb** 207.2	83 Bismuth **Bi** 208.98	84 Polonium **Po** (210)	85 Astatine **At** (210)	86 Radon **Rn** (222)

1s
2p
3p
4p
5p
6p
p

64 Gadolinium **Gd** 157.25	65 Terbium **Tb** 158.93	66 Dysprosium **Dy** 162.50	67 Holmium **Ho** 164.93	68 Erbium **Er** 167.26	69 Thulium **Tm** 168.93	70 Ytterbium **Yb** 173.04	71 Lutetium **Lu** 174.97

96 Curium **Cm** (247)	97 Berkelium **Bk** (247)	98 Californium **Cf** (251)	99 Einsteinium **Es** (254)	100 Fermium **Fm** (257)	101 Mendelevium **Md** (258)	102 Nobelium **No** (255)	103 Lawrencium **Lr** (260)

CHEMISTRY
FOR THE
Health Sciences

George I. Sackheim

Chemistry Instructor,
St. Francis Hospital School of Nursing, Evanston
Associate Professor Emeritus of Chemistry,
University of Illinois at Chicago Circle;
formerly Lecturer School of Health Sciences,
Michael Reese Hospital and Medical Center, Chicago
Coordinator of Biological and Physical Sciences, School of Nursing,
Michael Reese Hospital and Medical Center, Chicago;
Science Instructor, School of Nursing,
Presbyterian-St. Luke's Hospital, Chicago

Dennis D. Lehman

Professor of Chemistry,
Loop College, Chicago;
Visiting Professor of Chemistry,
Northwestern University, Evanston
Lecturer in Biochemistry,
Northwestern University Medical School, Chicago

CHEMISTRY
FOR THE
Health Sciences

**FIFTH
EDITION**

MACMILLAN PUBLISHING COMPANY
NEW YORK

Collier Macmillan Publishers
London

Macmillan Publishing Company
866 Third Avenue, New York, New York 10022

Collier Macmillan Canada, Inc.

Library of Congress Cataloging in Publication Data

Sackheim, George I.
  Chemistry for the health sciences.

  Includes bibliographies and index.
1. Chemistry. 2. Medicine. I. Lehman, Dennis D.
II. Title. [DNLM: 1. Chemistry. 2. Medicine. QD 33
*S*121c]
QD33.S13 1985   540   83-25149
ISBN 0-02-405140-3

Printing: 2 3 4 5 6 7 8   Year: 5 6 7 8 9 0 1 2 3

ISBN 0-02-405140-3

Preface
to the Fifth Edition

This textbook of chemistry is designed primarily for first-year students in various health-related programs—nursing, dietetics, laboratory technology, inhalation therapy, dental hygiene, dental assisting, medical assisting, dental technology, and other health-service technologies. Emphasis is placed on *practical* aspects of inorganic chemistry, organic chemistry, and biochemistry. Theoretic topics are dealt with only as an aid to understanding bodily processes in the human.

Unit One, "Inorganic Chemistry," stresses relationships with the life processes dealt with in Unit Three, "Biochemistry." Included are discussions of the following topics:

Acids, bases, salts, and electrolytes, as related to acid-base balance and electrolyte balance in the body

Oxidation-reduction, as related to biologic oxidation-reduction reactions taking place in the mitochondria of cells

Solutions, for understanding the solvent action involved in digestion

Colloids, for understanding the particular nature and properties of proteins, amino acids, and nucleic acids

Covalent compounds, as related to the types of bonds that must be broken and rearranged in the formation of high-energy phosphate bonds

Emulsions, for understanding the need for emulsification of fats before digestion

Nuclear chemistry and radioactivity, for understanding the biologic effects of radiation on cells and organs

Unit Two, "Organic Chemistry," introduces the various classes of organic compounds—hydrocarbons, alcohols, ethers, aromatic compounds, and heterocyclic compounds. In addition, the text discussion relates such compounds to carbohydrates, fats, proteins, vitamins, and hormones.

Unit Three, "Biochemistry," deals with the chemical and molecular basis of life itself. It endeavors to explain the various chemical processes taking place in the body during its normal as well as its abnormal metabolism. The role of ATP, the principal direct source of energy for the body, is stressed throughout the various chapters on metabolism. The formation and decomposition of this compound, and the energies involved, serve to indicate the very complex processes that take place "normally." The role of coenzymes, such as CoA, is also emphasized, to show the role these substances play in metabolic cycles. Discussions of excesses and deficiencies of vitamins and hormones are designed to demonstrate the involved interrelationships in the body's metabolic processes. In the chapter on heredity the authors have endeavored to combine chemistry with the molecular basis of life, as evidenced by the many recent advances in our understanding of DNA structure and of the replication of DNA and RNA.

An outline appears at the beginning of each chapter, indicating the topics to be discussed and, in general, how they are interrelated. The summary at the end of each chapter is also designed to help the reader identify the particular important aspects of the subject matter. The student who wishes to know more about any specific topic will find additional information in the references appended to each chapter. Also at the end of each chapter is a set of questions, which may be used for oral review or assigned as homework. Answers to odd-numbered questions appear at the end of the book.

New to the fifth edition are

(not in order of importance nor in sequence)
Thioesters, thiols, phosphate esters
Sources of hydrocarbons
Octane ratings
Normality and titration
Polar vs nonpolar liquids
Parts per million
Milliequivalents per liter
Diffusion and active transport
Balancing oxidation-reduction equations
Hydrogen peroxide; superoxides
Hypothermia and hyperthermia
Measurement of pressure
Molar gas volumes
Acid rain
Empirical and molecular formulas
Sizes of ions
Energy sublevels in atomic structure
Update on topics involving radioactivity
Update on actions of vitamins
Plasma substitutes
Plasma lipids
Hyperalimentation
Additional material on gluconeogenesis
Additional material on enzyme activity including induced-fit theory

Additional material on glycoproteins, electrophoresis, eicosanoids pro-
stacyclin, thromboxanes, leukotrienes
Material on cell membranes including fluid-mosaic model
Comparison of sweetness of compounds
Additional material on hydroquinones and coenzyme Q
Redrawing of aromatic compounds with greater emphasis on bond angles
New Material on isozymes, allosteric enzymes, zymogens.

A comprehensive set of laboratory experiments (Sackheim–Lehman, *Laboratory Chemistry for the Health Sciences,* Macmillan Publishing Company, New York) has been designed to implement and supplement the various topics in the textbook. These experiments are keyed to specific chapters and, when performed, will aid the student in understanding the fundamental concepts involved. Also available to the instructor is a helpful *Answer and Test Manual for Chemistry for the Health Sciences* (Macmillan Publishing Company, New York).

G. I. S.
D. D. L.

Acknowledgments

Many reviewers have given us invaluable criticism in the four editions prior to this one, and we would like to thank them again here. For their comments specifically for this fifth edition the authors would like to thank Professors Ronald Chriss, Western Connecticut State College (Danbury, Connecticut); Ronald DiStefano, Northampton County Community College (Bethlehem, Pennsylvania); Brodie T. Estes, Memphis State University (Memphis, Tennessee); Jack Grogan, West Georgia College (Carrollton, Georgia); Morris Lieff and Arthur Lurie, County College of Morris (Dover, New Jersey); David F. McCormick, Sinclair Community College (Dayton, Ohio); Richard J. Margelis, Kalamazoo Valley Community College (Kalamazoo, Michigan); Theodore Richerzhagen, Walla Walla Community College (Walla Walla, Washington); and Don Roach, Miami-Dade Community College (Miami, Florida).

Special thanks to Mrs. Fay E. Bennett, R.N., B.S., M.A., who gave freely of her time in reviewing the text and suggesting improvements in content.

Contents

UNIT I
Inorganic Chemistry

1	Units of Measurement	2
2	Properties of Matter	13
3	Structure of Matter	28
4	Radioactivity	42
5	Chemical Bonding	72
6	Chemical Equations and Reactions	90
7	The Gaseous State	102
8	Oxygen and Other Gases	117
9	Oxidation-Reduction	131
10	Water	141
11	Liquid Mixtures	158
12	Ionization	186
13	Acids and Bases	192
14	Salts	204

UNIT II
Organic Chemistry

15	Introduction to Organic Chemistry	214
16	Hydrocarbons	221
17	Alcohols and Ethers	240
18	Other Organic Compounds	250

19   Aromatic Compounds   269
20   Heterocyclic Compounds   286

Unit III
Biochemistry

21   Carbohydrates   298
22   Lipids   322
23   Proteins   346
24   Enzymes   370
25   Digestion   386
26   Carbohydrate Metabolism   396
27   Metabolism of Fats   416
28   Metabolism of Proteins   425
29   Body Fluids: Urine   436
30   Body Fluids: The Blood   448
31   Vitamins   479
32   Hormones   503
33   Heredity   526

APPENDICES

A   Exponential Numbers   546
B   Functional Groups   548
C   Glossary   549

ANSWERS TO ODD-NUMBERED QUESTIONS   553

INDEX   577

CHEMISTRY
FOR THE
Health Sciences

UNIT I
Inorganic Chemistry

1 Units of Measurement

CHAPTER
OUTLINE

The Metric System and the International System
Mass and Weight
Fundamental Units
Derived Units

Conversion Units
Density
Specific Gravity
Temperature Scales

The Metric System and the International System

We use measurements every day of our lives. We measure gasoline by the gallon and milk by the quart; we buy meat by the pound and pay for postage by the ounce. A recipe may call for a cup of flour, a tablespoonful of butter, and $\frac{1}{4}$ teaspoonful of salt. In chemistry, all measurements are made in the metric system or in its expanded modernized version, the Systeme Internationale (SI). The main advantage of the metric system or SI is that it is a decimal system; that is, the units are all multiples of ten of larger or smaller units. In the English system there is no such common number. Recall that there are 3 feet in a yard, 4 quarts in a gallon, and 16 ounces in a pound.

Mass and Weight

The mass of an object is a measure of the amount of matter it contains. The weight of an object depends on the pull of gravity. Mass remains constant regardless of location, whereas weight can vary slightly from place to place on the surface of the earth. For our purposes, however, we will use the terms mass and weight interchangeably.

Fundamental Units

The fundamental unit of length in both the SI and the metric system is the meter. A **meter** is a little longer than a yard. The meter was originally defined as one ten-millionth of the distance of a meridian from the equator to the North Pole on a line passing through Paris. The standard meter was later defined as the length between two marks on a platinum-irridium bar kept at the temperature of melting ice and stored at the International Bureau of Weights and Measures near Paris. Subsequently the standard meter was redefined in terms of the orange-red wavelengths of light emitted by the element krypton-86. In October 1983 the General Conference on Weights and Measures defined the meter as the distance light travels in a vacuum in 1/299,792,458 of a second. The word meter is abbreviated as **m**.

The fundamental SI unit of mass (weight) is the **kilogram**. In the metric system the kilogram is also the fundamental unit of mass (weight), but the basic laboratory unit is the **gram**, abbreviated as **g**. A gram is $\frac{1}{454}$ of a pound.

The SI unit of volume is the **cubic meter**, abbreviated m^3.

The basic unit of volume in the metric system is the **liter** (usually spelled out or abbreviated as **L** or **l**). A liter is approximately equal to a quart.

The basic units most commonly used in medicine are the meter, the gram, and the liter. For this reason, these are the units used throughout this text.

Derived Units In both the SI and metric system, prefixes are used to designate various multiples or submultiples. The most commonly used prefixes are as follows:

milli- (abbreviated m), which means one thousandth   (0.001)
centi- (abbreviated c), which means one hundredth   (0.01)
deci- (abbreviated d), which means one tenth   (0.1)
kilo- (abbreviated k), which means one thousand   (1000)

Thus, a centidollar is 0.01 dollars, or one cent; a kilometer (km) is one thousand meters, or 1000 m; a centigram (cg) is 1/100 of a gram, or 0.01 g. Likewise, a milliliter (ml) is 0.001 L (see Table 1–1). Another unit of volume is the cubic centimeter (cm^3); 1 cm^3 is equal to 1 ml, so these two units may be used interchangeably. Although the term cubic centimeter is abbreviated as cm^3 by chemists, the older abbreviation cc is still in use medically.

Other prefixes used are mega- (abbreviated M), which means one million, and micro- (abbreviated μ or mc), which means one millionth. Thus a Mci (megacurie) means 1 million Ci and a μg or mcg (microgram) means

TABLE 1-1. Metric Conversions

Weight	
1 g = 1000 mg	one gram = one thousand milligrams
1 g = 100 cg	one gram = one hundred centigrams
1 g = 10 dg	one gram = ten decigrams
1 kg = 1000 g	one kilogram = one thousand grams

Length	
1 m = 1000 mm	one meter = one thousand millimeters
1 m = 100 cm	one meter = one hundred centimeters
1 m = 10 dm	one meter = ten decimeters
1 km = 1000 m	one kilometer = one thousand meters

Volume	
1 L = 1000 ml	one liter = one thousand milliliters
1 L = 100 cl	one liter = one hundred centiliters
1 L = 10 dl	one liter = ten deciliters
1 kl = 1000 L	one kiloliter = one thousand liters

0.000001 g. Note that the letter m indicates both meter and milli-; however, when used by itself, it indicates meters.

Conversion Units Frequently we need to convert from one system of measurement to another (see Figure 1–1 and Table 1–2). This will no longer be necessary when the United States is fully converted to the SI or to metric system. The procedure is the same when converting from one system to another or within the English system. Consider, for example, the following English units:

$$12 \text{ in.} = 1 \text{ ft}$$

$$3 \text{ ft} = 1 \text{ yd}$$

$$1760 \text{ yd} = 1 \text{ mile}$$

FIGURE 1-1. Comparison of English and metric units ($\frac{1}{2}$ scale).

TABLE 1-2. English-Metric Conversion Factors

1 in. = 2.54 cm
1 lb = 454 g
2.2 lb = 1 kg
1.06 qt = 1 L

FIGURE 1-2. Use of metric units in various medical examples. (a) Courtesy of Merck Sharp & Dohme; (b) Courtesy of E. R. Squibb & Sons, Inc.; (c) Courtesy of Smith Kline & French Laboratories; (d) Courtesy of Travenol Laboratories, Inc.; (e) Courtesy of Becton-Dickinson, Division of Becton Dickinson and Company, Rutherford, New Jersey 07070.)

Units of Measurement

When asked to convert 6 ft to inches, many students merely multiply by 12. However, mathematically, the correct procedure is to multiply by the conversion unit 12 in./1 ft so that the result is correct both numerically and in units.

$$6 \text{ ft} = 6 \text{ ft} \times \frac{12 \text{ in.}}{1 \text{ ft}} = 72 \text{ in.}$$

Likewise, to convert 3.58 m to millimeters (mm), first recall that there are 1000 mm in a meter. The procedure is to multiply by 1000 mm/1 m. The unwanted units cancel, leaving the answer in millimeters, as desired.

$$3.58 \text{ m} = 3.58 \text{ m} \times \frac{1000 \text{ mm}}{1 \text{ m}} = 3580 \text{ mm}$$

(Note that if the 3.58 m were divided by the conversion unit of 1000 mm/1 m the units would not cancel, indicating an error in computation.)

When converting 20 in. to centimeters, the conversion factor 1 in. = 2.54 cm should be used (see Table 1–2). Thus

$$20 \text{ in.} = 20 \text{ in.} \times \frac{2.54 \text{ cm}}{1 \text{ in.}} = 50.8 \text{ cm}$$

Likewise, when converting 55 lb to kilograms, the conversion factor 2.2 lb = 1 kg should be used. Thus

$$55 \text{ lb} = 55 \text{ lb} \times \frac{1 \text{ kg}}{2.2 \text{ lb}} = 23 \text{ kg}$$

Density   The density of an object helps to characterize it physically and is defined as its mass (or weight) divided by its volume (see Figure 1–3). Density may be expressed by the following formula

$$D = \frac{M}{V}$$

where D is the density, M is the mass, and V the volume. Density must have units of mass and volume such as g/ml, g/cm^3, lb/ft^3, mg/L, or others.

EXAMPLE 1–1. What is the density of the mercury in a thermometer if 31.2 g of it occupy 2.29 ml?

$$D = \frac{M}{V}$$

$$= \frac{31.2 \text{ g}}{2.29 \text{ ml}} = 13.6 \frac{\text{g}}{\text{ml}}$$

Inorganic Chemistry   **6**

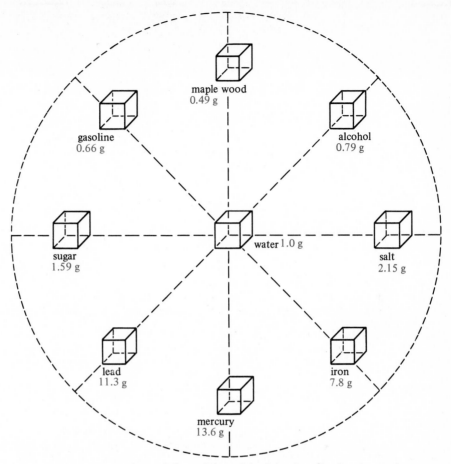

FIGURE 1-3. A comparison of the weights of 1 ml (or 1 cm³) of various substances.

EXAMPLE 1-2. Alcohol has a density of 0.80 g/ml. How much will 100 ml of it weigh?

$$D = \frac{M}{V}$$

$$M = D \times V$$

$$= 0.80\,\frac{g}{ml} \times 100\ ml = 80\ g \quad\blacksquare$$

Specific Gravity   Specific gravity (Sp.Gr.) is defined as the weight of an object compared to the weight of an equal volume of water, or also as the density of an object compared to the density of water (which is 1 g/ml). Specific gravity may be expressed mathematically as

$$\text{specific gravity} = \frac{\text{density of object}}{\text{density of water}}$$

Units of Measurement   **7**

EXAMPLE 1–3. The density of mercury is 13.6 g/ml. What is its specific gravity?

$$\text{specific gravity} = \frac{\text{density of object}}{\text{density of water}} = \frac{13.6 \text{ g/ml}}{1 \text{ g/ml}} = 13.6$$

Note that the specific gravity and the density (in the metric system) have the same number, but density has units whereas specific gravity does not. Thus, if an object has a density of 1.5 g/ml, its specific gravity will be 1.5; likewise, an object of specific gravity 0.75 will have a density of 0.75 g/ml. ■

The specific gravity of normal human urine ranges from 1.003 to 1.030. Values outside this range are of diagnostic value. For example, the urine of a person suffering from diabetes mellitus contains large amounts of sugar and thus will have a specific gravity greater than normal. Conversely, a person suffering from diabetes insipidus will have a urine specific gravity close to 1.000 because of the large amount of water being excreted (see page 438).

Temperature Scales

Temperature is a measure of the availability of heat or cold, or in simpler terms, of how hot or cold a substance is. It can be measured by means of a thermometer. When we speak of body temperature as being 98.6° or when we say that the outside temperature is 80° or 40° or even 2° below zero, we are usually speaking in terms of degrees Fahrenheit (F) even though we may not express the unit itself. In chemistry, the Celsius or centigrade (C) and the Kelvin (K) temperature scales are commonly used. Let us see first how the Celsius and the Fahrenheit temperature scales compare with one another.

If a Fahrenheit and a Celsius thermometer are placed in a mixture of ice and water, the reading on the Fahrenheit scale will be 32° and the reading on the Celsius scale 0° (see Figure 1–4)—that is, 32°F corresponds to 0°C. These temperatures indicate the freezing point of water. They also indicate the melting point of ice.

Next, if the same two thermometers are placed in boiling water at one atmosphere pressure, the reading on the Fahrenheit scale will be 212° and the reading on the Celsius scale will be 100°. These temperatures indicate the boiling point of water.

Thus, there is a 180-degree difference between the boiling and the freezing points of water on the Fahrenheit scale (212° to 32°) and a 100-degree difference between the boiling and freezing points of water on the Celsius scale (100° to 0°). The difference between the freezing points of water on the Fahrenheit and Celsius scales is 32° (32° − 0°).

This information may be combined into the following formulas.

$$°F = \frac{9}{5}°C + 32° \quad \text{and} \quad °C = \frac{5}{9}(°F - 32°)$$

boiling point of water — 212° → 100° — 373

180 scale divisions

100 scale divisions

100 scale divisions

freezing point of water — 32° → 0° — 273

Fahrenheit

Celsius (centigrade)

Kelvin

FIGURE 1-4. Comparison of Fahrenheit, Celsius, and Kelvin temperature scales.

The first formula is used to change Celsius temperatures to the corresponding Fahrenheit readings; the second formula is used to do the reverse, to change Fahrenheit readings to Celsius. Note that the first formula may be changed to the second by subtracting 32° from both sides and then dividing by $\frac{9}{5}$.

EXAMPLE 1-4. Change 80°C to °F.
Using the formula $°F = \frac{9}{5}°C + 32°$

$$°F = \frac{9}{5}(80°) + 32°$$

$$= 144° + 32°$$

$$= 176°$$

Thus,

$$80°C = 176°F \qquad ■$$

EXAMPLE 1-5. Change 50°F to °C.
Using the formula $°C = \frac{5}{9}(°F - 32)$

$$°C = \tfrac{5}{9}(50° - 32°)$$

$$= \tfrac{5}{9}(18°)$$

$$= 10°$$

Thus,

$$50°F = 10°C \qquad ■$$

A Kelvin thermometer will indicate the freezing point of water as 273 K and the boiling point of water as 373 K. Temperatures on the Kelvin scale are given as numbers only, without the degree sign. Why pick 273 K for the freezing point of water? Why not some even number? This temperature was selected so that zero on the Kelvin scale would represent the lowest temperature it is possible to reach. This temperature, 0 K, is also called **absolute zero.**

There are 100 units between the boiling and freezing points of water on the Kelvin scale (373 K − 273 K), just as there were on the Celsius scale. The difference between the freezing points of water on the Kelvin and Celsius scales is 273 (273 − 0). This information may be combined into the following formula:

$$K = °C + 273$$

EXAMPLE 1-6. Change 37°C to K.
Using the formula $K = °C + 273$

$$K = 37 + 273$$

$$= 310$$

Thus,

$$37°C = 310 \text{ K} \qquad ■$$

Summary
The SI units of length, mass (weight), and volume are the meter (m), the kilogram (kg), and the cubic meter (m³), respectively. The units of length, weight, and volume in the metric system are the meter (m), the gram (g), and the liter (L) respectively. Prefixes in common use in the metric system are the following: milli- (1/1000), centi- (1/100), deci (1/10), kilo- (1000).

Density is defined as mass divided by volume, or $D = M/V$.

Specific gravity is defined as the density of a substance compared to the density of water.

Although Fahrenheit and Celsius temperature scales are in common use, the Celsius (centigrade) temperature scale is the one used almost exclusively in scientific measurements.

To convert Fahrenheit temperatures to Celsius, use the formula $°C = \tfrac{5}{9}(°F - 32°)$. To convert Celsius temperature to Fahrenheit, use the formula $°F = \tfrac{9}{5}°C + 32°$. To convert Celsius temperature to Kelvin temperature, use the formula $K = °C + 273$.

Questions and Problems

A

1. Body temperature is 98.6°F. What is it in Celsius?
2. Which patient has a higher fever, one with a temperature of 101°F or one with a temperature of 38.2°C?
3. At the top of a certain mountain, water boils at 85°C. What is the Fahrenheit boiling point? the Kelvin?
4. If the water in a pressure cooker boils at 250°F, what will be the Celsius boiling point? the Kelvin?
5. Compare the following units: ml and cm^3.
6. What is the SI standard of length? the metric? the English?
7. What is the SI standard of mass and of volume? the metric?
8. What do the following prefixes indicate: milli-, deci-, kilo-, centi-?
9. What do the following abbreviations indicate: g, cm, mm, kl, m?
10. Convert the following:

    (a) 87.6 mm =   m   (b) 2.5 L =   ml
    (c) 375 ml =   L   (d) 1.76 g =   mg
    (e) 30.6 m =   dm   (f) 394 cg =   g
    (g) 16.4 cm =   m   (g) 0.54 kl =   L
    (i) 1.02 g =   kg   (j) 500 cm^3 =   ml

11. Convert the following (answers to one decimal place):

    (a) 20 in. =   cm   (b) 22 lb =   kg
    (c) 19.4 kg =   lb   (d) 63.5 cm =   in.
    (e) 10 cm =   in.   (f) 50 kg =   lb
    (g) 5 ft 4 in. =   cm   (h) 176 lb =   kg

B

12. A patient is 5 ft 10 in. tall and weighs 160 lb. What is his height in centimeters and his weight in kilograms?
13. The following information was recorded for a patient: height 152.5 cm, weight 68 kg, temperature 37.2°C. What would be the readings in inches, pounds, and degrees Fahrenheit?
14. What is the density of a medication if the contents of a filled 2-ml syringe weigh 2.50 g?
15. Normal urine has a density between 1.003 g/ml and 1.030 g/ml. Assuming a value of 1.020 g/ml, what will be the weight of a 250-ml sample of urine?
16. An object has a specific gravity of 3.06. What is its density in the metric system?
17. Mercury has a density of 13.6 g/ml. What volume will 200 g of it occupy?
18. An order for a medication reads: "Give 1.5 mg per kilogram of body weight." How much medication should be given to a patient weighing 165 lb?
19. What do the following mean in terms of known units: kilowatts, milliseconds, megacuries, microamperes?
20. An infant weighs 7000 g. How many kilograms does the infant weigh? How many pounds?
21. A rectangular object is 25 cm tall, 15 cm wide, and 10 cm deep. What is its volume in cubic centimeters, liters, and kiloliters?
22. Using Figure 1–3, what is the specific gravity of lead? Salt?
23. Compare weight and mass.
24. An order for a medication reads: "Give 0.04 ml per kilogram of body weight." How much medication should be given to a patient weighing 110 lb?
25. An order for a medication reads: "Give 0.6 mg per kilogram of body weight." How much medication should be given to a patient weighing 131 lb? Give the answer to the closest whole number of milligrams.

References DICKSON, T. R. *Introduction to Chemistry,* 4th ed. John Wiley & Sons, Inc., New York, 1983, Chapter 1.

EBBING, DARRELL D. *General Chemistry.* Houghton Mifflin Co., Boston, 1984, Chapter 1.

MILLER, FRANCIS MARION. *Chemistry, Structure and Dynamics.* McGraw Hill Book Co., New York, 1984, Chapter 1.

MORTIMER, CHARLES E. *Chemistry,* 5th ed. Wadsworth Pub. Co., Belmont, Calif., 1983, Chapter 1.

PETRUCCI, RALPH H. and ROBERT K. WISMER, *General Chemistry with Qualitative Analysis.* Macmillan Publishing Company, New York, 1983, Chapter 1.

RAYNER-CANHAM, GEOFFREY and MARK VAN ROODE. *Foundations of Chemistry.* Addison-Wesley Publishing Co., Reading, Mass., 1983, Chapter 2.

SACKHEIM, GEORGE I. *Chemical Calculations,* 12th ed. Series B. Stipes Publishing Co., Champaign, Ill., 1983, Chapter 2.

STOKER, H. STEPHEN. *Introduction to Chemical Principles.* Macmillan Publishing Company, New York, 1983, Chapter 3.

2 Properties of Matter

CHAPTER
OUTLINE

What Is Matter?
States of Matter
Changes of State
Properties of Matter
  Physical Properties
  Chemical Properties
  Comparison of Physical and Chemical
    Properties
Energy
  Kinetic Energy

Potential Energy
Transformation of Energy
Conservation of Energy and Matter
Measurement of Energy
Composition of Matter
  Elements
  Compounds
  Mixtures

What Is Matter? Matter is anything that occupies space and has weight. Everything we see or feel is matter, as well as many things we cannot see or feel. Such things as trees, food, machinery, and soil are examples of matter we can see and feel. Air is an example of matter we cannot see, yet we know that it is all around us. However, not all matter is of the same type. Matter can be classified as solid, liquid, or gas.

States of Matter A piece of iron is an example of matter in the solid state. A bar of iron has a definite shape, a shape that cannot be easily changed. The volume of the piece of iron (the amount of space that it occupies) is a definite volume; it cannot easily be changed. Also, the piece of iron does not flow.

When a pint of water is poured from a container of one shape into a container of another shape, the water (a liquid) assumes the shape of the new container as far as it fills it. However, the volume of the water remains the same—1 pt—regardless of the shape of the container into which it is poured (see Figure 2–1).

When air is pumped into an empty bottle, the air occupies all of the space and also takes the shape of the container. Forcing more air into the bottle will increase the pressure, but the air will still occupy all of the space and take the shape of the container. If the air is transferred to another bottle of different shape and size, again the air will occupy all of the space and take the shape of the container.

Figure 2-1. The same quantity (1 pint or approximately 500 ml) of water in variously shaped containers.

In most solids, the particles are closely adhering and tightly packed in a highly ordered system. The motion of the particles is highly restricted. (Figure 2–2a). These factors account for the fact that solids have a definite shape and resist changes in that shape. Tight packing also accounts for incompressibility of solids. Heating allows the particles in a solid to move about slightly. Therefore, most solids expand on heating.

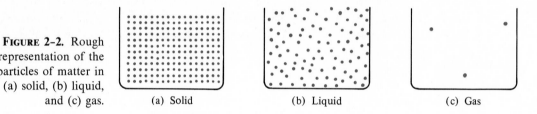

Figure 2-2. Rough representation of the particles of matter in (a) solid, (b) liquid, and (c) gas.

(a) Solid (b) Liquid (c) Gas

In liquids, the particles are moderately ordered (but still in contact with each other) and farther apart than the particles in solids (see Figure 2–2b). This loose structure accounts for the fact that liquids flow and have no definite shape. The particles in a liquid are close enough to resist compression. Liquids expand slightly on heating.

In gases, the motion of the particles is unrestricted so that the particles are independent of one another and are relatively very far apart (see Figure 2–2c). This independence allows gases to assume any shape or volume, to be compressed or expanded.

Some solids have a high density (gold, 19.3 g/ml), whereas others have a low density (cork, 0.2 g/ml). Many liquids have a relatively low density (water, 1 g/ml; gasoline, 0.66 g/ml), but some such as mercury (13.6 g/ml) have a high density. All gases have a very low density, expressed in the units grams per liter (g/L) (air, 1.3 g/L; hydrogen, 0.09 g/L). In summary:

1. Solids have a definite shape and a definite volume, do not flow, and have particles that are closely adhering (interacting) and tightly packed in a highly ordered system. The motion of the particles in solids is highly restricted so that solids generally are incompressible. Most solids expand slightly when heated and may exhibit high or low density.
2. Liquids have no definite shape, do have a definite volume, flow, have particles that are relatively close to one another and are moderately

ordered with some interaction, and may have high or low density. Liquids are incompressible and expand slightly when heated.

3. Gases have no definite shape and no definite volume, flow, and have particles whose motion is unrestricted so that they are independent and relatively far apart. Gases have a low density, are highly compressible, and expand greatly when heated.

Changes of State   Consider a piece of solid material. It consists of particles in a definite arrangement, as indicated in the preceding section. These particles are not motionless—they vibrate about fixed points. As heat is added to the solid, the temperature rises (see Figure 2–3,A). Because of the increased temperature, the rate of vibration increases and the particles move slightly farther apart. Eventually, a point is reached when the vibrating particles can no longer retain their orderly arrangement. When this occurs, the solid begins to melt and becomes a liquid. The temperature at which this occurs is called the **melting point** of the solid. As more heat is added, more of the solid melts. All of the heat being added is used to change the state from solid to liquid. This is indicated by plateau B on Figure 2–3, showing that there is a constant temperature while the solid is changing to a liquid (melting).

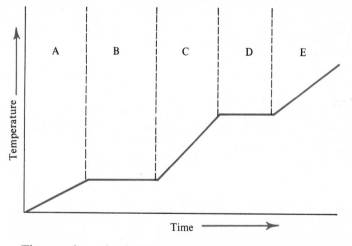

FIGURE 2–3. Temperature-time diagram. Section A indicates heating of the solid; section B, a change of state from solid to liquid; section C, heating of the liquid; section D, a change of state from liquid to gas; section E, heating of the gas.

The number of calories required to change 1 g of solid to liquid at the melting point is called the **heat of fusion.** The heat of fusion of ice is 80 cal/g.

After all of the solid has melted, additional heat causes the temperature of the liquid to rise (Figure 2–3,C). The particles move faster and also move farther apart. Soon a point is reached at which the particles move far enough apart to become independent of one another. When this occurs, the liquid changes to a gas; it boils. The temperature at which this occurs is called the **boiling point** of the liquid. As more heat is added, more of the liquid boils but all of the heat being added is used to change the state from liquid to gas. Thus the temperature remains constant during boiling (Figure 2–3,D).

Properties of Matter   **15**

The number of calories required to change 1 g of liquid to gas at the boiling point is called the **heat of vaporization.** The heat of vaporization of water is 540 cal/g. Water has a very high heat of vaporization. Steam will therefore cause a much more severe burn than boiling water because of its much higher heat content. Once all the liquid has boiled, additional heat increases the temperature of the gas (Figure 2–3,E).

The reverse steps are also possible. A gas can be cooled to become a liquid. Further cooling of that liquid changes it into a solid.

In general, then, matter can usually be changed from one state to another merely by changing its temperature. Such changes are called **physical changes.** A physical change is one in which no new substance is produced, although there may be a change of state or density, or both.

However, not all substances can be changed from solid to liquid to gas merely by changing the temperature. For example, a piece of wood bursts into flame when heated sufficiently; it does not become liquid. Dry ice changes from solid to gas without becoming a liquid.

Other examples of physical changes are dissolving salt in water, breaking a sheet of glass, and freezing water. In each of these changes, no new substance has been produced. Each substance retains its own properties. Note that in the last example there has been a change both in state and density, since the density of water is 1.00 g/ml and that of ice 0.917 g/ml.

The other type of change that matter can undergo is called a **chemical change.** A chemical change is one in which one or more substances disappear and a new substance or new substances are formed. The new substance or substances have entirely different properties than the original substance or substances.

Burning a piece of wood is an example of a chemical change. New substances—ash and smoke—are produced. These substances have properties different from those of the original piece of wood. Chemical changes are also involved in cooking food and in digestion.

Properties of Matter

One portion of matter can be distinguished from another by means of its properties. These distinguishing properties of matter may be classified into two main types: **physical properties** and **chemical properties.**

Physical Properties

Physical properties include color, odor, taste, solubility in water, density, hardness, melting point, and boiling point. These physical properties can serve to identify a substance, although not all of these properties may be necessary for the identification. For example, when we say that the color of a substance is white, we automatically eliminate all substances that are not white. Next, if we say that the white substance is odorless, we can eliminate all white objects that have an odor, leaving a smaller number of substances that are both white and odorless. If we continue to eliminate in this manner by using additional physical properties, such as density, hardness, melting point, and boiling point, eventually only one substance will fit all of these properties—the substance we are trying to identify.

Chemical Properties   Properties such as reacting (or not reacting) in air, reacting (or not reacting) with an acid, or burning (or not burning) in a flame are chemical properties. A substance can be identified by means of its chemical properties, but it is usually much simpler to do so by means of the physical properties.

Comparison of Physical and Chemical Properties   A physical property tells what a substance *is*—it is white or it is green; it is odorless or it has a sharp odor; it is hard or it is soft. A chemical property tells what a substance *does*—it burns or it does not burn; it reacts with an acid or it does not react with an acid, and so on.

Energy   Energy is defined as the ability to do work. The muscles in our bodies get their energy from the chemical reactions that take place in the muscle cells. The heat energy necessary to keep our bodies at a temperature of 98.6°F or 37°C comes from the oxidation of the foods we eat. The electrical energy we use in our homes comes from burning a fuel or from atomic energy. Energy exists in several forms—heat, light, electrical, mechanical, sound, chemical, and atomic. Energy may be classified int two categories: **kinetic energy** and **potential energy.**

Kinetic Energy   Kinetic energy is energy of motion; that is, energy that is doing something now, such as heat energy obtained from burning wood, light energy from an incandescent lamp, mechanical energy from a motor, and atomic energy from a nuclear reactor.

Potential Energy   Potential energy is stored energy, energy not associated with motion. Examples of potential energy are a dry cell (which can supply electrical energy when it is connected to something), food (which supplies energy to our bodies when it is metabolized), and water at the top of a waterfall (which becomes kinetic energy that can supply mechanical energy as it falls to the bottom).

   Chemical energy is a form of potential energy. Most chemical reactions involve changes in heat energy. If heat is given off during a chemical reaction, that reaction is said to be **exothermic.** If heat is absorbed during a chemical reaction, that reaction is said to be **endothermic.**

Transformation of Energy   Energy may be transformed from one form into another. Thus, burning a piece of coal changes its potential energy into heat (kinetic) energy. The heat energy thus produced might be used to boil water, which produces large amounts of steam. The steam might be used to drive a generator to produce electrical energy. In turn, this electrical energy might be used to drive a motor (mechanical energy), produce light in a fluorescent lamp (light energy), operate a radio (sound energy), or operate a toaster (heat energy).

   The sun produces energy by nuclear reactions and radiates this energy to the earth. Plants on the earth pick up the light energy from the sun during the process of photosynthesis and produce compounds that contain chemical energy. When humans eat these compounds in the plants, their bodies convert the chemical energy into heat energy and mechanical energy.

Conservation of Energy and Matter

The **law of conservation of energy** states that energy is neither created nor destroyed during a chemical reaction. Energy can be changed from one form to another, but the total amount of energy remains the same regardless of what form the energy is changed into.

The **law of conservation of matter** states that during a chemical reaction matter is neither created nor destroyed. This means that the total weights of substances before they react should be the same as the weights of the products after they react. For example, if a candle is placed in a sealed container, a certain weight will be obtained for both the candle and the container. If the candle is lit and allowed to burn (inside the sealed container) and if it is weighed as it continues to burn, the weight will be found to remain the same even though part of the candle is disappearing and several gaseous products are being produced. The same is true for a camera flashbulb before and after it is fired. Other experiments performed under very carefully controlled conditions have produced similar results—that is, the sum of the weights after a reaction is the same as the sum of the weights before a reaction.

In the early twentieth century Albert Einstein stated that matter and energy were interchangeable. That is, under certain conditions, matter could be changed into energy or energy into matter. These changes do not occur under the conditions of an ordinary chemical reaction, so that the laws of conservation of energy and conservation of matter are still used. However, these laws may be combined into one overall law, which states that matter and energy cannot be created or destroyed but they can be converted from one to the other.

Measurement of Energy

Heat is the most common form of energy; all other forms of energy can be converted into heat energy. The unit of heat energy is the **calorie,** which is defined as the amount of heat required to raise the temperature of 1 g of water one degree Celsius. The calorie is abbreviated as cal. It is a rather small unit of heat.

A larger unit of heat, the kilocalorie† is equal to 1000 cal. The kilocalorie is abbreviated as kcal. The kilocalorie is used when measuring the heat energy of the body and for nutritional values of foods.

Another unit of heat is the joule (abbreviated J); 1 cal equals 4.18 J. Calories are used primarily in medical work, whereas joules (and kilojoules) are used in chemical work.

There are three principal kinds of foods that produce energy in the body: carbohydrates, fats, and proteins. The oxidation of 1 g of carbohydrate pro-

---

† In the past people in the field of nutrition used the words "large Calorie," which they abbreviated Cal for the kilocalorie. This usage is confusing and now obsolete. The word kilocalorie states clearly what the measurement is—1000 cal—and cannot be confused with the calorie by an oversight in capitalization.

duces 4 kcal, the oxidation of 1 g of fat produces 9 kcal, and that of 1 g of protein produces 4 kcal.

The number of calories produced by a chemical reaction may be calculated in terms of the amount of water that can be heated from one temperature to another by using the following formula

number of calories = number of grams of water
$$\times \text{ change in temperature in } °C \times \text{ specific heat of water}$$

where the specific heat of water is 1 cal/g°C.

EXAMPLE 2-1. How many calories are produced during oxidation (burning) of a piece of food if the heat is sufficient to warm 2000 g of water from 20°C to 38°C?

number of calories = number of grams of water
$$\times \text{ change in temperature in } °C \times \text{ specific heat of water}$$

$$= 2000 \text{ g} \times (38 - 20)°C \times 1 \frac{\text{cal}}{\text{g}°C}$$

$$= 36,000 \text{ cal} = 36 \text{ kcal}$$

EXAMPLE 2-2. How much carbohydrate must be oxidized in the body to produce 36 kcal? How much fat? Protein?

Since the oxidation of 1 g of carbohydrate produces 4 kcal, it will require $\frac{36}{4}$ g, or 9 g, of carbohydrate to produce 36 kcal.

Since the oxidation of 1 g of fat produces 9 kcal, it will require $\frac{36}{9}$ g or 4 g of fat.

Since the oxidation of 1 g of protein produces 4 kcal, as did carbohydrates, it will require 9 g of protein.

TABLE 2-1. Caloric Values of Some Foods

Food	Portion	Kilocalories
Milk, whole	1 cup	160
Cheese, cheddar	1 ounce	115
Hamburger, broiled	3 ounces	245
Almonds, shelled, whole kernels	1 cup	850
Carrots, cooked	1 cup	91
Potato chips, 2-in. diameter	10 chips	115
Orange juice, fresh	1 cup	115
Bread, white, toasted	1 slice	70
Brownies, with nuts	1 brownie	95
Cola drink	12 ounces	145

Composition of Matter

All matter can be divided into three classes, depending upon the properties of the material being considered. These three classes are **elements, compounds,** and **mixtures.**

Properties of Matter

Elements   Elements are the building blocks of all matter. An element can be defined as a substance that cannot be broken down into any simpler substance by ordinary chemical means. There are more than 100 known elements. The names of some of these elements, such as oxygen, hydrogen, iron, carbon, copper, mercury, and uranium, are probably familiar. The names of some of the rarer elements, such as cesium, einsteinium, molybdenum, and xenon, may not be familiar. Many elements are in common industrial use. Consider iron in steel, germanium in transistors, and tungsten in incandescent light bulbs.

Because an element cannot be broken down into anything simpler by ordinary chemical means, it must contain only one type of substance.

Elements can be classified into two main types: metals and nonmetals. Each has its own specific properties.

CLASSIFICATION   **Metals** conduct heat and electricity. They have a luster (a shiny surface) similar to that of silver and aluminum. Metals reflect light. Some metals are ductile (they can be drawn out into a thin wire). Some metals are malleable (they can be pounded out into thin sheets). Some metals have a high tensile strength. Metals such as iron, copper, and silver are solid at room temperature, but mercury is a liquid.

Nonmetals usually do not conduct heat and electricity very well. They have little luster and seldom reflect light. Nonmetals frequently are brittle. They cannot be pounded into thin sheets (they are not malleable) and cannot be drawn into thin wires (they are not ductile). Nonmetals may be solids at room temperature (carbon and sulfur), liquid at room temperature (bromine), or gaseous at room temperature (oxygen and nitrogen). There are many more metallic elements than nonmetallic; see the periodic table inside the front cover. Among the nonmetals are the noble gases, which are gases at room temperature. They are relatively unreactive and were formerly called inert or rare gases. Among the noble gases are the elements helium, neon, and krypton.

SYMBOLS FOR THE ELEMENTS   Each element can be identified by a symbol that represents that element. The symbol C stands for the element carbon, S for sulfur, and O for oxygen. In these instances, the symbol is the first letter of the name of the element. Because conflicts would arise if the first letter were to be used for every

TABLE 2-2. Symbols for Some Elements

Symbol Using First Letter of Name	Symbol Using First Two Letters of Name	Symbol Using First Letter and One Other Letter in the Name	Symbol based on Latin Name
C (carbon)	Ca (calcium)	Cl (chlorine)	Cu (copper—cuprum)
H (hydrogen)	Al (aluminum)	Zn (zinc)	Na (sodium—natrium)
O (oxygen)	Ni (nickel)	Mg (magnesium)	Ag (silver—argentum)
N (nitrogen)	Ne (neon)	As (arsenic)	Au (gold—aurum)
I (iodine)	Br (bromine)	Mn (manganese)	Sn (tin—stannum)
S (sulfur)	Si (silicon)	Cr (chromium)	Fe (iron—ferrum)
P (phosphorus)	Co (cobalt)	Cd (cadmium)	Pb (lead—plumbum)

element, the first two letters are used for some elements, such as Ca for calcium and Al for aluminum. Or the symbol may use the first letter and one other letter to suggest a sound that is apparent in the name, such as Zn for zinc and Cl for chlorine. Note that when two letters are used to form a symbol, the first letter is capitalized and the second letter is small.

The symbols for some elements are based upon their Latin names. Ag, the symbol for silver, comes from the Latin word **argentum.** Fe, the symbol for iron, comes from the Latin word **ferrum.** Table 2-2 lists the symbols and names of various elements based on these categories.

ELEMENTS PRESENT IN THE HUMAN BODY

Table 2-3 lists the elements necessary for life, the symbols for these elements, and their functions in the body.

Compounds   When an electric current is passed through a container of water, the water is decomposed into two gases, each having its own set of properties. One gas is hydrogen and the other is oxygen (see Figure 2-4). If sugar is placed in a test tube and heated strongly, drops of water will collect at the top of the test tube while pieces of carbon will remain at the bottom. Both of these changes are chemical changes; that is, the original substance has disappeared and

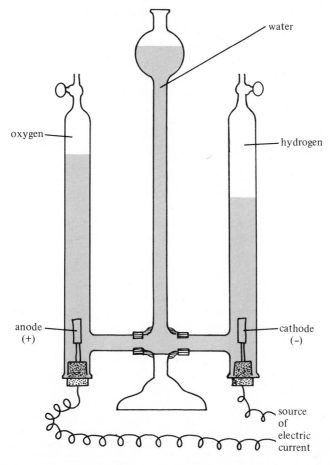

water

oxygen

hydrogen

anode (+)

cathode (−)

source of electric current

FIGURE 2-4. Electrolysis of water.

Properties of Matter

TABLE 2-3. Elements of Life

Element	Symbol	Function
		Major components of molecules found in humans
Oxygen	O	Required for water and organic compounds
Carbon	C	Required for organic compounds
Hydrogen	H	Required for water and organic compounds
Nitrogen	N	Required for many organic compounds, and for all protein
Sulfur	S	Required for some protein and some organic compounds
		Nutritionally important elements required in amounts greater than 100 mg/day
Calcium	Ca	Required for bones and teeth; necessary for certain enzymes, nerve muscle · function, hormonal actions, cellular motility, and clotting of the blood
Phosphorus	P	Required for bones and teeth; necessary for high-energy compounds, nucleoproteins, nucleic acids, phospholipids, and some proteins
Magnesium	Mg	Required for many enzymes; necessary for energy reactions requiring ATP
Sodium	Na	Principal positive extracellular ion
Potassium	K	Principal positive intracellular ion
Chlorine	Cl	Principal negative ion
		Trace elements necessary for humans
Iodine	I	Required for thyroid hormones
Fluorine	F	Required for bones and teeth; inhibitor of certain enzymes
Iron	Fe	Required for hemoglobin and many enzymes
Magnesium	Mg	Required for many enzymes
Copper	Cu	Required for many enzymes, for the synthesis of hemoglobin, and for normal bone formation
Zinc	Zn	Required for many enzymes; related to action of insulin; essential for normal growth and reproduction
Manganese	Mn	Required for some enzymes acting in the mitochondria; essential for normal bone structure, reproduction, and normal functioning of central nervous system
Cobalt	Co	Required for vitamin B_{12}
Molybdenum	Mo	Required for some enzymes
Chromium	Cr	Related to action of insulin
Selenium	Se	Essential for growth and fertility of animals; closely related to action of vitamin E
		Trace elements required for animal nutrition but having no known essential function in humans
Arsenic	As	
Cadmium	Cd	
Nickel	Ni	
Silicon	Si	
Tin	Sn	
Vanadium	V	

some new substances have been formed. Both sugar and water are classified as compounds, as are such other substances as salt, boric acid, carbon dioxide, and ether. Both water and sugar can be broken down into other substances by chemical means. Compounds, then, are substances that can be broken down into simpler substances by chemical means. Compare this definition with that of elements, which cannot be broken down into simpler substances by ordinary means.

Take a crystal of sugar from a sugar bowl. Examine it carefully. List its physical and chemical properties. Take another crystal of sugar from the sugar bowl and again list its physical and chemical properties. The properties are identical, as are the pieces of sugar. That is, the sugar in a bowl of sugar is homogeneous; it is the same throughout.

If a sample of sugar is analyzed, it will be found to contain carbon, hydrogen, and oxygen. The percentage of carbon in a portion of sugar can be calculated by weighing the piece of sugar as it is and again after heating it until nothing is left but carbon. Repeating this procedure with another portion of sugar will yield the same percentage of carbon. Likewise, analysis of several portions of sugar would give identical results for the percentage of oxygen and for the percentage of hydrogen. The analysis of many samples of water gives a constant percentage of oxygen and hydrogen. The result of examining many different compounds for the percentages of their components can be stated as the **law of definite proportions**—compounds have a definite proportion or percentage by weight of the substances from which they were made.

It has already been mentioned that compounds have properties that are entirely different from those of the substances from which they were made. That is, water, a compound, has entirely different properties from the oxygen and hydrogen it is composed of.

Compounds, then, have the following characteristics:

1. They can be separated into their component substances by chemical means.
2. They are homogeneous in composition.
3. They have a definite proportion by weight of the substances from which they were made.
4. They have different properties from those of the substances from which they were made.

Mixtures If a few crystals of salt are dissolved in a cup full of water, a mixture of salt and water—or salt water—is produced. If a few more crystals of salt are added to that same salt water, a little stronger salt solution is produced. If a teaspoonful of salt is added to the cup and stirred until it is dissolved, an even stronger salt solution will be produced. The salt and water formed a mixture because they were placed together and stirred. The salt water made by dissolving different amounts of salt in water will have a varying composition, depending upon how much salt was added to the water. Thus, one property of a mixture is that it can have a variable composition or variable proportions. More water, more salt, or both salt and water can be added to change the strength of the mixture, but in each case salt water is produced.

The property of variable proportions is characteristic of any mixture. If sugar and sand are stirred together, a mixture is produced regardless of the amounts of each used. Likewise, sugar and iron filings can be mixed, and again, the proportion of iron filings to sugar does not alter the fact that it is a mixture.

The ingredients of any mixture can be separated from each other by such physical processes as evaporation and filtering. Salt can be separated from a salt-water mixture merely by evaporating the water. The sugar-sand mixture can be separated by placing both of them in water, stirring to dissolve the sugar, filtering the solution, and recovering the sand. The sugar can be recovered from the filtered solution by evaporating the water. A sugar-iron filings mixture can be separated by passing a magnet over the mixture. The magnet will attract the iron filings, leaving the sugar behind. Mixtures can also be separated by a process known as chromatography (see page 364).

Evaporation, chromatography, and separation by means of a magnet are examples of a physical change—one in which no new substance is produced. In each of these mixtures, the individual substances retained their own properties. There is no evidence of a chemical reaction because no new substance is produced. Thus, in the salt water mixture, the salt retains its own properties, as does the water. In the sugar-sand mixture each retains its own properties. The sugar and the sand can be recognized separately under a microscope.

In summary, then, mixtures have the following characteristics:

1. They have no definite proportion or composition.
2. They can be separated into their component substances by physical means.
3. They retain the properties of the individual substances from which they were made.

Mixtures may be either homogeneous or heterogeneous in composition. **Homogeneous** means the same composition throughout. **Heterogeneous** means different composition throughout. Let us consider two of the mixtures already discussed, the salt water and the sugar-sand mixtures.

Samples of salt water are found to be identical from the top, from the middle, and from the bottom of a container of salt water. That is, the salt water mixture is homogeneous. It is of the same composition throughout.

Now consider a mixture of sugar and sand. Samples from different parts of the mixture, when examined carefully under a microscope or with a magnifying glass, would not appear to have the same composition. That is, a mixture of sugar and sand is heterogeneous.

A mixture of two or more solids is heterogeneous. One solid can be distinguished from another, even if they are ground together in making the mixture. On the other hand, a solution is a homogeneous mixture. When a substance is dissolved in a liquid such as water, the mixture becomes the same throughout; it is homogeneous.

Although both the saltwater and sugar-sand mixtures contained two different substances, mixtures can be made from any number of substances. Note the word *substances*. It can mean either elements or compounds. That is, a mixture can be composed of two (or more) elements (powdered iron and powdered sulfur), two (or more) compounds (sugar and salt), or both elements and compounds (iodine and water).

Summary   Matter is anything that occupies space and has weight. Matter can exist in the solid, the liquid, or the gaseous state. These states of matter are interchangeable and depend primarily upon temperature. Physical properties of matter describe what a substance is; chemical properties describe what a substance does.

Energy is the ability to do work. The two types of energy are kinetic, the energy of motion, and potential or stored energy. The law of conservation of energy states that energy may be transformed from one type to another but cannot be created or destroyed. The law of conservation of matter states that matter cannot be created or destroyed. These two laws may be combined into one stating that matter and energy cannot be created or destroyed but can be converted from one to the other.

The calorie is the unit of heat energy and is the amount of heat required to raise the temperature of 1 g of water 1°C. One kilocalorie (kcal) equals 1000 cal.

Matter may be divided into three categories: elements, compounds, and mixtures.

Elements are substances that cannot be broken down into simpler substances by ordinary means. Elements are homogeneous in composition. Elements are either metals or nonmetals. Each element may be represented by a symbol.

Compounds can be separated into their component substances by chemical means, are homogeneous in composition, have a definite proportion by weight of their component substances, and have different properties from those of the substances from which they were made.

Mixtures have no definite proportions or composition, can be separated into their component substances by physical means, and retain the properties of the individual substances from which they were made. Mixtures can be made from two or more substances. Mixtures of solids are heterogeneous; mixtures made by dissolving a substance in a liquid are homogeneous in composition.

Questions and Problems

A

1. Compare the properties of solids, liquids, and gases as to
   - (a) Definite shape
   - (b) Definite volume
   - (c) Density
   - (d) Motion of particles
   - (e) Compressibility
   - (f) Expansion upon heating
2. Which of the following properties are physical and which are chemical?
   - (a) Odor
   - (b) Reactivity
   - (c) Taste
   - (d) Boiling point
   - (e) Flammability
   - (f) Density
   - (g) Color
   - (h) Melting point
3. Define heat of vaporization; heat of fusion.
4. Which of the following substances are elements, which are compounds, and which are mixtures?
   - (a) Milk
   - (b) Zinc
   - (c) Mercury
   - (d) Paint
   - (e) Carbon
   - (f) Water
   - (g) Air
   - (h) Table salt
5. Distinguish between potential energy and kinetic energy.

6. State the laws of conservation of energy, conservation of matter, conservation of matter and energy.
7. How many calories are required to change the temperature of 500 g of water from 15°C to 27°C? How many grams of protein must be oxidized to produce this energy?
8. Which of the following processes involves a physical change and which a chemical change?

(a) Breaking glass
(b) Burning wood
(c) Boiling water
(d) Digesting food
(e) Distilling mercury
(f) Electrolysis of water
(g) Winding a clock
(h) Souring of milk

9. Which *must* be homogeneous: elements, compounds, or mixtures? Which may be?
10. What elements do the following symbols represent?

(a) O
(b) N
(c) Fe
(d) K
(e) Na
(f) Cl
(g) H
(h) F
(i) S
(j) Ag
(k) Al
(l) Cr

11. What are the symbols for the following elements?

(a) Magnesium
(b) Calcium
(c) Iodine
(d) Carbon
(e) Phosphorus
(f) Zinc
(g) Copper
(h) Bromine
(i) Mercury
(j) Boron
(k) Silver
(l) Manganese

12. Why are gases compressible?
13. Can all substances be changed from solid to liquid to gas? Explain.
14. Which particular element is required for

(a) Clotting of the blood
(b) Thyroid hormones
(c) Formation of all protein
(d) Vitamin B_{12}

15. Which elements are required for

(a) Action of insulin
(b) Formation of bones and teeth
(c) Synthesis of hemoglobin

B 16. Why does the temperature remain constant while a liquid is boiling?
17. What happens to the particles when a solid melts?
18. What is an exothermic reaction? Give an example.
19. Why do gases and liquids flow whereas solids do not?
20. Why do solids have a definite shape whereas liquids and gases do not?
21. Which is larger, a joule or a calorie?
22. Which expands more when heated—a solid, liquid, or gas? Why?
23. Compare the properties of metals and nonmetals.

References BOWEN, H. J. M. *Trace Elements in Biochemistry*. Academic Press, Inc., New York, 1966.

DICKERSON, R. E. Chemical evolution and the origin of life. *Scientific American,* **239**:70–86 (Sept. 1978).

DICKSON, T. R. *Introduction to Chemistry,* 4th ed. John Wiley & Sons, Inc., New York, 1983 Chapter 2.

EBBING, DARRELL D. *General Chemistry*. Houghton Mifflin Co., Boston, 1984, Chapter 2.

FRIEDEN, E. The chemical elements of life. *Scientific American,* **227:**52–60 (July 1972).

MILLER, FRANCIS MARION. *Chemistry, Structure and Dynamics*. McGraw Hill Book Co., New York, 1984, Chapter 2.

PETRUCCI, RALPH H. and ROBERT K. WISMER. *General Chemistry with Qualitative Analysis*. Macmillan Publishing Company, New York, 1983, Chapter 1.

RAYNER-CANHAM, GEOFFREY and MARK VAN ROODE. *Foundations of Chemistry*. Addison-Wesley Publishing Co., Reading, Mass., 1983, Chapter 1.

STOKER, H. STEPHEN. *Introduction to Chemical Principles*. Macmillan Publishing Company, New York, 1983, Chapter 4.

TOTESON, DANIEL C. Lithium and mania. *Scientific American,* **244:**167–174 (April 1981).

3 Structure of Matter

CHAPTER
OUTLINE

The Atom
   Size
   Weight
Inside the Atom
Fundamental Particles
Atomic Weight
Atomic Number
Mass Number

Numbers of Neutrons in the Nucleus
Structure of the Atom
Isotopes
Arrangement of the Electrons in the
   Atom
Energy Sublevels
Noble Gases
The Periodic Table

The Atom

The symbol of an element not only represents that element, it also represents one atom of that element. But what is an atom? We have all heard of atoms in connection with atomic bombs, "splitting the atom," and atomic power.

Consider a bar of iron. Iron is an element. It has certain properties. Cutting the bar in half produces two pieces of iron. Both pieces have the same properties as the original bar. Continued cutting produces smaller and smaller pieces, all with identical properties. In time, we could theoretically arrive at the smallest piece of iron attainable. This smallest piece of iron is an atom—an atom of iron. If this atom of iron were cut in two, particles with different properties would be produced. It would no longer be iron. Thus, an **atom** can be defined as the smallest portion of an element that retains all of the properties of the element.

A piece of iron is made up of many atoms of iron, a piece of copper of many atoms of copper, and a piece of silver of many atoms of silver. The atoms of one element differ from those of another and so give characteristic properties of each element. Atoms are called building blocks of the universe. A chemist uses different kinds of atoms to build chemical compounds just as the different letters of the alphabet are used to form words. Since there are more than 100 elements, there are more than 100 different kinds of atoms.

Size

Although an atom is extremely small, its size can be accurately measured. An atom has a diameter of approximately one hundred-millionth of a centimeter (1/100,000,000 cm). Because an atom is so small, one hundred trillion of them (100,000,000,000,000) could be placed on the head of a pin. And the head of a pin itself is a tiny object; it measures only about 1/25 in. in diameter.

Weight

An atom is extremely small; therefore, it is not surprising that an atom weighs very little. In fact, it would take 18 million billion billion (18,000,000,000,000,000,000.000,000) hydrogen atoms to weigh 1 oz.

Inside the Atom

The early chemists believed that the atom was solid and indivisible, that it could not be broken down into any simpler substances. Modern theory states that the atom is composed of a small, heavy nucleus with particles surrounding it at relatively great distances. Thus an atom is composed mostly of empty space, that space being between the nucleus and the surrounding particles.

If the nucleus of an atom could be expanded so that it was about 400 ft in diameter, the closest surrounding particle would be 4000 miles away. Between that nucleus and the closest particle would be empty space, 4000 miles of it. Actually, over 99.9 percent of the volume of an atom is empty space.

Fundamental Particles

Atoms are considered to be made primarily of three fundamental particles, the **proton**, the **electron**, and the **neutron**.† The proton (p) has a charge of positive one ($+1$) and mass (weight) of approximately one atomic mass unit (amu).‡ Protons are located inside the nucleus of the atom. The electron (e) has a negative charge (-1) and a mass (weight) of 1/1837 amu. Electrons are located outside the nucleus of the atom. The neutron (n) has no charge; it is neutral, as the name implies. It has a mass (weight) of approximately 1 amu. Neutrons are located inside the nucleus (see Table 3-1). In addition to these three fundamental particles there are many, many more particles—among them the positron, the meson, and the neutrino—but a discussion of these is beyond the scope of this book.

TABLE 3-1

Particle	Symbol	Charge	Approximate Mass (Weight), amu	Location in the Atom
Proton	p or p^+	$+1$	1	Inside nucleus
Electron	e or e^-	-1	1/1837	Outside nucleus
Neutron	n or n^0	0	1	Inside nucleus

† Theoretic physicists now believe that electrons are fundamental particles but protons and neutrons are made of even smaller particles called quarks. However, in this discussion we shall assume that protons, neutrons, and electrons are all fundamental particles.

‡ One atomic mass unit (amu) has a mass (weight) of 1.6605×10^{-24} g. A proton has a mass of 1.6726×10^{-24} g or 1.0073 amu. A neutron has a mass of 1.67495×10^{-24} g of 1.0087 amu. An electron has a mass of 9.1095×10^{-28} g or 5.5×10^{-4} amu. The actual masses of the fundamental particles are cumbersome to deal with, so we use the amu. For simplicity, as indicated in Table 3-1, we will assume that the proton and the neutron each have a mass (weight) of 1 amu and that the electron has a negligible mass.

Structure of Matter

Atomic Weight	One atom cannot be weighed even on the most sensitive weighing device. However, the weights of individual atoms can be determined accurately by weighing large numbers of them. As would be expected, the weights of individual atoms are infinitesimal. But the chemist is not as interested in the exact weights of atoms as in their relative weights. The relative weight of an atom is called its **atomic weight.** The chemist uses atomic weights rather than exact weights. Atomic weights are easier to use than the exact weights, and they are just as accurate because they can be determined very precisely.

What does the term **relative weight** mean? The chemist has arbitrarily given the carbon-12 atom (see page 32) a weight of 12.0000 amu.† The weights of atoms of all other elements can then be compared with this weight. Thus, if an atom of an element is exactly twice as heavy as the carbon-12 atom, that element is assigned a relative weight, or atomic weight, of 24.0000. For our purposes, we will usually use the atomic weights as whole numbers, ignoring the decimal values. Thus, the atomic weight of carbon-12 is 12, that of oxygen is 16, and that of sodium is 23. For precise work, however, the exact atomic weights must be used.

The atomic weights of all the elements are listed in the periodic table inside the front cover and also in the chart inside the back cover.

Atomic Number	Each element has a given atomic number that represents that element and no other. The atomic number indicates the number of protons in the nucleus of an atom of that element. However, since all atoms are electrically neutral, there must be as many electrons (negative charges) as protons (positive charges). Therefore, the atomic number also tells the number of electrons in the atom, these electrons being located outside the nucleus.

The atomic number is written as a subscript to the left of the symbol. Thus, $_6C$ indicates the carbon atom has an atomic number of 6.

Mass Number	The mass number of a nucleus is equal to the total number of protons and neutrons in that nucleus. The mass number is always a whole number.

The mass number is written as a superscript to the left of the symbol. Thus, $_{6}^{12}C$ indicates a carbon atom with an atomic number of 6 and a mass number of 12.

Number of Neutrons in the Nucleus	Because the weight of the electron is quite small (1/1837 that of the proton or the neutron) and because only the electrons are located outside the nucleus of the atom, practically all the weight of the atom is located in its nucleus. The atomic number of an element indicates the number of protons in its nucleus. Knowing that each proton weighs 1 amu, you can calculate the total weight of these protons. The rest of the weight of the atom must be due to the neutrons in the nucleus. Knowing that each neutron weighs 1 amu, you can calculate the number of neutrons present in the nucleus.

† In 1961, by international agreement, the atomic weights of the elements were based upon the carbon-12 atom having a relative weight of 12.0000 amu. Previously, the atomic weights had been based upon oxygen at 16.0000 amu.

For example, if the atomic number of an element is 5, there must be five protons in the nucleus of the atom and also five electrons outside the nucleus. If the mass number of that element is 11, the number of neutrons may be calculated as follows: since the five protons weigh 5 amu and the whole atom weighs 11 amu, the neutrons in it must weigh 6 amu. Knowing that each neutron weighs 1 amu, the number of neutrons must be 6. **The number of neutrons can be found by subtracting the atomic number of an element from its mass number.**

Structure of the Atom

What does the atom look like? The simplest atom, the hydrogen atom, has the atomic number 1 and a mass number of 1. The atomic number indicates one proton inside the nucleus of this atom; it also indicates one electron outside that nucleus. The number of neutrons can be calculated by subtracting the atomic number (1) from the mass number (1); thus, there are no neutrons in the nucleus of a hydrogen atom. The hydrogen atom can be represented as follows:

$1\,p$
$0\,n$
$1\,e$

hydrogen, atomic number 1, mass number 1, $^{1}_{1}\text{H}$

The circle represents the nucleus of the atom, the letter p the protons, e the electrons, and n the neutrons.

The element helium—atomic number 2 and mass number 4—has two protons in the nucleus and two electrons outside that nucleus. The number of neutrons is two (atomic number subtracted from mass number). The helium atom can be represented as follows:

$2\,p$
$2\,n$
$2\,e$

helium, atomic number 2, mass number 4, $^{4}_{2}\text{He}$

The sodium atom—atomic number 11 and mass number 23—has 11 protons in its nucleus, 11 electrons outside its nucleus, and 12 neutrons (23 − 11) in its nucleus.

$11\,p$
$12\,n$
$11\,e$

sodium, atomic number 11, mass number 23, $^{23}_{11}\text{Na}$

The uranium atom—atomic number 92 and mass number 238—has in its nucleus 92 protons and 146 neutrons. Outside the nucleus are 92 electrons.

$92\,p$
$146\,n$
$92\,e$

uranium, atomic number 92, mass number 238, $^{238}_{92}\text{U}$

Isotopes The periodic chart at the front of the book indicates that the element chlorine has an atomic number of 17 and an atomic weight of 35.5 (to one decimal place). According to the discussion in the previous paragraphs, the chlorine atom should have 17 protons in its nucleus, 17 electrons outside its nucleus, and 18.5 neutrons (35.5 − 17) in its nucleus. However, a neutron is a fundamental particle so that there can never be a fraction of a neutron. How can this problem be resolved?

The answer is that there are two types of chlorine atoms. One chlorine atom has a mass number of 35 and the other has a mass number of 37. (Chlorine with a mass number of 36 does not exist in nature.) Both of these types of atoms of chlorine have an atomic number of 17. These two varieties of chlorine are termed **isotopes.** Isotopes are defined as atoms of an element having the same atomic numbers but different mass numbers. The first isotope of chlorine—atomic number 17 and mass number 35—has 17 protons in its nucleus, 17 electrons outside its nucleus, and 18 neutrons (35 − 17) in its nucleus. The second isotope of chlorine—atomic number 17 and mass number 37—has 17 protons in its nucleus, 17 electrons outside its nucleus, and 20 neutrons (37 − 17) in its nucleus.

The atomic weight is the average weight of all the isotopes. If the two isotopes of chlorine, mass numbers 35 and 37, were present in equal amounts, the atomic (average) weight would be 36. However, since the atomic weight is listed as 35.5, the isotope of mass number 35 must be the predominant one because the atomic weight is closer to 35 than to 37.

The element carbon—atomic number 6—has three isotopes. Their mass numbers are 12, 13, and 14. They all have atomic number 6, which means that they all have six protons in their nucleus and six electrons outside their nucleus. The isotope of mass number 12 has six neutrons in its nucleus; the isotope of mass number 13 has seven neutrons in its nucleus; and the isotope of mass number 14 has eight neutrons in its nucleus. Carbon-12 is the most abundant since the atomic weight of carbon is 12.011, indicating small amounts of the other isotopes.

three isotopes of carbon

Isotopes have been defined as atoms of an element having the same atomic number but different mass numbers; therefore isotopes of an element must have the same number of protons and electrons but different numbers of neutrons.

Inorganic Chemistry

Most of the known elements have isotopes. Some have only two, whereas others have many more. In addition to the naturally occurring isotopes, there are many more artificially prepared isotopes. These isotopes will be discussed in the chapter on radioactivity (Chapter 4). In general, isotopes have identical chemical properties because they contain the same number of electrons as well as protons. However, isotopes have different physical properties.

Arrangement of the Electrons in the Atom

There is a definite order to the arrangement of electrons in atoms. The electrons are located in **energy levels.** An energy level represents a volume occupied by an electron cloud (Figure 3–1). For our purpose, we shall use the terms electron cloud and energy level interchangeably.

FIGURE 3–1. Electron clouds.

The maximum number of electrons in each energy level may be calculated from the formula $2n^2$, where n is the number of the energy level counting out from the nucleus. Thus, the first energy level holds a maximum of two electrons (if $n = 1$, $2n^2 = 2$); the second energy level holds a maximum of eight electrons (if $n = 2$, $2n^2 = 8$), and the third energy level has a maximum of 18 electrons. However, as will be discussed later in this chapter, the maximum number of electrons in any outer energy level is always eight.

The first energy level must be completely filled before electrons can begin filling the second energy level; the second energy level must be completely filled before electrons can begin filling the third energy level.

The element hydrogen—atomic number 1 and mass number 1—has one proton and no neutrons in its nucleus and one electron outside of its nucleus. This one electron can go into the first energy level so that the hydrogen atom may be represented as follows

hydrogen, atomic number 1, mass number 1

The curved line indicates the first energy level.

The element helium—atomic number 2 and mass number 4—has two protons and two neutrons in its nucleus. The helium atom has two electrons outside its nucleus. These two electrons can go into the first energy level, which can hold a maximum of two electrons, as shown.

helium, atomic number 2, mass number 4

The lithium atom—atomic number 3 and mass number 7—has three protons and four neutrons in its nucleus. Outside of its nucleus it has three electrons. Two of these electrons can go into the first energy level. The third electron must go into the second energy level because the first energy level can hold only two electrons.

$$\binom{3\,p}{4\,n}\ \Big)2\,e\Big)1\,e$$

lithium, atomic number 3, mass number 7

The element sodium—atomic number 11 and mass number 23—has 11 protons and 12 neutrons in its nucleus and 11 electrons outside its nucleus. The first energy level can hold two electrons and the second energy level eight electrons, so that the one remaining electron must go into the third energy level. Therefore, the structure of the sodium atom is as follows:

$$\binom{11\,p}{12\,n}\ \Big)2\,e\Big)8\,e\Big)1\,e$$

sodium, atomic number 11, mass number 23

Table 3–2 lists the progression of atomic numbers and the electron arrangement in the first 18 elements. The arrangement of the electrons for the heavier elements does not follow the simple rules mentioned previously and will not be discussed in this text.

Energy Sublevels

An energy level is composed of sublevels, differing from one another in their spatial arrangement. The sublevels are composed of atomic orbitals, also called orbitals. The rules relating to sublevels are as follows:

EACH ENERGY LEVEL HAS ONE *s* SUBLEVEL CONTAINING ONE *s* ORBITAL.
BEGINNING WITH THE SECOND ENERGY LEVEL, EACH ENERGY LEVEL CONTAINS A *p* SUBLEVEL, WHICH CONSISTS OF THREE *p* ORBITALS.
BEGINNING WITH THE THIRD ENERGY LEVEL, EACH ENERGY LEVEL CONTAINS A *d* SUBLEVEL, WHICH CONSIST OF FIVE *d* ORBITALS.
BEGINNING WITH THE FOURTH ENERGY LEVEL, EACH ENERGY LEVEL CONTAINS AN *f* SUBLEVEL, WHICH CONSISTS OF SEVEN *f* ORBITALS.
EACH ORBITAL CAN CONTAIN NO MORE THAN TWO ELECTRONS.
EACH GROUP OF ORBITALS MUST BE COMPLETELY FILLED BEFORE ELECTRONS CAN BEGIN TO FILL THE NEXT ONE.

This may be represented as follows:

Sublevels	s	p	d	f
Number of orbitals	1	3	5	7
Total number of electrons possible	2	6	10	14

If only the s sublevel is filled, there is a total of 2 electrons.

If the s and p sublevels are filled, there is a total of 8 electrons.

If the s, p, and d sublevels are filled, there is a total of 18 electrons.

If the s, p, d, and f sublevels are filled, there is a total of 32 electrons.

Recall that the maximum number of electrons in the first, second, third, and fourth energy levels is 2, 8, 18, and 32, respectively.

The orbitals are filled in a very definite sequence, as indicated in the following chart:

```
7s   7p
6s   6p   6d
5s   5p   5d   5f
4s   4p   4d   4f
3s   3p   3d
2s   2p
1s
```

The order of filling the orbitals can be found by reading diagonally upward in the direction indicated by the arrows. Thus the orbitals are filled in the order: $1s$, $2s$, $2p$, $3p$, $4s$, $3d$, $4p$, and so on.

TABLE 3–2. Electron Arrangements for the First 18 Elements

Element	Symbol	Atomic Number	Electron Arrangement		
			First Energy Level	Second Energy Level	Third Energy Level
Hydrogen	H	1	1		
Helium	He	2	2		
Lithium	Li	3	2	1	
Beryllium	Be	4	2	2	
Boron	B	5	2	3	
Carbon	C	6	2	4	
Nitrogen	N	7	2	5	
Oxygen	O	8	2	6	
Fluorine	F	9	2	7	
Neon	Ne	10	2	8	
Sodium	Na	11	2	8	1
Magnesium	Mg	12	2	8	2
Aluminum	Al	13	2	8	3
Silicon	Si	14	2	8	4
Phosphorus	P	15	2	8	5
Sulfur	S	16	2	8	6
Chlorine	Cl	17	2	8	7
Argon	Ar	18	2	8	8

EXAMPLE 3-1. Hydrogen, $_1$H, has only one electron. This electron must fill the lowest energy sublevel, the $1s$ orbital, so the hydrogen atom is indicated as $1s^1$, which means one electron in the s orbital of the first energy level. ∎

EXAMPLE 3-2. Helium, $_2$He, has two electrons. Both of these electrons can go into the $1s$ orbital since this orbital can hold a total of two electrons. Thus, helium may be indicated as $1s^2$, meaning two electrons in the s orbital of the first energy level. ∎

EXAMPLE 3-3. Lithium, $_3$Li, has a total of three electrons. The $1s$ orbital can hold only two electrons, or $1s^2$. The remaining electron must go into the next available orbital, the $2s$ orbital so that the electron arrangement for lithium is $1s^22s^1$ where the $2s^1$ indicates one electron in the s orbital of the second energy level. ∎

EXAMPLE 3-4. For beryllium, $_4$Be, there is a total of four electrons. The first orbital, the $1s$, can hold two electrons, or $1s^2$. The next orbital, the $2s$, can also hold two electrons or $2s^2$, so that the electron arrangement for beryllium is $1s^22s^2$. ∎

EXAMPLE 3-5. For boron, $_5$B, there is a total of five electrons. The first orbital, the $1s$, can hold two electrons or $1s^2$. The second orbital, the $2s$, can also hold two electrons or $2s^2$. The fifth electron must go into the next available orbital, the $2p$, or $2p^1$, so that the electron arrangement for boron is $1s^22s^22p^1$. ∎

EXAMPLE 3-6. For fluorine, $_9$F, there is a total of nine electrons. The first orbital can hold two electrons, or $1s^2$. The second orbital can also hold two electrons or $2s^2$. The remaining five electrons go into the $2p$ orbitals since there are three of these $2p$ orbitals and each orbital can hold two electrons. Thus, the electron arrangement for fluorine is $1s^22s^22p^5$. ∎

EXAMPLE 3-7. For potassium, $_{19}$K, there is a total of 19 electrons. The $1s$ orbital can hold 2 electrons and the $2s$ orbital can also hold 2 electrons. The $2p$ orbitals can hold 6 electrons, making a total 10 electrons so far. The next orbital to be filled is the $3s$, which can hold 2 electrons. Then comes the $3p$ orbitals, which can hold a total of 6 electrons, making a grand total of 18 electrons so far. The one remaining electron must go into the next orbital in order, the $4s$, so the electron arrangement for potassium is $1s^22s^22s^63s^23p^64s^1$. ∎

EXAMPLE 3-8. Cobalt, $_{27}$Co, has a total of 27 electrons. The $1s$ orbital can hold 2 electrons, or $1s^2$. The $2s$ orbital can also hold 2 electrons or $2s^2$, and the $2p$ orbitals can hold 6 electrons or $2p^6$. The $3s$ orbital can hold 2 electrons, $3s^2$, and the $3p$ orbitals can hold 6 electrons or $3p^6$. The total number of electrons placed in orbitals so far is 18, with 9 more to be placed. The next orbital in order is the $4s$, which can hold 2 electrons or $4s^2$ followed by the $3d$ orbitals, which can hold up to 10 electrons. Therefore, the remaining 7 electrons can go into the $3d$ orbitals or $3d^7$, so that the electron arrangement for cobalt is $1s^22s^22p^63s^23p^64s^23d^7$. ∎

Noble Gases   The noble (inert) gases are unreactive because they have an outer energy level of eight electrons (except for helium, which requires only two electrons

TABLE 3–3. The Noble Gases

| Symbol | Atomic Number | Energy Levels | | | | | |
		1	2	3	4	5	6
He	2	2					
Ne	10	2	8				
Ar	18	2	8	8			
Kr	36	2	8	18	8		
Xe	54	2	8	18	18	8	
Rn	86	2	8	18	32	18	8

to fill its outer energy level). Eight electrons in the outer energy level corresponds to filled *s* and *p* orbitals, which in turn leads to great stability. Table 3–3 compares the electron arrangements of the noble gases.

The Periodic Table

Toward the end of the nineteenth century, chemists noted many similarities between elements and tried to group them into certain families with similar properties and reactions. This was the beginning of the periodic table.

The modern periodic table places the elements according to the number and arrangement of the electrons in the atom. Look at the abbreviated periodic table shown in Figure 3–2 and the complete periodic table inside the front cover of this book. Note that the table is divided into horizontal and vertical columns. Each box in the table represents one element. There are over 100 known elements; thus, there are over 100 different kinds of atoms, each having its own place in the periodic table. The vertical columns are called **groups** or **families** and are numbered with Roman numerals. The horizontal rows are called **periods** and are numbered with Arabic numbers.

Each box on the chart contains a symbol with a number above and below that symbol. The name of the element is given above the symbol. Consider the box with the symbol O in it:

| 8 |
| Oxygen |
| O |
| 16.00 |

The symbol O represents the element oxygen. The atomic number of the element (8) is given above the name. Below the symbol is the atomic weight, 16.00.

Under group IA of the periodic chart are such elements as hydrogen (H), lithium (Li), and sodium (Na). The electron arrangement of these atoms is given in Table 3–4. Note that they all have one electron in their outermost energy level. All are listed under group IA. (A-group elements are commonly called main-group elements.)

Structure of Matter   **37**

FIGURE 3-2. Abbreviated periodic table.

TABLE 3-4

	First Energy Level	Second Energy Level	Third Energy Level
Hydrogen	1		
Lithium	2	1	
Sodium	2	8	1

Consider the elements beryllium (Be) and magnesium (Mg). Each of these elements has two electrons in its outermost energy level; they are in group IIA. Likewise, in group IIIA the elements aluminum (Al) and boron (B) have three electrons in their outermost energy level. In group VIIA the elements fluorine (F) and chlorine (Cl) each have seven electrons in their outermost energy level.

In general, the A-group number corresponds to the number of electrons in the outermost energy level. The principal exception to this rule is group 0 at the far right of the table. This group contains the noble gases. The noble gases all have eight electrons in their outer energy level except for helium, which contains only two (because the first energy level is filled when it contains two electrons).

The electrons in the outermost energy level are called **valence electrons.** The elements in a group (family) have similar chemical properties because they have the same number of valence electrons. We will see that elements in the same group form similar compounds and frequently can substitute for each other.

The B-group elements are called "transition" elements. They are all metals and usually have two electrons in their outer energy level.

Reading horizontally, in period 1 there are only two elements, hydrogen and helium. Both of these elements have an electron or electrons in the first energy level only. In period 2 and period 3 there are eight elements, all of which have one or more electrons in their outer energy level, the second and third energy level, respectively. In period 4 there are 18 elements, all having electrons in their fourth energy level.

Another generalization, then, is that the period corresponds to the number of energy levels in the atom. Thus, the element oxygen—group VIA and period 2—has six electrons in its outer energy level (from group VIA) and two energy levels (from period 2). The element vanadium (symbol V) is in group VB, period 4. Vanadium has two electrons in its outer energy level (B-group elements usually have two electrons in their outer energy level) and 4 energy levels (from period 4).

Summary   Atoms have an extremely small size and weight. The weights of all atoms are compared to that of the carbon-12 atom, which has been assigned a weight of 12.0000 amu. These relative weights are called atomic weights.

The atom is composed of a nucleus containing protons and neutrons and of electrons surrounding that nucleus. Both protons and neutrons weigh 1 amu; elec-

Structure of Matter   **39** trons weigh practically nothing. Almost the entire weight of the atom is therefore in its nucleus.

The atomic number of an element indicates the number of protons inside the nucleus of an atom of that element and also the number of electrons outside that nucleus.

The number of neutrons may be found by subtracting the atomic number of an element from its mass number.

Isotopes are atoms having the same atomic number but different mass numbers. Most elements have isotopes; some have two, others have several.

The electrons are located in electron clouds or energy levels. The first energy level holds a maximum of two electrons, the second a maximum of eight electrons, and the third energy level a maximum of 18 electrons.

The first electron energy level must be filled before electrons can begin filling the second. The second energy level must be filled before electrons can begin filling the third energy level.

Electron energy levels are composed of sublevels, which in turn consist of orbitals. Each orbital can hold a maximum of two electrons. The order of filling the orbitals is $1s$, $2s$, $2p$, $3s$, $3p$, $4s$, $3d$, and so on.

The noble gases each have eight electrons in their outer energy level with the exception of helium, which has only two.

The periodic table lists all of the elements in the order of their atomic numbers. The vertical columns are called groups and the horizontal rows are called periods. The A-group number indicates the number of electrons in the outer energy level; the B-group elements are called transition elements. They all are metals and usually have two electrons in their outer energy level; the period indicates the number of energy levels.

Questions and Problems

A

1. Diagram the following atoms showing protons, neutrons, and electrons in each energy level and sublevel.

Symbol	Atomic Number	Mass Number
N	7	14
Be	4	9
F	9	19
S	16	32
Ne	10	20
Si	14	28

2. Diagram the structures of the following isotopes showing electrons in each energy level.

Symbol	Atomic Number	Mass Number
H	1	1,2,3
O	8	16,17,18
Mg	12	24,25,26
N	7	13,14
Ne	10	20,22

3. Using the periodic table inside the front cover of this book, predict the number of electrons in the outer energy level and also the number of energy levels in the following elements:
   (a) Beryllium (Be)   (b) Phosphorus (P)   (c) Bromine   (Br)
   (d) Calcium   (Ca)   (e) Rubidium   (Rb)   (f) Arsenic   (As)

Inorganic Chemistry

(g) Radium   (Ra)   (h) Zirconium   (Zr)   (i) Manganese (Mn)
(j) Actinium (Ac)   (k) Radon   (Rn)

4. How do isotopes differ from one another with respect to chemical properties? physical properties?

5. What is an atom?

6. State the mass, charge, and location in the atom of the three fundamental particles.

7. Where is the mass of the atom concentrated?

8. What are the vertical columns in the periodic table called?

9. What are the horizontal rows in the periodic table called?

10. In general the elements in the periodic table are listed in order of increasing atomic weights, but there are exceptions. Give two examples.

B 11. Are all A-group elements metals? all B-group elements?

12. Group 0 contains what type of elements?

13. In which part of the periodic chart are the metals located? the nonmetals? the noble gases?

14. Elements 93 through 106 have been prepared synthetically. Are they all transition elements?

15. What are valence electrons? noble gases?

16. Chlorine consists of two isotopes of mass numbers 35 and 37 amu. If both isotopes were present in equal amounts, what would be the atomic weight of chlorine? If 75 percent of the lighter isotope and 25 percent of the heavier isotope were present, what would be the atomic weight?

17. Why do elements in the same group have similar chemical properties?

18. An atom of an element contains 15 protons and 18 neutrons.
   (a) How many electrons does it have?   (b) What is its mass number?
   (c) What is its atomic number?   (d) In which group is it?
   (e) In which period is it?   (f) Is it a metal or nonmetal?
   (g) What is its symbol?

19. An element is located in group VIA, period 4. What can you tell about that element?

20. As new elements are prepared synthetically, will they fit into the existing periodic chart? Explain.

References DICKSON, T. R. *Introduction to Chemistry,* 4th ed. John Wiley & Sons, Inc., New York, 1983, Chapter 4.

EBBING, DARRELL D. *General Chemistry.* Houghton Mifflin Co., Boston, 1984, Chapters 2, 5, 6.

MILLER, FRANCIS MARION. *Chemistry, Structure and Dynamics.* McGraw Hill Book Co., New York, 1984, Chapters 6, 7.

MORTIMER, CHARLES E. *Chemistry,* 5th ed. Wadsworth Publishing Co., Belmont, Calif., 1983, Chapter 4.

PETRUCCI, RALPH H. and ROBERT E. WISMER. *General Chemistry with Qualitative Analysis,* Macmillan Publishing Company, New York, 1983, Chapter 2.

RAYNER-CANHAM GEOFFREY and MARK VAN ROODE. *Foundations of Chemistry.* Addison-Wesley Publishing Co., Reading, Mass., 1983, Chapter 3.

SACKHEIM, GEORGE I. *Chemical Calculations,* 12th ed. Series B. Stipes Publ. Co., Champaign, Ill., 1983, Chapter 9.

STOKER, H. STEPHEN. *Introduction to Chemical Principles.* Macmillan Publishing Company, New York, 1983, Chapters 5, 9.

4 Radioactivity

CHAPTER OUTLINE

Discovery of Radioactivity
Types of Radiation Produced by a
    Radioactive Substance
    Alpha Particles
    Beta Particles
    Gamma Rays
    Other Types of Radiation
Nuclear Reactions
Natural and Artificial Radioactivity
Units of Radiation
Detection and Measurement of Radia-
    tion
Radioisotopes
Half-Life
Radioisotopes in Medicine
    Iodine-131, Iodine-123
    Technetium-99m
    Cobalt-60, Cobalt-52

Other Radioisotopes
Radioimmunoassay
X-Ray Therapy
Diagnostic Instrumentation
    X-Ray Scanners
    Xeroradiography
    Ultrasonography
    N Radiography
    MRI
Biologic Effects of Radiation
    Protection
Sources of Radiation
Nuclear Energy
    Nuclear Fission
    Chain Reactions
    Nuclear Reactors
    Fusion

Discovery of Radioactivity

In 1896 a French physicist, Henri Becquerel (1852–1908), found that uranium crystals had the property of "fogging" a photographic plate that had been placed near those crystals. This fogging took place even though the photographic plate was wrapped in black paper. By placing crystals of uranium on a photographic plate covered with black paper and then developing the plate, he obtained a self-photograph of the crystals. Becquerel concluded that the uranium gave off some kind of radiation or rays that affected the photographic plate. Figure 4-1 illustrates an autoradiograph* of a radioactive bone section.

Substances like uranium that spontaneously give off radiation are called **radioactive. Radioactivity** is the property that causes an element to emit radiation. This radiation comes from the nucleus of the atom.

* See Appendix C, Glossary for terms followed by asterisks.

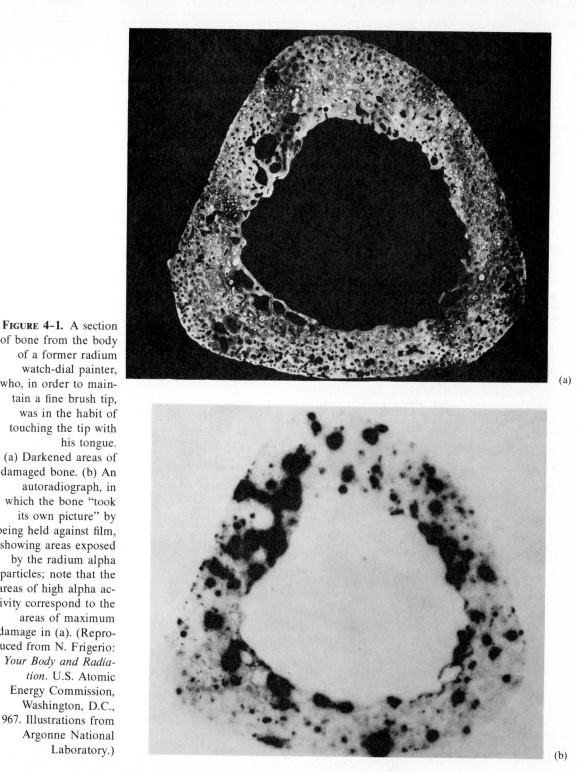

FIGURE 4-1. A section of bone from the body of a former radium watch-dial painter, who, in order to maintain a fine brush tip, was in the habit of touching the tip with his tongue. (a) Darkened areas of damaged bone. (b) An autoradiograph, in which the bone "took its own picture" by being held against film, showing areas exposed by the radium alpha particles; note that the areas of high alpha activity correspond to the areas of maximum damage in (a). (Reproduced from N. Frigerio: *Your Body and Radiation.* U.S. Atomic Energy Commission, Washington, D.C., 1967. Illustrations from Argonne National Laboratory.)

(a)

(b)

Radioactivity

Types of Radiation Produced by a Radioactive Substance

The following experiment was performed to study the radiations produced by a radioactive element (Figure 4–2). A piece of radium was placed at the bottom of a thick lead well. The purpose of the lead was to absorb all the radiation except that going directly upward. The escaping radiation was allowed to fall on a photographic plate. When these radiations were passed through a strong electrostatic field, three different areas showed up on the photographic plate. This indicated that there were actually three different kinds of radiation. These were called alpha, beta, and gamma.

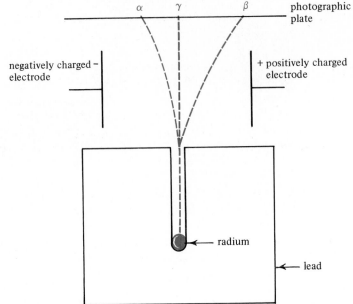

FIGURE 4-2. Radium emits radiation that an electrostatic field separates into alpha (α) and beta (β) particles and gamma (γ) rays.

Alpha Particles

Alpha particles (α particles) are attracted toward the negative electrostatic field, which indicates that they are positively charged. Alpha particles consist of positively charged helium nuclei; that is, they consist of the nuclei of helium atoms (each of which contains two protons and two neutrons) and so they have a charge of $+2$. Alpha particles have a very low penetrating power. They can be stopped by a piece of paper or by a thin sheet of aluminum foil. Alpha particles are relatively harmless when they strike the body because they do not penetrate the outer layer of the skin. However, if a source of alpha particles is inhaled or ingested, or should get into the body through an open wound, then those particles can cause damage to the cells and to the internal organs.

Alpha particles result from the radioactive decay of heavy elements such as uranium and radium.

Beta Particles

Beta particles (β particles) are attracted toward the positive electrostatic field, which indicates that they consist of negatively charged particles. Beta particles consist of high-speed electrons that travel at a speed in excess of 100,000 miles per second. Note that beta particles (electrons) are produced in the nucleus by the transformation of a neutron into a proton and an electron. The electron is emitted as a beta particle and the proton remains in the nucleus. Beta particles (electrons) have a charge of -1.

Beta particles have a slight penetrating power. They pass through a sheet of paper but can be stopped by heavy clothing. When beta particles strike the body, they penetrate only a few millimeters of skin and do not reach any vital organs. If a source of beta particles should be inhaled or ingested, those particles can also cause internal damage to the body cells and organs.

Note in Figure 4-2 that beta particles are deflected by the electrostatic field to a much greater extent than are the alpha particles. This indicates that beta particles have a much smaller mass than alpha particles.

Gamma Rays

Gamma rays (γ rays) are not affected by an electrostatic field because they have no charge. They are not particles at all. They have no mass. Gamma rays are a form of electromagnetic radiation similar to X rays. Gamma rays are very penetrating; they will pass through the body, causing cellular damage as they travel through (see page 63). Gamma rays are often emitted along with alpha or beta particles. Gamma rays originate from unstable atoms releasing energy to gain stability.

Other Types of Radiation

X rays are a form of electromagnetic radiation usually produced by man-made machines, whereas gamma rays are emitted by radioactive substances.

Neutrons are released from elements that undergo spontaneous fission. Their relatively large mass gives them great energy, and because they have no charge they readily penetrate the body. Neutrons are used in the treatment of cancer.

Nuclear Reactions

When the nucleus of an atom emits a ray, its atomic number and mass number may change. Such changes in the nucleus are called nuclear reactions.

In writing equations for nuclear reactions the following symbols are used:

1. The atomic number and the mass number are written to the left of the symbol of the element.

(mass number)

$$^{238}_{92}\text{U}$$

(atomic number)†

2. The alpha particle, which consists of a helium nucleus, is indicated as $^{4}_{2}\text{He}$.
3. The beta particle, which is an electron, is indicated as $^{0}_{-1}e$. (The beta particle has arbitrarily been assigned an atomic number of -1.)
4. The gamma ray, which is a radiation only, is indicated as γ.
5. The neutron is indicated as $^{1}_{0}n$.
6. The proton is indicated by $^{1}_{1}\text{H}$.

† Note that in the periodic table (inside front cover) the atomic number is above the symbol.

Radioactivity

7. The deuteron, which is the nucleus of a heavy hydrogen atom, is indicated by ^2_1H.

The following rules must be observed when writing nuclear reactions:

1. The sum of the atomic numbers on both sides of the equation must be the same.
2. The sum of the mass numbers on both sides of the equation must be the same.

When a uranium atom—atomic number 92 and mass number 238—loses an alpha particle, the nuclear reaction can be written as follows:

$$^{238}_{92}\text{U} \longrightarrow \alpha + ? \qquad \text{or} \qquad ^{238}_{92}\text{U} \longrightarrow {}^4_2\text{He} + X$$

where X is the product other than an alpha particle produced during the decomposition. The atomic number on the left side of the equation is 92 and on the right side it is 2, so that the atomic number of X must be 90. Likewise, the mass number on the left side of the equation is 238 and on the right side it is 4, so that the mass number of X must be $238 - 4$ or 234. Therefore, the reaction is written as follows:

$$^{238}_{92}\text{U} \longrightarrow {}^4_2\text{He} + {}^{234}_{90}X$$

Element 90 (from the periodic table in the front of the book) is thorium, symbol Th. The complete reaction therefore becomes

$$^{238}_{92}\text{U} \longrightarrow {}^4_2\text{He} + {}^{234}_{90}\text{Th}$$

indicating that, when uranium gives off an alpha particle, it changes into a new element, thorium. If a thorium atom should emit an alpha particle, the reaction could be written as

$$^{234}_{90}\text{Th} \longrightarrow {}^4_2\text{He} + Z$$

The atomic number of element Z must be 88 in order for the sum of the atomic numbers to be the same on both sides of the equation. Likewise, the mass number of element Z must be 230, so that the equation may be written as follows:

$$^{234}_{90}\text{Th} \longrightarrow {}^4_2\text{He} + {}^{230}_{88}Z$$

The element of atomic number 88 is radium, symbol Ra, so that the complete reaction may be written as follows:

$$^{234}_{90}\text{Th} \longrightarrow {}^4_2\text{He} + {}^{230}_{88}\text{Ra}$$

Thus, when an atom emits an alpha particle, its mass number decreases by 4 and its atomic number decreases by 2.

If a thorium atom, $^{234}_{90}\text{Th}$, emits a beta particle, $_{-1}^{0}\text{e}$, the following reaction takes place:

$$^{234}_{90}\text{Th} \longrightarrow {}^0_{-1}\text{e} + {}^{234}_{91}\text{Pa}$$

Therefore, when a thorium atom emits a beta particle, an isotope of protactinium (Pa) is produced. Note that the sum of the atomic numbers is the same on both sides of the equation, as is the sum of the mass numbers.

When an atom emits a beta particle, its mass number remains the same, but its atomic number increases by 1.

When an atom emits a gamma ray, there is no change in the atomic number or mass number because the gamma ray is not a particle. It has no mass and no charge. However, even though the same element is produced in the reaction, it has a slightly lower energy because of the energy carried away by the gamma ray

$$^{238}_{92}U \longrightarrow \gamma + {}^{238}_{92}U^*$$

where the * indicates a slightly lower energy.

Another way of indicating a loss of a gamma ray and the resulting change in energy is as follows:

$$^{99m}_{43}Tc \longrightarrow {}^{99}_{43}Tc + \gamma$$

where the "m" indicates a metastable (unstable) form of technetium, Tc. Thus, the unstable form of technetium emits a gamma ray and becomes a more stable (less energetic) isotope of technetium. ^{99m}Tc is used in various types of scans (see page 54).

Natural and Artificial Radioactivity

Some elements, such as uranium and radium, are naturally radioactive. Natural radioactivity may be defined as the spontaneous change of one element into another. Many of the heavier elements are naturally radioactive, whereas most of the lighter elements are naturally nonradioactive.

However, normally nonradioactive lighter elements can be changed into radioactive ones by bombardment with such particles as protons ($^1_1$H), neutrons ($^1_0$n), electrons ($_{-1}^0$e), or alpha particles ($^4_2$He). The radioactive substances so produced are called artificially radioactive. They may be produced in a nuclear reactor. If nitrogen ($^{14}_6$N) is bombarded with neutrons ($^1_0$n), the following nuclear reaction takes place:

$$^{14}_{7}N + {}^1_0n \longrightarrow {}^{14}_{6}C + {}^1_1H$$

The products are a radioactive isotope of carbon, ^{14}C, and a proton. Note that again the sum of the atomic numbers on both sides of the equation is the same; likewise the sum of the mass numbers.

Units of Radiation

Radiation is measured in terms of several different units, depending upon whether the measurement relates to a physical or a biologic effect.

The physical unit of radiation is a measure of the number of nuclear disintegrations occurring per second in a radioactive source. The standard unit is the **curie**,* which is defined as the number of nuclear disintegrations occurring per second in 1 g of radium; 1 curie equals 37 billion disintegrations per second. Smaller units are the millicurie (37 million disintegrations per second) and the microcurie (37 thousand disintegrations per second).

These smaller units are frequently used in describing the amount of radioactive fallout. The curie is not useful in biologic work because it simply indicates the number of disintegrations per second regardless of the type of radiation and regardless of the effect of that radiation upon tissue.

The **roentgen*** (abbreviated r) is a unit of radiation generally applied to X rays and gamma rays only. X rays and gamma rays produce ionization in air and also in tissue. The roentgen is defined as the intensity of X rays or gamma rays that produces 2 billion ion pairs (see page 63) in 1 ml of air. This is not the same for tissue as it is for air, so that the roentgen does not accurately indicate the amount of radiation on tissue.

The **rad*** (*r*adiation *a*bsorbed *d*osage) refers to the amount of radiation energy absorbed by tissue that has been radiated. One rad corresponds to the absorption of 100 ergs of energy per gram of tissue. An erg is a very small unit of energy. More than 40 million ergs are required to equal 1 cal. However, even though the erg is an extremely small unit of energy, the effect of 1 rad (100 ergs per gram) is important because of the ionization that the radiation produces in the cells.

The **rem*** (*r*ad *e*quivalent to *m*an) represents the amount of radiation absorbed by a human being. This unit of measure takes into consideration the difference in energy for various radioactive sources. A rem is the amount of ionizing radiation that, when absorbed by a human, has an effect equal to the absorption of 1 r. A smaller unit is the millirem, mrem.

Rem = Rad × Quality Factor, with the quality factor being larger for types of radiation that produce greater numbers of ions along the path of the radiation. Greater number of ions produced implies more damage to the individual cell.

LET (*l*inear *e*nergy *t*ransfer) is the amount of energy transferred to the atoms in a medium by radiation. Alpha particles with their large mass and slow speed, for example, impart much more energy over their path than do electrons. In general, the higher the LET of the radiation, the greater the injury for a given absorbed dosage. Gamma, and X rays and beta particles usually have low LETs whereas alpha particles and neutrons have high LET values.

Detection and Measurement of Radiation

The problem of detecting and measuring radiation is very important in medical work, particularly in the protection of personnel. One device used to detect radiation is the Geiger counter. This device consists of a glass tube containing a gas at low pressure through which runs a wire connected to a high voltage power supply. When the device is brought close to a radioactive substance, the radiation causes a momentary current to flow through the tube. A speaker is usually placed in the circuit to produce a click, indicating a momentary flow of current. Sometimes a counting device is connected to the tube to indicate the amount of radiation.

Scanners (see page 50) use another type of device, called a **scintillation counter,** to detect and measure radiation. This detector consists of a crystal of sodium iodide containing a small amount of thallium iodide. When the crystal is hit by radiation, it gives off a flash of light, a scintillation; hence the

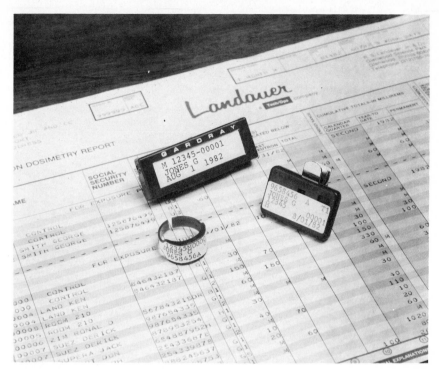

FIGURE 4-3. Film badge worn by X-ray technician. (Courtesy R. S. Landauer, Jr. & Co., Glenwood, IL.)

name. A counting device records these scintillations and the result is produced as a "scan."

X-ray technicians and others who work around radiation usually are required to wear film badges (see Figure 4-3). These badges indicate the accumulated amount of radiation to which they have been exposed. They contain a piece of photographic film whose darkening is directly proportional to the amount of radiation received. This film must be checked frequently to see how much radiation has been absorbed.

Radioisotopes

The isotopes produced artificially by bombardment with one of the various particles are called radioactive isotopes, or radioisotopes. Radioisotopes have the same chemical properties as nonradioactive isotopes of the same element because chemical properties are based upon electrons only, and isotopes of an element have identical electron structures. Thus, an organism cannot distinguish between normal carbon (^{12}C) and radioactive carbon (^{14}C).

If a plant is exposed to carbon dioxide containing radioactive ^{14}C, the resulting carbohydrates will contain radioactive carbon. The movement of the radioactive atoms as they proceed through the plant may be followed by means of a Geiger counter, a device that registers the presence of radioactive substances. Radioisotopes introduced into living organisms are called "tagged" atoms because their path can be followed readily as they move through the organism.

A radioisotope is usually indicated by its symbol and mass number only.

Radioactivity

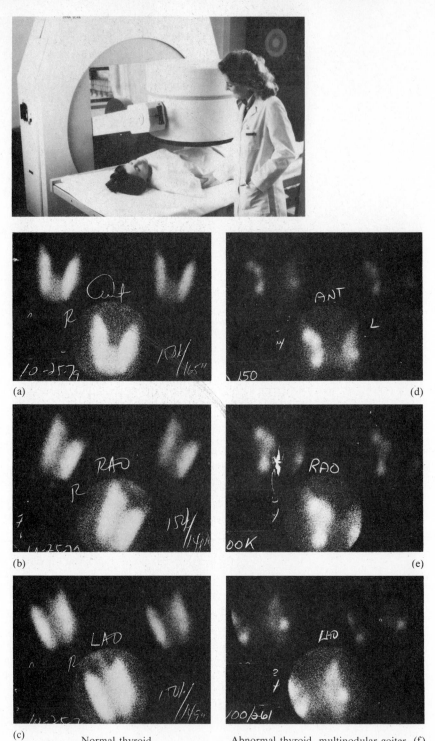

FIGURE 4-4. A scanner, an instrument used for depicting the distribution of radioactive material in the human body. (Courtesy Picker International, Northford, CT.)

(a)

(d)

(b)

(e)

(c)

(f)

FIGURE 4-5. Thyroid scans. (Courtesy Department of Nuclear Medicine, Michael Reese Hospital and Medical Center, Chicago, IL.)

Normal thyroid

Abnormal thyroid, multinodular goiter

The atomic number is not necessary because the symbol itself serves to identify the element. Some radioisotopes commonly used in medicine and in biochemistry are ^{131}I, ^{60}Co, ^{99m}Tc, ^{14}C, and ^{59}Fe (see page 53).

Radioisotopes are used medicinally in the diagnosis and treatment of various disorders of the human body. A medical tool called a scanner helps to locate malignancies (see Figure 4-4). A patient is given a selected radioisotope that will accumulate in the body area being studied. The scanner moves back and forth across that site and detects the difference in uptake between healthy and abnormal tissue. This information is fed to a receiver and recorder, when then produces a picture called a scan (see Figure 4-5). Proper interpretation of a scan can tell not only if there is a malignancy but where it is located and also its exact dimensions.

A new method, positron* emission transverse tomography (PETT) uses positron-emitting substances to trace biologically active chemicals through the brain. Positron-emitting elements used are ^{11}C, ^{15}O, ^{13}N, and ^{18}F. These elements have a short half-life, ranging from 2 min to 2 hr. Because of this short half-life (see following section), large amounts of these materials may be given with relatively small exposure to the patient. In addition, because of the short half-life, repeated measurements may be made effectively.

The PETT method allows glucose to be traced through the sensory sections of the brain. In one test, when volunteers were stimulated visually in only one eye, the region of the brain on the opposite side showed increased glucose usage. Similar tests are being performed for other senses, such as sound and smell. Not only can the change in glucose usage be determined but also the location of that usage can be pinpointed. PETT is also being used in detecting such disorders as epilepsy, heart disease, stroke, Parkinson's disease, and mental illnesses.

Half-Life

When a radioactive element gives off a particle, it changes or decays into another element. The rate of decay of all radioactive elements is not the same. Some elements decay rapidly, whereas others decay at an extremely slow rate. The half-life of a radioactive element is defined as the amount of time required for half of the atoms in a given sample to decay. Some radioactive elements have a half-life measured in terms of billions of years, whereas others are measured in fractions of a second.

The radioisotope ^{131}I has a half-life of approximately 8 days. Consider a 60-mg sample of ^{131}I. After 8 days (one half-life period of time) only half as much, or 30 mg, would be left. After another half-life period (a total of 16 days), only half of that amount, or 15 mg, of ^{131}I would be left. During every half-life period, half of the remaining amount decays.

This may be shown diagramatically in a decay curve in which the amount of radioactive material is plotted against elapsed time (Figure 4-6).

For medical work, a radioisotope must have a half-life such that it will remain in the body long enough to supply the radiation needed and yet not over expose the body to excess radiation. This requires either a relatively short half-life or rapid elimination from the body.

FIGURE 4-6. Decay curve for a radioactive substance, showing amount of ^{131}I versus time and half-life periods.

The half-life periods of several commonly used radioisotopes are listed in Table 4-1.

Radioisotopes of long half-life are very dangerous to the body. For example, radium has a half-life of 1590 years; therefore, if it is taken into the body, it continues to give off its radiation with practically no change in amount during the lifetime of that person. Radium, and also strontium-90 are members of group IIA in the periodic chart. This indicates that they act like calcium. They are easily taken up in the bones and not readily excreted.

Biologic half-life is the time taken for one half of an administered radio-active substance to be lost through biologic processes.

TABLE 4-1. Half-life Periods of Several Common Radioisotopes

Radioisotope	Half-Life	Radiation
^{99m}Tc	6 hr	γ
^{59}Fe	45 days	$\beta + \gamma$
^{198}Au	2.7 days	$\beta + \gamma$
^{131}I	8.0 days	$\beta + \gamma$
^{123}I	13 hr	$\beta + \gamma$
^{32}P	14.3 days	β
^{60}Co	5.3 yr	$\beta + \gamma$
^{14}C	5760 yr	β
^{3}H	12 yr	β

Radioisotopes in Medicine

When a radioisotope is to be used for diagnostic purposes, it must meet several criteria. Among them are the following: The radioactive element must be contained in a compound that will tend to concentrate in the area under study or in certain abnormal tissues. Since the presence of radiation is usually determined by an external counter or by a scan, a radioisotope emitting alpha particles is not generally used because such particles have too low a penetrating power to be detected outside the body. Beta-emitting radioisotopes must be located very close to the skin to be detected. Radioisotopes with gamma radiation are preferred.

The radioisotope selected should have a short half-life and should be in the form of a compound that will be eliminated from the body shortly after its diagnostic use is completed. Thus, the body will receive a minimum amount of radiation after the test is completed. In addition, the amount of radioisotope used should be as small as practicable.

When a radioisotope is to be used for therapy, external measurement is not as necessary, so that alpha as well as beta and gamma emitters may be used. In radiation therapy, selected cells or tissues are to be destroyed without damage to nearby healthy tissues. Thus, the given radioisotope should have the property of concentrating in the desired area and, preferably, should emit alpha or beta particles because these have limited penetrating power and will not damage adjacent tissues.

A radioimmunoassay technique measures the blood levels of an enzyme called CK BB. The blood levels of this enzyme increase after damage to the nervous system. This method allows rapid assessment of brain damage that can occur during a stroke.

Some of the many radioisotopes in common medical use are discussed in the sections that follow.

Iodine-131, Iodine-123

Iodine-131 and Iodine-123 are used in the diagnosis and treatment of thyroid conditions. The thyroid gland requires iodine to function normally. A patient suspected of having a thyroid disorder, is given a drink of water containing a small amount of ^{131}I (or ^{123}I) in the form of sodium iodide. If the thyroid is functioning normally, it should take up about 12 percent of the radioactive iodine within a few hours. This iodine uptake may be measured with a scan. If less than the normal amount of ^{131}I is taken up, the patient may have a hypothyroid condition. If the amount of ^{131}I taken up is greater than normal, a condition known as hyperthyroidism may exist.

For a typical thyroid scan, a dose of 50 μCi is administered orally. This amount of radiation gives 50 rads to the thyroid gland and 0.02 rad to the total body. Another method for a thyroid scan involves the use of ^{99m}Tc. This radioisotope has the following advantages: (1) 5 mCi of ^{99m}Tc administered intravenously give a dose of only 1 rad to the thyroid gland and 0.02 rad to the whole body; and (2) the scan can be performed 20 min after injection, rather than after a 24-hr wait as when ^{131}I is used.

In addition, ^{131}I is used for scans of the adrenal glands, the gallbladder, and the liver. ^{131}I is used to screen for impaired fat digestion and decreased intestinal absorption of fats. A normal result implies good pancreatic function. [131]I is employed therapeutically* in the treatment of hyperthyroidism and in cancer of the thyroid gland.

[125]I injected intravenously in the form of radioisotope-labeled fibrinogen is being used to detect deep thromboses.*

Technetium-99m

[99m]Tc (m for metastable) is one of the most widely used radioisotopes for various types of scans. Sodium pertechnate is used for brain scans and thyroid scans (see page 50); technetium sulfur colloid, for liver scans and bone marrow scans; technetium macroaggregates of albumin, for lung-perfusion scans; technetium pyrophosphate, for bone scans; technetium diethylene-triamine pentaacetic acid (DTPA), for renal scans; and technetium-labeled red blood cells, for pericardial studies. Technetium albuminate is used to scan the placenta for bleeding.

[99m]Tc is also used to measure blood volume. A sample of this radioisotope is injected into the bloodstream. A short while later a sample of blood is withdrawn and its radioactivity measured. By knowing the radioactivity of the ^{99m}Tc and the radioactivity present in the sample withdrawn, an accurate determination of the total blood volume may be obtained.

Cobalt-60, Cobalt-52

[60]Co gives off powerful gamma rays as well as beta particles. For treatment purposes, the beta particles are shielded out and only the gamma rays are used. [60]Co has a half-life of 5.3 years and is used as a substitute for radium

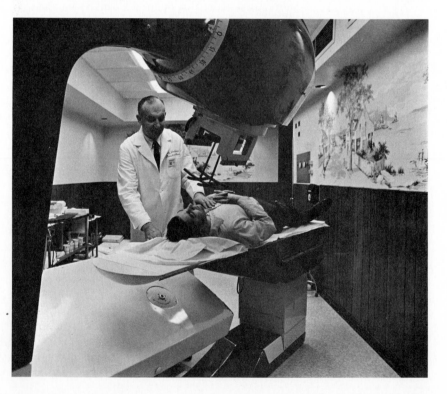

FIGURE 4-7. Cobalt machine in use. (Courtesy of University of Illinois Hospitals, Chicago, IL.)

because it is much cheaper and easier to handle. This radioisotope is employed in the treatment of many different types of cancer. Hospitals use large machines containing a cobalt "bomb" to supply gamma radiation directly to the cancer site (see Figure 4–7).

^{52}Co is used in the diagnosis of vitamin B_{12} malabsorption, a condition which might occur in pernicious anemia.

Other Radioisotopes Among the many other radioisotopes in medical use are xenon-133 (^{133}Xe) and krypton-81m (^{81m}Kr) for ventilation lung scans, selenium-75 (^{75}Se) for pancreas scans, and gallium-67 (^{67}Ga) for whole-body scans for tumors. ^{3}H is used to determine the total amount of water present in the body; ^{14}C has been employed to study the path of carbohydrates, fats, and protein in the body and their conversion into other substances; and gold-198 (^{198}Au) has been employed for the treatment of pleural and peritoneal metastases.*

Unlike ^{99m}Tc, which concentrates in damaged heart cells, thalium-201 (^{201}Tl) concentrates in normal heart muscle but not in abnormal tissue. Thus, damaged heart muscle areas show up on a scan as "cold spots." Cesium-129 (^{129}Cs) is used for scans on patients suspected of having acute myocardial infarction.*

Iron-59 (^{59}Fe) is used to measure the rate of disappearance of iron from the plasma, the plasma iron turnover rate, bone marrow function, the utilization of iron in red blood cell production, and to determine anemias caused by iron deficiency or chronic infections. The iron is usually injected as ferrous citrate, with blood samples being withdrawn at various intervals depending on the diagnostic test.

Strontium-85 (^{85}Sr) is used for bone scans. When used in conjunction with X rays, it is possible to diagnose fractures, metastatic bone diseases, osteomyelitis,* and neoplasm.* Since ^{85}Sr remains in the bone for a long period of time, it is possible to repeat the bone scan a month after the original test.

Chromium-51 (^{51}Cr), in the form of sodium chromate that has been tagged to albumin, is used to determine protein loss through the gastrointestinal tract. It is also used to determine the size, shape, and location of the spleen, and can be used in blood studies including plasma volume, red blood cell mass, and red blood cell survival time.

Phosphorus-32 (^{32}P) provides a useful means of determining eye tumors. It is not possible to biopsy the eye without loss of vision and destruction of the eye. Since ^{32}P uptake is greater in ocular tumors than in other areas of the eye, the location of a tumor can be pinpointed.

Rubidium-82 (^{82}Rb) shows promise for diagnosing heart defects. This radioisotope, with a half-life of 75 sec, is extracted from coronary blood by the heart muscle as if it were potassium.

Radioimmunoassay Radioimmunoassay (RIA) is a method of measuring the concentration of substances that are present in very small amounts in the blood. The procedure is based upon the body's ability to provide immunity against diseases.

When a foreign substance enters the bloodstream, the body produces antibodies to react with and neutralize the invading material. The foreign

Radioactivity

body, which causes the production of antibodies, is called an **antigen.** The reaction is

$$\text{antigen} + \text{antibody} \longrightarrow \text{antigen-antibody complex}$$

For each antigen there is a specific antibody. An antibody that protects against one disease will, in general, have no effect on other diseases.

Suppose an RIA is ordered for renin, an enzyme of the kidney. The laboratory will produce an artificially radioactive form of renin and also the specific antibody for that substance. As indicated in the previous paragraph, the antigen reacts with the antibody to form an antigen-antibody complex. However, in this case there are two antigens, the one present in the blood and the artificially radioactive one. Both can react with the antibody. The two antigen-antibody complexes are separated from the rest of the material. When the ratio of the radioactive complex to the nonradioactive complex is measured, the concentration of the antigen being determined may be calculated.

This method is capable of determining protein concentration as low as 10^{-9} g/ml. Concentrations of lower molecular weight compounds can be determined to within 10^{-12} g/ml.

Dying heart muscle releases MB isoenzyme, which is different from that produced by other types of cells. Radioimmunoassay for this isoenzyme can help diagnose heart attack in persons with chest pains.

X-Ray Therapy

X rays are a penetrating type of radiation, similar to gamma rays but of a lower energy. The amount of radiation and how deep it penetrates the tissue are adjustable in an X-ray machine, whereas these factors are generally fixed in a radioactive source such as Ra or ^{60}Co. X rays may be used for treatment of superficial skin conditions by adjusting the voltage of the machine so that it produces a "soft" or nonpenetrating radiation. Although more penetrating X rays have been used for the treatment of deep-seated malignancies, the cobalt machine (see Figure 4-7) is now widely utilized for the treatment of different types of cancer.

Another form of X-ray therapy involves the use of oxygen at pressures higher than atmospheric. This treatment is based upon the fact that cancer cells are almost three times as sensitive to destruction by X rays when the tissues are under 3 atmospheres (atm) pressure as they are at normal atmospheric pressure. This is not true for normal cells. The patient is placed in a chamber containing air at 3 atm pressure and then given X-ray treatments. This type of treatment is called hybaroxic cancer radiation.

X rays will not pass through bone and teeth as easily as through tissue, so dental X rays show the presence of cavities, advanced bone destruction, abscesses as well as the positions of normal and impacted teeth (see Figure 4-8).

Radiopaque substances are compounds that absorb X rays, thereby allowing body parts to become visible on film. One such radiopaque substance, barium sulfate ($BaSO_4$), is used to detect abnormalities in the stom-

FIGURE 4-8. Dental X rays. (a) Advanced bone destruction. (b) Root canal. (c) Root canal. (d) Bone destruction. (e) Caries. (f) Impacted molar. (g) Bone destruction. (h) Recurrent decay. (Courtesy of Dr. Norman Cohen, Chicago, IL.)

ach and esophagus. Barium sulfate, which is highly insoluble in water and is also nontoxic, is administered orally in the form of a suspension.

Diagnostic Instrumentation

X-Ray Scanners

In addition to X-ray machines, another type of instrument used is the CAT scanner (computerized axial tomography). This type of scanner rotates in a circle around the body and makes sharp, detailed records of narrow strips of a cross section of the body, each record yielding thousands of bits of information. All of the information is fed into a computer, which then produces a picture of the body section scanned. The results are available in minutes on television screens in black and white, or in color (see Figure 4–9). Even though the scanner makes many passes, the patient is exposed to about the same amount of radiation as with traditional X-ray equipment.

The use of the CAT scanner makes possible a detailed examination of any part of a patient's body for the detection of tumors of the brain, breast, kidney, lung, or pancreas. It can also detect abnormal cavities in the spinal cord and enlargements of such organs as the liver, spleen, and heart. In addition, this equipment allows examinations to be performed on an outpa-

FIGURE 4-9. (a) CAT scan of the abdomen demonstrating the liver, spleen, stomach, aorta and the upper pole of the left kidney. (b) CAT scan of the abdomen reveals the liver, including caudate and quadrate lobes, right adrenal gland, inferior vena cava, and aorta. (c&d) CAT scan of the abdomen at the level of the kidneys. (EMI MEDICAL INC., Northbrook, Illinois, Scans Courtesy of the Edward Mallinckrodt Institute of Radiology.)

(a)　　　(b)　　　(c)　　　(d)

tient basis, since no preparation is necessary. The examination may even be performed with the patient wearing clothing.

CAT scanners are also used to distinguish between benign and malignant lung tumors. A lung nodule that contains calcium absorbs more X radiation than the surrounding tissues and so appears darker on the "scan." It has been found that calcium-containing lung nodules are almost always benign.

Xeroradiography

In xeroradiography, conventional X-ray equipment is used to make the exposure (see Figure 4–10a). However, the image is produced by an entirely different process. In X-ray work, the image is produced on a piece of film by a photochemical process. In xeroradiography the image is produced on opaque paper by a photoelectric process. In contrast to X rays, the xeroradiographic process is dry and requires no darkroom.

Xeroradiography is applied principally to mammography* for early detection of breast cancer. It produces better resolution and makes the interpretation of soft tissue studies easier and more accurate (see Figure 4–10b). Xeroradiography is also useful in the search for foreign bodies, such as plastic, wood, and glass, that may not show up on a regular X ray.

Inorganic Chemistry **58**

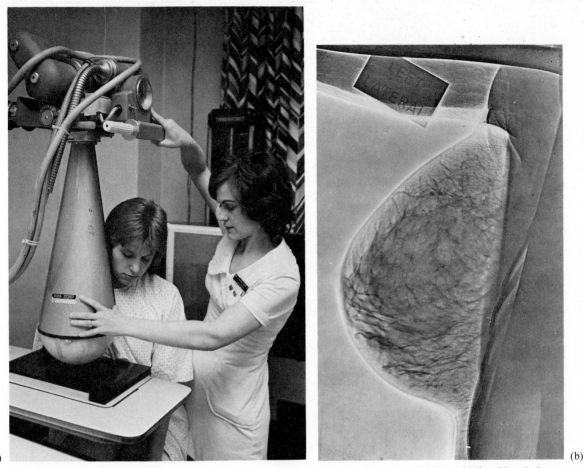

(a)

(b)

FIGURE 4-10. (a) Xeroradiography in use. (b) A mammograph. [(a) Courtesy of Miami Valley Hospital, Dayton, Ohio; (b) courtesy of X-ray Department, Michael Reese Hospital and Medical Center, Chicago, IL.]

Ultrasonography Ultrasonography employs very high frequency sound waves in place of X rays. Normal sound waves have a frequency range from 20 to 20,000 hertz* (Hz). Ultrasound frequencies are those above 20,000 Hz. Those used in diagnostic ultrasound range from 1,000,000 to 15,000,000 Hz (1 to 15 MHz).

Ultrasound waves are sent into the body, and the reflected waves are picked up, analyzed, and displayed on an oscilloscope. Photos of the image may also be taken (see Figure 4–11).

N Radiography N radiography is similar to X radiography except that it uses a beam of neutrons rather than X rays. However, unlike X rays, which interact with the electron cloud around the atomic nucleus, neutrons are absorbed and scattered by atomic nuclei. Whereas X rays go through tissue like a needle, fast neutrons, because of their great mass, smash their way through, producing a wide track of particles, which in turn create ionization in their paths. The

Radioactivity   **59**

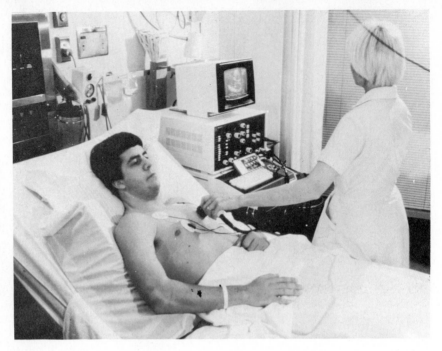

FIGURE 4-11. A gentle touch with an Advanced Technology Laboratories ultrasound scan head provides a detailed moving image of the heart for noninvasive diagnosis of cardiovascular disorders. The patient's electrocardiographic reading is being monitored simultaneously. (Courtesy of Advanced Technology Laboratories, a Squibb company.)

effect of neutron bombardment on tumors is greater than with X rays, whereas the effect on normal tissue is not significantly different. In addition, patients receive less radiation with neutrons than with X rays.

N radiation has another advantage over X rays. Recall that the more oxygenated a tissue, the greater the effect of radiation on it (see page 56). As a tumor grows, it tends to become short of oxygen because it is outgrowing its supply of that vital element. This shortage of oxygen, hypoxia, in turn, diminishes the effectiveness of X-ray treatment. However, lack of oxygen does not protect the tumor from the effects of neutron radiation.

N radiation is most effective against those cancers that resist X rays and gamma rays from cobalt machines. Such cancers frequently occur in the mouth, stomach, colon, and uterus. Like X rays, neutrons are less effective in treating deep-seated malignancies.

MRI MRI (magnetic resonance imaging) is a noninvasive method of following biochemical reactions in both cells and entire organs under normal physiological conditions. The principle of MRI, in general, is that a sample is placed in a strong magnetic field and subjected to radio waves of a frequency appropriate to the nucleus of the element being studied. For biochemical work, ^{31}P and ^{13}C are frequently used. In chemical work, this method is called NMR, nuclear magnetic resonance.

With MRI it is possible to follow changes in phosphate compounds during skeletal muscle contraction and even in heart muscle itself. Changes in heart muscle caused by oxygen deprivation can now be studied.

MRI is used to scan for brain damage in newborns that have suffered asphyxia or similar problems. MRI can detect brain damage due to strokes and heart attacks within minutes after an attack rather than the hours or days needed in a CAT scan. The opportunities of MRI with its advantage of not using potentially dangerous radiation such as X rays is just beginning to be investigated. However, MRI poses a potential hazard to patients with pacemakers and artificial metal joints.

Biologic Effects of Radiation

Externally, alpha and beta particles are relatively harmless to humans since they have slight penetrating power (see Figure 4-13). Gamma rays, with their great penetrating power, have a very definite effect upon the body. If a radioactive substance is taken inside the body, it is the alpha particles that are most harmful.

Protection

Shielding, distance, and limiting exposure are the only effective preventative methods against radiation exposure.

Exposure to external radiation may be controlled by increasing the distance between the body and the source of the radiation. The amount of radiation received varies inversely as the square of the distance; therefore, doubling the distance from a radioactive source permits the body to receive only one fourth as much radiation. Shielding material, such as lead, when placed between the body and the radioactive source will also protect the body against radiation. This is the reason that dentists and dental assistants

(a)   (b)

FIGURE 4-13. Changes in pigmentation of skin due to beta burns. (a) A burn area on the neck of a Rongelap native one month after accidental exposure to radiation in 1954. (b) The same burn area one year after the accident, showing complete recovery. (Reproduced from N. Frigerio: *Your Body and Radiation*. U.S. Atomic Energy Commission, Washington, D.C., 1967. Illustrations from Brookhaven National Laboratory.)

stand behind a lead shield when taking X rays. They also should shield patients by using lead aprons across their bodies. Clothing or plastic will offer protection against beta emitters.

EXAMPLE 4-1. A nurse receives an exposure of 20 mrem when standing 3 ft from a radioactive source. What will be the exposure at a distance of (a) 6 ft? (b) 10 ft?

Since exposure to radiation varies inversely with the square of the distance, we can use the relationship

$$\frac{\text{exposure at distance 1}}{\text{exposure at distance 2}} = \frac{(\text{distance 2})^2}{(\text{distance 1})^2}$$

(a) Exposure at distance 1 is 20 mrem; distance 1 is 3 ft and distance 2 is 6 ft. Exposure at distance 2 is unknown, or x.

$$\frac{20 \text{ mrem}}{x} = \frac{(6 \text{ ft})^2}{(3 \text{ ft})^2}$$

$$\frac{20 \text{ mrem}}{x} = \frac{36 \text{ ft}^2}{9 \text{ ft}^2}$$

Cancelling ft² and cross multiplying, we have

$$36x = 180 \text{ mrem}$$

$$x = 5 \text{ mrem}$$

(b) Distance 2 is now 10 ft, so

Inorganic Chemistry

$$\frac{20 \text{ mrem}}{x} = \frac{(10 \text{ ft})^2}{(3 \text{ ft})^2}$$

$$\frac{20 \text{ mrem}}{x} = \frac{100 \text{ ft}^2}{9 \text{ ft}^2}$$

$$100x = 180 \text{ mrem}$$

$$x = 1.8 \text{ mrem} \qquad \blacksquare$$

Radiologists, and others working with radioactive material, must wear protective gloves and handle the material with long tongs to avoid direct contact with the body.

Another factor to consider is the length of time of the exposure. The shorter the time that any individual is exposed to radiation, the less dosage will be absorbed.

Radioactive wastes must be disposed of in specially marked containers and they should be handled with care.

Persons in regular contact with radioactive material or radiation must wear film badges or other types of detectors (see page 49), and these must be checked periodically for exposure to radiation.

Radiation can strike the molecules within the cell. Since water is the most abundant cellular molecule, we will consider the effects of radiation on such a molecule. Radiation may knock an electron from a water molecule, or it may remove a hydrogen ion from a water molecule, as indicated in the following equations:

$$H_2O \xrightarrow{\text{radiation}} e^- + H_2O^+$$

$$H_2O \xrightarrow{\text{radiation}} H^+ + OH^-$$

In each case a pair of ions, an ion-pair, is produced (see page 48). That is, radiation causes ionization within the cells. Ionization within the cell can disrupt the chemical processes going on inside that cell. Ionization can alter DNA. As a result, some cells may die or fail to multiply but other cells will continue to live and reproduce. Because of the alteration in DNA, there may be genetic changes (mutations) that can show up in future generations. Large amounts of radiation may also produce cataracts, sterility, and leukemia. Exposure to radiation lessens life expectancy. Rapidly dividing tissue is highly susceptible to radiation. For this reason unnecessary radiation to growing children and pregnant women should be avoided. However, since cancerous cells are also rapidly dividing, they too should be highly susceptible to radiation. Hence, cancerous cells are radiated because they are more susceptible to radiation than are normal cells.

Exposure to large amounts of radiation can cause "radiation sickness." The symptoms are gastrointestinal disturbances (nausea, vomiting, diarrhea, general body weakness), a drop in red and white blood cell counts, loss of hair, extensive skin damage, and ulcerative sores that are difficult to heal. Extremely large doses of radiation (over 5,000 rads) are fatal.

Radioactivity

TABLE 4–2. LD_{50}^{30} Values
(in rads)

Dog	244
Human	450
Monkey	546
Rabbit	751
Rat	796
Bacteria	100,000
Viruses	1,000,000

The lethal effects of radiation can be expressed in terms of the dosage that will kill 50 percent of an exposed population within 30 days. The dosage is abbreviate LD_{50}^{30}. Typical values of LD_{50}^{30} for various organisms are listed in Table 4–2. Note the inverse relationship between the complexity of an organism and its tolerances to damage by radiation. Table 4–3 indicates the biologic effects of increasing amounts of radiation on rats, and Table 4–4 indicates the symptoms in humans.

The National Council on Radiation Protection and Measurement and the International Commission on Radiological Protection have set the following radiation standards:

1. A dose not exceeding 0.5 rem (500 mrem) per year of whole-body exposure for individual members of the general population.
2. An average dose to the general population not exceeding 0.17 rem (170 mrem) per year, whole-body radiation.
3. A dose not exceeding 5 rem per year, whole-body exposure for radiation workers.

It is also recommended that actual exposures to radiation be kept as low as possible.

TABLE 4–3. Effect of Radiation on Rats

Number of Roentgens	Time Period	Results
10	—	Genetic changes
50	—	Shortened lifespan
100	30 days	Cataracts; leukemia
500	10–14 days	Destruction of spleen, sternum, bone marrow; disappearance of leukocytes and platelets; decrease in gamma globulin
1,000	4–6 days	Failure of intestinal system; loss of intestinal mucosa; bacterial invasion; no antibodies present; no immunity
10,000	1–2 days	Severe body burns
100,000	1–2 hr	Destruction of central nervous system

TABLE 4-4. Symptoms in Humans Due to Exposure to Acute Whole-Body Radiation

Dosage (rads)	Symptoms (for 50% of population)
50–100	Decrease in circulating lymphocytes
120	Anorexia
170	Nausea
210	Vomiting
242	Diarrhea

Sources of Radiation

The body receives radiation externally from three principal sources: natural background radiation, medical radiation, and fallout and radioactive wastes. Background radiation comes from space and from radioactive material present in the soil, in the air, in water, and in the building materials of our houses. The average natural background radiation in the United States is 120 to 150 mrem per year. Global fallout contributes about 4 mrem per year and radiation from occupational sources about 1 to 2 mrem per year, which is about the same as that received from a television set.

The amount of diagnostic medical radiation varies with the type and frequency of medical treatment. The average in the United States is 70 mrem per year. However, X-ray photographs of specific parts of the body may give that body part a very high amount of radiation. Fluoroscopy produces an even greater amount of radiation. Table 4-5 indicates the amount of radiation received during selected types of medical treatment.

TABLE 4-5. Amount of Radiation Received During Various Types of Medical Treatment

Type of Treatment	Average Exposure (in mrem)
Chest X ray	27
Abdomen X ray	620
Diagnostic upper GI series	1,970
Dental X ray	910
^{131}I thyroid scan	10,000–20,000 (to thyroid)
^{99m}Tc thyroid scan	1,500 (to thyroid)
Radium implant treatment	3,000–8,000

Nuclear Energy

Some people believe that nuclear power is the answer to the world's energy problems. Others say that it is too dangerous to use and should be outlawed. What is nuclear power? How can the nucleus of an atom produce such tremendous amounts of energy? We shall discuss these topics under two general headings—nuclear fission and nuclear fusion.

Nuclear Fission

When bombarded with neutrons, the nuclei of several heavy elements split into smaller pieces. Such a process is called **fission.** * ^{235}U can be split by a neutron into smaller pieces such as strontium and xenon, accompanied by

Radioactivity

the release of more neutrons and a tremendous amount of energy. When this reaction takes place, the sum of the masses of the products is less than the masses of the reactants. That is, nuclear reactions do not obey the law of conservation of mass. They do, however, obey the combined law of conservation of mass and energy. The amount of mass that disappears is converted into an equivalent amount of energy. This amount of energy may be calculated by using Einstein's equation

$$E = mc^2$$

where E is the amount of energy, m the loss in mass, and c is a constant, the speed of light. When m is in kilograms, and c is in meters per second, E is in joules.

Consider the fission of ^{235}U, written in equation form, with weights of reactants and products also being indicated:

$$\underset{\text{(kg)} \quad 1.0087}{^{1}_{0}n} + \underset{234.9934}{^{235}_{92}U} \longrightarrow \underset{93.9154}{^{94}_{38}Sr} + \underset{138.9179}{^{139}_{54}Xe} + \underset{3(1.0087)}{3^{1}_{0}n} + \text{energy}$$

Total mass of reactants	236.0021 kg
Total mass of products	235.8594 kg
Loss in mass	0.1427 kg

Using Einstein's equation, $E = mc^2$

$$E = 0.1427 \text{ kg} \times (3.00 \times 10^8 \text{ m/sec})^2$$

$$= 1.28 \times 10^{16} \text{ joules}$$

This is equivalent to 3 million million kcal, a tremendous amount of energy.

Chain Reactions Note in the above reaction that, when a neutron strikes a uranium nucleus, three more neutrons are produced. If each of these three neutrons strikes another uranium nucleus, then nine more neutrons will be produced. This process keeps on building up as more and more uranium nuclei undergo fission. Such a reaction, called a **chain reaction,*** can sustain itself, producing more and more energy (see Figure 4–14). However, a minimum amount of uranium nuclei (called the critical mass) must be present for a chain reaction to occur.

In an atomic bomb, the chain reaction is uncontrolled, producing a tremendous explosion. If the chain reaction is controlled, large amounts of useful energy are available. Devices that control nuclear chain reactions are called **reactors.**

Nuclear Reactors A nuclear reactor, Figure 4–15 uses a fissionable isotope such as ^{235}U or ^{239}Pu as its fuel. Control rods, made of cadmium or boron steel, which absorb neutrons, are used to control the reaction. When inserted into the reactor, these rods absorb neutrons and slow down the rate of the reaction. When pulled part way out, they allow the rate of the reaction to increase by absorbing fewer neutrons. Surrounding the fissionable material is a modera-

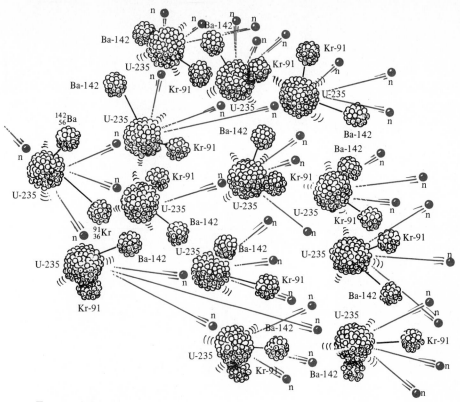

FIGURE 4-14. Chain reaction.

tor such as water or graphite, which slows down the neutrons produced during fission.

The energy produced during fission is primarily in the form of heat. A heat transfer system removes heat from the core of the reactor and transfers this heat to a steam-generating unit.

Naturally, because of the intense radiation in the reactor, there must be sufficient shielding to protect personnel from radiation. Also, safety equipment is designed to shut down the reactor in case of a malfunction or radiation leakage.

Fusion   The sun and other stars produce their energy by a process called **fusion.*** In this process, small nuclei are combined to form larger ones. In the sun, the overall reaction is the combination of hydrogen to form helium, with the subsequent release of incredible amounts of energy. Note that fusion is the opposite of fission. Fusion is the combination of small nuclei to make larger ones; fission is the splitting of a larger nucleus into smaller ones. It has been said that fusion is the energy source of the future. Fusion produces more energy than a comparable fission reaction, and with less radioactive by-products to be disposed of. The fuel for a fusion reaction, deuterium, an

Radioactivity   **67**

vent and head spray

steam dryer lifting lug

steam dryer assembly

steam separator assembly

steam outlet

feedwater inlet

feedwater sparger

core spray inlet

low pressure coolant injection inlet

core spray line

core spray sparger

top guide

core shroud

jet pump assembly

control blade

fuel assemblies

core plate

jet pump/recirculation water inlet

recirculation water outlet

vessel support skirt

shield wall

control rod drives

in-core flux monitor

control rod drive hydraulic lines

FIGURE 4-15. Nuclear reactor. (Courtesy of General Electric.)

isotope of hydrogen, comes from seawater and is relatively plentiful. What has prevented the production of fusion reactors?

The answer lies in the fact that, in order for a fusion reaction to work, temperatures in excess of 100 million °C must be produced. Also, suitable containers for the fusion reaction have not been designed in a workable form.

When a fusion reaction is produced in the laboratory, it will probably be the following:

$$\,^2_1\text{H} + \,^3_1\text{H} \longrightarrow \,^4_2\text{He} + \,^1_0 n + \text{energy}$$

isotopes of
hydrogen

The explosion of a hydrogen bomb is an example of an uncontrolled fusion reaction.

Summary

Radioactivity is the property of emitting radiation from the nucleus of an atom. The three types of radiation are alpha, beta, and gamma. Alpha particles are positively charged helium nuclei. Beta particles are high-speed electrons and are negatively charged. Gamma rays are a high-energy form of electromagnetic radiation and have no charge or mass.

In nuclear reactions both the sum of the atomic numbers and mass numbers on both sides of an equation are the same. In addition to naturally occurring radioactive substances, artificially radioactive substances may be prepared by bombardment with such particles as protons, neutrons, and alpha particles.

A scanner helps to locate malignancies by moving back and forth across the site being studied and detecting the radiation in each area over which it travels. The radiation comes from radioisotopes, which are selected to accumulate at the desired body part.

The half-life of a radioisotope is the amount of time required for half of its atoms to decay. For medical work, a radioisotope must have a half-life long enough to give the body part the radiation it needs and short enough that it will not give the body too much radiation within a reasonable period of time.

Radioisotopes are used in the diagnosis and treatment of various disorders in the body—^{131}I for thyroid conditions, ^{32}P for eye tumors, ^{99m}Tc for scans, and ^{60}Co for radiation therapy.

X rays are a type of radiation similar to gamma rays. The penetrating powers of X rays may be controlled, whereas those of gamma rays may not, X-ray treatment, combined with high-pressure oxygen, has had some success in the treatment of cancer.

The units of radiation are the curie, the roentgen, the rad, and the rem. The roentgen applies primarily to X rays. The rem is the unit most commonly used in relation to the body.

Radiation produces ionization within the cells, causing some type of damage. Small amounts of radiation produce genetic changes, larger amounts cause a shortened lifespan. Very large amounts of radiation may cause death within a short period of time.

X rays are harmful to the body because of the effects produced by the radiation, so care should be taken to avoid unnecessary exposure. Fluoroscopy produces even more radiation than X-ray photographs.

Nuclear fission involves the splitting of a large nucleus into smaller ones with large amounts of energy being produced. Nuclear fusion involves the combining of small nuclei into larger ones, with the release of tremendous amounts of energy.

Questions and Problems

A

1. What are alpha particles? beta particles? gamma rays?
2. Define the term *half-life*.
3. Balance the following equations:
   (a) $\,^9_4\text{Be} + \,^4_2\text{He} \longrightarrow \,^1_0 n + \,?$
   (b) $\,^{27}_{13}\text{Al} + \,^1_0 n \longrightarrow \,^4_2\text{He} + \,?$
   (c) $\,^{30}_{15}\text{P} \longrightarrow \,^0_{-1}e + \,?$

Radioactivity

4. What is artificial radioactivity?

5. What are radioisotopes? Give one use for ^{14}C, ^{131}I, and ^{59}Fe.

6. If 100 mg of ^{32}P is present on a certain day, approximately how much will be present 2 months later?

7. If 2 mg of ^{99m}Tc are present at 8 A.M. Monday, approximately how much was present at 2 A.M. on the preceding Sunday?

8. How may radiation be detected?

9. What are X rays used for?

10. What are the units of radiation?

11. List some of the physiologic effects of radiation.

12. What may be done to minimize the effects of radiation on the body?

13. From where does the body receive external radiation?

14. Describe the use of a scanner. Name one radioisotope used in scans and indicate where it may be used.

15. How may blood volume be determined?

16. What is xeroradiography? For what purposes is it used?

17. What is ultrasonography?

18. Compare criteria for selection of radioisotopes for diagnostic and therapeutic uses.

19. How does the CAT scanner work?

20. What are the values of radiation dosage for the general population? For radiation workers?

21. Explain changes in atomic number and mass number when an atom emits an alpha particle. a beta particle. a gamma ray.

B 22. What does the "m" in ^{99m}Tc stand for?

23. Compare nuclear fission with nuclear fusion.

24. How does a nuclear power plant produce energy?

25. Where does the energy of nuclear fission come from? How can the amount of energy of this type of reaction be calculated?

26. What is a chain reaction?

27. What is PETT? How is it used medically?

28. What is a scintillation counter?

29. What is radioimmunoassay? For what purposes is it being used?

30. What is a radiopaque substance? Where is it used?

31. How does radiation produce ion pairs? What effect can they have on cells?

32. What do the numbers in LD^{30}_{50} indicate?

33. If a nurse standing 2 ft from a patient with a radium implant receives an exposure of 32 mrem, what would be the exposure level at the foot of the bed 8 ft away?

References   DICKSON, T. R. *Introduction to Chemistry,* 4th ed. John Wiley & Sons, Inc., New York, 1983, Chapter 14.

EBBING, DARRELL D. *General Chemistry.* Houghton Mifflin Co., Boston, 1984, Chapter 22.

MCQUARRIE, DONALD A. and PETER A. ROCK. *General Chemistry.* W. H. Freeman Co., New York, 1984, Chapter 24.

MILLER, FRANCIS MARION. *Chemistry, Structure and Dynamics.* McGraw Hill Book Co., New York, 1984, Chapter 27.

MORTIMER, CHARLES E. *Chemistry,* 5th ed. Wadsworth Publishing Co., Belmont, Calif., 1983, Chapter 25.

PETRUCCI, RALPH H. and ROBERT E. WISMER, *General Chemistry with Qualitative Analysis.* Macmillan Publishing Company, New York, 1983, Chapter 23.

PYKETT, IAN L. NMR imaging in medicine. *Scientific American,* **246:**78–88 (May 1982).

SACKHEIM, GEORGE I. *Chemical Calculations,* 12th ed., Series B. Stipes Publishing Co., Champaign, Ill., 1983, Chapter 24.

SHULMAN, R. G. NMR stectroscopy of living cells. *Scientific American,* **248:**86–93 (Jan. 1983).

STOKER, H. STEPHEN *Introduction to Chemical Principles.* Macmillan Publishing Company, New York, 1983, Chapter 17.

UPTON, ARTHUR C. The biological effects of low level ionizing radiation. *Scientific American,* **246:**41–49 (Feb. 1982).

5 Chemical Bonding

CHAPTER
OUTLINE

Molecules
Stability of the Atom
Symbols and Formulas
Electron-Dot Structures
Formation of Ions
Size of Ions
Ionic Bonds
Polyatomic Ions
Naming Ionic Compounds
Covalent Bonds
Nonpolar and Polar Covalent Bonds
Naming Covalent Compounds

Strengths of Bonds
Oxidation Numbers
  Calculating Oxidation Numbers from
    Formulas
  Writing Formulas from Oxidation
    Numbers
Molecular Weight
  Calculating the Molecular Weight
    (Formula Weight) of a Compound
  Percentage Composition
  The Mole
Empirical and Molecular Formulas

Molecules   A molecule is a combination of two or more atoms. These atoms may be of the same elements, as in the oxygen molecule (O_2), or of different elements, as in the hydrogen chloride molecule (HCl). A more complicated molecule is that of glucose, $C_6H_{12}O_6$. What holds the atoms together in a molecule? Atoms are held together by bonds that may be classified into two main types—ionic and covalent.

Stability of the Atom   Most atoms are considered stable (nonreactive) when their highest (outer) energy level is filled to eight. The noble gases—neon, argon, krypton, xenon, and radon—all have eight electrons in their highest energy level. They are stable. One exception to this rule of eight (the octet rule) is helium, which is stable even though it has only two electrons in its outer energy level since that energy level (the first) can hold only two electrons.

Atoms that do not have eight outer electrons may lose, gain, or share their valence electrons with other atoms in order to reach a more stable structure with lower chemical potential energy. This process of rearrangement of the valence electrons is responsible for chemical reactions between atoms.

72

Symbols and Formulas

A symbol not only identifies an element but also represents one atom of that element. Thus, the symbol Cu designates the element copper and also indicates one atom of copper (the number 1 begins understood and not written). Two atoms of copper are designated as 2Cu.

A formula consists of a group of symbols that represents the elements present in a substance. It also indicates one molecule of that substance. Thus the formula NaCl indicates that the compound (sodium chloride) consists of one atom of sodium (Na) and one atom of chlorine (Cl).

If there is more than one atom of an element present in a compound, subscripts (lower numbers) are used to indicate how many atoms of each element are present. In the compound HNO_3 (nitric acid) there is one atom of hydrogen (H), one atom of nitrogen (N), and three atoms of oxygen (O), all of which make up one molecule of HNO_3. In the compound $K_2Cr_2O_7$ there are two atoms of potassium (K), two atoms of chromium (Cr), and seven atoms of oxygen making up one molecule of potassium dichromate, $K_2Cr_2O_7$.

To designate more than one molecule of that substance, a number (a **coefficient**) is placed in front of the formula for that substance. For example, $2HNO_3$ indicates two molecules of HNO_3; $6K_2Cr_2O_7$ indicates six molecules of $K_2Cr_2O_7$.

The formula O_2 indicates one molecule of oxygen with the 1 being understood. This molecule consists of two atoms of oxygen. The formula H_2 indicates one molecule of hydrogen. This molecule consists of two atoms of hydrogen. Both O_2 and H_2 are called **diatomic molecules** because they are made up of two atoms of those elements. Other examples of diatomic molecules are N_2, Cl_2, Br_2, and I_2.

Molecules may also be **monatomic**; that is, they consist of only one atom. Examples of such monatomic molecules are neon (Ne), and Argon (Ar). Molecules of other elements such as sulfur, S_8, are **polyatomic**; they contain several atoms in their molecules.

Be very careful in distinguishing between 2O and O_2. The 2O represents two atoms of oxygen that are not combined; they are separate, independent atoms; O_2 represents one molecule of oxygen, which consists of two atoms of oxygen that are chemically combined with a covalent bond between them. (Two molecules of oxygen would be shown as $2O_2$.) This note of caution applies to other diatomic molecules as well.

Electron-Dot Structures

The electron-dot structure of an atom (also called a Lewis structure) is an abbreviated representation for the structure of that atom. In this system, the nucleus and all of the energy levels except the outer one are represented by the symbol for that element. Each valence electron is indicated by a dot. For example, the element sodium (symbol Na, atomic number 11) has its nucleus surrounded by 11 electrons—2 in the first energy level, 8 in the second energy level, and 1 in the third (outer) energy level. The electron-dot structure for the sodium atom is Na·, with the dot representing the one valence electron and the symbol Na representing the remainder of the atom. Carbon, atomic number 6, has the electron configuration $2e) 4e)$. The electron-dot representation for carbon is

$$\cdot \overset{\displaystyle \cdot}{\underset{\displaystyle \cdot}{\text{C}}} \cdot$$

Argon, atomic number 18, has the electron configuration of $2e) 8e) 8e)$. The electron-dot structure for argon is

$$: \overset{\displaystyle \cdot\cdot}{\text{Ar}} :$$

Formation of Ions

Figure 5-1 indicates the electron-dot structures of the elements in the first three periods of the periodic chart. Consider the sodium atom with the electron structure $2e) 8e) 1e)$. If the sodium atom loses its one outer electron, it will reach a noble gas structure of eight electrons in its outer energy level. Such a noble gas structure has great stability.

^{1} H•							^{2} He••
^{3} Li•	^{4} Be••	^{5} B••	^{6} C••	^{7} N••	^{8} O••	^{9} F••	^{10} Ne••
^{11} Na •	^{12} Mg••	^{13} Al••	^{14} Si••	^{15} P••	^{16} S••	^{17} Cl••	^{18} Ar••

FIGURE 5-1. Electron-dot structures of the first 18 elements.

When a sodium atom loses an electron, it becomes a positively charged particle called a sodium ion. This reaction may be written as

$$\text{Na} \cdot - 1e \longrightarrow \text{Na}^+$$

or, with the electron-dot being understood,

$$\text{Na} - 1e \longrightarrow \text{Na}^+$$

where the positive sign indicates a charge of $+1$ on the sodium ion. (Note that the number 1 is understood and not written.) The charge on the sodium ion is positive because the sodium ion still has eleven protons in its nucleus but now has only ten electrons outside that nucleus.

Likewise, the aluminum atom, which has the electron structure of $2e) 8e) 3e)$, loses all three outer electrons when it forms an aluminum ion with a charge of $+3$ (written above the symbol as $3+$).

$$\text{Al} : - 3e \longrightarrow \text{Al}^{3+} \qquad \text{or simply} \qquad \text{Al} - 3e \longrightarrow \text{Al}^{3+}$$

A metal that has one valence electron forms an ion with a $1+$ charge; a metal with two valence electrons forms an ion with a $2+$ charge, and so on. The positive charge on a metallic ion is equal to the number of electrons lost by the metal.

Elements that have six or seven outer electrons tend to gain electrons to reach a stable configuration of eight. Such elements are called nonmetals. (Most elements having four or five outer electrons are also nonmetals. These will be discussed separately under covalent bonds.)

Consider the element chlorine, 2e) 8e) 7e). The chlorine atom will tend to gain one electron to fill its outer energy level to eight, reaching a stable (noble gas) structure. Chlorine will thus form an ion with a charge of -1, or omitting the dots,

$$Cl + 1e \longrightarrow Cl^-$$

Since the ion has one more electron than the atom, it will have a charge of -1, again with the 1 being understood and not written.

Likewise, the sulfur atom, 2e) 6e), can gain two electrons to form an ion with a charge of -2.

$$S + 2e \longrightarrow S^{2-}$$

The S^{2-} ion has a full outer energy level, a noble gas structure.

An atom that has either lost or gained electrons in its outer energy level is called an **ion.** Ions formed from a metal will have a positive charge equal to the number of electrons lost. Ions formed from nonmetals will have a negative charge equal to the number of electrons gained.

Positive ions are attracted toward a negatively charged electrode called a cathode. Such ions are called **cations.** Likewise, negative ions are attracted toward a positively charged electrode, an anode. These ions are called **anions.** Common cations in body fluids are the sodium ion, Na^+, the potassium ion, K^+, and the calcium ion, Ca^{2+}. The chloride ion, Cl^-, is the most common anion in body fluids.

Size of Ions

When a metal loses an electron (or electrons), the positive charge on the nucleus is greater than the negative charge in the electron energy levels, so that the nucleus pulls in the electrons and thus decreases the size. That is, for metals, the ionic radius is less then the atomic radius.

When a nonmetal gains an electron (or electrons), the positive charge on the nucleus is less than the negative charge in the electron energy levels; thus the nucleus cannot hold the electrons as tightly as before. Therefore, for nonmetals, the ionic radius is greater than the atomic radius.

Figure 5-2 illustrates the relative sizes of several atoms and their corresponding ions.

Ionic Bonds

When a sodium atom (Na) combines with a chlorine atom (Cl) to form a sodium chloride molecule (NaCl), the sodium atom loses one electron to form a positively charged sodium ion (Na^+). At the same time the chlorine atom gains that one electron to form a negatively charged chloride ion (Cl^-). The reaction is

$$Na \cdot + : \ddot{Cl} : \longrightarrow Na^+ + : \ddot{Cl} : ^- \qquad \text{or} \qquad Na + Cl \longrightarrow Na^+ + Cl^-$$

The positively charged sodium ion and the negatively charged chloride ion will be attracted to each other and will be held together by the electrostatic attraction of their charges (opposite charges attract each other). This type of bonding is called an **ionic bond.** An ionic bond results from the

Chemical Bonding

	Ia	IIa	IIIa	IVa	Va	VIa	VIIa	O
1	H							He
2	Li, Li$^+$	Be, Be^{2+}	B	C	N	O, O^{2-}	F, F$^-$	Ne
3	Na, Na$^+$	Mg, Mg^{2+}	Al, Al^{3+}	Si	P	S, S^{2-}	Cl, Cl$^-$	Ar

FIGURE 5-2. Atomic and ionic sizes of some elements.

transfer of an electron or electrons from one atom to another with the formation of ions that attract one another.

Another example of a transfer of electrons from a metal to a nonmetal is in the reaction between magnesium (Mg) and chlorine (Cl_2, here written as two Cl's),

or

$$Mg + 2Cl \longrightarrow Mg^{2+} + 2Cl^-$$

where the positively charged magnesium ion and the negatively charged chloride ions are held together by ionic bonds. (Again each ion has a completed outer energy level of eight.)

Polyatomic Ions

A group of atoms that stay together and act as a unit in a chemical reaction is called a **polyatomic ion**. A polyatomic ion acts as if it were a simple ion. Table 5-1 indicates the name, formula, and charge of several common polyatomic ions.

TABLE 5-1. Common Polyatomic Ions

Name	Formula and Charge
Sulfate	SO_4^{2-}
Nitrate	NO_3^-
Phosphate	PO_4^{3-}
Carbonate	CO_3^{2-}
Hydroxide	OH^-
Bicarbonate	HCO_3^-
Ammonium	NH_4^+

Inorganic Chemistry

Naming Ionic Compounds Compounds that contain ions are called ionic compounds. As shall be discussed later, ionic compounds or electrolytes fall into three categories—acids, bases, and salts.

Ionic compounds that contain only two types of elements are called **binary** compounds. To name binary compounds, the following system is used:

> name of positive ion   stem of negative ion + *ide*

Note that the names of all binary compounds end in the letters *ide*. The stem is the first part of the name of the element forming the negative ion. Stems for some common elements are listed in Table 5–2.

TABLE 5-2. Stems for Some Common Elements

Element	Stem	Element	Stem
Oxygen	ox	Nitrogen	nitr
Chlorine	chlor	Sulfur	sulf
Bromine	brom	Carbon	carb
Iodine	iod	Phosphorus	phosph

EXAMPLE 5-1. What is the name of the compound $CaBr_2$?

The name of the positive ion, which is always written first in an ionic compound, is calcium. The negative ion comes from Br, the element bromine. The stem for bromine is **brom**. The ending is **ide**. Thus the name of $CaBr_2$ is **calcium bromide.** ∎

EXAMPLE 5-2. What is the name of the compound KCl?

The name of the positive ion is potassium. The stem of the negative ion, from the element chlorine, Cl, is **chlor.** The ending is **ide.** The name is **potassium chloride.** ∎

For ionic compounds containing polyatomic ions, the following system of naming is used:

> name of positive ion   name of polyatomic ion

EXAMPLE 5-3. Name the compound $MgSO_4$.

The positive ion is **magnesium.** The name of the SO_4 polyatomic ion, from table 5–1, is **sulfate.** Thus, $MgSO_4$ is called **magnesium sulfate.** ∎

One exception of the rule for naming binary compounds is in the compound NH_4Cl where the NH_4 polyatomic ion is treated as if it were a simple positive ion. Thus the compound NH_4Cl is treated as if it were a binary compound and is called ammonium chloride.

Covalent Bonds Ionic bonding results from the loss or gain of electrons. However, there is another method by which atoms can be bonded together. This is by the sharing of electrons (covalent bonding).

Chemical Bonding

In the chlorine molecule, Cl_2, each of the two chlorine atoms has seven outer electrons. In this case both atoms will share electrons so that each will have a completed outer energy level of eight electrons. Diagram 5–1 shows two chlorine atoms with their electrons so situated that each has eight electrons around it.

$$:\overset{..}{\underset{..}{Cl}}\cdot \ + \ \cdot\overset{..}{\underset{..}{Cl}}: \ \longrightarrow \ \text{Cl} \ \text{Cl} \tag{5–1}$$

Note that each atom has a noble gas structure, with either outer electrons. Each of the chlorine atoms is sharing one electron with the other. The bond that holds these two atoms together is called a covalent bond. Note that in the chlorine molecule, Cl_2, there has been no electron loss or gain and so there are no chloride ions present. This is one of the primary differences between ionic and covalent bonds. In compounds containing ionic bonds, ions are present, whereas in compounds containing covalent bonds no ions are present.

The covalent bond between the two chlorine atoms may be indicated by a short line, or Cl—Cl, with the electrons being understood and not written.

Covalent bonds may also be formed between atoms of different elements. In compounds containing covalent bonds, each atom usually has eight electrons around it, since eight electrons in the outer energy level represent a stable structure. An exception to this rule (see page 72) is hydrogen, which in compounds has only two electrons around it. (Recall that the first energy level can hold only two electrons.)

The compound carbon tetrachloride, CCl_4, may be diagrammed as in (5–2)

$$\text{or} \qquad \begin{array}{c} Cl \\ | \\ Cl-C-Cl \\ | \\ Cl \end{array} \tag{5–2}$$

The compound ammonia, NH_3, may be represented as in Diagram 5-3

$$\text{or} \qquad \begin{array}{c} H \\ | \\ H-N-H \end{array} \tag{5–3}$$

In carbon tetrachloride there are four covalent bonds, one between each of the chlorines and the carbon. In ammonia there are three covalent bonds. Note that in these structures each element has eight electrons around it, except for hydrogen, which has only two.

Since metals tend to lose electrons, they usually do not form covalent compounds. Thus, we can say that most covalent compounds are formed between nonmetals having four, five, six, or seven outer electrons.

The compound carbon dioxide, CO_2, may be represented as (5–4)

$$\text{or} \qquad O{=}C{=}O \tag{5–4}$$

In carbon dioxide there are two double covalent bonds present. In the previous examples, single covalent bonds were present, representing one shared pair of electrons. Single covalent bonds are also called **single bonds.** A double covalent bond (also called a **double bond**) represents two shared pairs of electrons. A triple covalent bond (**triple bond**) represents three shared pairs of electrons, as in the compound nitrogen, N_2, structure (5–5)

$$: N (\!:\!:\!) N : \qquad \text{or} \qquad N \equiv N \qquad\qquad (5\text{–}5)$$

Note that in CO_2 and in N_2 there are eight electrons around each atom.

Nonpolar and Polar Covalent Bonds

Consider the compound Cl_2 or Cl—Cl. There is a single bond representing a pair of shared electrons between the two chlorine atoms. The two chlorines are identical and so the electrons should be shared equally between them. Such a type of bond is called a **nonpolar covalent bond.**

In the compound HCl, or H—Cl, the single bond again represents a shared pair of electrons. However, this pair of electrons is not shared equally. Let us see why.

Electronegativity is the attraction of an atom for electrons. The greater the electronegativity, the greater the attraction for electrons; the lower the electronegativity the less the attraction for electrons. Table 5–3 indicates the electronegativities of some elements.

TABLE 5-3. Electronegativities of Various Elements

F	4.0	Br	2.8	H	2.1
O	3.5	C, S	2.5	Ca	1.0
N, Cl	3.1	I	2.4	Na	0.9

Again consider the HCl molecule. Chlorine is more electronegative than hydrogen and so attracts the shared electrons more strongly. Thus, the shared pair of electrons will be closer to the chlorine than to the hydrogen, or

$$\text{H} : \overset{..}{\underset{..}{Cl}} : \qquad \text{which may also be represented as} \qquad \overset{\delta^+}{\text{H}}\ \overset{\delta^-}{\text{Cl}}$$

where the δ sign (Greek delta) indicates a partial charge. So, one end of the HCl molecule has a partial positive charge and the other end a partial negative charge. Note, however, that there are no ions formed, only partial charges. Such a type of bond is called a **polar covalent bond.** Thus, with equally shared electrons, as between like atoms or between atoms of equal electronegativity, nonpolar covalent bonds are formed. When atoms of different electronegativity form a covalent bond, such a bond is always polar.

Another example of a compound containing a polar covalent bond is water, H_2O. Its structure is

$$\text{H} : \overset{..}{\underset{..}{O}} : \qquad \text{or} \qquad \overset{\delta^+}{\text{H}} - \overset{\delta^-}{\text{O}}\diagdown_{\text{H}^{\delta^+}}$$
$$\text{H}$$

Because oxygen is more electronegative than hydrogen, it becomes the negative end of the molecule. The hydrogens are at the positive end. The polar nature of the water molecule will be discussed in more detail in Chapter 10.

However, a nonpolar molecule may contain polar bonds. Consider the compound CCl_4 whose partial charges are indicated in structure (5-6)

$$Cl-\overset{\overset{\displaystyle \overset{\delta^-}{Cl}}{|}}{\underset{\underset{\displaystyle \underset{\delta^-}{Cl}}{|}}{C}}\overset{\delta^-}{-}Cl \qquad\qquad (5\text{-}6)$$

The bonds between the carbon and each chlorine are polar. But, there is no negative end to the molecule and no positive end. Rather, the outer part is negative and the inner part positive (partially). So, the molecule is nonpolar. In general, symmetrical molecules are nonpolar even though they may contain polar bonds.

Naming Covalent Compounds

Covalent binary compounds have names ending in *ide*, as do ionic binary compounds. To name covalent binary compounds, the following system is used:

prefix + name of first element   prefix + stem of second element + *ide*

Note that this system is similar to that for ionic compounds except that, for covalent compounds, prefixes are used, whereas no prefixes are used in naming ionic compounds. The prefixes in common use are

mono—1   di—2   tri—3   tetra—4   penta—5

However, the prefix mono is usually understood and not written.

EXAMPLE 5-4. Name the covalent compound CCl_4.
The name of the first element is carbon. There is only one carbon atom indicated in the formula, so the prefix is mono (understood and not written). The second element is chlorine, stem **chlor** (see Table 5–3). Since there are four chlorines indicated in the formula, the prefix is **tetra**. The ending as with all binary compounds is **ide**; so, the name is **carbon tetrachloride**. ∎

EXAMPLE 5-5. Name the covalent compound P_2O_3.
By following the previous example and using the prefixes **di** and **tri**, respectively, the name is **diphosphorus trioxide**. ∎

Strengths of Bonds

Consider Table 5-4 of the melting points of several ionic and covalent compounds. In general, compounds containing ionic bonds have higher melting points than do compounds containing covalent bonds. That is it takes more energy (heat) to separate the particles in ionic compounds than it does in covalent compounds. Although the bonds holding ionic compounds to-

TABLE 5-4. Melting points of Various Substances

Ionic Compound	Melting Point (°C)	Covalent Compound	Melting Point (°C)
Sodium chloride, NaCl	800	Glucose, $C_6H_{12}O_6$	146
Calcium chloride, $CaCl_2$	782	Carbon tetrachloride, CCl_4	−23
Zinc oxide, ZnO	1975	Urea, NH_2CONH_2	133

gether are generally weaker than those holding covalent compounds together, ionic compounds contain many more bonds than covalent compounds. Covalent substances, such as a diamond, which do contain a network of covalent bonds, have extremely high melting points.

Water solutions of ionic compounds conduct electricity (they are electrolytes) because they contain ions. Water solutions of covalent compounds do not contain ions and do not conduct electricity.

Most ionic compounds are soluble in polar solvents such as water. Most covalent compounds are insoluble in polar solvents.

Most ionic compounds are insoluble in nonpolar solvents such as benzene. Many covalent compounds are soluble in nonpolar solvents.

Molten ionic compounds conduct electricity because they contain ions. Molten covalent compounds contain no ions and do not conduct electricity.

Oxidation Numbers

For ionic compounds, the oxidation number, sometimes called the *charge* of an element, is equal to the number of electrons lost or gained and so is the same as the charge on the ion. That is, in sodium chloride, Na^+Cl^-, the oxidation number of sodium is +1 and that of chlorine −1. In the compound $MgBr_2$, where the magnesium ion has a charge of 2+ and each bromide ion a charge of 1−, the oxidation number of magnesium is +2 and that of each bromine −1.

For covalent compounds, where electrons are shared and not transferred, oxidation numbers are assigned to elements using the following rules:

1. All elements in their free state have an oxidation number of zero.
2. The oxidation number of oxygen is −2 (except in peroxides where it is −1).
3. The oxidation number of hydrogen is +1.
4. The sum of oxidation numbers in all compounds must equal zero. (That is, all compounds are electrically neutral).
5. All elements in group IA have an oxidation number of +1.

Table 5-5 indicates the oxidation numbers of various elements.

Calculating Oxidation Numbers from Formulas

As has been previously mentioned, the sum of the oxidation numbers in any compound must equal zero. Let us find the oxidation number of zinc in zinc oxide, ZnO. Note that the oxidation number of oxygen, as listed in Table 5-5, is −2. Writing the formula of the compound with the known oxidation number above

$$\overset{?}{Zn} \; \overset{-2}{O} \; = 0$$

Chemical Bonding   **81**

TABLE 5-5. Oxidation Numbers of Elements[a]

Positive Oxidation Numbers			Negative Oxidation Numbers		
Name and Symbol		Oxidation Number	Name and Symbol		Oxidation Number
Hydrogen	H^+	$+1$	Chloride	Cl^-	-1
Sodium	Na^+	$+1$	Bromide	Br^-	-1
Potassium	K^+	$+1$	Iodide	I^-	-1
Silver	Ag^+	$+1$	Sulfide	S^{2-}	-2
Calcium	Ca^{2+}	$+2$	Oxide	O^{2-}	-2
Magnesium	Mg^{2+}	$+2$			
Aluminum	Al^{3+}	$+3$			
Ammonium	NH_4^+	$+1$			
Iron	Fe^{2+} and Fe^{3+}	$+2$ and $+3$			
Copper	Cu^+ and Cu^{2+}	$+1$ and $+2$			
Tin	Sn^{2+} and Sn^{4+}	$+2$ and $+4$			

[a] Note that some elements, such as copper, tin, and iron, have more than one oxidation number.

we see that the oxidation number of the Zn must be $+2$ in order for the sum of the oxidation numbers to be zero.

Next let us find the oxidation number of Mn in potassium permanganate, $KMnO_4$. From the table we see that the oxidation number of K is $+1$ and that of O is -2. Therefore, four oxygens will have a total oxidation number of $4(-2)$, or

$$\overset{+1 \ +(?) \ +4(-2) = 0}{KMn \quad O_4}$$

In order for the sum of the oxidation numbers to be zero, the oxidation number of Mn must be $+7$.

Now consider the compound diarsenic trisulfide, As_2S_3. The oxidation number of S from the table is -2. Therefore, three S's will have a total oxidation number of $3(-2)$

$$\overset{? \quad +3(-2) = 0}{As_2 \quad S_3}$$

In order for the sum of the oxidation numbers to be zero, the total oxidation number of the As atoms must be $+6$. However, this value of $+6$ applies to two As atoms, so that the oxidation number of each As is $+3$.

Writing Formulas from Oxidation Numbers To write the formula of a compound formed between calcium and chlorine, look up the oxidation numbers of these elements in Table 5–5 and write them above the symbols

$$\overset{+2 \ -1}{CaCl}$$

Note that the sum of the oxidation numbers is not zero so that this is not the correct formula for the compound. An easy method for obtaining the correct formula is to use a system of crisscrossing the oxidation numbers

Inorganic Chemistry   **82**

$$\overset{+2}{Ca}\diagdown\overset{-1}{Cl}\downarrow$$

Thus the formula of the compound between calcium and chlorine is $CaCl_2$. (Note that the subscript 1 is always understood and never written.) In this compound the sum of the oxidation numbers ($+2$ for the calcium and -2 for the two chlorines) does equal zero.

To write the formula for the compound formed between magnesium and the phosphate ion we first write the oxidation numbers above the symbols and then crisscross them

$$\overset{+2}{Mg}\diagup\overset{-3}{PO_4}$$

so that the formula is $Mg_3(PO_4)_2$, where the sum of the oxidation numbers now equals zero ($+6$ from three Mg's and -6 from two PO_4's). The parentheses around the PO_4^{3-} ion indicate that the ion occurs more than once in the formula. If the ion occurs only once in a compound, parentheses are not necessary. Thus, in the compound between the sodium ion (oxidation number $+1$) and the nitrate ion (oxidation number -1), the formula is simply written as $NaNO_3$.

When the positive and negative oxidation numbers are equal, the formula is correctly written without subscripts. The compound formed between calcium (oxidation number $+2$) and the sulfate ion (oxidation number -2) is $CaSO_4$ since the sum of the oxidation numbers is already zero.

Occasionally, when both positive and negative oxidation numbers are even numbers, the formula of the compound can be simplified by dividing by 2. Thus, the compound formed between tin (oxidation number $+4$) and the sulfate ion (oxidation number -2) may be written as

$$\overset{+4}{Sn}\diagup\overset{-2}{SO_4}$$

or $Sn_2(SO_4)_4$, which may be simplified to $Sn(SO_4)_2$.

Molecular Weight

The molecular weight or formula weight of any compound is the sum of the atomic weights† of all of the atoms present in one molecule of that compound. The molecular weight of sodium bromide, NaBr, is 103, which represents the sum of the atomic weight of sodium (23) plus that of bromine (80). (See Table of Atomic Weights inside back cover.)

Calculating the Molecular Weight (Formula Weight) of a Compound

To find the molecular weight (M.W.) of a compound, add the atomic weights of all of the atoms that are present in that compound. In the compound H_2O, the molecular weight can be calculated by adding the weight of two atoms of hydrogen and one atom of oxygen.

$$
\begin{array}{lr}
\text{2 hydrogen atoms (atomic weight 1)} & 2 \times 1 \;\; = \;\; 2 \\
\text{1 oxygen atom (atomic weight 16)} & 1 \times 16 = 16 \\
\hline
& \text{molecular weight} = 18
\end{array}
$$

† Atomic weights are usually rounded off to the closest whole number.

The molecular weight of glucose, $C_6H_{12}O_6$, can be calculated as follows:

6 carbon atoms (atomic weight 12) $6 \times 12 = 72$
12 hydrogen atoms (atomic weight 1) $12 \times 1 = 12$
6 oxygen atoms (atomic weight 16) $6 \times 16 = 96$
molecular weight $= 180$

The molecular weight of calcium phosphate, $Ca_3(PO_4)_2$, can be calculated as follows:

3 calcium atoms (atomic weight 40) $3 \times 40 = 120$
2 phosphorus atoms (atomic weight 31) $2 \times 31 = 62$
8 oxygen atoms (atomic weight 16) $8 \times 16 = 128$
molecular weight $= 310$

Percentage Composition   The percentage composition of a compound can be calculated from the relative atomic weights of the elements present in that compound. Consider the compound $Ca_3(PO_4)_2$, calcium phosphate whose molecular weight was found to be 310 (see previous paragraph). Of this weight, 120 was calcium, 62 phosphorus, and 128 oxygen. Then

$$\%Ca = \frac{\text{weight of calcium in compound}}{\text{weight of compound}} \times 100 = \frac{120}{310} \times 100 = 38.7\%$$

$$\%P = \frac{\text{weight of phosphorus in compound}}{\text{weight of compound}} \times 100 = \frac{62}{310} \times 100 = 20.0\%$$

$$\%O = \frac{\text{weight of oxygen in compound}}{\text{weight of compound}} \times 100 = \frac{128}{310} \times 100 = 41.3\%$$

$$\text{total} = 100\%$$

The Mole   We measure distances on earth in terms of miles. However, this unit is far too small for distances to the stars. In that case, we need a much larger unit, the light year. So, too, chemists need a larger unit to weigh molecules, since individual molecules are too small to measure even with the most sensitive equipment. Such a unit, the **mole** (abbreviated mol) is defined as the number of atoms in 12.000 g of ^{12}C. One mole† of anything—molecules, atoms, ions, electrons—always contain the same number of particles, 6.02×10^{23} (602,000,000,000,000,000,000,000). This large number is called **Avogadro's number.**

One mole of any substance has a weight, in grams, equal to its molecular (or atomic) weight. That is

1 mol of water, H_2O,   contains 6.02×10^{23} molecules and weighs 18 g
1 mol of carbon, C,   contains 6.02×10^{23} atoms   and weighs 12 g
1 mol of glucose, $C_6H_{12}O_6$, contains 6.02×10^{23} molecules and weighs 180 g

† Note that the word mole is a "counting word" like dozen.

Inorganic Chemistry   **84**

Note that H_2O and $C_6H_{12}O_6$ are molecules; so we deal with Avogadro's number of molecules. Carbon, C, represents an atom; so we deal with Avogadro's number of atoms.

EXAMPLE 5-6. How much does 1 mol of NH_3, ammonia, weigh? How many molecules are present in 1 mol of ammonia?

The molecular weight of ammonia is 17 (N = 14 and each H = 1). So, 1 mol of NH_3 weighs 17 g. By definition, 1 mol of any substance contains Avogadro's number of particles, so 1 mol of NH_3 contains 6.02×10^{23} molecules. ∎

EXAMPLE 5-7. How much will 2 mol of NH_3 weigh?

If 1 mol of NH_3 weighs 17 g, 2 mol will weigh 34 g. We can write this mathematically as follows, using the conversion factor $1 \cdot mol\ NH_3 = 17$ g:

$$2\ \text{mol NH}_3 \times \frac{17\ \text{g NH}_3}{1\ \text{mol NH}_3} = 34\ \text{g NH}_3 \qquad ∎$$

EXAMPLE 5-8. A container holds 45 g sugar, $C_6H_{12}O_6$ (molecular weight 180). How many moles of sugar are present?

Since the molecular weight of sugar is 180, 1 mol sugar weighs 180 g. Using this latter figure as a conversion factor,

$$45\ \text{g sugar} \times \frac{1\ \text{mol sugar}}{180\ \text{g sugar}} = 0.25\ \text{mol sugar} \qquad ∎$$

EXAMPLE 5-9. How many molecules are present in 27 g water, H_2O (molecular weight 18)?

We know that 1 mol of any substance contains Avogadro's number of particles, 6.02×10^{23}. So, first we have to convert grams of water to moles of water (1 mol of water weighs 18 g) and then moles of water to molecules of water (1 mol of water contains 6.02×10^{23} molecules).

$$27\ \text{g H}_2\text{O} \times \frac{1\ \text{mol H}_2\text{O}}{18\ \text{g H}_2\text{O}} = 1.5\ \text{mol H}_2\text{O}$$

$$1.5\ \text{mol H}_2\text{O} \times \frac{6.02 \times 10^{23}\ \text{molecules H}_2\text{O}}{1\ \text{mol H}_2\text{O}} = 9.03 \times 10^{23}\ \text{molecules H}_2\text{O}$$

∎

Empirical and Molecular Formulas

An **empirical (simplest) formula** represents the relative number of each type of atom present in each molecule of a given compound.

A **molecular formula** represents the actual number of atoms present in each molecule of a given compound.

The empirical formula for both acetylene and benzene is CH, indicating one atom of carbon for each atom of hydrogen in both compounds. The molecular formula for acetylene is C_2H_2 and that of benzene C_6H_6. Note that in both of these compounds the ratio of carbons to hydrogens is 1:1.

Chemical Bonding

The empirical formula does not always represent the actual number of atoms present and so cannot represent the molecular weight. The molecular formula is always a simple integral multiple (1, 2, 3, etc.) of the empirical formula.

EXAMPLE 5-10. A compound contains 11.2 percent hydrogen and 88.8 percent oxygen. What is its empirical formula? If its molecular weight is 18, what is its molecular formula?

Step 1. *Assume that 100 g of the compound are present.* If there are 100 g of compound present, there will be 11.2 g of hydrogen (11.2 percent of 100 g) and also 88.8 g of oxygen (88.8 percent of 100 g).

Step 2. *Convert grams to moles.*

$$\text{For hydrogen} - 11.2 \text{ g} \times \frac{1 \text{ mol}}{1.0 \text{ g}} = 11.2 \text{ mol}$$

$$\text{For oxygen} - 88.8 \text{ g} \times \frac{1 \text{ mol}}{16 \text{ g}} = 5.6 \text{ mol}$$

Step 3. *Find the empirical formula by dividing by the smaller number of moles.*

$$\text{For hydrogen} - \frac{11.2 \text{ mol}}{5.6 \text{ mol}} = 2$$

$$\text{For oxygen} - \frac{5.6 \text{ mol}}{5.6 \text{ mol}} = 1$$

The ratio of 2 mol hydrogen to 1 mol oxygen gives the empirical formula of H_2O.

Step 4. *Find the molecular formula by dividing the weight of the empirical formula into the molecular weight and multiplying that number by the empirical formula.*

The weight of H_2O = 18 (H = 1, O = 16). The molecular weight is 18, so the ratio of 18/18 = 1, and thus in this case the empirical formula is also the molecular formula. ∎

EXAMPLE 5-11. A compound of molecular weight 56 contains 85.6 percent carbon, and 14.4 percent hydrogen. What is its empirical formula? its molecular formula?

Step 1.
$$\text{Carbon} - 85.6 \text{ g} \times \frac{1 \text{ mol}}{12 \text{ g}} = 7.1 \text{ mol}$$

$$\text{Hydrogen} - 14.4 \text{ g} \times \frac{1 \text{ mol}}{1 \text{ g}} = 14.4 \text{ mol}$$

Step 2.
$$\text{For carbon} - \frac{7.1 \text{ mol}}{7.1 \text{ mol}} = 1$$

$$\text{For hydrogen} - \frac{14.4 \text{ mol}}{7.1 \text{ mol}} = 2$$

Note that the number of moles is rounded off to whole numbers because in step 1 the exact atomic weights are not used.

Step 3. The empirical formula is CH_2.

Step 4. The weight of CH_2 is 14. The molecular weight was given as 56. 56/14 = 4, so the molecular formula is $C_4H_8(CH_2)_4$. ∎

EXAMPLE 5-12. A compound of molecular weight 270 contains 17.0 percent sodium, 47.4 percent sulfur, and 35.6 percent oxygen. What is its molecular formula?

Step 1.

$$\text{Sodium—17.0 g} \times \frac{1 \text{ mol}}{23 \text{ g}} = 0.74 \text{ mol}$$

$$\text{Sulfur—47.4 g} \times \frac{1 \text{ mol}}{32 \text{ g}} = 1.5 \text{ mol}$$

$$\text{Oxygen—35.6 g} \times \frac{1 \text{ mol}}{16 \text{ g}} = 2.2 \text{ mol}$$

Step 2.

$$\text{For sodium—}\frac{0.74 \text{ mol}}{0.74 \text{ mol}} = 1$$

$$\text{For sulfur—}\frac{1.5 \text{ mol}}{0.74 \text{ mol}} = 2$$

$$\text{For oxygen—}\frac{2.2 \text{ mol}}{0.74 \text{ mol}} = 3$$

Step 3. The empirical formula is NaS_2O_3.

Step 4. The weight of the empirical formula is $135(23 + 2 \times 32 + 3 \times 16)$. The given molecular weight is 270. $270/135 = 2$, so the molecular formula is $Na_2S_4O_6$.

■

Summary　　Molecules are combinations of two or more atoms. Atoms are held together in molecules by ionic or covalent bonds.

A symbol for an element not only identifies that element but also represents one atom of that element. A formula consists of a group of symbols that represent the elements present in a substance.

The number of outer electrons determines the chemical properties of the atom. Atoms are most stable when they have eight electrons in their outer energy level.

The electron-dot structure of an element uses the symbol of that element to represent the nucleus and all of the electrons except those in the outer energy level. Each outer electron is represented by a dot placed near the symbol.

Metals have one, two, or three outer electrons and tend to lose all those electrons to form positively charged ions. Nonmetals with six or seven outer electrons tend to gain electrons to fill their outer energy level to eight, thereby forming ions with a negative charge. Positively charged ions are called cations; negatively charged ions are called anions.

The ionic radius of a metal is less than that of the corresponding atom; the ionic radius of a nonmetal is greater than that of the corresponding atom.

When a metal loses an electron to form a positively charged ion and a nonmetal gains that electron to form a negatively charged ion, these ions are held together by the attraction of their charges. This type of bonding is called ionic bonding.

A polyatomic ion is a group of atoms that acts as a unit in a chemical reaction.

Ionic binary compounds are named by writing the name of the positive ion and then the stem of the negative ion with the ending *ide*. Ionic compounds containing polyatomic ions are named by writing the name of the positive ion and then the name of the polyatomic ion.

Nonmetals may also share electrons to complete their outer energy level. Such a bond is called a covalent bond. In a covalent bond no ions are formed. In forming covalent bonds, each element has eight electrons around it, except for hydrogen, which has only two.

Covalent compounds in which a pair of electrons is shared either between two identical atoms or between two atoms of equal electronegativity contain nonpolar covalent bonds. Covalent compounds containing bonds between atoms of different electronegativity contain polar covalent bonds.

Covalent compounds are named by writing a prefix and the name of the first element; then writing a prefix, the stem of the second element, and the ending *ide*.

For ionic compounds, the oxidation number is the same as the charge on the ion. For covalent compounds the oxidation number is an arbitrary number based on unequal sharing of electrons. The oxidation number of oxygen is -2 and that of hydrogen $+1$. In all compounds the sum of the oxidation numbers must equal zero.

In writing the formula of a compound from a table of oxidation numbers, the values of the oxidation numbers are crisscrossed. Care must be taken to note when the oxidation numbers are divisible by 2 so that the formula can be simplified.

The molecular weight of a compound is equal to the sum of the atomic weights of the atoms present in that compound. One mole of any substance contains Avogadro's number (6.02×10^{23}) particles.

An empirical (simplest) formula represents the relative number of each type of element present in a given compound.

A molecular formula represents the actual number of atoms present in each molecule of a given compound.

Questions and Problems

A

1. What is a molecule?
2. What are valence electrons? What effect do they have on the properties of an atom?
3. What is means by the term *electron-dot structure?*
4. Give the electron-dot structures for the following elements (use periodic table):
   (a) Phosphorus   (b) Oxygen   (c) Hydrogen
   (d) Neon   (e) Nitrogen   (f) Aluminum
5. What electron configuration does an element usually need to reach maximum stability?
6. What is an ion? What type of elements form positively charged ions? Negatively charged?
7. What type of bond consists of ions held together by the attraction of their charges?
8. What is an anion? cation? Give an example of each.
9. Name the following ionic compounds: (a) KI (b) $CaSO_4$ (c) ZnS (d) $NaNO_3$ (e) $AlCl_3$
10. Define *covalent bond*. Compare ionic and covalent bonds.
11. Draw the electron-dot structures for the following covalent compounds:
    (a) H_2 (b) HCl   (c) H_2S
    (d) PH_3 (e) CH_4 (f) N_2
12. What is a polyatomic ion? Give two examples.
13. What is a single covalent bond? double bond? triple bond? Give an example of each.
14. What is a nonpolar covalent bond? a polar covalent bond? Give an example of each.
15. Name the following covalent compounds: (a) PCl_3 (b) SO_2 (c) N_2O_5 (d) CS_2 (e) ICl
16. Write the formulas for the compounds formed from the following ion pairs:
    (a) H^+ and SO_4^{2-} (b) Fe^{2+} and Cl^- (c) Cu^+ and I^-
    (d) Ca^{2+} and PO_4^{3-} (e) Ba^{2+} and HCO_3^- (f) Mg^{2+} and NO_3^-
    (g) Ca^{2+} and S^{2-} (h) Al^{3+} and CO_3^{2-}
17. Write the formulas for the compounds formed between the following: silver

ions and sulfate ions; potassium ions and bicarbonate ions; ammonium ions and sulfide ions; hydrogen ions and nitrate ions.

18. Calculate the oxidation number for *each* atom of the underlined element (consult Table 5-1 for charges and Table 5-5 for oxidation numbers).
    (a) $K\underline{Cl}O_4$ (b) $Na\underline{N}O_2$ (c) $\underline{Fe}_2O_3$ (d) $\underline{As}_2S_5$
    (e) $H_4\underline{P}_2O_7$ (f) $K_2\underline{Cr}_2O_7$ (g) $\underline{Ra}(HCO_3)_2$ (h) $(\underline{NH}_4)_2S$

19. What do the following symbols or formulas indicate: H_2, 2H, CO_2, CO?

20. Calculate the molecular weight of each of the following compounds (use atomic weights as whole numbers).
    (a) $NaNO_3$ (b) KBr   (c) $Ca(HCO_3)_2$ (d) $C_{12}H_{22}O_{11}$ (e) $C_{57}H_{110}O_6$

21. What is the difference between an empirical formula and a molecular formula? Can they ever be the same?

22. Calculate the empirical formula for a compound containing 31.9 percent potassium, 28.9 percent chlorine, and 39.2 percent oxygen.

23. Which is larger, a metallic atom or its corresponding ion? Why? a nonmetallic atom?

24. Why would water solutions of ionic compounds be expected to conduct electricity?

B 25. Explain how a nonpolar molecule may contain polar bonds.

26. Why is fluorine the most electronegative element?

27. What is the predominant cation in extracellular body fluids? in intracellular body fluids?

28. What is the predominant anion in extracellular body fluids? in intracellular body fluids?

29. How can you tell whether a covalent bond will be polar or nonpolar?

30. Why does a diamond have such a high melting point? What type of bonds does it have?

31. Why is the oxidation number of sodium +1 rather than +2 or −1?

32. Can elements have more than one oxidation number? Explain.

33. Can both elements in a binary compound have a positive oxidation number? Explain.

34. When writing the formula of a binary compound, is the first element always a metal? a nonmetal? Is the second element always a metal? a nonmetal?

35. Do all covalent bonds consist of atoms having eight electrons around them? Explain.

36. What is the empirical formula and the molecular formula for a compound of molecular weight 284 that contains 43.7 percent phosphorus and 56.3 percent oxygen?

References   DICKSON, T. R. *Introduction to Chemistry,* 4th ed. John Wiley & Sons, Inc., New York, 1983, Chapter 5.

MORTIMER, CHARLES E. *Chemistry,* 5th ed. Wadsworth Publishing Co., Belmont, Calif., 1983, Chapter 6.

PETRUCCI, RALPH H. and ROBERT E. WISMER. *General Chemistry with Qualitative Analysis.* Macmillan Publishing Company, New York, 1983, Chapters 9, 10.

RAYNER-CANHAN, GEOFFREY and MARK VAN ROODE. *Foundations of Chemistry.* Addison-Wesley Publishing Co., Reading, Mass., 1983, Chapter 4.

SACKHEIM, GEORGE I. *Chemical Calculations,* 12th ed., Series B. Stipes Publishing Co., Champaign, Ill., 1983, Chapter 11.

Stoker, H. Stephen. *Introduction to Chemical Principles.* Macmillan Publishing Company, New York, 1983, Chapter 10.

6 Chemical Equations and Reactions

CHAPTER
OUTLINE

Chemical Equations
    Balancing Chemical Equations
Types of Chemical Reactions
Equilibrium Reactions
    Equilibrium Constant
    Le Chatelier's Principle
    Effect of Concentration
    Effect of Temperature
    Effect of a Catalyst

Interpreting Chemical Equations
Reaction Rates
    Nature of Reacting Substances
    Temperature
    Concentration
    Catalyst
    Surface Area

Chemical Equations

When an electrical current (energy) is passed through water (a process known as **electrolysis**) hydrogen gas and oxygen gas are produced. The chemist uses symbols and formulas to describe this chemical reaction.

$$H_2O + \text{energy} \longrightarrow H_2\uparrow + O_2\uparrow$$

The arrow is used instead of an equal sign and is reads as "yields" or "produces." The plus sign on the right side of the equation is read as "and." A plus sign on the left side of the equation is read as "reacts with." The materials that react are called the **reactants.** The reactants are written on the left side of the equation. The substances that are produced are called the **products.** They are written on the right side of the equation. An arrow pointing downward after a substance indicates that that substance is a precipitate; that is, it is an insoluble solid, one that settles out of a reaction mixture. An arrow pointing upward after a substance indicates that that substance is a gas. The energy involved in the reaction may be written in words on the left (or right) side of the equation; it may be indicated above the arrow, or it may be indicated by the symbol Δ (Greek delta). The use of a catalyst may be shown above or below the arrow.

A chemical equation must be balanced before any specific interpretation can be made about that reaction. For example, if we wish to know how much oxygen will be required to metabolize a given amount of a particular carbohydrate, we must first set up a balanced equation for the reaction.

Balancing Chemical Equations

Note that the chemical equation shown below does not contain the same number of hydrogen and oxygen atoms on each side of the arrow. To be balanced, a chemical equation must contain the same number of atoms of each element on both sides of that equation. Thus equation (6–1) is *not* balanced.

$$H_2O + \text{energy} \longrightarrow H_2\uparrow + O_2\uparrow \quad \text{(unbalanced)} \quad (6\text{–}1)$$

In balancing a chemical equation, you must not change the subscripts (the lower numbers after the symbols) because doing so would change either the reactants or the products, thus changing the meaning of the reaction. Instead, place coefficients in front of the symbols and formulas to indicate how many atoms or molecules of each are needed.

In the equation $H_2O \rightarrow H_2 + O_2$, there are two hydrogen atoms on each side of the equation. There is one oxygen atom on the left side and two oxygen atoms on the right side of the equation. To get two atoms of oxygen on the left side of the equation (in order to balance the two oxygen atoms on the right side), place a 2 in front of the H_2O. The 2 cannot be placed as a subscript after the O in H_2O because then another substance would be represented, not water. The 2 cannot be placed between the H and the O because this also would change the meaning of the formula. Therefore, place the 2 in front of the H_2O.

$$2H_2O + \text{energy} \longrightarrow H_2\uparrow + O_2\uparrow \quad \text{(unbalanced)}$$

However, now there are four hydrogen atoms on the left side of the equation ($2H_2$'s). In order to get four hydrogen atoms on the right side of the equation, place a 2 in front of the H_2. There are already two oxygen atoms on each side of the equation. Thus the balanced equation is as follows:

$$2H_2O + \text{energy} \longrightarrow 2H_2\uparrow + O_2\uparrow \quad \text{(balanced)}$$

This balanced equation now shows that two molecules of water, on electrolysis, yield two molecules of hydrogen gas and one molecule of oxygen gas.

When aluminum metal reacts with sulfuric acid, the products are hydrogen gas, H_2, and aluminum sulfate, $Al_2(SO_4)_3$. The unbalanced equation for this reaction is

$$Al + H_2SO_4 \longrightarrow Al_2(SO_4)_3 + H_2\uparrow + \Delta \quad \text{(unbalanced)} \quad (6\text{–}2)$$

Equation (6–2) is not balanced because there are more aluminum atoms on the right side of the equation than on the left side. The same is true for the sulfur and oxygen atoms. To balance an equation of this type, pick out the most complicated-looking formula and assume that one molecule of it is present. The most complicated-looking formula in the above equation is $Al_2(SO_4)_3$. Assuming that one molecule of it is produced, then there are two atoms of aluminum on the right side of the equation. To balance this, place a 2 in front of the Al on the left side of the equation. (For simplicity, we will omit the Δ sign from all the equations that follow.)

$$2Al + H_2SO_4 \longrightarrow Al_2(SO_4)_3 + H_2\uparrow \quad \text{(unbalanced)}$$

Next note that there are three SO_4 groups in the molecule of $Al_2(SO_4)_3$. There then must be three SO_4 groups on the left side of the equation. To get these three groups place a 3 in front of the H_2SO_4.

$$2Al + 3H_2SO_4 \longrightarrow Al_2(SO_4)_3 + H_2\uparrow \quad \text{(unbalanced)}$$

To complete the equation, note that there are now six hydrogen atoms on the left side of the equation (in the $3H_2$'s). Therefore, there must be six hydrogen atoms on the right side, so place a 3 in front of the H_2.

$$2Al + 3H_2SO_4 \longrightarrow Al_2(SO_4)_3 + 3H_2\uparrow \quad \text{(balanced)}$$

Now the equation is balanced. There are two aluminums, six hydrogens, three sulfurs, and twelve oxygens (or $3SO_4$'s) on each side of the equation.

When sulfur is burned in excess oxygen, sulfur trioxide is produced. When this reaction is written in equation form, it becomes equation (6–3).

$$S + O_2 \longrightarrow SO_3 \quad \text{(unbalanced)} \qquad (6\text{–}3)$$

Following the balancing procedure, pick out the most complicated compound and take one molecule of it. Thus, in equation (6–3) take one molecule of SO_3. This molecule contains one atom of sulfur. There is already one atom of sulfur on the left side of the equation. There are three atoms of oxygen on the right side of the equation and only two on the left side. However, there is no *whole* number that can be placed in front of the O_2 to make three oxygen atoms on that side of the equation. If a 2 is placed there, there will be four atoms of oxygen. In this case, then, instead of selecting one molecule of the most complicated compound, select two molecules of it.

$$S + O_2 \longrightarrow 2SO_3 \quad \text{(unbalanced)}$$

Then, in order to balance two sulfur atoms on the right side of the equation, start with two sulfur atoms on the left side.

$$2S + O_2 \longrightarrow 2SO_3 \quad \text{(unbalanced)}$$

Next, the right side of the equation contains six oxygen atoms and so must the left side. Place a 3 in front of the O_2 in order to have six oxygen atoms on that side of the equation. The equation then is balanced.

$$2S + 3O_2 \longrightarrow 2SO_3 \quad \text{(balanced)}$$

Types of Chemical Reactions Chemical reactions can be divided into **combination reactions, decomposition reactions, single replacement or substitution reactions,** and **double displacement or metathesis reactions.** These are illustrated in Table 6–1. Note that the example equations are written as balanced equations.

TABLE 6-1. Chemical Reactions

Type	General Equation	Example
Combination	$A + B \longrightarrow AB$	$C + O_2 \longrightarrow CO_2$ $2S + 3O_2 \longrightarrow 2SO_3$
Decomposition	$AB \longrightarrow A + B$	$2HgO \longrightarrow 2Hg + O_2\uparrow$ $2KClO_3 \longrightarrow 2KCl + 3O_2\uparrow$
Single replacement	$A + BC \longrightarrow AC + B$ or $A + BC \longrightarrow BA + C$	$Zn + CuSO_4 \longrightarrow ZnSO_4 + Cu$ $Cl_2 + 2NaBr \longrightarrow 2NaCl + Br_2$
Double displacement	$AB + CD \longrightarrow AD + CB$	$Na_2SO_4 + BaCl_2 \longrightarrow 2NaCl + BaSO_4\downarrow$ $FeS + 2HCl \longrightarrow FeCl_2 + H_2S\uparrow$

Other types of chemical reactions include equilibrium reactions (see following paragraphs) and oxidation–reduction reactions (see Chapter 9).

Equilibrium Reactions

Many times when two or more reactants unite to form a certain number of products, these products themselves unite to reform the original reactants. Reactions of this type are called **reversible reactions.** They are indicated by double arrows $\rightleftharpoons$ showing that the reaction may proceed in either direction depending upon the conditions that exist.

If we start with a mixture of N_2 and H_2, at a given temperature and pressure (with a catalyst) we will soon have some NH_3 formed. As more NH_3 is formed, it will begin to decompose into N_2 and H_2, or

$$N_2 + 3H_2 \rightleftharpoons 2NH_3$$

When the rates of formation and decomposition become equal, a chemical **equilibrium** exists. This does not mean that all reaction has stopped; it merely means that the rate of decomposition is the same as the rate of formation so that the composition remains constant. An equilibrium may be defined as a dynamic state in which the **rate of the forward reaction is equal to the rate of the reverse reaction.**

Two examples of equilibrium reactions in the body are

$$HCO_3^- + H^+ \rightleftharpoons H_2CO_3 \rightleftharpoons CO_2 + H_2O$$

and

$$\text{hemoglobin} + \text{oxygen} \rightleftharpoons \text{oxyhemoglobin}$$

Equilibrium Constant

Consider the following general equilibrium reaction.

$$A + B \rightleftharpoons C + D$$

The **law of mass action** states that the rate of a chemical reaction is proportional to the concentration of the reacting substances. So, for the above reaction, rate forward $= k_1[A][B]$ where k_1 is a proportionality constant and the brackets, [ ], indicate concentrations in the units moles per liter. Like-

Chemical Equations and Reactions   **93**

wise, the rate of the reverse reaction $= k_2[C][D]$ where k_2 is another proportionality constant.

At equilibrium, the rate of the forward reaction is equal to the rate of the reverse reaction, so

$$k_1 \times [A] \times [B] = k_2 \times [C] \times [D]$$

whence

$$\frac{[C] \times [D]}{[A] \times [B]} = \frac{k_1}{k_2} = K_{eq}$$

where K_{eq} is the equilibrium constant (since the ratio of two constants k_1/k_2 is itself another constant).

In general, the equilibrium constant, K_{eq}, equals the product of the concentrations of the products divided by the product of the concentrations of the reactants, each concentration raised to the power indicated by its coefficient in the equation. So, for the reaction $4A + 3C \rightleftharpoons 2D + F$, we have

$$K_{eq} = \frac{[D]^2[F]}{[A]^4[C]^3}$$

EXAMPLE 6-1. In the conversion of glucose to vitamin C, the following equilibrium reaction takes place.

$$\underset{\text{gluconic acid}}{C_5H_{11}O_5COOH} \rightleftharpoons \underset{\text{hydrogen ion}}{H^+} + \underset{\text{gluconate ion}}{C_5H_{11}O_5COO^-}$$

If the equilibrium concentrations in moles per liter are $C_5H_{11}O_5COOH$, 0.10; H^+, 3.7×10^{-3}; $C_5H_{11}O_5COO^-$, 3.7×10^{-3}, calculate the value of K_{eq}.

Using the formula

$$K_{eq} = \frac{[H^+][C_5H_{11}O_5COO^-]}{[C_5H_{11}O_5COOH]}$$

$$K_{eq} = \frac{(3.7 \times 10^{-3})(3.7 \times 10^{-3})}{0.10}$$

$$= 1.4 \times 10^{-4} \qquad\qquad \blacksquare$$

EXAMPLE 6-2. In the manufacture of wood alcohol (page 241), the following equilibrium reaction occurs: $CO + 2H_2 \rightleftharpoons CH_3OH$. At equilibrium, the concentrations in moles per liter are CO, 0.025; H_2, 0.050; CH_3OH, 0.12. Calculate the value of K_{eq}.

$$K_{eq} = \frac{[CH_3OH]}{[CO][H_2]^2} = \frac{(0.12)}{(0.025)(0.050)^2} = 1.9 \times 10^3 \qquad \blacksquare$$

In general, a large value of K_{eq} indicates an equilibrium that has been shifted far to the right, whereas a small value indicates one shifted to the left.

Inorganic Chemistry

Le Chatelier's Principle

Le Chatelier's principle states that **if a stress is applied to a reaction at equilibrium, the equilibrium will be displaced in such a direction as to relieve that stress.** Thus, if we apply a stress such as a change in concentration or temperature, we should be able to predict the results of such a stress upon the given equilibrium.

Effect of Concentration

Let us see what will be the effect upon the equilibrium and upon the equilibrium constant if we add more A to a mixture of A, B, C, and D. The reaction is

$$A + B \rightleftharpoons C + D$$

Increasing the concentration of a reactant increases the number of collisions between reactant molecules so that the rate of the forward reaction is greater than the rate of the reverse reaction. The system is no longer in equilibrium. However, as the reactant molecules are used up, the rate of the forward reaction will decrease and the rate of the reverse reaction will increase until a new equilibrium is established. That is, the addition of more A will cause a stress that the reaction will tend to oppose by using up more A, thus shifting the equilibrium to the right. Since the equilibrium constant depends upon temperature only, the addition of more A will have no effect upon it. Thus, the addition of more A increases the amount of products; likewise for the addition of more B to the equilibrium mixture. In accordance with Le Chatelier's principle, removal of a product (or products) should also shift the equilibrium to the right.

Consider the enzyme-catalyzed reaction

$$CO_2 + H_2O \rightleftharpoons H_2CO_3$$

Carbon dioxide is a waste product produced in the cells. As the CO_2 flows into the blood, its concentration increases and so, according to Le Chatelier's principle, the equilibrium shifts toward the right, producing more H_2CO_3. In the lungs, as carbon dioxide is exhaled, the equilibrium is shifted to the left, again according to Le Chatelier's principle.

Effect of Temperature

In the reaction

$$4HCl + O_2 \rightleftharpoons 2H_2O + 2Cl_2 + heat$$

heat is liberated when the reaction proceeds to the right and is absorbed when it proceeds to the left.

If we raise the temperature of this reaction mixture at equilibrium, the reaction will tend to go in a direction to relieve this stress. That is, as the temperature is raised, the equilibrium will shift to the left, favoring the reaction which tends to absorb this heat. Conversely, as the temperature is lowered, the reaction speeds more to the right for the production of more heat to relieve the new stress.

Effect of a Catalyst

The addition of a catalyst will speed up the forward reaction but will speed up the reverse reaction equally. Thus, all that is accomplished is that the

they lower activation energy

Chemical Equations and Reactions

system reaches equilibrium much sooner. The equilibrium reached is the same as would have been reached if no catalyst had been used. Again we note that temperature is the only thing that affects the equilibrium constant, so naturally a catalyst will have no effect on it.

Interpreting Chemical Equations

A balanced chemical equation specifies a great deal of quantitative information. Consider balanced equation (6-4):

$$2H_2 + O_2 \longrightarrow 2H_2O \qquad (6\text{-}4)$$

Equation (6-4) indicates that two molecules of H_2 react with one molecule of O_2 to produce two molecules of H_2O. Note that the numbers are the same as the coefficients (numbers in front of the substances) in the balanced equation. That is why the equation must be balanced before doing any type of calculation.

Equation (6-4) may also be interpreted in terms of moles—2 mol of H_2 react with 1 mol O_2 to produce 2 mol H_2O.

We can substitute molecular weights in grams for moles in equation 6-4. Thus the equation can be represented as

$$2H_2 + \qquad O_2 \qquad \longrightarrow 2H_2O$$

$$2 \text{ molecules} + 1 \text{ molecule} \longrightarrow 2 \text{ molecules}$$

$$2 \text{ mol} + \qquad 1 \text{ mol} \qquad \longrightarrow 2 \text{ mol}$$

$$2(2 \text{ g}) + \qquad 32 \text{ g} \qquad \longrightarrow 2(18 \text{ g})$$

Note that the law of conservation of mass must be satisfied.

EXAMPLE 6-3. Given the balanced equation

$$C_6H_{12}O_6 + 6O_2 \longrightarrow 6CO_2 + 6H_2O + 686 \text{ kcal}$$

how many moles of CO_2 will be produced from 3.5 mol of $C_6H_{12}O_6$?
We note from the balanced equation that 1 mol of $C_6H_{12}O_6$ yields 6 mol of CO_2. Using this as a conversion factor,

$$3.5 \text{ mol } C_6H_{12}O_6 \times \frac{6 \text{ mol } CO_2}{1 \text{ mol } C_6H_{12}O_6} = 21 \text{ mol } CO_2 \qquad \blacksquare$$

EXAMPLE 6-4. Using the balanced equation in Example 6.3, how many grams of water will be produced from the reaction of 0.50 mol $C_6H_{12}O_6$?
The balanced equation indicates that 1 mol of $C_6H_{12}O_6$ yields 6 mol of H_2O so that

$$0.50 \text{ mol } C_6H_{12}O_6 \times \frac{6 \text{ mol } H_2O}{1 \text{ mol } C_6H_{12}O_6} = 3 \text{ mol } H_2O$$

Then, recalling that 1 mol of H_2O weighs 18 g, we obtain

$$3 \text{ mol } H_2O \times \frac{18 \text{ g } H_2O}{1 \text{ mol } H_2O} = 54 \text{ g } H_2O \qquad \blacksquare$$

EXAMPLE 6-5. Using the balanced equation in Example 6-3, how much energy will be produced from the complete combustion of 0.5 moles $C_6H_{12}O_6$?

The balanced equation indicates that complete oxidation of 1 mol of $C_6H_{12}O_6$ yields 686 kcal, so

$$0.50 \text{ mol } C_6H_{12}O_6 \times \frac{686 \text{ kcal}}{1 \text{ mol } C_6H_{12}O_6} = 343 \text{ kcal} \qquad \blacksquare$$

Reaction Rates   Some chemical reactions proceed at a slow rate. Iron, for example, rusts very slowly. Wood takes years to decay. On the other hand, some chemical reactions proceed more rapidly. Coal burns steadily and quickly. Concrete begins to set within a few hours. Some chemical reactions not only occur rapidly, they take place almost instantaneously. Consider the violent explosion of dynamite. Within a fraction of a second, the complete reaction has taken place.

In order for a chemical reaction to occur between two substances, their molecules must collide (interact) with sufficient energy to overcome any force of repulsion between the electron clouds.

The minimum amount of energy required for a collision to produce a successful reaction is called the **activation energy*** (Figure 6–1).

FIGURE 6-1. A catalyst increases the rate of a reaction by lowering the activation energy so that more reactant molecules collide with enough energy to surmount the lower energy barrier.

What determines the speed of a chemical reaction? The speed of a chemical reaction depends upon several factors: (1) the nature of the reacting substances, (2) the temperature, (3) the concentration of the reacting substances, (4) the presence of a catalyst, and (5) the surface area and the intimacy of contact of the reacting substances.

Nature of Reacting Substances   When a solution of sodium sulfate (Na_2SO_4) is mixed with a solution of barium chloride ($BaCl_2$), a white precipitate of barium sulfate ($BaSO_4$) is formed immediately.

Chemical Equations and Reactions   **97**

$$Na_2SO_4 + BaCl_2 \longrightarrow 2NaCl + BaSO_4\downarrow \qquad (6\text{-}5)$$

Equation (6-5) can be rewritten to show the ions of which these salts consist.

$$2Na^+ + SO_4^{2-} + Ba^{2+} + 2Cl^- \longrightarrow 2Na^+ + 2Cl^- + BaSO_4\downarrow$$

Next, as in any algebraic equation, cancel the sodium ions and the chloride ions from both sides of equation (6-5) leaving the net equation

$$Ba^{2+} + SO_4^{2-} \longrightarrow BaSO_4\downarrow$$

This is an example of an ionic reaction—the reaction between ions. Many of the reactions taking place in the body are of this type.

Consider, however, the reaction between hydrogen (H_2) and oxygen (O_2) to form water (H_2O). This reaction proceeds very slowly, even at a temperature of 200°C unless a spark is introduced into the mixture.

$$2H_2 + O_2 \xrightarrow{\text{spark}} 2H_2O$$

In this reaction, it is necessary for the bonds between the hydrogen atoms in the hydrogen molecules to be broken. Also, the bonds between the oxygen atoms must be broken before the reaction can occur. This is an example of a reaction in which covalent bonds must be broken and new ones formed. In general, such reactions proceed much more slowly than ionic reactions.

Temperature   As the temperature rises, the speed of a chemical reaction increases because at higher temperatures the molecules move faster and therefore collide more often. Thus even a slight change in temperature may affect the speed of a reaction with noticeable results.

A patient who has a fever of only a few degrees has an increased pulse rate and also an increased respiratory rate. Reactions taking place throughout the body proceed at an accelerated rate.

When the temperature of the human body drops, the various metabolic processes slow down considerably. This fact is of great importance, for example, during open-heart surgery when the temperature of the body is lowered considerably.

A drop in body temperature of 2 to 3°F causes uncontrolled shivering as the body tries to generate heat by muscle activity. Death from exposure occurs when the body temperature drops below 78°F. Victims who fall overboard in water whose temperature is near freezing may survive only a short time unless they are rescued or wearing the proper type of insulated coverings. A person who has been "chilled" in such an accident should be given dry clothing and warmed as soon as possible. Warm liquids are helpful in increasing body temperature as are "sugars." Contrary to popular belief, alcohol is not helpful in such a situation because it dilates blood vessels, allowing cold blood to flow more rapidly to the vital organs.

Concentration   The concentration of a reactant is the amount present in a given unit of volume. The more of a given material present in a certain volume, the greater its concentration. Greater concentration produces faster reactions because there are more molecules than can react.

A patient with a respiratory disease can breathe more easily when using a nasal catheter with oxygen because the concentration of the oxygen in the lungs is increased. This increased concentration increases the speed of oxygen uptake, making breathing easier for the patient.

Catalyst   When a protein substance is placed in water and heated, a hydrolysis reaction (see page 355) proceeds at an extremely slow speed. If a strong acid is added to the mixture, the reaction proceeds at a much faster rate. The acid is not used up (that is, it is not changed chemically). Its presence merely increases the speed of the reaction. Any substance that increases the speed of a reaction without itself being changed chemically is called a catalyst.

Catalysts function to increase the rate of a reaction because they provide a pathway with a lower activation energy.* Many of the chemical reactions used in industry would not be practical without a catalyst. They would take too long to be of commercial use (see diagram on page 97).

The body uses catalysts to enable its chemical reactions to proceed at a rapid pace. Those catalysts present in the body are called **enzymes.** During digestion, for example, the food undergoes many chemical changes, each under the influence of a specific enzyme. There are also **inhibitors** that slow down rather than speed up chemical reactions.

Surface Area   The speed of a chemical reaction also depends upon the amount of surface area present in the reacting substances. Although a pile of flour is quite harmless, the same flour in the form of dust can cause a dangerous explosion. This effect is due to the tremendous amount of surface area of the dust. This large surface area can then react rapidly with the oxygen in the air to cause an explosion.

Many medications are given in the form of finely divided suspended solids. In this manner, more surface area means more rapid absorption in the body.

Increasing the concentration of the reacting substances may also be considered as increasing the amount of surface area.

Summary   A chemical equation uses symbols and formulas to represent a chemical reaction. The substances on the left side of the equation are called reactants and those on the right side products. An arrow pointing upward indicates a gas; an arrow pointing downward indicates a precipitate.

To balance a chemical equation, pick out the most complicated-looking compound and assume that one molecule of it is present. Then proceed back and forth adding coefficients in front of the reactants and products until the number of atoms of each type on each side of the equation is the same.

Chemical Equations and Reactions   **99**

The four types of chemical reactions and their general equations are

Combination	$A + B \longrightarrow AB$
Decomposition	$AB \longrightarrow A + B$
Single replacement	$A + BC \longrightarrow AC + B$
	or
	$A + BC \longrightarrow BA + C$
Double displacement	$AB + CD \longrightarrow AD + CB$

An equilibrium reaction is a dynamic state in which the rate of the forward reaction is equal to the rate of the reverse reaction.

Le Chatelier's principle states that, if a stress is applied to a reaction at equilibrium, the equilibrium will be displaced in such a direction as to relieve that stress.

The speed of a chemical reaction depends upon the nature of the reacting substances, upon the temperature, upon the concentration of the reacting substances, upon the presence of a catalyst, and upon the surface area of the reacting substances.

Questions and Problems

A

1. Balance the following equations:
   (a) $Mg + O_2 \longrightarrow MgO$
   (b) $Zn + HCl \longrightarrow ZnCl_2 + H_2$
   (c) $C + O_2 \longrightarrow CO_2$
   (d) $NaCl + AgNO_3 \longrightarrow AgCl + NaNO_3$
   (e) $ZnSO_4 + NaOH \longrightarrow Zn(OH)_2 + Na_2SO_4$
   (f) $Fe + O_2 \longrightarrow Fe_3O_4$
   (g) $Mg + AgNO_3 \longrightarrow Mg(NO_3)_2 + Ag$
   (h) $Al(OH)_3 + H_2SO_4 \longrightarrow Al_2(SO_4)_3 + H_2O$
2. Label each of the reactions in question 1 as to type.
3. What factors determine the rate of a chemical reaction? Indicate at least one practical application of each factor.
4. Calculate the percentage composition of each compound in question 1 (answers to one decimal place).
5. What is a mole? What does 1 mol of $C_{12}H_{22}O_{11}$ weigh?
6. How many moles are present in 500 g $CaCO_3$? How many molecules?
7. Given the balanced equation $Zn + H_2SO_4 \longrightarrow ZnSO_4 + H_2$, how many moles of H_2 can be produced from 2.5 mol Zn?
8. How many grams of $ZnSO_4$ can be produced from 0.54 mol H_2SO_4 according to the equation in question 7?
9. Define equilibrium. What does Le Chatelier's principle state?
10. Calculate the value of K_{eq} for the reaction $A + 2B \rightleftharpoons 3C$ if the molar concentrations are A, 1.0; B, 1.5; and C, 0.80.

B

11. How much will 6.02×10^{23} atoms of Ne weigh?
12. How many moles of $Fe_2(SO_4)_3$ are present in 6.00×10^{-5} g?
13. How many molecules are present in 5 mol H_2O? how many atoms?
14. Why must an equation be balanced before weight calculations can be made?
15. How many grams of S will react with oxygen to yield 2.5 mol SO_3?
    $2S + 3O_2 \longrightarrow 2SO_3$

Inorganic Chemistry

16. Calculate K_{eq} for the reaction $N_2 + 3H_2 \rightleftharpoons 2NH_3 +$ heat if the molar concentrations are N_2, 5.0; H_2, 2.0; NH_3, 50.0.
17. How may the reaction in question 16 be shifted to the right? to the left?
18. What effect will a change of temperature have on the equilibrium in question 16?
19. Why does an increase in the concentration of a reactant increase the rate of the forward reaction?
20. What effect does a catalyst have upon an equilibrium? Why?
21. Is a reaction at equilibrium static or dynamic? Explain.

References

DICKSON, T. R. *Introduction to Chemistry,* 4th ed. John Wiley & Sons, Inc., New York, 1983, Chapters 3, 6.

EBBING, DARRELL D. *General Chemistry.* Houghton Mifflin Co., Boston, 1984, Chapter 3.

MCQUARRIE, DONALD A. and PETER A. ROCK. *General Chemistry.* W. H. Freeman Co. New York, 1984, Chapters 3, 4.

MILLER, FRANCIS MARION. *Chemistry, Structure and Dynamics.* McGraw Hill Book Co., New York, 1984, Chapter 3.

PETRUCCI, RALPH H. and ROBERT E. WISMER. *General Chemistry with Qualitative Analysis.* Macmillan Publishing Company, New York, 1983, Chapters 4, 5.

RAYNER-CANHAN, GEOFFREY and MARK VAN ROODE. *Foundations of Chemistry.* Addison-Wesley Publishing Co., Reading, Mass., 1983, Chapters 5, 8.

SACKHEIM, GEORGE I. *Chemical Calculations,* 12th ed., Series B. Stipes Publishing Co., Champaign, Ill., 1983, Chapters 4, 7, 8.

STOKER, H. STEPHEN. *Introduction to Chemical Principles.* Macmillan Publishing Company, New York, 1983, Chapters 6–8.

7 The Gaseous State

CHAPTER OUTLINE

General Properties
The Kinetic Molecular Theory
Measurement of Pressure
The Gas Laws
    Boyle's Law
    Charles' Law
    Pressure–Temperature Relationship
    Combined Gas Laws

Dalton's Law
Graham's Law
Henry's Law
Molar Gas Volumes
Air Pollution
    Gases
The Ozone Layer

General Properties

In Chapter 2 we saw that gases have no definite shape, no definite volume, and a low density. Gases have a much greater volume than an equal mass of solid or liquid. For example, 1 g of liquid water occupies 1 ml and 1 g of solid water (ice) occupies nearly 1 ml, but 1 g of water vapor (at 0°C and 1 atm pressure) occupies nearly 1250 ml. These and other properties of gases can be explained in terms of the kinetic molecular theory.

The Kinetic Molecular Theory

The principal assumptions of the kinetic molecular theory are as follows:

1. Gases consist of tiny particles called molecules.
2. The distance between the molecules of a gas is very great compared to the size of the molecules themselves (that is, the volume occupied by a gas is mostly empty space).
3. Gas molecules are in rapid motion and move in straight lines, frequently colliding with each other and with the walls of the container.
4. Gas molecules do not attract each other.
5. When molecules of a gas collide with each other or with the walls of the container, they bounce back with no loss of energy. Such collisions are said to be perfectly elastic.
6. The average kinetic energy of the molecules is the same for all gases at the same temperature. The average kinetic energy increases as the temperature increases and decreases as the temperature decreases.

Let us see how the various properties of gases can be explained in terms of this theory.

1. If the distance between molecules is very great compared to the size of the molecules themselves, the molecules will occupy only a small fraction of that volume so the density will be very low.

2. If the molecules are moving rapidly in all directions, they can fill any size container. They can keep on moving until they hit a wall of the container or until they hit each other and bounce back; that is, the gas will have no definite volume and no definite shape.

3. If the molecules of a gas strike the walls of a container, they should exert a pressure on that wall. And, since the molecules are moving in all directions, they should exert a pressure equally in all directions. Gases do just this.

4. If a bottle of ether is opened in a room, the odor is soon apparent in all parts of that room; that is, the molecules of ether gas diffuse into the air (a mixture of gases). According to the kinetic molecular theory, there is a great deal of empty space between the molecules of a gas so that the ether molecules (or any other gas) can diffuse into the spaces between the air molecules.

5. We can show that the collisions must be perfectly elastic by means of a reverse type of reasoning. Suppose that the collisions between molecules were not perfectly elastic; that is, some energy was lost upon collisions with each other and with the walls of the container. Eventually, the gas molecules would have so little energy left that they would settle to the bottom of the container. However, gases never settle. Therefore, the collisions between the molecules themselves and the walls of the container must be perfectly elastic.

6. Since gas molecules are so far apart, it should be possible to force them closer together by increasing the pressure; that is, gases should be compressible, as indeed they are.

Measurement of Pressure

Pressure is measured by a barometer, one form of which is shown in Figure 7-1. A glass tube about 1 yd long is filled with mercury and the open end inverted into a dish of mercury. The mercury falls in the tube, leaving a

FIGURE 7-1. Pressure is measured by a barometer.

The Gaseous State

vacuum above it, until the pressure exerted by the air just balances the mercury column in the tube. Thus the atmospheric pressure is expressed as being equal to so many millimeters of mercury or the height of the column from A to B.

One unit of pressure is the torr, named after the Italian scientist Torricelli who invented the barometer. One torr is the pressure exerted by 1 mm of mercury at sea level.

Standard pressure is 1.00 atm and will support a column of mercury 760 mm tall. Standard pressure may be expressed in many different units. Among these are the following:

760 mm Hg	29.92 in. Hg	1.013×10^5 pascals (Pa)
76.0 cm Hg	14.7 lb/in.^{2}	101.3 kilopascals (kPa)
760 torr		

The Gas Laws

Boyle's Law

If the volume of a gas is reduced, the molecules will have less space in which to move. Therefore, they will strike the walls of the container more often and cause a greater pressure.

The relationship between the volume of a given quantity of a gas and its pressure is expressed by **Boyle's law,** which states that the volume occupied by a gas is inversely proportional to the pressure, if the temperature remains constant.

This may be illustrated by Figure 7–2, a graph of pressure versus volume. Note that as the pressure increases the volume of the gas decreases and as the pressure decreases the volume of the gas increases.

In normal breathing, the diaphragm moves downward, allowing the lungs to expand. The increased volume in the lungs causes the pressure in the lungs to drop slightly. Since air always flows from an area of high pressure to one of lower pressure, air flows into the lungs. When the diaphragm moves upward, the volume of the lungs decreases and the pressure of the air inside the lungs increases. Now the air flows out of the lungs (again from an area of high pressure to one of lower pressure).

A direct application of Boyle's law may be seen in a chest respirator, (see

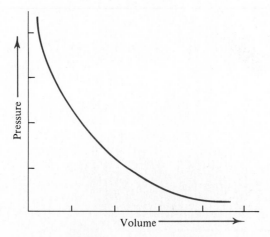

FIGURE 7-2. Graph illustrating Boyle's law; pressure and volume are related inversely.

FIGURE 7-3. Chest respirator in use. (Courtesy of LIFECARE, 5505 Central Ave., Boulder, CO. 80301.)

Figure 7-3) a machine used in the treatment of patients with respiratory difficulties. When the pressure inside of the respirator is decreased, the air in the lungs expands, forcing the diaphragm down. When the pressure in the respirator is increased, the volume of air in the lungs is decreased, allowing the diaphragm to move upward again. This alternate increase and decrease in pressure enables the patient to breathe even though he or she cannot control the movement of the diaphragm muscles.

Another example of Boyle's law is in the use of a sphygmomanometer, a device used to measure blood pressure. When the rubber bulb is squeezed, the volume of air in that bulb is decreased and its pressure is increased. This increased pressure is transmitted to the cuff (see Figure 7-4).

FIGURE 7-4. Sphygmomanometer, an instrument that makes use of Boyle's law to measure blood pressure. (Courtesy Methodist Hospital School of Nursing, Peoria, IL.)

Boyle's law may be stated mathematically as

$$P_1 V_1 = P_2 V_2 \quad \text{(at constant temperature)}$$

where P_1 and P_2 are the initial and final pressure, and V_1 and V_2 the initial and final volumes, respectively. Pressures are usually expressed in millimeters of mercury (mm Hg). Recall that 760 mm Hg equals 1 atm pressure.

EXAMPLE 7-1. What volume will 500 ml of gas initially at 25°C and 750 mm Hg occupy when conditions change to 25°C and 650 mm Hg?

Note first that the temperature is constant so that we can use Boyle's law. Note also that P_1 is 750 mmHg, V_1 is 500 ml, and P_2 is 650 mm Hg. Then, using $P_1 V_1 = P_2 V_2$, we have

$$750 \text{ mm Hg} \times 500 \text{ ml} = 650 \text{ mm Hg} \times V_2$$

Dividing by 650 mm Hg we have

$$\frac{750 \text{ mm Hg} \times 500 \text{ ml}}{650 \text{ mm Hg}} = V_2 \quad \text{and} \quad V_2 = 577 \text{ ml} \quad \blacksquare$$

EXAMPLE 7-2. A gas exerts a pressure of 858 mm Hg when confined in a 5-L container. What will be the pressure if the gas is confined in a 10-L container at constant temperature?

Again using $P_1 V_1 = P_2 V_2$

$$858 \text{ mm Hg} \times 5 \text{ L} = P_2 \times 10 \text{ L}$$

$$P_2 = 429 \text{ mm Hg} \quad \blacksquare$$

Charles' Law   When gases are heated, they expand; when gases are cooled, they contract. The relationship between volume and temperature is expressed by Charles' law, which states that the volume of a fixed quantity of a gas is directly proportional to its Kelvin temperature, if the pressure remains constant. Recall that Kelvin (absolute) temperature is Celsius temperature plus 273 (see page 10).

Charles' law may be explained in terms of the kinetic molecular theory. As the temperature of a gas is increased, the molecules move faster and strike the walls of the container more often. However, if the pressure is to be kept constant, then the volume must increase; that is, the higher the temperature, the greater the volume of a gas, at constant pressure, and vice versa.

A direct application of Charles' law may be seen in such equipment as an incubator. When air comes in contact with the heating element, it expands and becomes lighter. This lighter air rises, causing a circulation of warm air throughout the incubator.

Charles' law may be expressed mathematically as

$$\frac{V_1}{T_1} = \frac{V_2}{T_2} \quad \text{(at constant pressure)}$$

Inorganic Chemistry   **106**

where V_1 and V_2 are the initial and final volumes and T_1 and T_2 the initial and final temperatures, respectively, all temperatures Kelvin.

EXAMPLE 7-3. A gas occupies 368 ml at 27°C and 600 mm Hg. What will be the volume of that gas at 127°C and 600 mm Hg?

We note that pressure is constant so that we can use Charles' law. Also note that V_1 is 368 ml, T_1 is 27° + 273° or 300 K, and T_2 is 127° + 273° or 400 K. Then, using

$$\frac{V_1}{T_1} = \frac{V_2}{T_2}$$

$$\frac{368 \text{ ml}}{300 \text{ K}} = \frac{V_2}{400 \text{ K}}$$

$$V_2 = 491 \text{ ml}$$

EXAMPLE 7-4. At constant pressure 200 ml of gas at 35°C is cooled to −20°C. What will be its new volume?

Here V_1 is 200 ml, T_1 is 35° + 273° or 308 K, and T_2 is −20° + 273° or 253 K. Then, using

$$\frac{V_1}{T_1} = \frac{V_2}{T_2}$$

$$\frac{200 \text{ ml}}{308 \text{ K}} = \frac{V_2}{253 \text{ K}}$$

$$V_2 = 164 \text{ ml}$$

Pressure–Temperature Relationship

Another relationship may be expressed between the pressure exerted by a gas and its temperature. These two factors are directly proportional. That is, as the temperature of a gas increases, the pressure increases, and vice versa, if the volume remains constant.

A common application of this relationship is the autoclave, a device used in hospitals for sterilization (see Figure 7–5). The normal temperature of steam is 100°C, but in an autoclave it may rise as high as 120°C because of the increased pressure. This higher temperature is sufficient to destroy any microorganisms that may exist in the material being autoclaved.

Combined Gas Laws

Boyle's law refers to the volume of a fixed quantity of a gas at constant temperature; Charles' law refers to the volume of such a gas at constant pressure. However, frequently none of these factors is constant. In such a case we use the combined gas laws, which may be stated mathematically as

$$\frac{P_1 V_1}{T_1} = \frac{P_2 V_2}{T_2}$$

EXAMPLE 7-5. What volume will 250 ml of gas at 27°C and 800 mm Hg occupy at STP? (STP means standard temperature and pressure, 0°C and 760 mm Hg or 760 torr, where the units "mm Hg" and "torr" are commonly used interchangeably.) Using

$$\frac{P_1 V_1}{T_1} = \frac{P_2 V_2}{T_2}$$

$$\frac{800 \text{ mm Hg} \times 250 \text{ ml}}{300 \text{ K}} = \frac{760 \text{ mm Hg} \times V_2}{273 \text{ K}}$$

$$V_2 = 239 \text{ ml}$$

Dalton's Law Dalton's law refers to a mixture of gases rather than to a pure gas. Dalton's law states that, in a mixture of gases, each gas exerts a partial pressure proportional to its concentration. For example, if air contains 21 percent oxygen, then 21 percent of the total air pressure is exerted by the oxygen. Normal air pressure of 1 atm will support a mercury column 760 mm high. The partial pressure of the oxygen in the air would be 21 percent of 760 mm, or 0.21 × 760 mm, or 160 mm.

Dalton's law may be explained in terms of the kinetic molecular theory. Since there is no attraction between gas molecules, each kind of molecule strikes the walls of the container the same number of times per second as if it were the only kind of molecule present. That is, the pressure exerted by each gas (its partial pressure) is not affected by the presence of other gases. Each gas exerts a partial pressure proportional to the number of molecules of that gas (proportional to its concentration).

Gases always flow from an area of higher partial pressure to one of lower partial pressure. An example of the diffusion of gases caused by a difference in partial pressures is found in our own bodies (see Figure 7-6). The partial pressure of oxygen in the inspired air is 158 mm. The partial pressure of oxygen in the alveoli* is 104 mm. Therefore, oxygen passes from the lungs into the alveoli (from a higher partial pressure to a lower one). From the alveoli the oxygen diffuses into the venous blood (from a partial pressure of 104 mm to one of 40 mm). This diffusion of oxygen into the venous blood in the lungs changes the venous blood into arterial blood, in which the partial pressure of oxygen is 95 mm. When the arterial blood reaches the tissues, where the partial pressure of oxygen is 40 mm, oxygen diffuses to those tissues (again from a higher partial pressure to a lower one). When the arterial blood loses oxygen to the tissues, its oxygen partial pressure drops to 40 mm and it becomes venous blood, which returns to the lungs to begin the cycle anew.

Conversely, in the tissues the partial pressure of the carbon dioxide is 50 mm and in the arterial blood it is 40 mm, so that carbon dioxide diffuses out of the tissues into the blood. When the arterial blood picks up carbon dioxide (and at the same time loses oxygen) it becomes venous blood with a carbon dioxide partial pressure of 45 mm. This venous blood, in turn, loses carbon dioxide to the alveoli where the carbon dioxide partial pressure is

FIGURE 7-6. Diagram showing oxygen and carbon dioxide (CO_2) flow and partial pressures in body.

FIGURE 7-7. Intermittent partial pressure breathing apparatus. (Courtesy Methodist Hospital School of Nursing, Peoria, IL.)

40 mm. From the alveoli the carbon dioxide passes into the lungs (from a partial pressure of 40 mm to one of 0.3 mm) and then is exhaled.

Use is made of Dalton's law in the intermittent partial pressure breathing apparatus, which fills the patient's lungs by increasing the partial pressure of the gas being inhaled (see Figure 7-7).

Graham's Law   If a container of ammonia and a container of ether are opened simultaneously, a person standing at the far end of the room will notice the odor of ammonia before that of the ether. Both gases will diffuse through the air but ammonia has a molecular weight of 17 and ether a molecular weight of 74. Lighter molecules diffuse faster than heavier ones. This relationship was stated by Graham as, "The rates of diffusion of gases are inversely proportional to the square roots of the molecular weights" (or inversely proportional to the square roots of their densities).

$$\frac{\text{rate of diffusion gas}_1}{\text{rate of diffusion gas}_2} = \sqrt{\frac{\text{molecular weight gas}_2}{\text{molecular weight gas}_1}}$$

Henry's Law   Carbonated drinks are made by dissolving carbon dioxide, under pressure, in a given liquid. When the container is opened, the pressure is released and bubbles of carbon dioxide escape.

This relationship is expressed in terms of Henry's law, which states, "The solubility of a gas in a liquid at a given temperature is proportional to the

Inorganic Chemistry   **110**

FIGURE 7-8. Treatment in hyperbaric chamber. (Courtesy of intensive care building of Edgewater Hospital, Chicago, IL.)

pressure of that gas." That is, more gas dissolves at higher pressures and less at lower pressures.

Oxygen should be more soluble in blood at pressures above normal. Hybaroxic* (hyperbaric) chambers, chambers in which air pressures are two to three times normal, are used in the treatment of cancer (see page 56), and for victims of scuba diving accidents. Decompression sickness can occur in any individual who has been breathing compressed gas at depths greater than 30 ft. Flying within 24 hr of diving can precipitate illness after an otherwise safe decompression (see Figure 7–8).

Deep-sea divers are subject to pressures far above normal and so can have greater amounts of dissolved gases in their blood stream. This condition might lead to the "bends" (see page 125).

Molar Gas Volumes   The volume occupied by 1 mol of any gas at STP (*s*tandard *t*emperature and *p*ressure, 0°C and 760 mm Hg) is 22.4 L. However, this volume may be used only at STP. If a gas is at some other temperature or pressure, its volume must first be converted to STP before the molar gas volume can be used.

> **EXAMPLE 7-6.** How many moles of O_2 gas are present in 5.6 L at STP? Since 1 mol of a gas at STP occupies 22.4 L, then
>
> $$5.6 \text{ L} \times \frac{1 \text{ mol}}{22.4 \text{ L}} = 0.25 \text{ mol } O_2$$ ■

> **EXAMPLE 7-7.** What volume will 1.50 mol CH_4 gas occupy at STP?
>
> $$1.50 \text{ mol} \times \frac{22.4 \text{ L}}{1 \text{ mol}} = 33.6 \text{ L at STP}$$ ■

> **EXAMPLE 7-8.** At STP 2.50 g of a gas occupies 500 ml. What is the molecular weight of that gas?

The Gaseous State   **111**

First we must convert the volume to liters.

$$\frac{2.50 \text{ g}}{500 \text{ mL}} \times \frac{1000 \text{ mL}}{1 \text{ L}} = \frac{5.00 \text{ g}}{1 \text{ L}}$$

Then using the conversion factor 1 mol occupies 22.4 L,

$$\frac{5.00 \text{ g}}{1 \text{ L}} \times \frac{22.4 \text{ L}}{1 \text{ mol}} = \frac{112 \text{ g}}{1 \text{ mol}}$$

That is, 1 mol of the gas weighs 112 g, so the molecular weight is 112. ■

Air Pollution

Air pollutants may be gases such as sulfur dioxide, nitrogen oxides, ozone, hydrocarbons, and carbon monoxide, or they may be particulate matter such as smoke particles, asbestos, and lead aerosols.*

Concentrations of pollutants in the air are often expressed as parts per million (ppm), where 1 ppm corresponds to one part pollutant to 1 million parts air.

Concentrations of pollutants at levels far below 1 ppm can have an adverse effect upon human life. For example, 0.2 ppm sulfur dioxide in the atmosphere leads to an increased death rate and 0.02 ppm peroxybenzoyl nitrate (a constituent of smog) causes severe eye irritation.

The word *smog* is derived from the words *smoke* and *fog* and is characterized by air that contains lung and eye irritants along with reduced visibility. Smog frequently occurs during a thermal inversion. Normally, warm air near the ground surface rises and carries away pollutants. However, during a thermal inversion, the air near the surface is cooler than the air above it and so remains at the surface, keeping the air pollutants down at that level.

Gases

The principal source of three gaseous pollutants—carbon monoxide, hydrocarbons, and nitrogen oxides—is the automobile, which is also the source of such particulate matter in the air as asbestos (from brake linings) and lead aerosols (from leaded gasoline). Tobacco smoke is a source of carbon monoxide as well as particulate matter (ash): fossil-fuel-powered electrical generating stations are also a major source of air pollutants such as sulfur dioxide.

Each pollutant poses a different threat to human life.

1. **Carbon monoxide** is a deadly poison that interferes with the transportation of oxygen by the blood by competing with oxygen for the iron-binding sites in hemoglobin. Low concentrations of this gas, such as are found in automobiles, garages, downtown streets during rush hours, and space-heated rooms, cause impairments of judgment and vision. Evidence has shown that intermittent exposure to carbon monoxide at low levels of concentration may cause strokes and hypertension in susceptible individuals. High concentrations of carbon monoxide may cause headache, drowsiness, coma, respiratory failure, and death.

2. **Nitrogen oxides** are just as dangerous a pollutant as carbon monoxide, even though environmental groups do not stress them equally. The first effects of nitrogen oxides upon humans is an irritation of the eyes and respiratory passages. Concentrations of 1.6 to 5 ppm of nitrogen dioxide for a

1-hr exposure cause increased airway resistance and diminish diffusing capacity of the lungs. Concentrations of 25 to 100 ppm cause acute but reversible bronchitis and pneumonitis.* Concentrations above 100 ppm are usually fatal, with death resulting from pulmonary edema.*

Nitrogen dioxide, NO_2, can react with water to form nitric acid, a constituent of "acid rain."

3. **Oxides of sulfur** cause acute airway spasm and poor airway clearance in all people and exert a deadly effect upon patients already disabled by lung disease. Concentrations of 8 to 10 ppm cause immediate throat irritation, and concentrations of 20 ppm cause immediate coughing.

Particulate matter absorbs sulfur dioxide, and the resulting tiny particles may get into the small air passages in the lungs, causing spasms and destruction of cells. Particles of the smallest size penetrate deepest into the lungs and remain there the longest.

Sulfur dioxide, SO_2, is oxidized in the air to sulfur trioxide, SO_3. Sulfur trioxide can react with the moisture in the air to form sulfuric acid, another constituent of acid rain.

Why is acid rain so detrimental? It can react with calcium carbonate, which is found in marble and in mortar. Many famous marble sculptures around the world are rapidly deteriorating because of the acid in the air. The mortar between the bricks is also affected by acid rain and is slowly being dissolved, leaving the bricks with very little to hold them together.

Acid rain also affects trees and fruits and vegetables with considerable commercial consequences.

4. **Cigarette and tobacco smoke** is one of the most dangerous types of air pollution. Smokers inhale large amounts of carbon monoxide, tars, and particulate matter. People around smokers are also exposed to these same pollutants. Evidence has shown that expectant mothers who smoke have smaller babies who have a higher infant mortality rate than those of nonsmokers. Smokers also have a greater chance of developing lung cancer, emphysema,* and cardiovascular disease (see Figure 7–9).

5. **Ozone** is formed by the action of sunlight on oxygen and is normally present in the atmosphere in extremely small amounts. Ozone reacts with hydrocarbon emissions and with oxides of nitrogen to form peroxyacyl nitrates, which are the eye irritants of smog. Since ozone is produced by the action of sunlight, its levels in the air are usually lower at night than during the day.

Los Angeles-type smog is primarily a photochemical phenomenon because many of the changes that take place in the air pollutants occur because of the action of sunlight upon the substances mentioned previously.

The Ozone Layer Ozone is found in a layer 20 to 50 km (12 to 30 miles) above the earth's surface. Ozone is formed by the reaction of the sun's high-energy ultraviolet radiation upon oxygen molecules in the upper air.

$$3O_2 \underset{\text{radiation}}{\overset{\text{ultraviolet}}{\rightleftharpoons}} 2O_3$$

The Gaseous State   **113**

FIGURE 7-9. (a) Normal lung tissue and lung tissue darkened by deposits from smoking and air pollution. (b) The darkened area shows the distention of small airways, which is characteristic of emphysema. (Courtesy Chicago Lung Association, photo by Milton Regier; lung tissue provided by David W. Cugell, M.D., Northwestern University.)

This layer, called the *ozone layer,* filters out most of the sun's high-energy ultraviolet radiation. This type of radiation is detrimental to life, and therefore the ozone layer serves a vital function. If the ozone layer is reduced or eliminated, the effect on life would be catastrophic.

There are two principal threats to the ozone layer:

1. Chlorofluorocarbons, used in aerosol spray cans, in refrigeration, and in air conditioners.
2. Oxides of nitrogen.

Chlorofluorocarbons are widely used in air conditioning and refrigeration units and in aerosol spray cans because they are volatile,* chemically unreactive, and liquefy under pressure. In the atmosphere, they gradually diffuse upward into the stratosphere where they can react with the ozone layer and reduce the amount of ozone present. Even if the ozone layer is depleted by only a small amount, the result would be a marked increase in skin cancer, caused by the dangerous ultraviolet radiation from the sun reaching the earth's surface. For this reason, it has been recommended that the use of chlorofluorocarbons in aerosol cans be limited and eventually replaced by other substances that (1) will not affect the ozone layer and (2) will not have an adverse effect on life.

Inorganic Chemistry

Oxides of nitrogen such as NO and NO_2 are formed in the exhaust of automobiles and planes. In the lower levels of the atmosphere, although these compounds are detrimental to human health, they pose no threat to the ozone layer because they do not remain in the atmosphere long enough to rise into the stratosphere. However, supersonic and military planes do inject large amounts of oxides of nitrogen into the ozone layer because they fly at such great altitudes. This is one reason why the use of supersonic planes has not been greatly expanded.

Summary

The properties of gases may be explained in terms of the kinetic molecular theory, which states that (1) gases are composed of tiny particles called molecules, (2) the distances between molecules of a gas are very great compared to the size of the molecules themselves, (3) gas molecules move rapidly in straight lines, (4) gas molecules do not attract each other, (5) collisions between molecules and between the molecules and the walls of the container are perfectly elastic, and (6) the average kinetic energy of the molecules is the same for all gases at the same temperature.

Pressure is measured by means of a barometer. Standard pressure is 1 atm and will support a column of mercury 760 mm tall.

Boyle's law states that the volume of a fixed quantity of a gas is inversely proportional to the pressure if the temperature remains constant. Boyle's law may be expressed mathematically as $P_1V_1 = P_2V_2$.

Charles' law states that the volume of a fixed quantity of a gas is directly proportional to its Kelvin temperature if the pressure remains constant. Charles' law may be stated mathematically as $V_1/T_1 = V_2/T_2$.

The combined gas laws may be stated mathematically as $P_1V_1/T_1 = P_2V_2/T_2$.

Dalton's law states that in a mixture of gases each gas exerts a partial pressure proportional to its concentration.

Gases flow from an area of high partial pressure to one of lower partial pressure.

Graham's law states that the rates of diffusion of gases are inversely proportional to the square roots of their molecular weights.

The molar gas volume is 22.4 L at STP. It is the volume occupied by 1 mol of any gas under those conditions.

Air pollutants may be gases such as carbon monoxide, ozone, nitrogen oxides, and sulfur oxides, and they also may be particulate matter such as smoke particles, asbestos, and lead aerosols. Each pollutant poses a different threat to human life.

Questions and Problems

A

1. Explain in terms of the kinetic molecular theory (a) why gases have a low density, (b) why gases are compressible, (c) why gases do not settle, (d) why gases diffuse into each other, (e) why gases have no definite shape or volume, (f) Charles' law, and (g) Boyle's law.
2. What volume will 800 ml of neon gas initially at 25°C and 720 mm Hg occupy at 25°C and 680 mm Hg?
3. Calcualte the pressure necessary for 1.50 L of oxygen at 13°C and 675 mm Hg to occupy 1.75 L at 13°C.
4. What would be the change in volume of 200 ml of oxygen at 27°C and 600 mm Hg when the temperature rises to 227°C at 600 mm Hg?
5. When 3.00 ft³ of hydrogen at 40°C and 1.15 atm pressure are cooled to −40°C and 1.15 atm what will the volume be?
6. What volume will 250 ml of carbon dioxide gas at 15°C and 900 mm Hg occupy at STP (0°C and 760 mm Hg)?

7. Explain how a chest respirator enables a person whose lungs are paralyzed to breathe.
8. Explain how an autoclave works in terms of the appropriate gas law.
9. Why does carbon dioxide pass from the blood to the lungs instead of vice versa?
10. Explain why oxygen flows to the tissues and carbon dioxide from the tissues instead of vice versa?
11. Which gas will diffuse faster: methane, CH_4, or ammonia, NH_3?
12. Arrange the following gases in order of increasing rates of diffusion: H_2, O_2, NH_3, CO_2, SO_2, C_2H_6, Ar, and He.
13. What are the principal sources of air pollution?
14. What are the hazards of cigarette smoking?
15. What threats to life are caused by (a) oxides of nitrogen, (b) ozone, (c) carbon monoxide, (d) oxides of sulfur, (e) particulate matter?

B 16. Explain in terms of the kinetic molecular theory why gases exert a pressure.
17. Why do gases exert pressure equally in all directions?
18. Why are collisions between molecules elastic?
19. Explain how a sphygmomanometer works.
20. Explain why air flows into and out of the lungs.
21. Explain in terms of the kinetic molecular theory why gases exert a partial pressure proportional to the concentration.
22. Define Henry's law. What use is made of this law in the treatment of cancer?
23. Explain "the bends" in terms of Henry's law.
24. What is "smog"? What are its effects?
25. Explain how a barometer works.
26. What does a "falling barometer" indicate in terms of weather conditions?
27. How many moles of CO_2 are present in 2.8 L at STP?
28. What volume will 0.75 mol of C_2H_2 gas at STP occupy?
29. What is "acid rain" and why is it harmful?
30. At STP 1.65 g of a gas occupy 224 ml. What is the molecular weight of that gas?
31. Why is the ozone layer so important? What substances might affect it?

References DICKSON, T. R. *Introduction to Chemistry,* 4th ed. John Wiley & Sons, Inc., New York, 1983, Chapter 9.

EBBING, DARRELL D. *General Chemistry.* Houghton Mifflin Co., Boston, 1984, Chapter 4.

McQUARRIE, DONALD A. and PETER A. ROCK. *General Chemistry.* W. H. Freeman and Company, New York, 1984, Chapter 5.

MILLER, FRANCIS MARION. *Chemistry, Structure and Dynamics.* McGraw-Hill Book Co., New York, 1984, Chapter 5.

MORTIMER, CHARLES E. *Chemistry,* 5th ed. Wadsworth Publishing Co., Belmont, Calif., 1983, Chapter 8.

PETRUCCI, RALPH H. and ROBERT E. WISMER. *General Chemistry with Qualitative Analysis.* Macmillan Publishing Company, New York, 1983, Chapter 5.

RAYNER-CANHAN, GEOFFREY and MARK VAN ROODE. *Foundations of Chemistry.* Addison-Wesley Publishing Co., Reading, Mass., 1983, Chapter 9.

SACKHEIM, GEORGE I. *Chemical Calculations,* 12th ed., Series B. Stipes Publishing Co., Champaign, Ill., 1983, Chapter 6.

STOKER, H. STEPHEN. *Introduction to Chemical Principles.* Macmillan Publishing Company, New York, 1983, Chapter 12.

8 Oxygen and Other Gases

CHAPTER OUTLINE

Oxygen
  Occurrence
  Combustion
  Preparation
  Uses
Hydrogen peroxide

Superoxide
Ozone
  Preparation
  Properties and Uses
Nitrous Oxide
Noxious Gases

Oxygen

Occurrence

Oxygen is the most abundant element on the earth's surface. Air contains about 21 percent free oxygen. The oceans and lakes on the earth's surface consist of about 80 percent oxygen in the combined state. The earth's crust consists of about 50 percent oxygen, combined mostly with silicon. Oxygen compounds comprise most of the weight of plants and animals.

Properties

At room temperature oxygen is a colorless, odorless, tasteless gas. It is slightly heavier than air and is slightly soluble in water.

PHYSICAL PROPERTIES

The method of preparation illustrated in Figure 8–1 shows that oxygen does not dissolve appreciably in water. If it were soluble in water, it could not be collected by this method. However, a small amount of oxygen does dissolve in water. This amount, though small, is of very definite importance to marine life. It is this small amount of dissolved oxygen that enables fish and other aquatic animals to "breathe."

The density of oxygen is 1.43 g/L. The density of air is 1.29 g/L. Therefore, oxygen is slightly heavier than air. When oxygen is collected in the laboratory, it is kept in covered bottles with the mouth upward.

When cooled sufficiently, oxygen forms a pale blue liquid that boils at $-182.5°C$. Further cooling produces a pale blue solid, which freezes at $-218.4°C$.

CHEMICAL PROPERTIES

Oxygen is a moderately active element at room temperature but is extremely active at higher temperatures. It combines with almost all elements to produce a class of compounds called oxides.

117

FIGURE 8-1. Laboratory preparation of oxygen. The reaction is $2KClO_3 \xrightarrow[\text{heat}]{MnO_2} 2KCl + 3O_2\uparrow$.

$$2Mg \quad + \quad O_2 \quad \longrightarrow \quad 2MgO$$

magnesium   oxygen   magnesium
                                          oxide

$$C \quad + \quad O_2 \quad \longrightarrow \quad CO_2$$

carbon   oxygen   carbon
                                        dioxide

The reaction between oxygen and some other substance is an example of **oxidation.** Common examples of oxidation are the rusting of iron, the burning of a candle, and the decay of wood. Oxidation also occurs in living plant and animal tissues. These oxidation reactions are able to occur rapidly at relatively low temperatures because of the presence of specific catalysts called enzymes. An example of such a reaction occurring in the human body is the oxidation of glucose, a simple sugar, to carbon dioxide and water.

$$C_6H_{12}O_6 + 6O_2 \xrightarrow{\text{enzymes}} 6CO_2 + 6H_2O + energy$$

glucose   oxygen   carbon   water
                                                    dioxide

(This reaction is greatly oversimplified. As will be discussed later, when glucose is oxidized to carbon dioxide and water in the body, there are many intermediate steps involved, each with its own particular enzyme.)

Combustion Wood, coal, and gas burn, that is, undergo combustion, in the presence of oxygen. Combustion may be defined as a rapid oxidation in which heat and light are produced, usually accompanied by a flame. Oxygen supports combustion (that is, substances burn in oxygen), but oxygen itself does not burn.

Combustion is usually thought of in terms of a reaction with oxygen. However, oxygen is not absolutely necessary for a combustion reaction. When powdered iron and sulfur are heated together in a test tube, a rapid reaction occurs in which heat and light are given off. This is also a combustion reaction even though no oxygen is involved.

SPONTANEOUS COMBUSTION

When iron combines with the oxygen of the air, it rusts, continuously liberating a small amount of heat as the reaction continues. The total amount of liberated heat, however, will be the same as that which would have been liberated had the iron been burned in oxygen. That is, the total amount of heat produced is the same regardless of whether the reaction proceeds rapidly or slowly.

This is the principle underlying spontaneous combustion, which can be defined as a slow oxidation that develops by itself into combustion. How is such a process possible? If rags containing a "drying oil" such as boiled linseed oil are placed in a dry container without adequate ventilation, the oil will slowly combine with the oxygen in the air, liberating a small amount of heat during the process. Without ventilation the heat will not be dissipated, especially since rags are such poor conductors of heat. As the oxidation proceeds, more and more heat will be liberated until a sufficient amount accumulates to start the rags burning. This is spontaneous combustion.

If such rags had been placed in a closed container, the oxidation would not continue after the oxygen supply was used up. Likewise, if the rags were hung in a place where freely circulating air could carry away the heat, no spontaneous combustion could occur.

FIRE PREVENTION AND CONTROL

Care should be taken in handling and storing flammable liquids such as ether and alcohol. Where smoking is allowed, nonflammable receptacles should be provided for the butts. One frequent cause of fires is throwing lighted cigarettes into a wastebasket. Oily rags and mops should be stored in well-ventilated fireproof lockers to avoid the danger of spontaneous combustion.

In case a fire should occur, how can it be extinguished? There are two methods of putting out a fire—removing the oxygen from the burning material or lowering the temperature of the burning substance below its kindling point.

One type of fire extinguisher contains carbon dioxide gas under pressure (see Figure 8–2). This type of extinguisher has several advantages. The carbon dioxide is extremely cold and lowers the temperature of the burning substance. A large amount of carbon dioxide, which is heavier than oxygen, surrounds the burning area, keeping out the oxygen. For these reasons the carbon dioxide should be directed at the base of the flame. This type of extinguisher is recommended for electrical fires because the carbon dioxide does not conduct electricity. It is also used for oil and gasoline fires because it shuts off the oxygen supply and at the same time lowers the temperature. When a fire is extinguished, the carbon dioxide disappears into the air so that it does not have to be cleaned up along with the material that was burning. A cylinder of carbon dioxide holds a large volume of the gas under pressure and thus has a great capability in fire fighting.

Carbon tetrachloride (CCl_4) was formerly used in fire extinguishers but its use for this purpose has been outlawed because (1) its vapors are toxic and (2) a hot fire converts it to phosgene ($COCl_2$), a poisonous gas.

Oxygen and Other Gases

FIGURE 8-2. Carbon dioxide fire extinguisher. (Courtesy of The Ansul Co., Marinette, WI.)

Preparation

LABORATORY METHODS

One very common method for preparing oxygen in the laboratory is by heating potassium chlorate, $KClO_3$ (see Figure 8–1). The reaction is as follows:

$$2KClO_3 \xrightarrow{\text{heat}} 2KCl + 3O_2\uparrow$$

It takes a considerable amount of heat to produce oxygen by this method because the potassium chlorate must be heated to its melting point (370°C) before it gives off oxygen.

However, when manganese dioxide (MnO_2) is added to the potassium chlorate, oxygen is evolved from the heated mixture at a much lower temperature and at a more rapid rate. The manganese dioxide acts as a catalyst in this reaction—a catalyst increases the speed of the reaction but does not take part in it. The presence of a catalyst in a reaction is indicated over the arrow in the equation for that reaction.

$$2KClO_3 \xrightarrow[\text{heat}]{MnO_2} 2KCl + 3O_2\uparrow$$

Oxygen may also be produced in the laboratory by the electrolysis of water.

$$2H_2O \xrightarrow{\text{electricity}} 2H_2\uparrow + O_2\uparrow$$

Inorganic Chemistry   **120**

The commercial source of oxygen is the air, an inexhaustible supply as long as we have trees and other green plants, both on land and in the water. When air is cooled to a low enough temperature under compression, it becomes a liquid. Liquid air, like ordinary air, consists mostly of nitrogen and oxygen. Liquid nitrogen boils at $-196°C$. Liquid oxygen boils at $-182.5°C$. When liquid air is allowed to stand, the nitrogen boils off first (because of its lower boiling point) leaving almost pure oxygen behind. Liquid oxygen is stored in steel cylinders under high pressure.

Uses

MEDICAL USES

Oxygen is necessary to life. When oxygen is taken into the lungs, it combines with the hemoglobin of the blood to form a compound called oxyhemoglobin (see page 461). The blood carries the oxyhemoglobin to the tissues where oxygen is released. This oxygen then reacts with the food products in the cells, producing energy. At the same time, carbon dioxide is produced and carried back to the lungs where it is exhaled. Blood going to the tissues (arterial blood) contains oxyhemoglobin and has a characteristic bright red color. Blood coming from the tissues (venous blood) does not contain oxyhemoglobin, so it has a characteristic reddish purple color.

Patients with lung diseases, such as pneumonia, frequently do not have enough functioning lung tissue to pick up sufficient oxygen from the air. These patients are given a mixture of oxygen and air to breathe instead of air alone. Then, because of the higher partial pressure of oxygen, a small functioning area can pick up more oxygen than it could if air alone were breathed in. Therefore, the patient can breathe and live until the diseased area is cured and returns to normal. The oxygen may be administered by nasal cannula or mask (see Figures 8–3 and 8–4). Oxygen is given to patients with lung cancer to help them adjust to a decreased lung area.

Living tissues require oxygen. Without it they soon die. However, if the temperature is lowered sufficiently, tissues can survive with very little oxygen. At normal body temperature, $98.6°F$, the brain is extremely sensitive to a lack of oxygen. However, it too can live for a longer period of time without oxygen if its temperature is lowered. But how low is low when we are talking about body temperature?

In one form of surgery used to repair ruptured blood vessels in the brain, the body temperature is dropped from normal to $86°F$ by means of an ice bath. At this temperature the heart can be stopped for about 15 min without damage to the body. However, brain surgery requires more time than the 15 min allowed. After the body temperature is lowered to $86°F$ and after the heart is stopped, a saltwater solution at $32°F$ is pumped directly into the main artery that feeds the brain. This cold solution lowers the brain's temperature to approximately $60°F$; at this temperature brain surgery may be completed without damage to either the brain or the body. After surgery, the heart is restarted and blood (carrying oxygen) again flows to the brain.

Hypothermia is also used for open-heart surgical procedures. The patient is placed on a plastic pad through which an iced solution is run in order to lower body temperature to $25°C$ or $20°C$ ($77°F$ or $68°F$). However, the

FIGURE 8-3. Nasal oxygen cannula. (Courtesy of Puritan-Bennett Corporation.)

main cooling is done through the bypass machine during the surgery. The heart itself is cooled by perfusion of coronary arteries with an iced solution, or packed in an ice solution. The temperature of the heart may be lowered to 5°C (41°F). Hypothermia of the organs is also necessary during transplant surgery.

Hyperthermia is a technique of using microwave radiation to raise the temperature of target cancer cells without harming nearby normal tissue.

Since oxygen supports combustion, an object such as a candle, which burns slowly in air, will burn very vigorously in oxygen. Therefore, a patient must not smoke or use matches in a room where oxygen is in use. The following precautions should also be taken

1. Electrical devices such as radios, televisions, electric shavers, and so on are likewise banned because of the danger that a spark from the equipment could cause a fire.
2. Electric signal cords should be replaced by a hand bell because of the danger of a spark.
3. Patients should not be given back rubs with alcohol or oil because of the danger of a fire. Instead, lotion or powder should be used.

Inorganic Chemistry

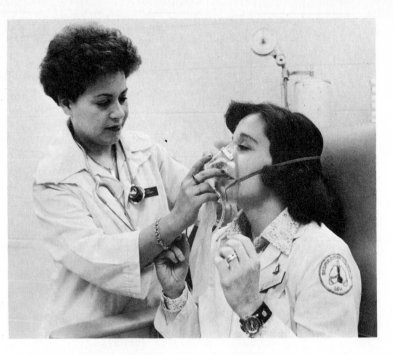

FIGURE 8-4. Aerosol mask. (Courtesy of Lutheran General Hospital, Park Ridge, IL.)

4. Oil or grease should never be applied to any part of the oxygen equipment. The nurse should take care not to have oil on her or his hands when manipulating the regulator of the oxygen tank.

Hypoxia* is a condition in which the body does not receive enough oxygen. In cases of hypoxia, oxygen must be administered to permit the body to function normally. Newborn babies who have difficulty in breathing are given oxygen containing a small amount of carbon dioxide. The carbon dioxide stimulates the respiratory center of the brain so that the rate of breathing increases, and the oxygen is picked up more rapidly and carried to the tissues.

During dental surgery when nitrous oxide is used as the anesthetic, oxygen must be administered along with the nitrous oxide to prevent asphyxiation (lack of oxygen). Firefighters who breathe large quantities of smoke may suffer from asphyxiation.* They are treated by breathing from an oxygen mask. Death by smoke inhalation during a fire is often the result of noxious material such as hydrogen cyanide, HCN, or phosgene produced by the burning of plastics.

A person who is under water for several minutes and becomes unconscious because of lack of oxygen is given oxygen in an effort to build up the oxygen concentration in the blood rapidly. Pilots and astronauts breathe oxygen through a face mask because of the decrease or lack of oxygen in the atmosphere around them, as do miners, deep sea divers, and smoke fighters.

In the hospital, oxygen under pressure (hybaroxic treatment) is administered in the treatment of cancerous tissues (see page 56), of patients with gangrene, and also of patients with carbon monoxide poisoning.

Oxygen and Other Gases   **123**

Another use of oxygen in the hospital is in the determination of the basal metabolic rate (BMR). Basal metabolism tests measure the energy production of the body by measuring the amount of oxygen a patient breathes during a specified period of time (usually 6 min). The BMR has been used as an indicator of thyroid function, but its use for this purpose has been largely supplanted by tests using [131]I (radioactive iodine).

One measure of the body's use of oxygen (pulmonary function) is the MET, derived from the word metabolism. One MET corresponds to the consumption of 1 ml of O_2 per minute for each kilogram of body weight (see Figure 8–5). Table 8–1 compares MET values for various activities.

TABLE 8-1. MET values

	MET
At rest	1
Walking 2 mph	3
Running 7 mph	12
Walking upstairs	15
Shoveling snow	7

FIGURE 8-5. A technician tests a man in the pulmonary function lab. (Courtesy of University of Illinois at Chicago.)

Inorganic Chemistry

Formerly, all premature infants were routinely given oxygen until respiratory sufficiency had been established (see Figure 8–6). Now it is known that, when the concentration of oxygen rises above 40 percent in the inspired air, premature infants develop retrolental fibroplasia, a disease that affects the eyes. This disease produces complete or nearly complete blindness due to separation and fibrosis of the retina.

COMMERCIAL USES Deep-sea divers who worked at great depths formerly were supplied air under pressure to enable them to breathe. However, this process introduced a difficulty in that the nitrogen in the air became much more soluble in the blood under the higher pressure. When the diver was taken out of the water too rapidly, this dissolved nitrogen became less soluble because of the decrease in pressure. When this happened, bubbles of nitrogen formed in the blood, causing a condition called the "bends." Unless the diver could be placed immediately in a compression chamber under high pressure, which then was gradually reduced to normal pressure, the results were generally fatal. Recall the similar effect of tiny bubbles being formed in a liquid when a bottle of warm carbonated beverage is opened.

FIGURE 8-6. Infant in isolette. (Courtesy of Augustana Hospital, Chicago, IL.)

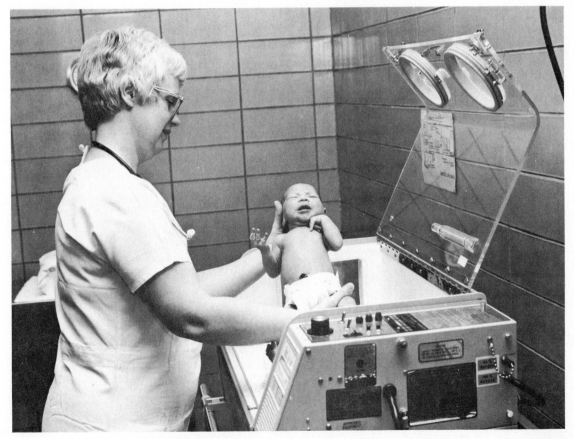

A newer method enabling the diver to breathe a mixture of oxygen and helium is now used. Helium is less soluble in the blood than is nitrogen and so decreases the chances of the bends occurring.

Industrially, oxygen is used in the operation of furnaces for production of iron and steel. It is also used in welding torches. These torches frequently use acetylene as their fuel. When acetylene is burned with oxygen, the heat produced is high enough to melt steel. Liquid oxygen (LOX) is used in rockets for launching satellites.

HYDROGEN PEROXIDE Another product besides water (H_2O) is possible between the elements hydrogen and oxygen. This compound is hydrogen peroxide, H_2O_2, produced by means of the following reactions:

$$Ba + O_2 \longrightarrow BaO_2$$

$$BaO_2 + H_2SO_4 \longrightarrow BaSO_4 + H_2O_2$$

Hydrogen peroxide is a pale blue, oily liquid that boils at 150°C and freezes at −0.89°C. It is very unstable and decomposes according to the following reaction:

$$2H_2O_2 \longrightarrow 2H_2O + O_2$$

This reaction is induced by light, and therefore hydrogen peroxide is usually stored in dark-colored bottles. A 3 percent solution of H_2O_2 is used as an antiseptic; a 30 percent solution is used as a bleach and as an oxidizing agent in chemistry laboratories.

The oxidation state of oxygen in water and in oxides is −2. The oxidation state of oxygen in the free state is 0. In peroxides, the oxidation state of the oxygen (the oxidation number) is −1.

Hydrogen peroxide is an intermediate product in the reduction of O_2 to H_2O in many cellular reduction reactions. Since hydrogen peroxide is toxic to living cells, it must be removed quickly before it can cause harm. The enzyme that catalyzes such a reaction is catalase (see page 379).

SUPEROXIDE When a metal reacts with oxygen, an oxide is formed.

$$2Al + 3O_2 \longrightarrow 2Al_2O_3 \quad \text{(aluminum oxide)}$$

When an active metal reacts with oxygen, a peroxide is formed.

$$2Na + O_2 \longrightarrow Na_2O_2 \quad \text{(sodium peroxide)}$$

When a very active metal reacts with oxygen, a superoxide is formed.

$$K + O_2 \longrightarrow KO_2 \quad \text{(potassium superoxide)}$$

In superoxides, the oxidation number of oxygen is −1/2. Superoxide ions exist in the human body and in some microrganisms. In the production of uric acid (page 440), superoxide ions are produced. Superoxide ions are formed during the oxidation of Fe^{2+} to Fe^{3+} in the hemoglobin molecule. Superoxide ions are also involved in the immune response and possibly in the aging process.

Both the superoxide ion (O_2^-) and hydrogen peroxide (H_2O_2) are very reactive substances and extremely dangerous to living cells; therefore, their removal is of great importance to the well-being of the organism. The superoxide ion is rapidly converted to O_2 and H_2O_2 by the enzyme superoxide dismutase. The H_2O_2 thus produced is decomposed into H_2O and O_2 by the enzyme catalase (page 379).

Ozone

Oxygen occurs most frequently as the diatomic molecule, O_2. However, it also exists as a triatomic molecule, O_3, called ozone. These two different forms of the element oxygen are called allotropic forms (see Figure 8–7). **Allotropic forms** of an element have different physical and chemical properties. Other elements that exist in allotropic forms are carbon, sulfur, phosphorus, tin, and lead.

Preparation

When air or oxygen is passed between two electrically charged plates, the volume decreases and a pale blue gas with a strong odor is formed. This gas is ozone. An equation for the formation of ozone is

$$3O_2 \rightleftharpoons 2O_3$$

The double arrow indicates an **equilibrium reaction,** one that proceeds in both directions.

Ozone is formed by the action of ultraviolet light from the sun upon the oxygen in the air. It is also formed in the air by electrical discharges (lightning). Ozone may also be found around high-voltage machinery where sparks convert some of the oxygen of the air into ozone.

The ozone layer in the upper atmosphere helps protect the earth from the harmful effect of the sun's ultraviolet radiation (see page 113).

Properties and Uses

Ozone is a colorless gas (or sometimes slightly blue) at room temperature. It has a very pungent odor, similar to that of garlic. It is heavier than oxygen and more soluble in water. Liquid ozone is blue. Ozone is a powerful oxidizing agent. The use of ozone is rather limited because of its poisonous nature and its instability. Ozone is irritating to the mucous membranes and it is quite toxic to the body except in extremely small amounts.

Ozone is not tolerated in industrial establishments in concentrations of more than 1 part per million (ppm), whereas carbon monoxide (CO) can be tolerated in strengths as high as 100 ppm. In other words, ozone is 100 times as poisonous as carbon monoxide. It is also 100 times as poisonous as hydro-

FIGURE 8-7. Scale models of oxygen and ozone molecules.

Oxygen molecule

Ozone molecule

Oxygen and Other Gases

gen sulfide (H_2S) and approximately 10 times as poisonous as hydrocyanic acid (HCN).

Ozone is not used medically for any purpose because it reaches a fatal concentration long before it can act in any useful way. However, the industrial use of ozone is increasing rapidly. It is a more powerful oxidizing agent than oxygen itself. Its usefulness as a bacteriocide,* a decolorizer, and a deodorizer is great when it is employed carefully and in sufficient strengths. Ozone is used in the rapid aging of wood, for rapid drying of varnishes and inks, in the treatment of water, and in the disinfection of swimming-pool water, but it should only be handled with great care by trained personnel.

Nitrous Oxide

Nitrous oxide, N_2O, is frequently used as a general anesthetic. It is a colorless gas with almost no odor or taste. It is heavier than air and has a relatively low solubility in blood. N_2O does not combine with hemoglobin and is carried dissolved in the bloodstream. It is excreted, unchanged, primarily through the lungs, but a small fraction may escape through the skin. It has been found that nitrous oxide can be useful in relieving the pain in heart attack victims by reducing the strain on the heart muscles.

Although N_2O is not flammable, it does support combustion, as does oxygen, so that care must be taken with its use.

The highest concentration of N_2O that can be safely given for the maintenance of anesthesia is 70 percent. Above this concentration hypoxia develops. However, at a concentration of 70 percent or less, N_2O is not potent enough for most patients, so additional drugs such as halothane or methoxyflurane are used to complete the anesthesia.

Nitrous oxide can react with the benzpyrene (page 275) in the air to produce mutagenic* substances. Large doses of vitamin E seem to protect mice and rats from these substances; however, humans do not benefit in the same way.

Noxious Gases

Carbon monoxide, CO, is a colorless, odorless, tasteless gas. It is nonirritating to the body but has a great affinity for hemoglobin. CO is poisonous because the hemoglobin forms such a strong bond with the gas that the blood is unable to carry sufficient oxygen to the tissues.

Vapors of carbon tetrachloride, CCl_4, are very toxic to the body because of the damaging effects upon both the liver and the kidneys. CCl_4 has been used as an anesthetic, as a cleaning fluid, in fire extinguishers, and for the management of hookworm infestations; however, because of its great toxicity and its carcinogenic* properties, its use has been banned by the U.S. Food and Drug Administration. Today carbon tetrachloride has no clinical use at all.

Chlorine is a greenish yellow gas with a very pungent odor. In neutral or acid solutions chlorine acts not only as a bacteriocide but also as a virucide* and amebicide.* It is less effective as a germicide in basic solution. Chlorine kills microorganisms in water and so is used for water purification. In large amounts, chlorine vapors are toxic because they react with and destroy lung tissues.

Sulfur dioxide is released into the air during the combustion of fossil fuels. Catalytic converters in automobiles change SO_2 to SO_3, which can then form sulfuric acid and other sulfates that are extremely harmful to human health.

Hydrogen sulfide, H_2S, is characterized by its distinctive odor of rotten eggs. H_2S is extremely poisonous, even more so than hydrogen cyanide (HCN), but its odor warns a person of its presence long before its concentration reaches lethal proportions. This is not true for HCN.

Summary

Oxygen is the most abundant element on the earth's surface. It is colorless, odorless, tasteless, slightly heavier than air, and very slightly soluble in water.

Oxygen combines with most elements to form a class of compounds called oxides. The reaction between oxygen and some other substances is an example of oxidation. Oxidation also occurs in plant and animal tissues in the presence of specific catalysts called enzymes.

Combustion is a rapid reaction with oxygen, one in which heat and light are produced, usually accompanied by a flame. Spontaneous combustion is a slow oxidation that develops by itself into combustion.

Fire extinguishers accomplish their work either by removing the oxygen from the burning substance or by lowering its temperature below its kindling point, or both.

Oxygen may be prepared in the laboratory by heating such compounds as potassium chlorate ($KClO_3$) or by the electrolysis of water.

Oxygen is prepared commercially from liquid air.

Oxygen is used medically in the treatment of various respiratory diseases. Oxygen is inhaled and carried to the tissues by the hemoglobin in the blood. Care must be taken to prevent fires in the room of a patient receiving oxygen therapy. This means no smoking or use of electrical devices, no alcohol or oil backrubs.

Asphyxiation (hypoxia) may be overcome by the administration of oxygen. Oxygen is used in the treatment of cancer for some patients and in the determination of basal metabolic rate.

Industrially, oxygen is used in welding, in the production of steel, and in rockets.

When oxygen reacts with an active metal, a peroxide is formed; when oxygen reacts with a very active metal, a superoxide is formed.

Ozone (O_3) is an allotropic form of oxygen (O_2). Ozone is a colorless gas with a pungent odor. It is very toxic to the body. Ozone is not used medically but has many industrial uses; it must be employed under carefully controlled conditions by trained personnel.

Nitrous oxide is used as a general anesthetic, usually in conjunction with another drug such as halothane or methoxyflurane.

Among the noxious gases are carbon monoxide, the vapor of carbon tetrachloride, chlorine, sulfur dioxide, and hydrogen sulfide.

Questions and Problems

A

1. When oxygen is collected in the laboratory, why is the bottle kept mouth upward?
2. List several physical properties of oxygen.
3. When elements combine with oxygen, what type of compound is produced?
4. What is combustion? How does it differ from spontaneous combustion?
5. What precautions should a nurse take in preventing fires?
6. Describe the operation of one type of fire extinguisher.
7. How can oxygen be prepared in the laboratory? Commercially?

8. How is oxygen carried to the tissues?
9. Discuss the medical uses of oxygen and also the hazards involved in oxygen therapy.
10. What causes retrolental fibroplasia? How can this disease be prevented?
11. Why is carbon dioxide sometimes given along with oxygen to newborn babies?
12. What is hypoxia?
13. What is the "bends," and how can it be overcome?
14. What is ozone? List some properties of this substance. How can it be prepared?
15. List the general properties of nitrous oxide. What precautions should be taken with its use?
16. Why must nitrous oxide be used at concentrations less than 70 percent? Why is it used in conjunction with other drugs?
17. Why is carbon monoxide poisonous?
18. Why is carbon tetrachloride dangerous?
19. Under what conditions is a solution of chlorine an effective germicide?
20. Why are chlorine vapors toxic to the body?
21. Compare the reactions of metals, active metals, and very active metals with oxygen.
22. Why is hydrogen peroxide usually stored in dark bottles?
23. What are the oxidation states of oxygen in free oxygen, an oxide, a peroxide, a superoxide?
24. Where are superoxides formed in the body? How are they removed?
25. How is hydrogen peroxide removed from living cells?

B
26. Compare the reaction involving the oxidation of glucose with photosynthesis.
27. Do all oxidation reactions require oxygen? Explain.
28. Why are fire extinguishers containing carbon tetrachloride no longer in use?
29. What causes the red color of blood?
30. Compare the use of a nasal catheter with the use of an oxygen tent.

References

CLOUD, P., and A. GIBOR. The oxygen cycle. *Scientific American,* **223**:110–123 (Sept. 1970).

DELWICHE, C. C. The nitrogen cycle. *Scientific American,* **223**:136–146 (Sept. 1970).

EBBING, DARRELL E. *General Chemistry.* Houghton Mifflin Co., Boston, 1984, Chapters 13, 14.

PETRUCCI, RALPH H. and ROBERT E. WISMER. *General Chemistry with Qualitative Analysis.* Macmillan Publishing Company, New York, 1983, Chapter 20.

WINDLE, W. F. Brain damage by asphyxia at birth. *Scientific American,* **221**:76–84 (Oct. 1969).

9 Oxidation-Reduction

CHAPTER
OUTLINE

Oxidation
Reduction
Oxidizing Agents and Reducing Agents
    Balancing Oxidation–Reduction Reactions

Importance of Oxidation–Reduction
    Antiseptic Effects
    Effects on Hair Protein
    Stain Removal

Oxidation

Oxidation may be defined as "a loss of electrons." Consider the electron-dot structures in reaction 9–1. The sodium atom has one outer electron. When the sodium atom loses this one electron, it forms a sodium ion with a +1 charge. This loss of an electron is defined as oxidation. Therefore, the sodium atom was oxidized.

$$Na\cdot + \overset{\cdot\cdot}{\underset{\cdot\cdot}{:Cl}}: \longrightarrow Na^+ + \overset{\cdot\cdot}{\underset{\cdot\cdot}{:Cl}}:^- \tag{9–1}$$

A second definition of oxidation states that it is an increase in oxidation number. Consider reaction 9–2.

$$2Na + Cl_2 \longrightarrow 2NaCl \tag{9–2}$$

An uncombined element has an oxidation number of zero. (See page 81 for a discussion of oxidation numbers.) The oxidation number of sodium in sodium chloride (NaCl) is +1 and that of chlorine −1. Therefore, reaction 9–2 may be written as follows

$$\overset{0}{2Na} + \overset{0}{Cl_2} \longrightarrow \overset{+1}{2Na} + \overset{-1}{2Cl}$$

where the upper numbers indicate the respective oxidation numbers of the substances. The sodium has changed in oxidation number from zero to +1, a gain. This is oxidation. The sodium atom was oxidized.

The cells in the body "burn" glucose producing carbon dioxide, water, and energy.

$$\underset{\text{glucose}}{\overset{0}{C_6H_{12}O_6}} + \overset{0}{6O_2} \longrightarrow \overset{+4}{6CO_2} + \overset{-2}{6H_2O} + \text{energy}$$

131

The oxidation number of each carbon atom in glucose is zero. The oxidation number of the carbon atom in carbon dioxide (CO_2) is $+4$.† Therefore, the carbon atom increased in oxidation number. A gain in oxidation number is oxidation; therefore, the carbon atom in glucose was oxidized, or it can be said that the glucose, which contains the carbon atom, was oxidized.

A third definition of oxidation is "addition of oxygen." Consider reaction 9–3, which involves the oxidation of formaldehyde to formic acid (this type of reaction will be discussed in Chapter 18).

$$\underset{\text{formaldehyde}}{HCHO} + [O] \longrightarrow \underset{\text{formic acid}}{HCOOH} \qquad (9\text{–}3)$$

Note that this reaction involves the addition of oxygen.

A fourth definition of oxidation involves the "removal of hydrogen." In reaction 9–4

$$\underset{\text{ethanol}}{CH_3CH_2OH} + [O] \longrightarrow \underset{\text{acetaldehyde}}{CH_3CHO} + H_2O \qquad (9\text{–}4)$$

ethanol is changed to acetaldehyde. This process is called oxidation because it involves the loss of hydrogen.

The following oxidation reactions take place in the body. They will be discussed in detail in the appropriate chapters on carbohydrates, fats, and proteins.

$$\text{carbohydrate} + O_2 \longrightarrow CO_2 + H_2O + \text{energy}$$

$$\text{fat} + O_2 \longrightarrow CO_2 + H_2O + \text{energy}$$

$$\text{protein} + O_2 \longrightarrow CO_2 + H_2O + \text{urea} + \text{energy}$$

Thus, oxidation may be defined as

1. An increase in oxidation number
2. A loss of electrons
3. A gain of oxygen
4. A loss of hydrogen

Reduction   Oxidation was defined as a loss of electrons and also as an increase in oxidation number. Reduction is the opposite of oxidation; that is, a gain of electrons and, therefore, a decrease in oxidation number. **Oxidation can never take place without reduction** because something must be able to pick up the electrons lost by the oxidized atom, ion, or compound. Free electrons cannot exist by themselves for very long.

In the reactions of sodium with chlorine

$$\overset{0}{2Na} + \overset{0}{Cl_2} \longrightarrow \overset{+1}{2Na} + \overset{-1}{2Cl}$$

† Refer to Chapter 5.

$$\underset{C_6 \quad H_{12} \quad O_6}{6(0) + 12(+1) + 6(-2) = 0} \qquad \text{and} \qquad \underset{C \quad O_2}{+4 + 2(-2) = 0}$$

Inorganic Chemistry   **132**

the sodium increased in oxidation number from 0 to +1. It was oxidized. At the same time, the chlorine decreased in oxidation number from 0 to −1. Therefore, the chlorine was reduced. Consider the structures in reaction 9–1 on page 131. The chlorine atom has seven outer electrons. It gains one electron to form the chloride ion with a charge of −1. This gain of an electron is called reduction. Thus, by either definition, the chlorine was reduced.

In the reaction of glucose with oxygen

$$\overset{0}{C_6H_{12}O_6} + \overset{0}{6O_2} \longrightarrow \overset{+4}{6CO_2} + \overset{-2}{6H_2O} + energy$$

glucose was oxidized because the carbon atoms changed in oxidation number from 0 to +4. However, at the same time, the oxygen changed from 0 to −2, a decrease in oxidation number. Therefore, the oxygen was reduced.

Since reduction is the opposite of oxidation, reduction can also be defined as a loss of oxygen or as a gain of hydrogen. Equations 9–5 and 9–6 illustrate reduction reactions that will be discussed in Chapter 18.

$$CH_3COOH + H_2 \longrightarrow CH_3CHO + H_2O \qquad (9\text{–}5)$$
$$\text{acetic acid} \qquad\qquad \text{ethanal}$$

$$CH_3COCH_3 + H_2 \longrightarrow CH_3CH(OH)CH_3 \qquad (9\text{–}6)$$
$$\text{acetone} \qquad\qquad \text{isopropyl alcohol}$$

Reaction 9–5 is reduction because it involves a loss of oxygen; reaction 9–6 is reduction because it involves a gain of hydrogen.

Thus, reduction is

1. A decrease in oxidation number
2. A gain of electrons
3. A loss of oxygen
4. A gain of hydrogen

Oxidizing Agents and Reducing Agents

In reaction 9–7

$$H_2 + PbO \longrightarrow Pb + H_2O \qquad (9\text{–}7)$$

$$\overset{0}{H_2} + \overset{+2\ -2}{PbO} \longrightarrow \overset{0}{Pb} + \overset{2(+1)-2}{H_2O}$$

the lead decreases in oxidation number from +2 to 0. Therefore, the lead was reduced. What reduced it? What supplied the electrons that it had to gain in order to decrease in oxidation number? The answer is that the hydrogen reduced it. The hydrogen supplied the electrons so that the lead could be reduced; therefore, hydrogen is called the **reducing agent.** The substance that causes the reduction of an element or compound is known as a reducing agent.

At the same time, the hydrogen gained in oxidation number from 0 to +1. Therefore, the hydrogen was oxidized. What oxidized it? What picked up the electrons that the hydrogen must have lost in being oxidized? The answer is that the PbO picked up these electrons; thus, the PbO is called the

Oxidation-Reduction

oxidizing agent. An oxidizing agent is defined as a substance that causes the oxidation of some element or compound.

Rewriting equation 9–7 and indicating what was oxidized, what was reduced, what the oxidizing agent was, and what the reducing agent was, we have the following

$$H_2 + PbO \longrightarrow Pb + H_2O$$

$$\begin{array}{cc} \text{oxidized} & \text{reduced} \\ \text{(reducing} & \text{(oxidizing} \\ \text{agent)} & \text{agent)} \end{array}$$

Another way of stating the same thing is to say that **whatever is oxidized is the reducing agent** and **whatever is reduced is the oxidizing agent.**

Balancing Oxidation–
Reduction Reactions

To balance a redox equation use the following rules:

1. Write the complete equation listing the oxidation numbers of all the elements (see page 82) and locate those elements that are changing their oxidation number.
2. Calculate the change in oxidation number and indicate this change below the equation.
3. Multiply the change in oxidation number for each atom by the total number of those atoms that are changing in oxidation number.
4. Find a least common multiple for the total increase and decrease in oxidation number.
5. Equate the increase and decrease in oxidation numbers, since they must always be equal.
6. Complete the remainder of the equation by adding the proper coefficients to make sure that there are the same number of each type of atom on each side of the equation.
7. Note that any element in the free state, that is, uncombined, has an oxidation number of zero.

EXAMPLE 9-1. Balance $H_2 + O_2 \longrightarrow H_2O$.
Step 1. *Write in all the oxidation numbers.*

$$\begin{array}{ccc} 0 & 0 & 2(+1) \; -2 \\ H_2 + O_2 & \longrightarrow & H_2 \quad O \end{array}$$

(Since the molecules of hydrogen and oxygen are uncombined, their atoms have an oxidation number of zero; from the table on page 82 we know that the oxidation number of oxygen in water is -2 and that of each hydrogen is $+1$).

Step 2. *Show the increase and decrease in oxidation numbers.*

Since the hydrogen is changing from an oxidation number of 0 to $+1$, there is an increase of 1 in oxidation number. The oxygen, in changing from an oxidation number of 0 to -2, decreases by 2 in oxidation number. These changes may be indicated in the equation as

$$\begin{array}{ccc} 0 & 0 & 2(+1) \; -2 \\ H_2 + O_2 & \longrightarrow & H_2 \quad O \end{array}$$

$$\begin{array}{c|c} \uparrow \text{1 for} & \text{2 for} \\ \text{each} & \text{each} \\ \text{atom} & \text{atom} \downarrow \end{array}$$

Inorganic Chemistry

where the upward pointing arrow indicates an increase in oxidation number and the downward pointing arrow a decrease in oxidation number.

Step 3. *Find the total change in oxidation number for each of the elements that is changing.*

The total increase in oxidation number for the hydrogen is 2 (1 for each of the hydrogens). The total decrease in oxidation number for the oxygen is 4 (2 for each of the oxygen). These total changes in oxidation number may be indicated as

$$\text{Total changes:} \quad \overset{0}{H_2} + \overset{0}{O_2} \longrightarrow \overset{2(+1)}{H_2} \overset{-2}{O}$$
$$\Big\uparrow 2 \qquad \Big\downarrow 4$$

Step 4. *The least common multiple (LCM) for an increase of 2 and a decrease of 4 is 4.*

Step 5. *Equate the increase in oxidation number with the decrease.*

The increase in oxidation number for the hydrogen (2) goes into the LCM twice, so we place a 2 in front of the H_2. The decrease in oxidation number for the O_2 (4) goes into the LCM once, so we place a 1 in front of the O_2 (no number in front of a formula designates 1). Thus, we have

$$2H_2 + O_2 \longrightarrow H_2O$$

where the total increase in oxidation number is now equal to the total decrease.

Step 6. *Complete the equation.*

Since we now have a total of 4 H's on the left side of the equation we must have 4 H's on the right side, so we place a 2 in front of the H_2O and then we have 4 H's on each side of the equation, or

$$2H_2 + O_2 \longrightarrow 2H_2O$$

We note that there are also 2 O's on each side of the equation, and it is therefore completely balanced. ∎

After you have tried several redox equations you will be able to combine many of these steps and save time in balancing.

Let us see what was *oxidized* and what was *reduced*. Since the definition of oxidation is an increase in oxidation number, the H_2 must have been oxidized because its oxidation number did increase (from 0 to 1 each). Also, the O_2 must have been reduced because it decreased in oxidation number (from 0 to −2 each). The H_2 was oxidized. What oxidized it? The O_2; so the O_2 is the oxidizing agent. The O_2 was reduced. What reduced it? The H_2; so the H_2 is the reducing agent.

$$\begin{array}{cc} H_2 & O_2 \\ \text{oxidized} & \text{reduced} \\ \text{reducing agent} & \text{oxidizing agent} \end{array}$$

EXAMPLE 9-2. Balance $KClO_3 \longrightarrow KCl + O_2$.

Listing the oxidation numbers we have

$$\overset{+1}{K} \overset{+5}{Cl} \overset{3(-2)}{O_3} \longrightarrow \overset{+1}{K} \overset{-1}{Cl} + \overset{0}{O_2}$$

Note that the Cl and the O are changing in oxidation number. The Cl, in changing from +5 to −1, exhibits a decrease of 6 in oxidation number. The O, in changing from −2 to 0, exhibits an increase of 2 in oxidation number of each of the O atoms present. Since there are three O atoms present, the total increase in oxidation number is 6. These changes may be indicated as

$$\text{Total changes:} \quad \overset{+5}{\text{K Cl}} \overset{3(-2)}{\text{O}_3} \longrightarrow \overset{-1}{\text{K Cl}} + \overset{0}{\text{O}_2}$$

$$\downarrow 6 \quad \uparrow 6$$

Because the increase in oxidation number here does equal the decrease, we need no LCM and so leave the left side of the equation as is.

Now to complete the equation. Since we have 1 KClO₃ on the left side of the equation we can have only 1 KCl on the right because the number of K's on each side of the equation must be the same and so must the number of Cl's. Since we have 3 O's on the left side of the equation we must have 3 O's on the right side; we get these by placing a $1\frac{1}{2}$ in front of the O_2 ($1\frac{1}{2} \times O_2 = 3O$). Thus we have

$$KClO_3 \longrightarrow KCl + 1\tfrac{1}{2}O_2$$

However, we can never have fractions of atoms or molecules in a chemical equation, so we multiply the whole equation by 2 to get

$$2KClO_3 \longrightarrow 2KCl + 3O_2$$

which is balanced because it contains the same number of each type of atom on each side of the equation.

What was reduced? An error made by many students is the statement that the chlorine was reduced because it decreased in oxidation number. It is true that a decrease in oxidation number is reduction, but the chlorine did not decrease in oxidation number, the Cl^{+5} decreased. This makes quite a difference as we shall see in the following paragraph.

What was oxidized? The O^{-2} was oxidized because it increased in oxidation number. If we had said that the oxygen was oxidized, that would have been incorrect because oxygen is a product of the reaction and not one of the original reactants.

Also the Cl^{5+}, since it was reduced, is the oxidizing agent and the O^{2-}, which was oxidized, is the reducing agent. ■

EXAMPLE 9-3. Balance $P + HNO_3 + H_2O \longrightarrow NO + H_3PO_4$.
We will combine a few of the steps to save space. Therefore, we have

$$\text{Total changes:} \quad \overset{0}{P} + \overset{+1}{H} \overset{+5}{N} \overset{3(-2)}{O_3} + \overset{2(1)}{H_2} \overset{-2}{O} \longrightarrow \overset{+2}{N} \overset{-2}{O} + \overset{3(+1)}{H_3} \overset{+5}{P} \overset{4(-2)}{O_4}$$

$$\uparrow 5 \qquad \downarrow 3$$

The LCM between an increase of 5 and a decrease of 3 is 15. The increase in oxidation number by the P (5) goes into the LCM three times, so we place a 3 in front of the P; the decrease in oxidation number by the N (3) goes into the LCM five times, so we place a 5 in front of the HNO₃ (to give us 5 N's) or

$$3P + 5HNO_3 + (\quad) H_2O \longrightarrow (\quad) NO + (\quad) H_3PO_4$$

Three P's on the left side of the equation must give 3 P's on the right, so we put a 3 in front of the H₃PO₄ to give us a total of 3 P's there. Five HNO₃ on the left side of the equation contain 5 N's, so we must have 5 N's on the right side, we get these by placing a 5 in front of the NO

Inorganic Chemistry

$$3P + 5HNO_3 + (\;\;)\,H_2O \longrightarrow 5NO + 3H_3PO_4$$

Now to complete the equation, let us balance the H's. There are 9 H's on the right side of the equation ($3H_3$). On the left side there are 5 H's in the HNO_3's, so we need 4 more, we get these by taking $2H_2O$ (4 H's), or

$$3P + 5HNO_3 + 2H_2O \longrightarrow 5NO + 3H_3PO_4$$

To check, let us see if the O's balance. There are $5 \times 3 + 2 \times 1 = 17$ O's on the left side and $5 \times 1 + 3 \times 4 = 17$ O's on the right side, so the equation is correctly balanced.

What was oxidized? The P, since it increased in oxidation number. Thus it is the reducing agent.

What was reduced? The N^{5+} (or we could say the HNO_3) was reduced because it decreased in oxidation number and, therefore, it is the oxidizing agent. ■

EXAMPLE 9-4. Balance

$$FeSO_4 + K_2Cr_2O_7 + H_2SO_4 \longrightarrow Fe_2(SO_4)_3 + Cr_2(SO_4)_3 + K_2SO_4 + H_2O$$

Since this equation is a little more complex than those we have studied previously, we will solve it carefully and slowly to see why we take each step. First, we will list the oxidation numbers, giving the whole (SO_4) polyatomic ion a charge of -2 instead of giving the separate oxidation numbers of the S and the O because we see that SO_4 occurs unchanged on both sides of the equation. Se we have

$$\begin{array}{cccccc} +2 & -2 & 2(+1)\,2(+6)\,7(-2) & 2(+1) & -2 \\ Fe & SO_4 + & K_2\;\;Cr_2\;\;O_7 \;+\; & H_2 & SO_4 \longrightarrow \end{array}$$
$$\begin{array}{cccccccc} & 2(+3)\,3(-2) & 2(+3)\,3(-2) & 2(+1)\,-2 & 2(+1)\,-2 \\ & Fe_2\;(SO_4)_3 \;+\; & Cr_2\;(SO_4)_3 \;+\; & K_2\;SO_4 \;+\; & H_2\;O \end{array}$$

We note that the Fe is changing from $+2$ to $+3$, which is an increase of 1, and the Cr is changing from $+6$ to $+3$, which is a decrease of 3 in oxidation number for each Cr or a total decrease of 6 in oxidation number for the 2 Cr's, or

$$\begin{array}{cccccc} +2 & 2(+6) & & 2(+3) & 2(+3) \\ FeSO_4 + & K_2Cr_2O_7 + & H_2SO_4 \longrightarrow & Fe_2(SO_4)_3 + & Cr_2(SO_4)_3 + K_2SO_4 + H_2O \\ \uparrow 1 & \downarrow 6 \end{array}$$

The LCM for an increase of 1 and a decrease of 6 in oxidation number is 6. Therefore, an increase of 1 (by the Fe) goes into the LCM six times, so we place a 6 in front of the $FeSO_4$; a decrease of 6 in oxidation number (by the Cr's in $K_2Cr_2O_7$) goes into the LCM once, so we place a 1 (understood) in front of the $K_2Cr_2O_7$, or

$$6FeSO_4 + K_2Cr_2O_7 + (\;\;)\,H_2SO_4 \longrightarrow$$
$$(\;\;)\,Fe_2(SO_4)_3 + (\;\;)\,Cr_2(SO_4)_3 + (\;\;)\,K_2SO_4 + (\;\;)\,H_2O$$

Now to complete the rest of the equation. Since there are 6 Fe's on the left side there must be 6 on the right; we get these by placing a 3 in front of the $Fe_2(SO_4)_3$ ($3Fe_2 = 6Fe$). Since there are 2 K's on the left side of the equation, there must be 2 on the right, and we get these by taking $1K_2SO_4$. Since there are 2 Cr's on the left side, there must be 2 on the right, and so we place a 1 in front of the $Cr_2(SO_4)_3$, or

$$6FeSO_4 + K_2Cr_2O_7 + (\;\;)\,H_2SO_4 \longrightarrow$$
$$3Fe_2(SO_4)_3 + Cr_2(SO_4)_3 + K_2SO_4 + (\;\;)\,H_2O$$

Now let us count the SO_4 groups on the right side of the equation. There are 9 in the $3Fe_2(SO_4)_3$ plus 3 in the $Cr_2(SO_4)_3$ plus 1 in the K_2SO_4, or a total of 13 SO_4's. We started with 6 SO_4's in the $6FeSO_4$ so we need 7 more; we get these by taking $7H_2SO_4$. These 7 H_2's on the left side must give 7 H_2's on the right, so we have 7 H_2O, or

$$6FeSO_4 + K_2Cr_2O_7 + 7H_2SO_4 \longrightarrow 3Fe_2(SO_4)_3 + Cr_2(SO_4)_3 + K_2SO_4 + 7H_2O$$

To check if the equation is correctly balanced, let us add up the O's on each side and see if the totals are the same.

Left Side		Right Side	
$6FeSO_4$	24 O's	$3Fe_2(SO_4)_3$	36 O's
$1K_2Cr_2O_7$	7 O's	$Cr_2(SO_4)_3$	12 O's
$7H_2SO_4$	28 O's	K_2SO_4	4 O's
		$7H_2O$	7 O's
	59 O's		59 O's

And so we see that the equation is correctly balanced. ■

What is the oxidizing agent? We know that the oxidizing agent is reduced, which means that it decreases in oxidation number. The Cr^{+6}, in going from $+6$ to $+3$, decreases in oxidation number, therefore, it is the oxidizing agent; or we might say that the $K_2Cr_2O_7$ is the oxidizing agent since the Cr^{+6} is a part of this compound and the rest of it does not change in oxidation number. Likewise, the reducing agent is the Fe^{+2} or the $FeSO_4$ (which is oxidized).

Oxidation and reduction reactions produce the energy the body needs to carry out its normal functions. Oxidation–reduction in the body involves either oxygen or hydrogen, or both.

Enzymes involved in oxidation–reduction reactions in the body are called oxidoreductases (see page 378). Many of these enzymes are present in the mitochondria (page 378).

Importance of Oxidation–Reduction

Antiseptic Effects

Because they are oxidizing agents, many antiseptics* have the property of killing bacteria. Among these is chlorine, which oxidizes organic matter and bacteria and so is used in the treatment of water to make it potable (see page 151). Calcium hypochlorite, $Ca(OCl)_2$, another commonly used oxidizing agent and bleaching powder, is used as a disinfectant for clothes and hospital beds. Table 9–1 lists some of the common antiseptics that are oxidizing agents.

Formaldehyde and sulfur dioxide are two reducing agents used in disinfecting rooms formerly occupied by patients with contagious diseases.

Effects on Hair Protein

Oxidizing and reducing agents denature protein by affecting the disulfide bonds (see page 357) of the amino acid cysteine. Use is made of this effect in "home permanents." Hair protein is primarily keratin, and keratin contains a large amount of cysteine. During the treatment, a reducing agent is used

TABLE 9-1. Antiseptic Agents

Formula	Name	Use
$3\%H_2O_2$	Hydrogen peroxide	Minor cuts and scratches
$KMnO_4$	Potassium permanganate	Treatment of infection in urethra and bladder
$KClO_3$	Potassium chlorate	Treatment of sore throat
I_2 in H_2O	Lugol's solution	Treatment of minor cuts
$NaOCl$	Sodium hypochlorite (Dakin's solution)	Treatment of wounds

Look

first. This substance breaks the disulfide bonds in the hair protein. The hair is then shaped with rollers. The new shape is "set" by using an oxidizing agent, which forms new disulfide bonds in the desired places. The hair will retain its new shape only until new hair grows out. Then the entire process has to be repeated.

Stain Removal Oxidizing agents and reducing agents are used to remove most stains that cannot otherwise be removed. Table 9–2 lists some of the common stain removers and indicates where they may be used safely.

TABLE 9-2. Stain Removers

Substance	Name	Function	Use
H_2O_2	Hydrogen peroxide	Oxidizing agent	Blood stains on cotton or linen
$KMnO_4$	Potassium permanganate	Strong oxidizing agent	Almost all stains on white fabrics except rayon ($KMnO_4$ stain must be removed, usually with oxalic acid)
$(COOH)_2$	Oxalic acid	Reducing agent	Rust spots and $KMnO_4$ stains
$NaOCl$	Javelle water	Oxidizing agent	Effective on almost all stains on cotton and linen (not to be used on wool or silk)
$Na_2S_2O_3$	Sodium thiosulfate	Reducing agent	Iodine and silver stains

Summary Oxidation is defined as a loss of electrons. Oxidation is also an increase in oxidation number, a combination with oxygen, or a loss of hydrogen.

Reduction is a gain of electrons. Reduction is also a decrease in oxidation number, a gain of hydrogen, or a loss of oxygen. Oxidation can never take place without reduction and vice versa.

Whatever is oxidized is called a reducing agent.

Whatever is reduced is called an oxidizing agent.

Oxidizing and reducing agents may be useful as antiseptics and also as stain removers.

Questions and Problems

A

1. In the following equations, indicate the oxidizing agent and the reducing agent:
   (a) $Cl_2 + 2KI \longrightarrow 2KCl + I_2$
   (b) $2Al + 3H_2SO_4 \longrightarrow Al_2(SO_4)_3 + 3H_2$
   (c) $Cu + 2AgNO_3 \longrightarrow Cu(NO_3)_2 + 2Ag$
   (d) $2H_2 + O_2 \longrightarrow 2H_2O$

Oxidation-Reduction **139**

2. In the following equations, what was oxidized and what was reduced?
   (a) $4Fe + 3O_2 \longrightarrow 2Fe_2O_3$ (b) $2S + 3O_2 \longrightarrow 2SO_3$
   (c) $Zn + 2HCl \longrightarrow ZnCl_2 + H_2$ (d) $CuO + H_2 \longrightarrow Cu + H_2O$
   (e) $MnO_2 + 4HCl \longrightarrow MnCl_2 + Cl_2 + 2H_2O$
3. Why can oxidation never take place without reduction?
4. List several substances that can be used to remove stains.

B 5. Give an example of oxidation involving (a) loss of electrons, (b) gain of oxygen, (c) loss of hydrogen.
6. Consider the following reaction: $2H_2 + O_2 \rightleftharpoons 2H_2O$. Does it involve oxidation–reduction in both directions? Are all oxidation–reduction reactions reversible?
7. Discuss oxidation–reduction in terms of disulfide bonds.
8. Balance the following oxidation–reduction reactions:
   (a) $Zn + HCl \longrightarrow ZnCl_2 + H_2$
   (b) $P + HNO_3 + H_2O \longrightarrow NO + H_3PO_4$
   (c) $MnCl_2 + NaOH + Br_2 \longrightarrow MnO_2 + NaCl + NaBr + H_2O$
   (d) $Mn(NO_3)_2 + NaBio_3 + HNO_3 \longrightarrow$
   $$HMnO_4 + Bi(NO_3)_3 + NaNO_3 + H_2O$$
9. In each of the equations in question 8, indicate what was oxidized, what was reduced, the oxidizing agent, and the reducing agent.

References   DICKSON, T. R. *Introduction to Chemistry,* 4th ed. John Wiley & Sons, Inc., New York, 1983, Chapter 13.

MCQUARRIE, DONALD A. and PETER A. ROCK. *General Chemistry.* W. H. Freeman and Company, New York, 1984, Chapter 24.

PETRUCCI, RALPH H. and ROBERT E. WISMER. *General Chemistry with Qualitative Analysis.* Macmillan Publishing Company, New York, 1983, Chapter 19.

SACKHEIM, GEORGE I. *Chemical Calculations,* 12th ed., Series B. Stipes Publishing Co., Champaign, Ill., 1983, Chapter 16.

STOKER, H. STEPHEN. *Introduction to Chemical Principles.* Macmillan Publishing Company, New York, 1983, Chapter 15.

10 Water

CHAPTER
OUTLINE

Importance
Physical Properties
Physical Constants Based on Water
Structure of the Water Molecule
Hydrogen Bonding
Evaporation
Boiling Point
Chemical Properties
   Electrolysis
   Stability
   Reaction with Metal Oxides
   Reaction with Nonmetal Oxides
   Reaction with Active Metals

Formation of Hydrates
Hydrolysis
Purification of Water
   Impurities Present in Water
   Distillation
   Boiling
   Sedimentation and Filtration
   Aeration
Hardness in Water
   Home Methods for Water Softening
   Commercial Water Softeners
Water Pollution

Importance

Water is one of the most important chemicals known. Without it neither animal nor plant life would exist. Humans can live for a few weeks without food, but only a few days without water. Almost three fourths of the earth's surface is covered by water. Rain, snow, sleet, hail, fog, and dew are manifestations of the water vapor present in the air.

Water is present on the solid part of the earth's surface as lakes, streams, waterfalls, and glaciers. The human body is approximately 50 percent water. Water is essential in the processes of digestion, circulation, elimination, and the regulation of body temperature. Indeed, every activity of every cell in the body takes place in a watery environment. Normally, in the body water intake equals water output. If water intake is greater than water output, a condition known as edema* results (see Figure 10–1). If water intake is less than output, dehydration occurs.

Water is important as a solvent. Many substances dissolve in water—sugar, salt, and alcohol, for example.

Physical Properties

Pure water is colorless, odorless, and tasteless. Tap water owes its taste to dissolved gases and minerals. Large amounts of water such as lakes and oceans appear blue owing to the presence of finely divided solid material and also to the reflection of the sky.

When water at room temperature is cooled, its volume contracts. However, water is an unusual liquid in that, after it is cooled to 4°C, further

141

FIGURE 10-1. Patient's leg showing pitting edema. (Courtesy Evanston Hospital, Evanston, IL.)

cooling produces an expansion in volume. When water freezes at 0°C, it expands even more, increasing in volume by almost 10 percent and decreasing in density. These changes on freezing explain why ice floats and why water pipes may burst when the water freezes. Expansion of water during frostbite explains the damage to the cells.

The density of water changes with the temperature. At 4°C water has its smallest volume and its maximum density, 1 g/ml. However, for all practical purposes, the density of water is given as 1 g/ml regardless of temperature, since the variation in density between 0° and 100°C is quite small.

Pure water boils at 100°C at 1 atm pressure. At lower pressures it boils at a lower temperature. In certain mountainous localities, water boils at 80°C because of the lower pressure. If more heat is applied to the water, it merely boils faster. The boiling point does not increase. When water boils at 80°C, there may not be sufficient heat to cook food. In this case, the food must be heated in a pressure cooker. This device increases pressure and so increases the boiling point of the water. The same principle is true in the autoclave where the increased pressure increases the boiling temperature.

For water to evaporate, a certain amount of heat is necessary. This amount of heat is approximately 540 cal/g. When water is placed on the skin, the heat it needs to make it evaporate comes from that skin. Therefore, the skin loses the heat and so is cooled. Likewise, the skin is cooled by the evaporation of perspiration (see page 145).

For ice to melt, the amount of heat required is 80 cal/g. When an ice pack is placed on the skin, the heat needed to melt the ice comes from the body, thus lowering the temperature of the body.

Physical Constants Based on Water

The freezing point of water (0°C or 32°F) and the boiling point of water at 1 atm pressure (100°C or 212°F) are the standard reference points for the measurement of temperature.

The weight of 1 ml of water at 4°C (its maximum density) is a standard of weight in the metric system—the gram. Specific gravity is based upon water. It is defined as the weight of a substance compared with the weight of an equal volume of water.

The calorie is defined as the amount of heat required to change the temperature of 1 g of water 1°C.

Structure of the Water Molecule

Pure water does not conduct electricity. This indicates that water is a covalent compound in which the atoms share electrons. Thus each hydrogen atom of the water molecule shares its one electron with the oxygen atom.

We might expect the oxygen and the hydrogen atoms in the water molecule to be arranged in a straight line such as HOH. However, laboratory evidence indicates that atoms in the water molecule are arranged in a nonlinear manner with the angle between the hydrogen atoms being approximately 105° (see page 79).

$$\text{H} \underset{x}{\overset{..}{\cdot}} \overset{..}{\underset{\cdot x}{\text{O}}} \!: \\ \text{H}$$

The X's represent the electrons of the hydrogen atom and the dots the electrons from the oxygen atom. However, the oxygen atom has a greater attraction for electrons than does the hydrogen atom. Therefore, the electrons will spend more of their time closer to the oxygen atom than to the hydrogen atom. This shifting of the electrons toward the oxygen atom will tend to give the oxygen atom a slight negative charge, whereas the hydrogen atoms have a slight positive charge. The structure and distribution of relative charges in the water molecule may be represented as

Molecules in which there is an unequal or uneven *distribution* of charges are called **polar molecules.** Water is a polar molecule. The polar nature of the water molecule is responsible for its property of dissolving many materials. When the ionic compound sodium chloride (NaCl) is placed in water, it dissolves partly because of the water molecule attracting the ions and pulling them apart (see Figure 10–2). Sodium chloride is a polar compound because of the uneven distribution of charges, Na^+Cl^-, within the molecule. A general rule is that polar compounds dissolve in polar liquids, and nonpolar compounds dissolve in nonpolar liquids. Nonpolar compounds generally do not dissolve in polar liquids. Carbon tetrachloride (CCl_4) and benzene (C_6H_6) are nonpolar liquids. Water is a polar liquid. As should be expected, carbon tetrachloride dissolves in benzene, but not in water. Likewise, benzene does not dissolve in water (see page 160).

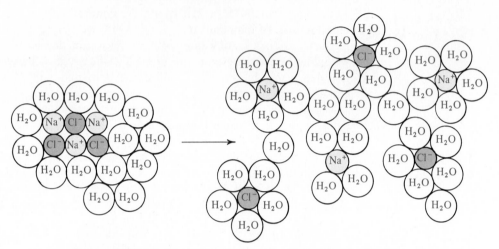

FIGURE 10-2. Model of the solution of sodium chloride (NaCl) in water. (Reproduced from J. E. Fernandez and R. D. Whitaker. *An Introduction to Chemical Principles.* Macmillan Publishing Co., New York, 1975.)

Hydrogen Bonding

Since water molecules are polar, we might expect the positive (hydrogen) end of one water molecule to attract the negative (oxygen) end of one or more other water molecules. This type of attraction is called **hydrogen bonding** and is a weak type of bonding which, as the name implies, always involves hydrogen (see Figure 10–3). The three-dimensional shapes of proteins as well as DNA and RNA are partially due to the presence of hydrogen bonds.

Hydrogen bonds also account for many of the unusual properties of water. In the following section we will see how this type of bonding can account for the abnormally low vapor pressure of water.

Evaporation

The particles in a liquid, such as water, are not held as tightly as those in a solid (see Figure 2–2), so they have some freedom of motion. When some of the surface molecules escape completely from the liquid, the process is called evaporation. As the temperature of the liquid rises, the molecules move faster so more of them can escape from the surface. Thus, the rate of evaporation increases as the temperature increases.

FIGURE 10-3. Hydrogen bonding in (a) water, (b) amino acids.

Evaporation requires energy. When water evaporates, it takes energy (540 cal/g) either from its surroundings or from the remaining water. When water is placed on the skin, it evaporates by taking heat from the body. That is, evaporation is a cooling process. Alcohol evaporates faster than water, so it has a greater cooling effect when placed on the skin. Thus, alcohol sponge baths lower body temperature faster than do water sponge baths.

Consider two containers of water, one open to the air and the other sealed (Figure 10-4). The water in the open container will continue to evaporate until none is left. However, the situation is different in the sealed container. As more and more of the surface molecules escape into the air above the liquid, some of those molecules will return to the liquid. Soon the rate of evaporation will equal the rate at which the gaseous molecules return to the liquid. This condition is known as an **equilibrium.** * The pressure exerted by the gaseous form of the liquid under equilibrium conditions is known as the **vapor pressure** of the liquid.

FIGURE 10-4. Evaporation takes place from the open container; equilibrium is established in the closed container, after which the amount of evaporation and condensation become equal.

Open water container

Sealed water container

TABLE 10-1. Vapor Pressure of Water

Temperature (°C)	Pressure (mm Hg)	Temperature (°C)	Pressure (mm Hg)
20	18	60	149
30	32	70	234
40	55	80	355
50	93	90	526
		100	760

TABLE 10-2. Vapor Pressures of Various Liquids at Room Temperature

Liquid	Pressure (mm Hg)
Water	18
Alcohol (ethyl)	44
Benzene	75
Acetone	177
Ether (ethyl)	442

Since the rate of evaporation increases as the temperature increases, the vapor pressure also increases as the temperature increases. Table 10–1 indicates the vapor pressure of water at various temperatures. Table 10–2 indicates the vapor pressures of various liquids at room temperature (20°C).

Because alcohol has a higher vapor pressure than water at the same temperature, alcohol will evaporate faster than water. Therefore, medications containing alcohol should be tightly closed when stored. If not, some of the alcohol will evaporate, thus changing the strength of that medication.

Water has a relatively low vapor pressure. Why? Recall that water molecules are held together by hydrogen bonds. In order for water to evaporate, not only must the surface molecules have enough energy to escape but they must also have enough energy to break the hydrogen bonds holding them together. So, the tendency to evaporate is low; hence the low vapor pressure.

Boiling Point   Both boiling and evaporation involve a change from the liquid to the gaseous state. In boiling, however, heat is applied directly whereas in evaporation heat is taken from the surroundings.

The boiling point of a liquid is defined as the temperature at which the vapor pressure of the liquid is equal to atmospheric pressure. For water, the temperature at which the vapor pressure equals 1 atm (760 mm Hg) is 100°C (see Table 10–1). Thus, at 1 atm pressure water boils at 100°C. If the atmospheric pressure is lower than 1 atm, water will boil at a correspondingly lower temperature. Conversely, at pressures above 1 atm, water boils at a temperature higher than 100°C. An autoclave (see page 107) uses this principle.

| Chemical Properties | When water undergoes electrolysis—that is, when an electric current is passed through it—hydrogen gas (H_2) and oxygen gas (O_2) are formed. The volume of hydrogen produced is twice that of oxygen. |

Electrolysis

$$2H_2O \xrightarrow[\text{current}]{\text{electric}} 2H_2\uparrow + O_2\uparrow$$

Stability

When water is heated to 100°C at 1 atm pressure, it boils and turns into a gas, steam. Even when the steam is heated to a high temperature, it does not decompose. The water molecule is extremely stable. There is very little decomposition of the water molecule even at a temperature of 1600°C.

Reaction with Metal Oxides

Water reacts with soluble metal oxides to form a class of compounds called **bases** (see Chapter 13). For example

$$CaO + H_2O \longrightarrow Ca(OH)_2$$
calcium   calcium hydroxide,
oxide   a base

$$Na_2O + H_2O \longrightarrow 2NaOH$$
sodium   sodium hydroxide,
oxide   a base

Reaction with Nonmetal Oxides

Water reacts with soluble nonmetal oxides to form a class of compounds called **acids** (see Chapter 13). For example

$$CO_2 + H_2O \longrightarrow H_2CO_3$$
carbon   carbonic
dioxide   acid

$$SO_3 + H_2O \longrightarrow H_2SO_4$$
sulfur   sulfuric
trioxide   acid

Reaction with Active Metals

When an active metal such as sodium or potassium is placed in water, a vigorous reaction takes place, with the rapid evolution of hydrogen gas. At the same time, a base is formed.

$$2Na + 2H_2O \longrightarrow 2NaOH + H_2\uparrow$$
sodium

Formation of Hydrates

When water solutions of some soluble compounds are evaporated, the substances separate as crystals that contain the given compound combined with water in a definite proportion by weight. Crystals that contain a definite proportion of water as part of their crystalline structure are called **hydrates.** The water contained in a hydrate is called **water of hydration** or **water of crystallization.**

Barium chloride crystallizes from solution as a hydrate containing two molecules of water. The formula for this hydrate is $BaCl_2 \cdot 2H_2O$. It is called barium chloride dihydrate. The dot in the middle of the compound indicates that two molecules of water have combined with one molecule of barium chloride. When the water of hydration is removed from a hydrate, the resulting compound is called **anhydrous** (meaning without water). When barium chloride dihydrate is heated, the water of hydration is driven off, leaving anhydrous barium chloride.

$$BaCl_2 \cdot 2H_2O \xrightarrow{\text{heat}} BaCl_2 + 2H_2O\uparrow$$

barium chloride   anhydrous
dihydrate   barium
           chloride

Substances that lose their water of hydration on exposure to air are called **efflorescent.** An example of an efflorescent hydrate is washing soda ($Na_2CO_3 \cdot 10H_2O$), sodium carbonate decahydrate. Substances that pick up moisture from the air are called **hygroscopic.** An example of a hygroscopic compound is calcium chloride ($CaCl_2$). A hygroscopic compound may be used as a drying agent because it will pick up and remove moisture from the air.

A hydrate of particular importance in the medical field is plaster of paris. When plaster of paris is mixed with water, it forms a hard crystalline compound called gypsum.

$$(CaSO_4)_2 \cdot H_2O + 3H_2O \longrightarrow 2(CaSO_4 \cdot 2H_2O)$$

plaster of paris (soft)   gypsum (hard)

Plaster of paris was formerly used extensively in preparing surgical casts (see Figure 10–5). It was spread on crinoline to form a bandage. When the bandage was to be used, it was placed in water, wrung out, and quickly

FIGURE 10–5. Cast being applied. (Courtesy Saint Joseph Hospital, Chicago, IL.)

TABLE 10-3. Properties of Water

Physical	Chemical
Colorless, except in deep layer, when it is greenish blue	Stable compound—not easily decomposed—at 1600°C about 0.3% dissociates
Odorless	
Tasteless	Reacts violently with sodium and potassium
At 1 atm, water freezes and ice melts at 0°C or 32°F	Reacts with metal oxides—CaO, for example—to form bases
At 1 atm, water boils and steam condenses at 100°C or 212°F	Reacts with non-metal oxides—SO_2, for example—to form acids
Water expands when it freezes to ice	When crystals are formed from aqueous solutions of certain substances, water and the solute combine to build crystals, which are called hydrates
Density at 4°C, 1.0 g/ml	
Specific heat, 1.0 cal/(g)(°C)	
Heat of vaporization, 540 cal/g	
Heat of fusion, 80 cal/g	

Source: F. J. Quick. *Introductory College Chemistry.* Macmillan Publishing Company, New York, 1965.

applied. Plaster of paris expands on setting, so that the cast may appear comfortable when applied but become too tight when it is set. Therefore, it is very important for the nurse to check the circulation to the body part to which a plaster cast has been applied.

A newer method of preparing surgical casts involves the use of knitted fiberglass fabric impregnated with a water-activated urethane resin. Exposure to moisture or water initiates a chemical reaction resulting in a rigid tape within a few minutes. These casts have the advantages that they are lighter than comparable plaster casts, they can be immersed in water, they are porous and allow free air circulation, and they are resistant to breakage.

Other hydrates are $MgSO_4 \cdot 7H_2O$, magnesium sulfate heptahydrate, commonly known as Epsom salts and $Na_2SO_4 \cdot 10H_2O$, sodium sulfate decahydrate, commonly known as Glauber's salts. Both of these hydrates are used as cathartics.*

Hydrolysis   When some salts are placed in water, hydrolysis occurs. Hydrolysis is the reaction of a compound with water. When ammonium chloride, a salt, is placed in water, some hydrolysis occurs according to the following equilibrium reaction.

$$NH_4Cl + H_2O \rightleftharpoons NH_4OH + HCl$$

| ammonium chloride | water | ammonium hydroxide | hydrochloric acid |

Note that hydrolysis in this example is the reverse of neutralization.

Hydrolysis occurs during the process of digestion of foods. For example, sucrose is hydrolyzed into glucose and fructose through the action of an enzyme.

Water   **149**

$$C_{12}H_{22}O_{11} + H_2O \xrightarrow{\text{enzyme}} C_6H_{12}O_6 + C_6H_{12}O_6$$

sucrose   glucose   fructose

Note that both glucose and fructose have the same formula, $C_6H_{12}O_6$. How two different compounds can have the same formula will be discussed in Chapter 21.

The hydrolysis of fats in the body yields fatty acids and glycerol. The hydrolysis of proteins yields amino acids. Specific enzymes are necessary for these hydrolytic reactions. They will be discussed in the appropriate chapters on fats and protein.

Purification of Water

Impurities Present in Water

Natural water contains many dissolved and suspended materials. Rain water contains dissolved gases—oxygen, nitrogen, and carbon dioxide—plus air pollutants (see page 112), suspended dust particles, and other particulate matter. Groundwater contains minerals dissolved from the soil through which the water has passed. It also contains some suspended materials. Seawater contains over 3.5 percent of dissolved matter, the principal compound being sodium chloride. Both sea- and groundwater also contain dissolved and undissolved pollutants.

Lake water or river water may appear clear when a glass full of it is held up to the light or it may at first contain suspended clay or mud, which tends to settle slowly, leaving what appears to be pure water. However, in both of these cases, the "clear" water may contain many bacteria and other microorganisms that can be quite harmful to the body. Their destruction or removal is necessary for the proper purification of water. Water may be purified by several processes. The most common are distillation, boiling, filtration, and aeration.

Distillation

Distillation is a process of converting water to steam and then changing the steam back to water again. In the laboratory, a "still" is used to prepare distilled water (see Figure 10–6). Impure water is placed in the flask at the left and then heated to boiling. As the water boils and changes into steam, it passes into a condenser, which consists of a long glass tube surrounded by another glass tube through which cold water runs. The cold water changes the steam in the condenser back into liquid water; this then runs out of the end of the tube into the receiving vessel at the right. The suspended and dissolved solids (including the bacteria) that were present in the impure water remain behind in the flask. They do not pass over into the condenser with the steam. The dissolved gases originally present in the impure water, however, do pass over with the steam. The usual practice is to discard the first few milliliters of distilled water coming from the condenser, since they will contain most of the dissolved gases.

Although distilled water is pure water, it is too expensive and the process too slow for large-scale use. The principal use of distilled water in the hospital is in the preparation of sterile solutions.

Boiling

Groundwater or contaminated water can usually be made safe for drinking by boiling it for at least 15 min. The boiling does not remove the dissolved

cooling water out

tap water

cooling water in

distilled water

FIGURE 10-6. A laboratory distillation apparatus.

impurities but does kill any bacteria that might be present. Freshly boiled water has a flat taste because of the loss of dissolved gases. The taste may be brought back to normal by pouring the water back and forth from one clean vessel to another. This process, called aeration, allows air to dissolve in the water again.

Sedimentation and Filtration   For large-scale use, water is first allowed to stand in large reservoirs where most of the suspended dirt, clay, and mud settle out. This process is called sedimentation. However, sedimentation is a very slow process. Put some finely divided clay in a graduated cylinder full of water, shake, and see how slowly the clay settles out. Commercially, a mixture of aluminum sulfate and lime is added to the water. These two chemicals combine to form aluminum hydroxide, which precipitates as a gelatinous (sticky) substance. As the sticky aluminum hydroxide settles out, it carries down with it most of the suspended material. The main advantage of this material is that it settles much more rapidly than does the suspended material by itself and so increases the rate of sedimentation.

After sedimentation, the water is filtered through several beds of sand and gravel to remove the rest of the suspended material. The water then is essentially free of suspended material. However, this process does not remove the dissolved material nor much of the bacteria originally present. The water must then be treated with chlorine to kill the bacteria before it is fit to drink.

Aeration   Water may be purified by exposing it to air for a considerable period of time. The oxygen in the air dissolves in the water and destroys the bacteria by the process of oxidation. The oxygen also oxidizes the dissolved organic material in the water so that the bacteria have no source of food. However, this

Water   **151**

process is slow and expensive because of the long time involved in exposing water to the air. Commercially, aeration is accomplished by spraying filtered chlorinated water into the air. This additional process also removes objectionable odors from the water.

Hardness in Water

When a small amount of soap is added to soft water, it forms copious suds. When a small amount of soap is added to hard water, it forms a precipitate or scum and no lather. What is the difference between soft water and hard water? Hard water contains dissolved compounds of calcium and magnesium. Soft water may contain other dissolved compounds, but these compounds do not cause hardness. The calcium and magnesium compounds (which cause the hardness) react with soap to form a precipitate, thus removing the soap from the water. More and more soap must be added until all the hardness is removed. Only then will the soap cause a lather. The reactions involved are as follows:

$$Ca^{2+} + Na \ (soap) \longrightarrow Ca \ (soap)\downarrow + 2Na^+$$

$$Mg^{2+} + Na \ (soap) \longrightarrow Mg \ (soap)\downarrow + 2Na^+$$

hardness   hardness   no hardness

The precipitated soap adheres to washed materials, making them rough so that they may irritate tender skin, or to washed hair, making it sticky and gummy (see Figure 10–7). Food cooked in hard water is likely to be tougher than that cooked in soft water because of the existence of additional miner-

FIGURE 10–7. When the hair is shampooed in hard water, curd clings to the hair strands, dulling their natural luster and interfering with their ability to reflect light. The hair strands on the left are stringy and not clean, due to the clinging hard water curd. Those on the right, washed in soft water, are radiant and clean. (Courtesy of Culligan Water Institute, Northbrook, IL.)

als. When hard water is boiled, some of the salts form a deposit on the inside of the container in which it is heated. Look inside an old teakettle at home and see the "boiler scale." Hard water must never be used to sterilize surgical instruments because the precipitated hardness will dull the cutting edges. (If iron compounds are present in water, they also will cause hardness.)

Detergents have replaced soaps for washing clothes because they do not precipitate in the presence of hardness in water.

Home Methods for Water Softening

Temporary hardness is hardness that can be removed by boiling. It is caused by the bicarbonates of calcium and magnesium. Boiling converts these to insoluble carbonates, thus removing part of the hardness.

$$Ca(HCO_3)_2 \xrightarrow{\text{heat}} CaCO_3\downarrow + CO_2\uparrow + H_2O$$

Other soluble compounds of calcium and magnesium cause permanent hardness. Permanent hardness cannot be removed by boiling.

Ammonia (ammonium hydroxide) is frequently used to soften water used in washing clothes and windows because it precipitates all temporary hardness and some of the permanent hardness. Borax, sodium tetraborate ($Na_2B_4O_7$), is also frequently used in the home as a laundry water softener. Its effect is similar to that of ammonia. Washing soda (Na_2CO_3), frequently used as a home-laundry water softener, removes both temporary and permanent hardness from the water. Trisodium phosphate, TSP (Na_3PO_4), which is another home-laundry water softener, has an action similar to that of washing soda. However, TSP is no longer recommended for laundry use because of the effects of phosphates on our lakes and streams.

Commercial Water Softeners

The preceding methods for water softening are practical for use in a home, but they are too expensive for large-scale commercial use. One commercial method used is the lime-soda process. In this process lime, $Ca(OH)_2$, and then soda, Na_2CO_3, are added to water to remove both temporary and permanent hardness.

Complex silicates called zeolites are also used commercially to remove both types of hardness from water. These zeolites, in the form of large granules, are placed in a cylindrical container and hard water is allowed to flow through that container (see Figure 10–8). As the water passes over the zeolites, the sodium ions in the zeolite replace the calcium and magnesium ions in the water. This process, called **ion exchange,** takes the calcium and magnesium ions out of the water and replaces them with sodium ions. Sodium ions do not cause hardness. The reactions involved are

$$Ca^{2+} + Na_2Z \longrightarrow CaZ + 2Na^+$$
$$\text{sodium} \qquad \text{calcium}$$
$$\text{zeolite} \qquad \text{zeolite}$$

$$Mg^{2+} + Na_2Z \longrightarrow MgZ + 2Na^+$$
$$\text{sodium} \qquad \text{magnesium}$$
$$\text{zeolite} \qquad \text{zeolite}$$

The zeolite in the cylinder will be gradually used up as more and more water is softened. However, the used zeolite may be regenerated and used over and over again. Many hospitals use this process for water softening. However, this type of softened water must be avoided by patients on low sodium diets.

Water that has been softened by the zeolite process still has dissolved minerals in it—the sodium compounds obtained by ion exchange. To prepare water comparable to distilled water, all soluble minerals must be removed. This may be accomplished by using a set of two different resins, one to remove the soluble metal (positive) ions and the other to remove the negative ions present in the water. If a sample of hard water is assumed to contain calcium chloride, $CaCl_2$, the dissolved mineral may be removed as follows

$$CaCl_2 + 2HY \longrightarrow 2HCl + CaY$$
$$\text{resin}$$

The HCl then reacts with the second resin, XNH_2

$$HCl + XNH_2 \longrightarrow XNH_3Cl$$
$$\text{resin}$$

Inorganic Chemistry

so that no ions (aside from those of the water itself) are left in the water. Such water is called **deionized** water. Although this process is inexpensive and quick, it will not remove bacteria or dissolved nonelectrolytes.

Water Pollution

What is polluted water? Strictly speaking, it is any water that is not pure. However, tap water contains many dissolved and suspended substances. It is not pure, yet it is not called polluted water. Any substance that prevents or prohibits the normal use of water is termed a **pollutant**. The signs of polluted water are usually quite obvious—oil and dead fish floating on the surface of a body of water or deposited along the shores, a bad taste to drinking water, a foul odor along a waterfront, unchecked growth of aquatic weeds along the shore, or tainted fish that cannot be eaten.

Water pollutants can be classified into several categories.

1. **Oxygen-demanding wastes.** Dissolved oxygen is required for both plant and animal life in a body of water. Anything that tends to decrease the supply of this vital element endangers the survival of the life forms. Oxygen-demanding wastes are acted upon by bacteria in the presence of oxygen, thus leading to a depletion of the dissolved oxygen. Oxygen-demanding pollutants include sewage and wastes from paper mills, food-processing plants, and other industrial processes that discharge organic materials into the water.

2. **Disease-causing agents.** Among the diseases that can be caused by pathogenic microorganisms present in polluted water are typhoid fever, cholera, infectious hepatitis, and poliomyelitis.

3. **Radioactive material.** Low-level radioactive wastes from nuclear power plants are sealed in concrete and buried underground. High-level radioactive wastes are initially stored as liquids in large underground tanks and later converted into solid form for burial in concrete. In either case, leakage can lead to pollution of nearby water supplies.

4. **Heat.** Although heat is not normally considered a pollutant of waterways, it does have a detrimental effect on the amount of dissolved oxygen. Thermal pollution results when water is used as a coolant for industrial plants and nuclear reactors and then returned to its source.

In addition to decreasing the amount of dissolved oxygen, thermal pollution also causes an increased rate of chemical reactions. The metabolic processes of fish and microorganisms are speeded up, increasing their need for oxygen, at a time when the supply of oxygen is diminishing. Higher water temperatures can also be fatal to certain forms of marine life.

5. **Plant nutrients.** Nutrients stimulate the growth of aquatic plants. This may lead to lower levels of dissolved oxygen. It may also lead to disagreeable odors when the large amount of plant material decays. Excessive plant growth is often unsightly and interferes with recreational use of water. Excess phosphorus in sewage comes from phosphate detergents and is one cause for this type of pollution.

6. **Synthetic organic chemicals.** In this category of pollutants are such substances as surfactants in detergents, pesticides, plastics, and food additives.

7. Inorganic chemicals and minerals. These pollutants come from industrial wastes as well as from runoff water from urban areas. One example of such a pollutant is mercury. It was once believed that metallic mercury was inert and settled to the bottom of a lake. It is now known that anaerobic bacteria in bottom muds are capable of converting this mercury into compounds that are poisonous. Another pollutant in this category is sulfuric acid, which is formed by the reaction of sulfur-containing ores with water and oxygen in the air. Salt is also a pollutant, which can occur when brine from oil wells is released into fresh water.

Summary

Water is one of the most important chemicals known. Pure water is a colorless, odorless, flat-tasting liquid that freezes at 0°C and boils at 100°C at 1 atm pressure. Water has its maximum density at 4°C. When water freezes, its volume increases by almost 10 percent.

Water is used as a solvent for many substances. Many chemical reactions take place only when the reactants are dissolved in water. The evaporation of water or perspiration from the skin is a cooling process because the skin provides (loses) the heat required to change the liquid to the vapor state. Water is the standard of reference for such physical constants as the temperature scale, specific gravity, the calorie, and the standard of weight in the metric system (the gram).

The water molecule is a covalent one with a hydrogen-oxygen-hydrogen angle of about 105°. Water is a polar liquid. Polar liquids usually dissolve polar compounds and nonpolar liquids dissolve nonpolar compounds.

The electrolysis of water yields hydrogen and oxygen gases. Water does not otherwise appreciably decompose into these gases, even when heated to 1600°C.

Water reacts with certain metal oxides to form bases; water reacts with certain nonmetal oxides to form acids. Water reacts with sodium and potassium to form hydrogen gas and a base. Water reacts with certain salts to form hydrates. Hydrates that lose their water of hydration on standing are called efflorescent. Substances that pick up moisture from the air are called hygroscopic.

Hydrolysis of a salt is the reaction of that salt with water, whereby the water molecule is split.

Water may be purified by distillation, by boiling, by sedimentation and filtration, and by aeration.

Hardness in water is caused by ions of calcium and magnesium (and iron). Temporary hardness is due to bicarbonates of calcium and magnesium. Temporary hardness can be removed by boiling. Permanent hardness cannot be removed by boiling. Hardness in water can be removed by using ammonia, washing soda, trisodium phosphate, lime-soda, or zeolite. Deionized water contains no contaminating ions and is frequently used in place of distilled water.

Water pollution may be caused by oxygen-demanding wastes, disease-causing agents, radioactive materials, heat, plant nutrients, synthetic organic chemicals, and inorganic chemicals and minerals.

Questions and Problems

A

1. Why is pure water flat tasting?
2. Why do lakes and oceans appear blue?
3. Why does ice float?
4. At what temperature does water have its maximum density?
5. Why use a pressure cooker at high altitudes?
6. How much heat is required to evaporate 10 g water from the skin?

7. Why is evaporation a cooling process?

8. Water is used as the standard of reference for which physical constants?

9. Diagram the structure of the water molecule. Why is the molecule polar?

10. Why does salt dissolve in water?

11. Will carbon tetrachloride (CCl_4), a nonpolar liquid, dissolve in water?

12. What type of compound is produced when water reacts with a metal oxide?

13. What type of compound is produced when water reacts with a nonmetal oxide?

14. What type of reaction occurs when a salt reacts with water?

15. Why purify water?

16. Describe the preparation of distilled water.

17. What effect does boiling have on water as far as purification is concerned? as far as the removal of impurities is concerned?

18. Of what importance are filtration and aeration of water?

19. What is a hydrate?

20. What reaction occurs when a hydrate is heated?

21. What is efflorescence?

22. What is a hygroscopic compound? For what purpose may it be used?

23. What causes temporary hardness in water? How may it be removed?

24. What causes permanent hardness in water? How may it be removed?

25. Describe the zeolite process for water softening.

26. What is deionized water and how may it be prepared?

27. What is polluted water? What signs indicate such a condition?

28. What diseases can be caused by polluted water?

29. A depletion of the oxygen content of water can be caused by what factors?

30. How are radioactive wastes disposed of? Why are precautions necessary?

31. What might be the effects of thermal pollution? What might cause this type of pollution?

32. Indicate several synthetic organic water pollutants. Where do they come from?

B 33. What causes the vapor pressure of a liquid? How is vapor pressure affected by temperature?

34. What effect does hydrogen bonding have on the boiling point of water? Explain.

35. How is the vapor pressure of a liquid related to its boiling point?

36. How is the boiling point of a liquid related to the atmospheric pressure?

37. Why is hydrolysis important in the human body?

38. Is hard water safe to drink? Explain.

39. Should zeolite-softened water be used by all persons? Explain.

References DICKSON, T. R. *Introduction to Chemistry,* 4th ed. John Wiley & Sons, Inc., New York, 1983, Chapter 10.

PETRUCCI, RALPH H. and ROBERT E. WISMER. *General Chemistry with Qualitative Analysis.* Macmillan Publishing Company, New York, 1983, Chapter 11.

RAYNER-CANHAN, GEOFFREY and MARK VAN ROODE. *Foundations of Chemistry.* Addison-Wesley Publishing Co., Reading, Mass., 1983, Chapter 10.

SOLOMON, A. K. The status of water within red blood cells. *Scientific American,* **224:**88–96 (Feb. 1981).

11 Liquid Mixtures

CHAPTER
OUTLINE

Solutions
  General Properties
  Solvents Other Than Water
  Factors Affecting Solubility of a Solute
  Importance of Solutions
  Strength of Solutions
  Special Properties of Solutions
  Isotonic Solutions
  Hypotonic Solutions
  Hypertonic Solutions
Suspensions

Colloids
  Size
  Adsorption
  Electrical Charge
  Tyndall Effect
  Brownian Movement
  Gels and Sols
  Dialysis
  Hemodialysis
Emulsions

Liquid mixtures may be divided into four types: solutions, suspensions, colloids, and emulsions. Each type has its own specific properties and uses.

Solutions

General Properties

A solution is a homogeneous mixture of two or more substances evenly distributed in each other. A liquid solution consists of two parts: the solid, liquid, or gaseous material that has dissolved, the **solute,** and a liquid material in which it has dissolved, the **solvent.**

When a crystal of salt is placed in water, which is then stirred, the crystal dissolves and a clear solution is formed. When more salt is added to this saltwater solution, it too dissolves, making the solution more concentrated than the previous one. Even more salt can be dissolved in the water to make it a much more concentrated salt solution. Thus, one of the properties of solutions is that they have a variable composition. Varying amounts of salt and water can be mixed to form various concentrations of saltwater solution.

When salt is dissolved in water to make a saltwater solution, the solution formed is clear and colorless. When sugar is dissolved in water, again a clear, colorless solution is formed. When copper sulfate is dissolved in water, it also forms a clear solution. However, the solutions formed with the salt and the sugar are colorless whereas that formed with copper sulfate is blue. Solutions are always clear. They may or may not have a color. Clear merely means that the solution is transparent to light.

When a salt solution is examined under a high-power microscope, it appears homogeneous. The same is true for a sugar solution. In general, all solutions are homogeneous. The solute cannot be distinguished from the solvent in a solution.

When a solution is allowed to stand undisturbed for a long period of time, no crystals of solute settle out, provided the solvent is not allowed to evaporate. This is another property of solutions—the solute does not settle out.

The salt in a saltwater solution may be recovered by allowing the water to evaporate; likewise, the sugar from a sugar solution. In general, solutions may be separated by physical means.

If a solution (such as saltwater) is poured into a funnel containing a piece of filter paper, the solution will pass through unchanged. That is, the particles in solution must be smaller than the openings in the filter paper.

The properties of solutions are summarized as follows. Solutions

1. Consist of a soluble material or materials (the solute) dissolved in a liquid (the solvent).
2. Have a variable composition.
3. Are clear.
4. Are homogeneous.
5. Do not settle.
6. May be separated by physical means.
7. Pass through filter paper.

Solvents Other Than Water

Solvents other than water are also used. One common solvent used in hospitals is alcohol. An alcohol solution used medicinally is called a tincture.* Tincture of iodine contains iodine dissolved in alcohol. Tincture of green soap contains potassium soap dissolved in alcohol.

Ether is an excellent solvent for fats and oils.

Factors Affecting Solubility of a Solute

TEMPERATURE

Most solid solutes are more soluble in hot water than in cold water. Figure 11-1 shows that KNO_3 becomes much more soluble as the temperature increases; however $Ce_2(SO_4)_3$ becomes less soluble with an increase in temperature, and NaCl shows little change in solubility. Gases such as HCl and SO_2 become less soluble with increasing temperature. The solubility of Br_2, a liquid, is practically unaffected by temperature.

PRESSURE

A change in pressure has no noticeable effect on solubility of a solid or liquid solute in a given solvent but will affect the solubility of a gaseous solute. The greater the pressure, the greater the solubility of a gas in a liquid.

SURFACE AREA

Although surface area does not affect the amount of solute that will dissolve, it does affect the rate of dissolution. The greater the amount of surface area, the quicker a solute will dissolve in a solvent. Thus, to make a solid solute dissolve faster we frequently powder it, thereby increasing the surface area.

STIRRING

The rate at which a solute dissolves can also be increased by stirring the mixture. The process of stirring brings fresh solvent in contact with the solute and so permits more rapid solution.

Therefore, to dissolve most solid solutes rapidly, the solute should be powdered and the mixture should be heated while it is stirred.

Liquid Mixtures   **159**

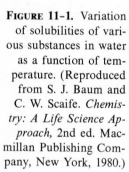

FIGURE 11-1. Variation of solubilities of various substances in water as a function of temperature. (Reproduced from S. J. Baum and C. W. Scaife. *Chemistry: A Life Science Approach,* 2nd ed. Macmillan Publishing Company, New York, 1980.)

NATURE OF SOLVENT

In general, polar liquids dissolve polar compounds and nonpolar liquids dissolve nonpolar compounds. Water is a polar liquid (see page 143) and dissolves polar compounds such as sodium chloride (NaCl).

Sometimes, in spite of all attempts a substance does not appreciably dissolve in water. If the substance is nonpolar, then it should not be expected to be soluble in water. But it should be soluble in a nonpolar liquid. Sometimes polar materials do not dissolve in water. These are called insoluble salts (see page 204).

Table 11-1 lists several polar and nonpolar liquids. Using this table we could predict that potassium iodide (KI), a polar compound, should be soluble in water and that most likely it would not be soluble in a nonpolar liquid

TABLE 11-1. Some Polar and Nonpolar Liquids

Polar Liquids		Nonpolar Liquids	
Name	Formula	Name	Formula
Water	H_2O	Benzene	C_6H_6
Methyl alcohol	CH_3OH	Carbon tetrachloride	CCl_4
Ethyl alcohol	C_2H_5OH	Ether	$C_2H_5OC_2H_5$

Inorganic Chemistry

such as benzene. Likewise we could predict that oils and waxes, which are nonpolar compounds, should be insoluble in water but soluble in ether (or other nonpolar liquids).

In addition to liquid solutions, there are also solid solutions. They usually consist of one metal dissolved in another while both are in the molten (liquid) state. Such a solid solution is called an **alloy.*** Some alloys are used in preparing replacements for such body parts as hip bones and knee joints.

A special type of alloy consists of a metal dissolved in mercury, a liquid metal. An alloy containing mercury is called an **amalgam.** If silver is dissolved in mercury, a silver amalgam is produced. This substance is used in dental work to fill a cavity in a tooth.

Importance of Solutions

During digestion, foods are changed to soluble substances so that they may pass into the bloodstream and be carried to all parts of the body. At the same time the waste products of the body are dissolved in the blood and carried to other parts of the body where they can be eliminated. Plants obtain minerals from the groundwater in which those minerals have dissolved.

Many chemical reactions take place in solution. When solid silver nitrate is mixed with solid sodium chloride, no reaction takes place because the movement of the ions in the solid state is highly restricted. However, when a solution of silver nitrate is mixed with a solution of sodium chloride, a precipitate of silver chloride is formed instantaneously. This reaction occurs because the ions in the solution are free to move and react with other ions.

Many medications are administered orally, subcutaneously, or intravenously as solutions.

Drugs must be in solution before they can be absorbed from the gastrointestinal (GI) tract. As you might expect, when drugs are taken in solution, such as syrups and elixirs, they are absorbed more rapidly than drugs in a solid form, such as tablets and capsules.

Strength of Solutions

DILUTE AND CONCENTRATED

When a few crystals of sugar are placed in a beaker of water, a *dilute* sugar solution is produced. As more and more sugar is added to the water, the solution becomes more *concentrated*. But when does the solution change from dilute to concentrated? There is no sharp dividing line. Dilute merely means that the solution contains a small amount of solute in relation to solvent. Concentrated merely means that the solution contains a large amount of solute in relation to solvent.

However, both dilute and concentrated are relative terms. A dilute sugar solution may contain 5 g of sugar per 100 ml of solution, whereas 5 g (the same amount) of boric acid per 100 ml of solution will produce a concentrated boric acid solution. That is, the terms dilute and concentrated usually have no specific quantitative meaning and so are not generally used for medical applications.

SATURATED

Suppose a small amount of salt is placed in a beaker of water. When the mixture is stirred, all the salt will dissolve. If more and more salt is added with stirring, a point will soon be reached where some of the salt settles to the bottom of the beaker. This excess salt does not dissolve even upon more rapid agitation. This type of solution is called a *saturated solution*. Some of the crystals are continually dissolving and going into solution. At the same time, the same amount of solute crystallizes out of the solution. This type of interchange, as you may remember, is called *equilibrium*.

Thus, a saturated solution may be defined as one in which there is an equilibrium between the solute and the solution. A saturated solution may also be defined as one that contains all the solute that it can hold under the given conditions.

UNSATURATED An unsaturated solution contains less of a solute than it could hold under normal conditions. Suppose that a saturated solution of glucose in a certain amount of water contains 25 g glucose. An unsaturated glucose solution would be one that contained an amount of glucose less than 25 g in the same amount of water. In an unsaturated solution, no equilibrium exists because there is no undissolved solute.

The terms saturated and unsaturated are relative terms. The same amount of two different solutes may produce entirely different types of solutions. For glucose, 5 g in 100 ml of water produces an unsaturated solution, whereas 5 g boric acid in 100 ml of water produces a saturated solution. Therefore, saturated and unsaturated solutions are relative terms and are not used for medical applications.

SUPERSATURATED Under certain conditions a solvent can be made to dissolve more solute than its saturated solution can hold under the same conditions. A supersaturated solution can be prepared by adding excess solute to a saturated solution, heating that mixture, filtering off the excess solute, and then allowing liquid to cool slowly. If this is done carefully, some excess solute will remain dissolved, thus forming a supersaturated solution. However, such a solution is very unstable. If one crystal of solute is added, or if the liquid is shaken vigorously, the excess solute will crystallize out immediately and a saturated solution will remain. The formation of gallstones involves the precipitation of cholesterol from a supersaturated solution.

PERCENTAGE SOLUTIONS The **weight-volume method** expresses the weight of solute in a given volume of solvent, usually water. A 10 percent glucose solution will contain 10 g glucose per 100 ml of solution. A 0.9 percent saline solution will contain 0.9 g sodium chloride per 100 ml of solution. The percentage indicates the number of grams of solute per 100 ml of solution.

EXAMPLE 11-1. Prepare 500 ml of 2 percent citric acid solution.

First let us calculate how much citric acid will be required. A 2 percent citric acid solution contains 2 g citric acid per 100 ml of solution. Therefore, in 500 ml solution there should be

$$500 \text{ ml} \times \frac{2 \text{ g citric acid}}{100 \text{ ml}} = 10 \text{ g citric acid}$$

To prepare the solution, the procedure is as follows:

1. Weigh out exactly 10 g citric acid.
2. Dissolve the 10 g citric acid in a small amount of water contained in a 500-ml graduated cylinder.
3. Add water to the 500-ml mark and stir.

Note the 10 g citric acid was dissolved in water and then diluted to the required volume—500 ml. It was *not* dissolved directly in 500 ml water. (If it had been, the final volume would have been more than 500 ml.) ■

EXAMPLE 11-2. A patient is given 1000 ml 0.9 percent NaCl intravenously. How many grams of NaCl did the patient receive?

$$0.9\% \text{ means } \frac{0.9 \text{ g NaCl}}{100 \text{ ml solution}} \quad \text{so}$$

$$1000 \text{ ml} \times \frac{0.9 \text{ g NaCl}}{100 \text{ ml}} = 9 \text{ g NaCl} \qquad ■$$

In clinical work involving dilute solutions, concentrations are sometimes expressed in terms of **milligram percent** (mg %), which indicates the number of milligrams of solute per 100 ml of solution. Milligram percent is also referred to as milligrams per deciliter (mg/dl). Table 30–1 lists the values of blood components in these units.

PARTS PER MILLION

Low concentrations may be expressed in the units *milligrams per liter* (mg/L). Another method of expressing low concentrations is **parts per million** (ppm). One part per million is equivalent to 1 mg/L. That is, if a solution has a concentration of 40 mg/L, its concentration may also be expressed as 40 ppm.

Parts per million are used to indicate the hardness of water and also to show the concentration of both common substances and pollutants in water and in air.

Extremely low concentrations of pollutants are expressed in the units **parts per billion,** which is equivalent to milligrams per 1000 L (mg/1000 L).

RATIO SOLUTIONS

Another method of expressing concentration is a ratio solution. A 1:1000 merthiolate solution contains 1 g merthiolate in 1000 ml solution. A 1:10,000 $KMnO_4$ solution contains 1 g $KMnO_4$ in 10,000 ml solution. The first number in the ratio indicates the number of grams of solute and the second number gives the number of milliliters of solution. As with percentage solutions, the solute is dissolved in a small amount of solvent (water) and then diluted to the desired volume.

Percentage and ratio solutions are frequently used by doctors, nurses, and pharmacists.

MOLAR SOLUTIONS

Molar solutions are used most frequently by chemists. A molar solution is defined as one that contains 1 mol (see page 84) of solute per liter of solution. A 1 molar (1 M) solution of glucose ($C_6H_{12}O_6$) will contain 1 mol glucose (180 g) in 1 L solution. As before, the solute is dissolved in a small amount of water and then diluted to the desired volume.

Liquid Mixtures   **163**

EXAMPLE 11-3. Prepare 3 L of 2 M (2 molar) KCl (molecular weight 74.5).

The problem calls for the preparation of 3 L of 2 M KCl or 3 L × 2 M KCl. Recall that molarity means moles per liter. So,

$$3\text{ L} \times 2\,M\text{ KCl} = 3\text{ L} \times \frac{2\text{ mol KCl}}{1\text{ L}} = 6\text{ mol KCl}$$

Then, since 1 mol KCl weighs 74.5 g,

$$6\text{ mol KCl} = 6\text{ mol KCl} \times \frac{74.5\text{ g KCl}}{1\text{ mol KCl}} = 447\text{ g KCl}$$

So, we take 447 g KCl, dissolve in water, and dilute to a total of 3 L. ∎

EXAMPLE 11-4. Prepare 500 ml 0.1 M NaOH (molecular weight 40).

The problem calls for 500 ml of 0.1 M NaOH, or 500 ml × 0.1 M NaOH. Changing molarity to moles per liter and also changing milliliters to liters, we have

$$500\text{ ml} \times \frac{1\text{ L}}{1000\text{ ml}} \times \frac{0.1\text{ mol NaOH}}{1\text{ L}} = 0.05\text{ mol NaOH}$$

Then, changing moles NaOH to grams NaOH,

$$0.05\text{ mol NaOH} \times \frac{40\text{ g NaOH}}{1\text{ mol NaOH}} = 2\text{ g NaOH}$$

Thus, we should dissolve 2 g NaOH in water and dilute to 500 ml. ∎

EXAMPLE 11-5. How many grams of glucose are present in 0.5 L of 2.0 M glucose solution? The molecular weight of glucose is 180.

Changing molarity to moles per liter, we have

$$0.5\text{ L} \times \frac{2.0\text{ mol glucose}}{1\text{ L}} = 1\text{ mol glucose}$$

Then, $1\text{ mol glucose} \times \dfrac{180\text{ g glucose}}{1\text{ mol glucose}} = 180\text{ g glucose}$ ∎

NORMAL SOLUTIONS

A 1 normal (1 N) solution contains one gram equivalent weight of solute per liter of solution. The gram equivalent weight of an acid can be calculated by dividing the weight of 1 mol of that acid by the number of replaceable hydrogens that it contains. For example, hydrochloric acid,

$$\text{HCl} \longrightarrow \text{H}^+ + \text{Cl}^-$$

contains one replaceable hydrogen. The grams equivalent weight of HCl is the weight of 1 mol (36.5 g) divided by 1, or 36.5 g.

The gram equivalent weight of sulfuric acid (H_2SO_4),

$$H_2SO_4 \longrightarrow 2H^+ + SO_4^{2-}$$

Inorganic Chemistry

is the weight of 1 mol of H_2SO_4 (98 g) divided by 2, or 49 g.

The gram equivalent weight of a base can be calculated by dividing the weight of 1 mol of that base by the number of OH^- groups it contains. The gram equivalent weight of sodium hydroxide (NaOH),

$$NaOH \longrightarrow Na^+ + OH^-$$

is the weight of 1 mol of NaOH (40 g) divided by 1, or 40 g.

The gram equivalent weight of calcium hydroxide $Ca(OH)_2$,

$$Ca(OH)_2 \longrightarrow ca^{2+} + 2OH^-$$

is the weight of 1 mol of $Ca(OH)_2$ (74 g) divided by 2, or 37 g.

EXAMPLE 11-6. Prepare 2 L of 1.5 N H_2SO_4.

The problem calls for the preparation of 2 L of 1.5 N H_2SO_4, or 2 L × 1.5 N H_2SO_4. Recall that N means gram equivalent weights per liter. So,

$$2\,L \times 1.5\,N\,H_2SO_4 = 2\,\cancel{L} \times \frac{1.5 \text{ gram equivalent weights } H_2SO_4}{\cancel{L}}$$

$$= 3 \text{ gram equivalent weights } H_2SO_4$$

According to the previous calculation, the gram equivalent weight of H_2SO_4 is 49 g, so

$$3 \cancel{\text{ gram equivalent weights } H_2SO_4}$$

$$\times \frac{49 \text{ g } H_2SO_4}{1 \cancel{\text{ gram equivalent } H_2SO_4}} = 147 \text{ g } H_2SO_4$$

So we take 147 g H_2SO_4, dissolve it in water, and dilute to a total of 2 L. ■

EXAMPLE 11-7. Prepare 100 ml of 0.2 N NaOH (molecular weight of 40).

The problem calls for 100 ml of 0.2 N NaOH or 100 ml × 0.2 N NaOH. Changing normality to gram equivalent weights per liter and also changing milliliters to liters, we have

$$100\,\cancel{\text{ml}} \times \frac{1\,\cancel{L}}{1000\,\cancel{\text{ml}}} \times \frac{0.2 \text{ gram equivalent weights NaOH}}{1\,\cancel{L}}$$

$$= 0.02 \text{ gram equivalent weights NaOH}$$

Then, changing gram equivalent weights NaOH to grams NaOH (1 gram equivalent weight of NaOH weighs 40 g),

$$0.02 \cancel{\text{ gram equivalent weights NaOH}}$$

$$\times \frac{40 \text{ g NaOH}}{1 \cancel{\text{ gram equivalent weight NaOH}}} = 0.8 \text{ g NaOH}$$

Thus we should dissolve 0.8 g NaOH in water and dilute to 100 ml. ■

Normality is a very common concentration unit used in a procedure called titration whereby the strength of an unknown acid or base may be determined (see page 198).

MEQ / L   Concentrations of ions in body fluids are frequently expressed in the units milliequivalents per liter, mEq/L (see page 452). One equivalent of an ion, 1 Eq, is defined as 1 mol multiplied by the value of the charge the ion carries. That is, 1 mol of sodium ions (Na^+) contains 1 Eq of sodium ions. One mole of calcium ions Ca^{2+}, contains 2 Eq of calcium ions and 1 mol of CO_3^{2-} ions contains 2 Eq of carbonate ions.

One milliequivalent (mEq) is 1/1000 of an equivalent.

EXAMPLE 11-8. A solution contains 0.045 mol Na_2CO_3/L. How many equivalents per liter and milliequivalents per liter of each ion are present?

$$Na_2CO_3 \longrightarrow 2Na^+ + CO_3^{2-}$$

According to the equation, 1 mol Na_2CO_3 yields 2 mol Na^+ and 1 mol CO_3^{2-}. So,

$$0.045 \text{ mol/L } Na_2CO_3 \longrightarrow 2 \times 0.045 = 0.090 \text{ mol } Na^+/L$$

$$0.090 \text{ mol/L } Na^+ = 0.090 \text{ Eq/L } Na^+$$

$$0.090 \text{ Eq/L } Na^+ = 0.090 \text{ Eq/L } Na^+ \times \frac{1000 \text{ mEq}}{1 \text{ Eq}} = 90 \text{ mEq/L } Na^+$$

Likewise,

$$0.045 \text{ mol/L } Na_2CO_3 \longrightarrow 0.045 \text{ mol/L } CO_3^{2-}$$

$$0.045 \text{ mol/L } CO_3^{2-} = 0.090 \text{ Eq/L } CO_3^{2-}$$

$$0.090 \text{ Eq/L } CO_3^{2-} \times \frac{1000 \text{ mEq}}{1 \text{ Eq}} = 90 \text{ mEq/L } CO_3^{2-} \quad \blacksquare$$

DILUTION OF   It is often necessary to prepare a weaker solution from a stronger (stock)
SOLUTIONS   solution. To do so, we must add water to the stock solution. But, how much water must be added? To answer this question we use the relationship

initial volume $\times$ initial concentration $=$ final volume $\times$ final concentration

where the initial volume is the amount of stock solution to be used, the initial concentration is the strength of the stock solution, the final volume is the amount of dilute solution to be prepared, and the final concentration is the strength of the dilute solution to be prepared.

EXAMPLE 11-9. Prepare 100 ml 0.9 percent saline solution from 10 percent saline solution.

Using the above formula where initial volume $= x$; final volume $=$ 100 ml; initial concentration $= 10$ percent; and final concentration $= 0.9$ percent

$$x \times 10\% = 100 \text{ ml} \times 0.9\%$$

$$x = \frac{100 \text{ ml} \times 0.9\%}{10\%} = 9 \text{ ml}$$

Thus, 9 ml of 10 percent saline solution should be diluted to a volume of 100 ml to prepare 100 ml of 0.9% saline solution. The solution could also be prepared by adding 91 ml of water to the 9 ml of 10 percent saline solution. ∎

OSMOLARITY   The osmotic pressure of a solution is expressed in terms of the osmolarity of a solution. Osmolarity* (osmol) is a measure of the number of particles in solution and will be discussed later in this chapter, under Osmotic Pressure.

Special Properties of Solutions

EFFECT OF SOLUTE ON BOILING POINT AND FREEZING POINT

Whenever a nonvolatile solute is dissolved in a solvent, the boiling point of the solution thus prepared is always greater than that of the pure solvent. Pure water boils at 100°C at 1 atm pressure. A solution of salt in water or a solution of sugar in water will boil at a temperature above 100°C.

Likewise, when a nonvolatile solute is dissolved in a solvent, the freezing point of the solution is always less than the freezing point of the pure solvent. The freezing point of water is 0°C. The freezing point of salt solution or sugar solution is always less than 0°C.

Use is made of these facts in the cooling system of automobiles. Antifreeze is added to the water in the car radiator to lower the freezing point so that the liquid will not freeze when the temperature drops below 32°F. The same material is used in some areas to raise the boiling point of the liquid in the automobile radiator—to prevent it from boiling over when the temperature rises.

SURFACE TENSION   Consider a water molecule in the center of a beaker of water (see Figure 11–2). This water molecule will be attracted in all directions by the water molecules around it. Next, consider a molecule at the surface of the water. This molecule is attracted sideways and downward, but it is not attracted very much by the air molecules above it. Therefore there is a net downward attraction on the surface water molecules. This downward pull on the sur-

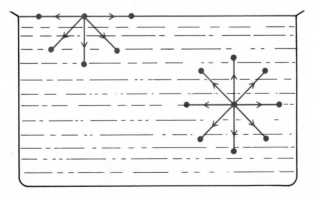

FIGURE 11–2. Surface tension of a liquid.

face molecules causes them to form a surface film. Surface tension may be defined as the force that causes the surface of a liquid to contract. Surface tension also is the force necessary to break this surface film. All liquids exhibit surface tension; the surface tension of water is higher than that of most liquids.

Surface tension is responsible for the formation of drops of water on a greasy surface. The surface film holds the drop in a spherical shape rather than letting it spread over the surface as a sheet of water.

Some medications designed for use on the tissues in the throat contain a very special surface active agent—one that will reduce the surface tension of the water. This surface active agent, called a **surfactant,** lowers the surface tension of the liquid so that it spreads rapidly over the tissues rather than collecting in the form of droplets with less "active" surface area. Soaps and detergents are surfactants.* Bile, which is secreted by the liver, contains bile salts, which act as surfactants. These surfactants help in the digestion of fats (page 388).

A lack of a surfactant in the lungs of premature infants causes respiratory distress syndrome (RDS), formerly called hyaline membrane disease. The surfactant is necessary to form a coating on the inner lining of the small air sacs (alveoli) in the lungs. If the surfactant is present in low amounts, or is not present at all, the surface tension in the alveoli rises, causing portions of the lung to collapse and producing respiratory distress.

The attraction of like molecules for each other is known as **cohesion;** the attraction of unlike molecules is known as **adhesion.** Water rises in a capillary tube because of surface tension and also because of the adhesion of the water molecules to the glass. This effect, known as **capillary action,** is used when drawing blood samples. Capillary action also accounts for the absorption of water by absorbent cotton and by paper towels.

VISCOSITY   Some liquids flow readily (water) whereas others (molasses) do not. A measure of the resistance to flow is called **viscosity*** (see page 353). Table 11-2 indicates the viscosities of several liquids compared to water, which is assigned a value of 1.00. Note the viscosity of blood compared to that of water.

As the temperature increases, liquids tend to flow more readily and so the viscosity decreases.

DIFFUSION   Diffusion, also known as passive transport, is the process whereby a substance moves from an area of its higher concentration to a region where it is less concentrated. That is, the molecules of the substance move from an area where they are crowded together and where molecular collisions are frequent to a region where they are less crowded and collisions will occur

TABLE 11-2. Relative Viscosities of Various Liquids at 20°C

Alcohol (ethyl)	1.20	Ether (ethyl)	0.23
Blood, male	4.71	Glycerol	1.490
Blood, female	4.46	Water	1.00

less often. The greater the difference in concentration between the two areas (the greater the concentration gradient), the faster will be the rate of diffusion. During diffusion, no source of energy is required.

For example, when a crystal of copper sulfate pentahydrate (a blue crystalline substance) is dropped into a cylinder of water, the blue color is soon observed in the water surrounding the crystal. After a while, the blue color may be seen extending upward from the crystal. The liquid at the bottom of the cylinder will be darker blue and the liquid above it will be lighter blue. After several hours the entire contents of the cylinder will be uniformly blue. That is, the solute particles from the crystal are uniformly distributed into all parts of the solution.

Gases will diffuse into one another. When a bottle of ether is opened the odor may soon be detected at a distance. Diffusion into a gas takes place more rapidly than diffusion into a liquid.

Another example of diffusion is the loss of perspiration from the body. The moisture flows from an area of high concentration (the skin) to one of lower concentration (the air). The higher the moisture content of the air (the lower the concentration gradient), the slower the rate of evaporation of moisture from the skin.

Passive transport (diffusion) occurs along a concentration gradient from an area of higher concentration to one of lower concentration with no energy being required.

Active transport occurs when a substance is moved against the concentration gradient, that is, from an area of low concentration to one of higher concentration. In this process energy is required. Active transport is responsible for the high concentration of potassium ions inside the cells compared to a much lower potassium ion concentration outside the cells. Active transport is also responsible for the low concentration of sodium ions inside the cells compared to a much higher sodium ion concentration outside the cells. The amount of energy required for active transport could be as much as 35 percent of the energy output of a resting cell.

OSMOSIS   When a diffusing substance is water and when the diffusion takes place through a semipermeable* or selectively permeable membrane, the process is called osmosis.

Osmosis may be defined as the diffusion of water (solvent) through a semipermeable membrane from a weaker solution (one containing less dissolved solute) to a stronger solution (one containing more dissolved solute). Osmosis may also be defined as the diffusion of water (solvent) down a concentration gradient from an area of high solvent concentration (a weak solution) to a region of low solvent concentration (a stronger solution).

Consider two salt solutions (one dilute and the other concentrated) separated by a semipermeable membrane, a selective membrane. The two solutions will tend to equalize in concentration. That is, the dilute one will tend to become more concentrated whereas the concentrated one will tend to become more dilute. How can they do this? There are two possibilities. First, osmosis can take place. That is, the solvent, water, can diffuse through the membrane from the weaker to the stronger solution (or from an area of high

FIGURE 11-3. Osmosis; prune in water.

solvent concentration to a region of lower solvent concentration). This process will continue until the two solutions have the same concentration.

The second possibility is that of diffusion. The solute will diffuse through the membrane from the stronger to the weaker solution (down the concentration gradient) until the two solutions have equal concentrations. Both osmosis and diffusion may occur at the same time, but not at the same rate. In general, osmosis occurs more rapidly than diffusion.

An example of osmosis that is quite common in the home can be observed by placing a dried prune in water (see Figure 11-3). The skin of the prune acts as a semipermeable membrane. Inside the prune are rather concentrated juices. The water surrounding the prune is certainly dilute in comparison to the juices inside. Thus there are two different concentrations of a solution separated by a semipermeable membrane, and osmosis can take place. In which direction? In osmosis the diffusion of solvent is from the weaker to the stronger solution. Therefore the water will diffuse into the prune, causing it to swell.

Another example of osmosis may be seen when a cucumber is placed in a strong salt solution (Figure 11-4). The skin of the cucumber acts as a semipermeable membrane. The liquid inside the cucumber is quite dilute in comparison to that of the salt solution. Therefore, osmosis takes place because solutions of two different concentrations are separated by a semipermeable membrane. The diffusion, again from dilute to concentrated, takes place from the cucumber into the solution. Thus the cucumber shrinks and becomes a pickle, again by the process of osmosis.

Sailors lost at sea die of dehydration if they drink salt water. In this case,

FIGURE 11-4. Osmosis; cucumber in salt water.

the seawater has a higher concentration of salts than the body fluids, so water diffuses out of the tissues and dehydration results.

In osmosis, water diffuses from a dilute to a concentrated solution. In **reverse osmosis,** the opposite is true. This reverse process can be brought about by applying hydrostatic pressure to the system and is a commercial method of purifying water.

OSMOTIC PRESSURE   Consider a beaker of water into which is placed a thistle tube with a semipermeable membrane over its end. Assume that the thistle tube contains sugar solution (see Figure 11-5). In which direction will osmosis take place? Osmosis will take place with the water diffusing into the thistle tube (from weaker to stronger solution). As the water diffuses into the thistle tube, the water level in the tube will rise. The rising water in the thistle tube will exert a certain amount of pressure, as does any column of liquid. The pressure exerted during the osmotic flow is called the osmotic pressure. This concept is of great importance in the regulation of fluid and electrolyte balance in the body (see page 466).

The osmotic pressure of a solution can be expressed in terms of **osmolarity*** and depends upon the number of particles in solution. The unit of osmolarity is the osmol. For dilute solutions, osmolarity is expressed in milliosmols (mosmol). Body fluids have an osmolarity of about 300 mosmol.

Osmolarity may be calculated from molarity as follows.

$$\text{osmolarity} = \text{molarity} \times \frac{\text{number of particles}}{\text{molecule of solute}}$$

thistle tube

sugar solution

semipermeable membrane

water

FIGURE 11-5. Osmotic pressure as shown by a thistle tube containing sugar solution that is placed in water.

Liquid Mixtures   171

EXAMPLE 11-10. What is the osmolarity of a 1 M glucose solution?

Glucose is a nonelectrolyte (see page 187); it is undissociated. That is, it produces no ions in solution. Therefore, one molecule of glucose yields one particle in solution. Thus,

$$\text{osmolarity} = \text{molarity} \times \frac{\text{number of particles}}{\text{molecule of solute}} = 1\,M \times 1 = 1 \text{ osmol} \quad \blacksquare$$

EXAMPLE 11-11. What is the osmolarity of 1 M NaCl solution?

Each NaCl yields two ions, Na^+ and Cl^-, in solution (see page 187). Thus,

$$\text{osmolarity} = 1\,M \times 2 = 2 \text{ osmol}$$

Therefore we should expect a 1 M NaCl solution to have twice the osmotic pressure of a 1 M glucose solution, as it does. $\quad \blacksquare$

EXAMPLE 11-12. What is the osmolarity of a 0.1 M Na_2SO_4 solution?

$$(Na_2SO_4 \longrightarrow 2\,Na^+ + SO_4^{2-})$$

Since each molecule of Na_2SO_4 yields three ions in solution

$$\text{osmolarity} = 0.1\,M \times 3 = 0.3 \text{ osmol} \quad \blacksquare$$

EXAMPLE 11-13. What is the osmolarity of physiologic saline solution whose concentration is 0.9 percent NaCl? (0.9 percent NaCl is equivalent to 0.15 M NaCl).

Since each NaCl yields two ions, Na^+ and Cl^-, osmolarity = 0.15 M $\times$ 2 = 0.30 osmol.

Then, changing osmol to milliosmol (1 osmol = 1000 mosmol),

$$0.30 \text{ osmol} = 0.30\,\cancel{\text{osmol}} \times \frac{1000 \text{ mosmol}}{1\,\cancel{\text{osmol}}} = 300 \text{ mosmol} \quad \blacksquare$$

EXAMPLE 11-14. What is the osmolarity of 5.5 percent glucose solution? (A 5.5 percent glucose solution is 0.305 M.)

Since glucose yields no ions in solution,

$$\text{osmolarity} = 0.305\,M \times 1$$

$$= 0.305 \text{ osmol} = 0.305\,\cancel{\text{osmol}} \times \frac{1000 \text{ mosmol}}{1\,\cancel{\text{osmol}}} = 305 \text{ mosmol} \quad \blacksquare$$

A cardioplegic solution is used for cardiac instillation during open heart surgery. This buffered solution contains the following electrolytes:

	mEq/L		mEq/L
Ca^{2+}	2.4	Na^+	120
Mg^{2+}	32	Cl^-	160
K^+	16	HCO_3^-	10

The osmolar concentration of this solution is 280 mosmol/L, and the pH† is approximately 7.8.

Isotonic Solutions

Two solutions that have the same solute concentration are said to be **isotonic.*** The normal salt concentration of the blood is approximately equal to 0.9 percent sodium chloride solution. The common name for 0.9 percent sodium chloride solution is **physiologic saline** solution. The blood and physiologic saline solution are isotonic—they have the same salt concentration. A 5.5 percent glucose solution is also approximately isotonic with body fluids.

Suppose that a red blood cell were placed in a small amount of physiologic saline solution. What would happen? The red blood cell is surrounded by its cell wall, which acts as a semipermeable membrane. Will osmosis take place? The answer is no, because there is no difference in concentration on either side of the semipermeable membrane. Actually, the water molecules move in both directions equally with no net change (see Figure 11–6). Thus, physiologic saline solution can be given intravenously to a patient without any effect on the red blood cells (see Figure 11–7). Physiologic saline is administered under the following conditions:

1. When the patient has become dehydrated.
2. When the patient has lost considerable fluid, as in the case of hemorrhage.
3. To prevent postoperative shock.

FIGURE 11-6. Red blood cell in isotonic solution.

Normal blood   Isotonic solution   Unchanged blood

Hypotonic Solutions

A **hypotonic** solution is one that contains a lower solute concentration than that of another solution. Distilled water and tap water are hypotonic when compared with blood.

Suppose that a red blood cell is placed in water (a hypotonic solution). What will happen? The salt concentration in the red blood cell is higher than that of the water. Therefore, osmosis will take place with the water diffusing into the red blood cell (from dilute to concentrated solution) (see Figure 11–8). The red blood cell thus enlarges until it bursts. This process of the bursting of a red blood cell because of a hypotonic solution is called **hemolysis.*** During hemolysis the blood is said to be **laked.*** Thus a hypotonic solution is *not* usually used for transfusions.

† pH will be discussed in Chapter 13.

FIGURE 11-7. Intravenous infusion with physiologic saline solution. (Courtesy St. Francis Hospital School of Nursing, Evanston, IL.)

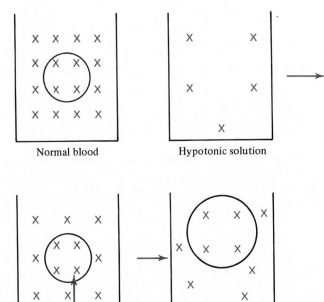

Normal blood

Hypotonic solution

Mixture of normal blood and hypotonic solution immediately after mixing

water flow

Corpuscle enlarges and may even rupture

FIGURE 11-8. Red blood cell in hypotonic solution.

Inorganic Chemistry

A **hypertonic*** solution is one that contains a higher solute concentration than that of another solution. A 5 percent sodium chloride solution or a 10 percent glucose solution is an example of a hypertonic solution when compared with blood.

Suppose a red blood cell is placed in a hypertonic solution. What will happen? The salt concentration in the red blood cell is less than that in the hypertonic solution. Therefore, osmosis will take place with the water diffusing out of the red blood cell (from dilute to concentrated) (see Figure 11–9). The red blood cell thus shrinks. This shrinking of the red blood cell in a hypertonic solution is called **crenation*** or **plasmolysis.***

Usually only isotonic solutions may be safely introduced into the bloodstream. Hypotonic solutions may cause hemolysis and hypertonic solutions may cause crenation.

Saline cathartics* such as magnesium sulfate, milk of magnesia, and magnesium citrate are absorbed from the large intestine slowly and incompletely. When these substances are ingested, a hypertonic solution is produced in the large intestine and water will flow from the tissue spaces into the intestinal tract until the solution is again isotonic with the body fluids. This additional water in the large intestine produces a watery stool that is easily evacuated. Therefore, by the continual use of cathartics a patient may become dehydrated. On the same basis, cathartics have been used to rid the body of excess fluid, although diuretics are now preferred for this purpose.

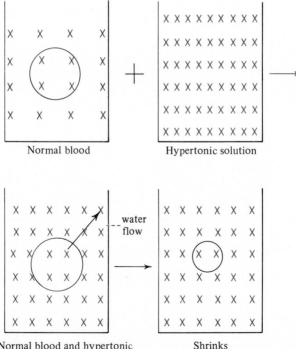

FIGURE 11-9. Red blood cell in hypertonic solution.

Normal blood

Hypertonic solution

water flow

Normal blood and hypertonic solution immediately after mixing

Shrinks

Suspensions

Suppose that some powdered clay is placed in water and vigorously shaken. A suspension of clay in water will be produced. This suspension will not be clear; it will be opaque. Upon standing, the clay will slowly settle. The composition of the suspension is actually changing as the clay settles out so that it is a heterogeneous mixture.

The clay is not dissolved in the water; it is merely distributed in it. When the suspension is poured into a funnel containing a piece of filter paper, only the water passes through the filter paper; the clay does not. Evidently the suspended clay particles are too large to pass through the holes in a piece of filter paper. Undoubtedly they will also be too large to pass through a membrane that has even finer openings (see Figure 11–10).

FIGURE 11–10. Relative sizes of solution, colloid, and suspension particles. Particles in solution are ions or molecules; colloidal particles consist of small clumps of molecules; suspension particles consist of large clumps of molecules.

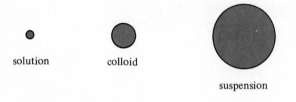

solution   colloid

suspension

Properties of suspensions are summarized as follows. Suspensions

1. Consist of an insoluble substance dispersed in a liquid.
2. Are heterogeneous.
3. Are not clear.
4. Settle.
5. Do not pass through filter paper.
6. Do not pass through membranes.

Some medications, such as milk of magnesia, are administered as a suspension. Many bottles of medication state on the label "shake before using." Most suspensions use water as the suspending medium, but procaine penicillin G, for example, is usually administered as an oil suspension.

A mist is a suspension of a liquid in a gas. Water droplets suspended in air are one example of a mist.

Patients having a decreased water content in their lungs usually have thickened bronchial secretions. To increase the water content of the lungs requires a higher-than-normal water content in the inspired air. A nebulizer is a device that generates an aerosol mist consisting of large water particles that can penetrate into the trachea and large bronchi. An ultrasonic nebulizer produces a supersaturated mist by means of ultrasonic sound waves. Such a mist is very effective in inhalation therapy because the particle size is small enough to reach the smallest bronchioles*. Also, the concentration of the mist is greater than that produced by other means.

Care must be taken in the use of a nebulizer to avoid (1) bacterial contamination in the water reservoir of the equipment (such bacteria will go directly into the bronchi) and (2) excess water being added to the patient's lungs.

Colloids The third class of liquid mixtures, called colloids, consists of tiny particles suspended in a liquid. We might ask, if these particles are suspended in a liquid, why aren't they suspensions? The answer is that these colloids behave quite differently from ordinary suspensions and have an entirely different set of properties.

Size When a colloid (or a colloidal dispersion as it is frequently called) is poured into a funnel containing filter paper, the colloid passes through the filter paper. This indicates that the colloidal particles are smaller than the openings in a filter paper. When a colloid is placed in a membrane, the colloidal particles do not pass through. Thus, colloidal particles are larger than the openings in the membrane.

We know that solutions pass through filter paper. They can also pass through certain types of membranes, whereas suspensions pass through neither. Therefore colloidal particles must be intermediate in size between solution particles and suspension particles. Colloidal particle sizes are measured in nanometers (nm) (1 nanometer is 0.000000001 m or one millionth of a millimeter). Colloidal particles range in size from 1 to 100 nm. Solution particles are smaller than 1 nm, whereas suspension particles are larger than 100 nm (see Figure 11–10).

Colloids have a tremendous amount of surface area because they consist of so many tiny particles. Consider a cube 1 cm on an edge. The volume of such a cube is 1 cubic centimeter (cm^3) and the surface area is 6 square centimeters (cm^2). (There are six faces to a cube, and each face has an area of 1 cm^2).

If the cube is cut in half the total volume of both pieces is still 1 cm^3. However, the total surface area has now increased to 8 cm^2 (cutting introduces two new faces each having an area of 1 cm^2). Cutting in half again still retains the volume of 1 cm^3. The surface area now is 10 cm^2. Continued cutting further increases the surface area.

When the size of the individual particle reaches colloidal size—approximately 10 nm—the total amount of surface area is about 60,000,000 cm^2. This tremendous surface area gives colloids one of their most important properties—adsorption.

Adsorption Adsorption is defined as the property of holding substances to a surface. Colloidal charcoal will adsorb tremendous amounts of gas. It has a selective adsorption, as do most colloids. Coconut charcoal is used in gas masks because it selectively adsorbs poisonous gases from the air. It does not adsorb ordinary gases from the air.

Several commonly used medications owe their use to their adsorbent properties. Charcoal tablets are administered to patients to aid indigestion. Kaolin, a finely divided aluminum silicate, is administered for the relief of diarrhea. Colloidal silver adsorbed on protein (Argyrol) has been used as a germicide.

Electrical Charge   Almost all colloidal particles have an electrical charge—either positive or negative. Why? Colloids selectively adsorb ions on their surface. If a colloid selectively adsorbs negative ions, it becomes a negatively charged colloid. If it adsorbs positive ions, it becomes a positively charged colloid.

Consider two negatively charged colloidal particles suspended in water. What would happen when these particles come close together? They would repel each other because of the repulsion of their like charges. Therefore, these colloidal particles will have little tendency to form large particles that would then settle out.

How can colloids be made to settle? Colloidal particles have an electrical charge that will repel all other similarly charged colloidal particles. However these charged particles *will* attract particles of opposite charge. Therefore, a negative colloid may be made to coagulate (begin to settle out) by adding to it positively charged particles.

Bichloride of mercury ($HgCl_2$) is a poisonous substance. When swallowed it forms a positive colloid in the stomach. The antidote for this type of poisoning is egg white, which is a negative colloid. These two oppositely charged colloids neutralize each other and coagulate in the stomach. The stomach must then be pumped out to remove the coagulated material. If this is not done, the stomach will digest the egg white, exposing the body once again to the poisonous substance.

Protein may also be coagulated by heat. Egg white—a colloidal substance—is quickly coagulated when heated.

The charge of a colloid may be determined by placing it in a U tube containing two electrodes. When a current is passed through the U tube each electrode will attract particles of opposite charge. A negative colloid will begin to accumulate around the positive electrode and a positive colloid around the negative electrode. The movement of electrically charged suspended particles toward an oppositely charged electrode is called **electrophoresis.** Electrophoresis is a slow process because the charged particles are not soluble and are much larger than the particles in solution (see page 458).

Tyndall Effect   When a strong beam of light is passed through a colloidal dispersion, the beam becomes visible because the colloidal particles reflect and scatter the light. This phenomenon is called the Tyndall effect (see Figure 11–11). The Tyndall effect may also be observed when a beam of sunlight passes through a darkened room. The dust particles in the air scatter the light so that the sun's rays become visible. The blue color of the sky is due to scattered light, as is the blue color of the ocean. However, we actually do not see the colloidal particles; we merely see the light scattered by them.

When a strong beam of light is passed through a solution, no Tyndall effect is observed because the solution particles are too small to scatter the light. Thus, the Tyndall effect is a way of distinguishing between solutions and colloids.

solution   colloid

FIGURE 11-11. Tyndall effect.

Dissolved particles in a solution are not large enough to scatter light.

Colloidal particles are large enough to scatter light.

Brownian Movement

When colloidal particles are observed with a transmission electron microscope, the particles are seen to move in a haphazard irregular motion called Brownian movement (see Figure 11–12).

What causes this irregular motion? It cannot be caused by the vibration of the slide on a microscope stand because the same motion can be observed when the microscope is mounted on a concrete pillar sunk deep into the earth. Brownian movement can be observed during the day or night, in the city and the country, in warm weather and cold weather, at high altitudes and low altitudes. The strangest characteristic of all is that this particular motion *never* ceases. It can be observed in containers that have been sealed for years. It has also been observed in liquid occlusions*—in quartz samples that have been undisturbed for perhaps millions of years.

Careful investigation by scientists established the fact that Brownian movement is not due to the colloidal particles themselves but rather to their bombardment by the molecules of the suspending medium. The molecules of the suspending medium are in continuous random motion. When these

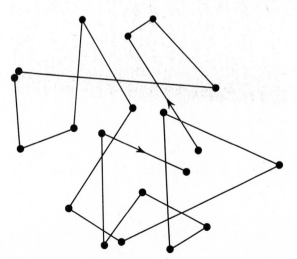

FIGURE 11-12. Brownian movement.

rapidly moving molecules of the medium strike the colloidal particles, they cause these particles to have the random motion characteristic of Brownian movement.

Gels and Sols   Colloidal dispersions may be subdivided into two classes. Where there is a strong attraction between the colloidal particle and the suspending liquid (water), the system is said to be **hydrophilic*** (water loving). Systems of this type are called **gels.** Gelatin in water is an example of such a system. Gels are semisolid and semirigid; they do not flow easily.

A colloidal system where there is little attraction between the suspended particles and the suspending water is called **hydrophobic*** (water hating). Systems of this type are called **sols.** They pour easily. A small amount of starch in water forms a sol. A hydrosol is a colloidal dispersion in water, while an aerosol is a colloidal dispersion in air.

If a gel, such as gelatin, is heated, it turns into a sol but returns to its original gel state on cooling. Protoplasm has the ability to change gel (in membranes) into sol and vice versa.

Dialysis   Dialysis is the separation of solute particles from colloidal particles by means of a semipermeable membrane. Recall that solute particles can pass through semipermeable membranes but colloidal particles cannot. Suppose that a colloidal starch suspension and sodium chloride solution are placed inside that type of membrane, which in turn is placed in a beaker of water. The starch is a colloid and cannot pass through the membrane. The salt is in solution and does pass through the membrane. This is an example of diffusion. The salt will continue to pass through the membrane until the salt concentration inside the membrane is the same as that in the water surrounding the membrane.

When this happens no more salt will be removed from the mixture inside the membrane. However, if the membrane is suspended in running water, soon all the salt will be removed from inside the membrane leaving behind only the starch—the colloid. This is dialysis—the separation of a solute from a colloid by means of a membrane (see Figure 11–13). Antitoxins* are prepared by this method. The impure material is placed inside a membrane suspended in running water. The soluble impurities flow out of the membrane leaving the pure antitoxin behind. The same process is used to prepare low-sodium milk. Milk is placed in a membrane suspended in running water. The soluble salt (sodium chloride) leaves the milk so that the remaining liquid is practically free from sodium compounds.

In the body the membranes in the kidneys allow the soluble waste material to pass through. The same membranes do not allow protein to pass through since proteins are colloids. In an average 150-lb adult, approximately 180 L of blood are purified daily.

Hemodialysis   Hemodialysis refers to the removal of soluble waste products from the bloodstream by means of a membrane. Purification of the blood can be accomplished in this way because soluble particles can diffuse through

Inorganic Chemistry   **180**

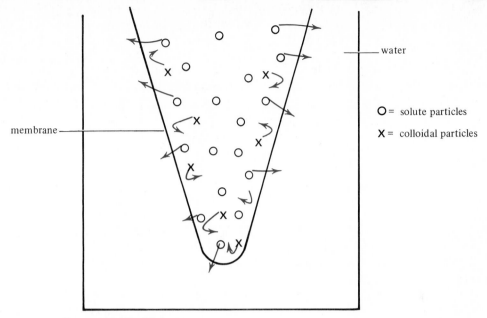

FIGURE 11-13. Dialysis.

water

O = solute particles

X = colloidal particles

membrane

dialysizing membranes whereas blood cells and plasma proteins cannot. When a patient has problems related to renal excretion, an artificial kidney machine may be used (see Figure 11–14). This machine applies the principles of hemodialysis.

The artificial kidney machine consists of a long cellophane tube, which is wrapped around itself to form a coil. This coil is immersed in a tempera-

FIGURE 11-14. Artificial kidney machine. (Courtesy of Michael Reese Hospital and Medical Center, Chicago, IL.)

ture-controlled solution whose chemical composition is carefully regulated according to the needs of the patient. The patient's blood is pumped through the coil, and the soluble end products of protein catabolism, water, and exogenous* poisons are removed from the blood. At the same time the blood cells and plasma proteins remain in the blood (recall that proteins, which are colloids, cannot pass through a membrane and here the cellophane acts as such a membrane). If the solution in which the coil is immersed has the same concentration of sodium ions as the blood, no net diffusion of sodium ions will take place. The same applies to other soluble substances in the bloodstream. That is, by regulating the composition of the solution, the waste products and unwanted material can be removed from the bloodstream.

A patient may remain on the artificial kidney machine 4 to 7 hr or even more. During this time the solution must be changed at intervals to avoid accumulation of waste products. Otherwise, the waste products would no longer continue to diffuse out of the blood. After passing through the coil, the blood is returned to the patient's veins.

As we might expect, the dialysate is mostly water. The kind of water used in its preparation is of utmost importance to the patient. If the water has been softened by the zeolite process (see page 153), it may contain too high a concentration of sodium ions (and so add sodium to the blood; see page 470). Improper levels of calcium and magnesium ions in the water may lead to metabolic bone diseases. Traces of copper in the water (from copper tubing in the equipment, copper pipes in the water supply, or copper sulfate used to kill algae in the water treatment plant) have caused fatalities in dialysis patients.

Emulsions

When two liquids are mixed, either they dissolve in each other or they do not. Two liquids that are soluble in each other are called **miscible.** Two liquids that do not dissolve in each other are called **immiscible.**

Suppose two immiscible liquids such as oil and water are poured together and then shaken vigorously. The oil forms tiny drops, which are suspended in the water. After a while the tiny drops come together to form larger drops; these soon rise to the top and separate from the water. This type of liquid mixture is called a **temporary emulsion**—emulsion because it consists of a liquid colloidally suspended in a liquid and temporary because it separates.

What are the properties of a temporary emulsion? First, as was just noted, it separates. Since it separates, it must be heterogeneous; its composition continues to change. Temporary emulsions, such as oil in water, are not clear. If placed in a funnel containing a piece of filter paper, they do not pass through the filter paper. Neither do they pass through any membrane.

A temporary emulsion such as oil and water separates because the oil drops attract one another to form larger drops, which soon rise to the top. However, suppose that each drop of oil were given a negative charge. Then the drops would not attract one another. They would not settle out; they would form a **permanent emulsion.** To give the oil drops an electrical charge we need an emulsifying agent. An emulsifying agent is a protective colloid that coats the suspended oil drops and prevents them from coming together. Permanent emulsions are not clear; they are homogeneous; they do not settle; they do not pass through either filter paper or membranes.

An example of a permanent emulsion is mayonnaise, which is an emulsion of oil in vinegar with egg yolk as an emulsifying agent. Milk is an emulsion of butterfat in water, with casein acting as the emulsifying agent. Soap acts as an emulsifying agent on grease and oils in water. Many medications are given in the form of emulsions, gum acacia being the most common emulsifying agent for the dispersion of fats.

Summary

Solutions consist of a solute and a solvent. Solutions are clear, homogeneous, have a variable composition, do not settle, may be separated by physical means, and pass through filter paper.

Factors affecting the solubility of a solute are temperature, pressure, surface area, agitation, and nature of the solvent.

Many chemical reactions take place in solution. Many medications are administered as solutions.

Solutions may be labeled as dilute or concentrated, as saturated or unsaturated, all of which are relative terms and do not indicate any definite amount of solute and solvent.

A percentage solution indicates the number of grams of solute per 100 ml of solution. A ratio solution indicates the number of grams of solute and the number of milliliters of solution. A molar solution indicates the number of moles of solute per liter of solution. A normal solution indicates the number of gram equivalent weights of solute per liter of solution.

Concentrations of ions in body fluids are frequently expressed in the units milliequivalents per liter (mEq/L).

When a nonvolatile solute is dissolved in a solvent, the boiling point is elevated and the freezing point depressed.

All liquids exhibit surface tension, which causes the surface molecules to form a surface film.

The movement of solute into a solvent or through a solution is called diffusion. The flow of solvent through a semipermeable membrane is called osmosis. The pressure exerted during osmosis is called the osmotic pressure. Osmotic pressure is expressed in terms of the osmolarity of the solution.

An isotonic solution has the same salt concentration as the blood and is used for transfusions.

A hypotonic solution has a solute concentration less than that of the blood. If injected into the bloodstream, a hypotonic solution can cause hemolysis—the bursting of the red blood cells.

A hypertonic solution has a solute concentration greater than that of the blood. If injected into the bloodstream, a hypertonic solution may cause crenation or plasmolysis—the shrinking of the red blood cells.

Suspensions consist of a nonsoluble solid suspended in a liquid medium. Suspensions are not clear; they settle out; they are heterogeneous; they do not pass through a filter paper; and they do not pass through a membrane.

Colloids consist of tiny particles suspended in a liquid. Colloids do not settle; they pass through filter paper but not through membranes; they adsorb (hold) particles on their surface; they have electrical charges, owing to the adsorption of charged particles (ions); they exhibit the Tyndall effect and Brownian movement.

Colloidal dispersions may be subdivided into two classes—sols and gels.

Dialysis is the separation of a solute from a colloid by means of a semipermeable membrane.

Hemodialysis refers to the removal of soluble waste products from the bloodstream by means of a membrane. When a patient has problems related to renal excretion, an artificial kidney machine may be used.

An emulsion consists of a liquid suspended in a liquid. An emulsion that settles is called a temporary emulsion. When an emulsifying agent is added to a temporary emulsion, it becomes a permanent emulsion.

Questions and Problems

A

1. Give specific directions for preparing
   (a) 100 ml of 5 percent boric acid solution.
   (b) a 1:300 $KMnO_4$ solution.
   (c) 2 L of 1 *M* NaCl solution.
   (d) 500 ml of 0.9 percent NaCl solution.
2. Define (a) osmosis; (b) dialysis; (c) adsorption; (d) osmotic pressure; (e) hypertonic solution; (f) diffusion; (g) saturated solution.
3. Why must an isotonic solution be used during a blood transfusion?
4. What factors affect the rate of solution of a solid solute?
5. List the general properties of solutions.
6. List the general properties of suspensions.
7. List the general properties of colloids.
8. List the general properties of emulsions.
9. What is the Tyndall effect?
10. What is Brownian movement?
11. What is surface tension?
12. How do colloids obtain their electrical charge?
13. What effect does a solute have on the boiling point and on the freezing point of a solution?
14. Explain how an artificial kidney machine functions.
15. Why must the solution in an artificial kidney machine be changed at intervals during use over a long time?
16. Why does diffusion take place more rapidly in a gas than in a liquid?
17. How may a temporary emulsion be changed into a permanent emulsion?
18. How can a colloid be made to settle? Explain.
19. Why do colloids pass through filter paper but not through membranes?
20. What is the size range of colloidal particles? solution particles? suspension particles?
21. What is meant by the term *tincture*?
22. Does pressure always affect the amount of a solute that will dissolve in a given solvent? Explain.
23. How can you tell whether a solution is saturated or unsaturated?
24. What is a nebulizer? For whatever purposes is it used in the hospital? What precautions should be taken with its use?
25. Why is the control of water important in hemodialysis? Would you expect control of temperature also to be important? Explain.
26. What is the difference between a sol and a gel? Give an example of each.
27. How can a supersaturated solution be prepared? Is it stable? Explain.

28. A patient is given 1500 ml of 10% glucose solution intravenously in a 24-hr period. How many grams of glucose did the patient receive per hour?

29. How many grams of NaCl are present in 100 ml of 0.5 M solution? (molecular weight of NaCl = 58.5)

30. A 0.125 M solution of $Al_2(SO_4)_3$ will contain how many milliequivalents per liter of each ion?

$$Al_2(SO_4)_3 \longrightarrow 2Al^{3+} + 3SO_4^{2-}$$

31. How would you prepare 1.5 L of 1.2 N KOH solution?

32. How would you prepare 50 ml of 0.25 N HNO_3 solution?

B   33. Which substance of those shown on Figure 11-1 has the greatest increase in solubility with an increase in temperature?

34. From Figure 11-1 calculate the number of grams of $NaNO_3$ that will dissolve in 500 g of water at 20°C.

35. What is an alloy? an amalgam? Give one medical use for each.

36. How does a percent solution compare with a milligram percent solution?

37. Give specific directions for preparing
   (a) 500 ml of 2% KI solution from 10% stock KI solution.
   (b) 200 ml of 1:100 solution from 1:10 stock solution.

38. What is a surfactant? Explain why surfactants are needed in the body.

39. What is adhesion? cohesion? capillary action? viscosity?

40. What is the purpose of a blood extender?

41. What is reverse osmosis? How does it work?

42. Explain how drinking salt water can cause dehydration.

43. Calculate the osmolarity of the following solutions:
   (a) 0.5 M sucrose solution
   (b) 0.1 M K_3PO_4 solution ($K_3PO_4 \longrightarrow 3K^+ + PO_4^{3-}$).
   (c) 10% glucose solution (0.55 M).

44. Upon what basis can the solubility of a solute in a solvent be predicted? Explain.

References   DICKSON, T. R. *Introduction to Chemistry,* 4th ed. John Wiley & Sons, Inc., New York, 1983, Chapter 11.

EBBING, DARRELL D. *General Chemistry.* Houghton Mifflin Company, Boston, 1984, Chapter 12.

LEVENSPIEL, O., and N. DE NEVERS. The osmotic pump. *Science,* **183:**157–160 (Jan. 18, 1974).

MCQUARRIE, DONALD A. and PETER A. ROCK. *General Chemistry.* W. H. Freeman and Company, New York, 1984, Chapter 14.

MORTIMER, CHARLES E. *Chemistry,* 5th ed., Wadsworth Publishing Co., Belmont, Calif., 1983, Chapter 10.

PETRUCCI, RALPH H. and ROBERT E. WISMER. *General Chemistry with Qualitative Analysis.* Macmillan Publishing Company, New York, 1983, Chapter 11.

RAYNER-CANHAN, GEOFFREY and MARK VAN ROODE, *Foundations of Chemistry.* Addison-Wesley Publishing Co., Reading, Mass., 1983, Chapter 10.

SACKHEIM, GEORGE I. *Chemical Calculations,* 12th ed., Series B. Stipes Publishing Co., Champaign, Ill., 1983, Chapter 18.

STOKER, H. STEPHEN. *Introduction to Chemical Principles.* Macmillan Publishing Company, New York, 1983, Chapter 13.

TANAKA, TOYUICHI. Gels. *Scientific American,* **244:**124–138 (Jan. 1981).

12 Ionization

CHAPTER OUTLINE

Conductivity of Solutions
Effect of Electrolytes on Boiling Points and Freezing Points
Theory of Ionization
Conductivity of Solutions of Electrolytes
Strong and Weak Electrolytes
Other Evidences of Ionization
Importance of Ions in Body Chemistry

Conductivity of Solutions

Figure 12–1 illustrates an apparatus designed to show whether a liquid will conduct electricity or not. When two metal plates called electrodes are immersed in a liquid and the current is turned on, the bulb will light if the liquid conducts a current. If a liquid does not conduct a current, the bulb will not glow at all.

battery

electrodes

solution to be tested

FIGURE 12–1. Conductivity apparatus.

It can be shown experimentally that the only water solutions that conduct electricity are those of acids, bases, and salts. The substances whose water solutions conduct electricity are called electrolytes. Substances whose water solution does not conduct electricity are called nonelectrolytes. Pure water is a nonelectrolyte, as is alcohol. Sugar solutions are also nonelectrolytes.

Effect of Electrolytes on Boiling Points and Freezing Points

Electrolytes have an unusual effect on the boiling point and the freezing point of a solution compared to the boiling point and the freezing point of the solvent itself. When a solid compound is dissolved in water, the resulting solution has a boiling point above 100°C. That is, solid solutes raise the boiling point of water. However, the results are considerably exaggerated if the solute is an electrolyte rather than a nonelectrolyte.

Consider a 1 M solution of an electrolyte such as sodium chloride and a 1 M solution of a nonelectrolyte such as sugar. The increase in the boiling point of the water containing the electrolyte sodium chloride will be approximately twice that for the water containing the nonelectrolyte sugar.

Likewise, the freezing point of the sodium chloride solution will be lowered approximately twice as much as that of the sugar solution.

Why do electrolytes conduct electricity? Why do they have an effect on the boiling point and freezing point of the solution?

Theory of Ionization

In 1887, a Swedish chemist, Svante Arrhenius, proposed a theory to explain the behavior of electrolytes in solution. The main points of his theory are as follows:

1. When electrolytes are placed in water, the molecules of the electrolyte break up into particles called ions. This process he called ionization.
2. Some of the ions have a positive charge, others a negative charge.
3. The sum of the positive charges is equal to the sum of the negative charges. That is, the original molecules were neutral so that the sum of the charges making up this molecule must also be neutral.
4. The conductance of electricity by solutions of electrolytes is due to the presence of ions.
5. Nonelectrolytes do not conduct electricity because of the absence of ions.
6. The effect of electrolytes on the boiling point and on the freezing point of a solution is due to the increased number of particles (ions) present in the solution.

Arrhenius proposed that an equilibrium exists between the ions and the nonionized molecules. This equilibrium may be represented by equation (12–1).

$$\text{NaCl} \rightleftharpoons \text{Na}^+ + \text{Cl}^- \qquad (12\text{–}1)$$

sodium chloride molecule   sodium ion   chloride ion

Arrhenius also proposed that the ionization should increase as the solution became more dilute. That is, in extremely dilute solutions, the electrolyte molecule would be almost completely dissociated (ionized).

Arrhenius's theory had to be modified as more information became available. Yet the modern theory of ionization retains most of his principles.

Arrhenius believed that the molecules of an electrolyte such as sodium chloride broke up into ions when placed in water. Later evidence proved conclusively that the sodium chloride existed as ions even in the solid state. When sodium chloride is formed from its elements, the sodium atom loses one electron to form a positively charged sodium ion. At the same time the chlorine atom gains one electron to form a negatively charged chloride ion. Thus, sodium chloride exists in an ionic state even in the solid state. When sodium chloride is dissolved in water, the ions are free to move around.

Solid sodium chloride consists of sodium ions and chloride ions bonded together by ionic bonds in a definite crystalline structure. These ions are held tightly in place and cannot move about to any great extent. Thus they are not free to conduct an electrical current, and solid sodium chloride does not conduct electricity. If sodium chloride is heated until it melts (about 800°C), the resulting liquid will conduct electricity because the ions have some freedom to move around.

Conductivity of Solutions of Electrolytes

When sodium chloride crystals are placed in water, the ions present in the crystal are free to move about in the solution. These positively and negatively charged ions will be attracted to oppositely charged electrodes. Thus, if two electrodes are connected to a battery and are placed in a sodium chloride solution, the solution will conduct electricity.

The positively charged sodium ions will be attracted to the negative electrode, the cathode. Ions attracted to a cathode are called cations. At the same time, the negatively charged chloride ions will be attracted to the positive electrode, the anode. Ions attracted toward an anode are called anions. This movement of ions through the solution consists of a flow of current. If a nonelectrolyte is placed in water, no ions are formed and no conductance takes place.

Strong and Weak Electrolytes

Acids are electrolytes. Yet all acids do not behave the same when placed in water. A dilute solution of hydrochloric acid (HCl) is a strong electrolyte. When it is placed under a conductivity apparatus, the bulb glows brightly. However, when a dilute solution of acetic acid ($HC_2H_3O_2$) is placed under the conductivity apparatus, the bulb glows dimly. This indicates that the acetic acid is a weak electrolyte. Likewise, sodium hydroxide (NaOH) solution is a strong electrolyte, whereas ammonium hydroxide (NH_4OH) is a weak electrolyte.

How can one acid or base be a strong electrolyte and another one be weak? What accounts for the difference between the types of electrolytes?

When hydrochloric acid or sodium hydroxide is placed in water, it dissociates (breaks up) almost completely into ions, as indicated by the arrows pointing in one direction only.

$$HCl \longrightarrow H^+ + Cl^-$$

$$NaOH \longrightarrow Na^+ + OH^-$$

Because these substances are just about completely ionized, they are called strong electrolytes.

However, some acids and bases when placed in water ionize only to a limited extent. They remain primarily as nonionized molecules. These substances maintain an equilibrium between the nonionized molecule and the ions with the equilibrium being far to the left, as indicated by the arrows.

$$HC_2H_3O_2 \rightleftharpoons H^+ + C_2H_3O_2^-$$

$$NH_4OH \rightleftharpoons NH_4^+ + OH^-$$

These substances are called weak electrolytes.

Thus the original Arrhenius theory is true for weak electrolytes but not for strong ones.

Other Evidences of Ionization   It has already been mentioned that the conductivity of solutions of electrolytes indicates the presence of ions. Likewise, the effect of electrolytes on the boiling point and the freezing point can be explained by the presence of ions. The change in the boiling point or freezing point depends on the number of particles present in solution. Sugar, $C_6H_{12}O_6$, contributes only one particle per molecule because it is not ionized. Sodium chloride, NaCl, contributes two particles—the two ions—and so should have twice the effect on the boiling point and the freezing point.

Another factor indicating the presence of ions is the instantaneous reaction of solutions of electrolytes. When a solution of sodium chloride (NaCl) is mixed with a solution of silver nitrate (AgNO₃), a white precipitate of silver chloride (AgCl) is formed instantaneously.

$$Na^+ + Cl^- + Ag^+ + NO_3^- \longrightarrow AgCl\downarrow + Na^+ + NO_3^-$$

The silver chloride is written as a molecule rather than as ions. This is because that substance precipitates, thus removing the ions from the solution.

When an acid reacts with a base, a salt and water are formed. If potassium hydroxide (KOH) is reacted with nitric acid (HNO₃), potassium nitrate and water are formed. The ionic reaction is as follows

$$K^+ + OH^- + H^+ + NO_3^- \longrightarrow K^+ + NO_3^- + H_2O$$

Potassium nitrate is a soluble salt, an electrolyte, which is ionized. Water is a nonelectrolyte; it is not ionized and is therefore written as a molecule.

Hydrolysis of salts (see page 205) may also be explained on the basis of ionization. When sodium acetate (NaC₂H₃O₂) is placed in water the acetate ion reacts with the water according to equation 12–2

$$\underset{\text{acetate ion}}{Na^+ + C_2H_3O_2^-} + H_2O \rightleftharpoons \underset{\text{acetic acid}}{HC_2H_3O_2} + Na^+ + OH^- \quad (12\text{--}2)$$

The acetic acid, being a weak acid, does not ionize appreciably to furnish any hydrogen ions and so is written as a molecule in the reaction (12–2). If the ions common to both sides of equation (12–2) (the sodium ions) are eliminated, the net reaction becomes

$$C_2H_3O_2^- + H_2O \rightleftharpoons HC_2H_3O_2 + OH^- \qquad (12\text{–}3)$$

That is, the acetate ion (which came from a weak acid) hydrolyzes (reacts with water) to form nonionized acetic acid, a weak electrolyte, leaving hydroxide ions in solution. Therefore, when sodium acetate is placed in water, hydroxide ions are formed, causing the solution to be basic. Note that ions from a strong acid or a strong base (see page 205) do not hydrolyze. Thus, the sodium ion in reaction (12–2) does not react with water and so can be eliminated from both sides of the equation, giving equation (12–3).

Importance of Ions in Body Chemistry

Ions play the chief role in the various processes that take place in the body. Many of the body's vital processes take place in the ionic state within the cell. Table 12–1 lists some of the more important ions that are found in the body.

TABLE 12–1. Ions Found in the Body

Calcium ion	Ca^{2+}	Necessary for clotting of the blood; for formation of milk curd during digestion in the stomach; for formation of bones and teeth; for action of muscle, including heart
Iron ion	Fe^{2+}	Necessary for formation of hemoglobin and cytochromes
Sodium ion	Na^+	Principal extracellular positive ion
Potassium ion	K^+	Principal intracellular positive ion
Chloride ion	Cl^-	Intracellular and extracellular negative ion
Bicarbonate ion	HCO_3^-	Extracellular negative ion
Iodide ion	I^-	Present in thyroid hormones
Ammonium ion	NH_4^+	Plays a role in maintaining body's acid-base balance
Phosphate ion	PO_4^{3-}	Plays an important role, along with calcium ions, in the formation of bones and teeth
Magnesium ion	Mg^{2+}	An important activator for many enzyme systems (See Table 2–2, page 22, for other ions necessary for enzymes.)

In addition, ions are necessary as part of the blood buffer system. They cause osmotic pressure in the cells and are necessary to control the contracting and relaxing of muscles. Ions are necessary to carry nerve impulses and help regulate the digestive processes (see pages 462 and 470).

Summary

Substances whose water solutions conduct electricity are called electrolytes. Soluble acids, bases, and salts are electrolytes. Solutions that do not conduct electricity are nonelectrolytes.

Electrolytes have an effect on the boiling and freezing point of a solution. This effect is due to the presence of ions.

Inorganic Chemistry **190**

Ionization (the formation of ions) accounts for the electrical conductivity of a solution. When a substance ionizes, the sum of the positive charges equals the sum of the negative charges. The positive ions, cations, are attracted toward the cathode (negative electrode) whereas the negative ions, the anions, are attracted toward the anode (positive electrode).

The modern theory of ionization considers that ions are already present in a crystalline salt and that these ions are released to move about when that substance is placed in solution.

Most salts are strong electrolytes because they are completely (strongly) ionized. Acids and bases that are strong electrolytes are highly ionized. Acids and bases that are poor electrolytes are weakly ionized.

The presence of ions is of great importance in the body in the maintenance of the electrolyte balance of the body fluids.

Questions and Problems

A

1. Describe a laboratory experiment to determine whether a substance is an electrolyte or not.
2. What effect does an electrolyte have on the boiling point of a solution? Why?
3. What effect does an electrolyte have on the freezing point of a solution? Why?
4. What effect does a nonelectrolyte have on the freezing point of a solution? Why?
5. State the main ideas of Arrhenius's theory of ionization.
6. How does the modern theory of ionization differ from that of Arrhenius?
7. How does an electrolyte conduct a current?
8. What is an anion? a cation?
9. What is a strong electrolyte? Give an example.
10. What is a weak electrolyte? Give an example.
11. List several ions necessary for the proper functioning of the body. What purpose does each ion serve?

B

12. When an insoluble salt is placed in water, will the mixture conduct electricity? Explain.
13. Compare the osmolarity of equal molar solutions of glucose and sodium chloride. What effect will these solutions have on the boiling point?
14. Explain why solid sodium chloride does not conduct electricity whereas molten sodium chloride does.
15. Compare reversible and irreversible reactions in terms of strong and weak electrolytes.

References

DICKSON, T. R. *Introduction to Chemistry,* 4th ed. John Wiley & Sons, Inc., New York, 1983, Chapter 11.

PETRUCCI, RALPH H. and ROBERT E. WISMER. *General Chemistry with Qualitative Analysis.* Macmillan Publishing Company, New York, 1983, Chapter 18.

SACKHEIM, GEORGE I. *Chemical Calculations,* 12th ed., Series B. Stipes Publishing Co., Champaign, Ill., 1983, Chapter 21.

13 Acids and Bases

CHAPTER
OUTLINE

Acids
Properties of Acids
Uses of Acids
Bases
Properties of Bases

Uses of Bases
Acid-Base Titration
Ionization of Water
pH

Acids

Acids may be defined as compounds that yield or donate hydrogen ions (H^+) in a water solution. Bronsted (a Danish chemist) **defined an acid as a substance that donates protons.** Note that a hydrogen ion results when a hydrogen atom loses its only electron, leaving a single proton, so that both definitions say essentially the same thing. That is, a hydrogen ion is a proton.

It is the hydrogen ions that are responsible for the particular properties of acids. Most people think of acids as being liquids. However, there are many solid acids; boric acid and citric acid are two common examples. The names and formulas of the most common acids are given in Table 13–1.

TABLE 13–1. Common Acids

Strong
HCl	Hydrochloric acid
H_2SO_4	Sulfuric acid
HNO_3	Nitric acid
H_2CO_3	Carbonic acid
H_3PO_4	Phosphoric acid
$HC_2H_3O_2$	Acetic acid

Weak

Properties of Acids

Acids yield hydrogen ions when placed in water solution.

$$HCl \longrightarrow H^+ + Cl^-$$
hydrochloric acid   hydrogen ion   chloride ion

$$H_2SO_4 \longrightarrow 2H^+ + SO_4^{2-}$$
sulfuric acid   hydrogen ions   sulfate ion

192

$$HNO_3 \longrightarrow H^+ + NO_3^-$$

nitric acid   hydrogen ion   nitrate ion

$$HC_2H_3O_2 \rightleftharpoons H^+ + C_2H_3O_2^-$$

acetic acid   hydrogen ion   acetate ion

Recall that strong acids are almost completely ionized in solution whereas weak acids are only partially ionized.

Solutions of acids have a sour taste. Lemon and grapefruit juices owe their sour taste to citric acid. Vinegar owes its sour taste to acetic acid. Sour milk owes its taste partly to lactic acid.

When acids react with certain compounds, these compounds change in color. Substances that change in color in the presence of acids are called **indicators.** One of the most common indicators for acids is litmus. Blue litmus turns red in the presence of an acid (in the presence of hydrogen ions). Another common indicator—phenolphthalein—turns from red to colorless in the presence of an acid.

Acids react with metal oxides and hydroxides to form water and a salt, for example

$$2HCl + MgO \longrightarrow H_2O + MgCl_2$$

acid   metal oxide   water   salt

$$H_2SO_4 + 2NaOH \longrightarrow 2H_2O + Na_2SO_4$$

acid   metal hydroxide   water   salt

The reaction of acids with certain metal hydroxides (called bases) is termed **neutralization.** That is, acids neutralize bases to form water and a salt.

The activity series of metals (Table 13–2) lists metals in order of decreasing activity. Note that hydrogen is classified with the metals. **Any metal above hydrogen in this series will replace the hydrogen from an acid. The**

TABLE 13–2. The Activity Series of the Metals

K	Potassium
Ca	Calcium
Na	Sodium
Mg	Magnesium
Al	Aluminum
Zn	Zinc
Fe	Iron
Sn	Tin
Pb	Lead
H	Hydrogen
Cu	Copper
Hg	Mercury
Ag	Silver
Au	Gold

farther above hydrogen a metal is in the activity series, the greater will be its tendency to replace hydrogen from an acid.

Acids react with any metal above hydrogen in the activity series to produce hydrogen gas and a salt, for example

$$Zn + H_2SO_4 \longrightarrow \underset{\text{salt}}{ZnSO_4} + H_2\uparrow$$

$$Mg + 2HCl \longrightarrow \underset{\text{salt}}{MgCl_2} + H_2\uparrow$$

These are examples of single replacement reactions—the metal replaces the hydrogen in the acid. Thus acids cannot be stored in containers made of these active metals. Iron is above hydrogen in the activity series and should replace hydrogen in an acid. Therefore, acids should not be allowed to come in contact with surgical or dental instruments, which are frequently made of stainless steel. Acids are usually stored in glass or plastic containers. Reactions involving acids are usually carried out in glass or plastic vessels.

Acids react with carbonates and bicarbonates to form carbon dioxide, water, and salts, for example

$$\underset{\text{acid}}{2HCl} + \underset{\text{carbonate}}{CaCO_3} \longrightarrow \underset{\text{salt}}{CaCl_2} + \underset{\substack{\text{carbonic} \\ \text{acid}}}{H_2CO_3}$$

and
$$H_2CO_3 \longrightarrow CO_2\uparrow + H_2O$$

$$\underset{\text{acid}}{HNO_3} + \underset{\text{bicarbonate}}{NaHCO_3} \longrightarrow \underset{\text{salt}}{NaNO_3} + \underset{\substack{\text{carbonic} \\ \text{acid}}}{H_2CO_3}$$

and
$$H_2CO_3 \longrightarrow H_2O + CO_2\uparrow$$

The stomach normally secretes hydrochloric acid (HCl), which is required for the digestion of protein (page 391). Emotional stress can lead to hyperacidity, too great an acid concentration in the stomach. Commercial **antacids** are available to react with the excess stomach acid. Among these are

Tums, which contains calcium carbonate ($CaCO_3$), magnesium carbonate ($MgCO_3$), and magnesium trisilicate ($Mg_2Si_3O_8$).
Maalox, which contains magnesium hydroxide [$Mg(OH)_2$], and aluminum hydroxide [$Al(OH)_3$] in suspension.
Rolaids, which contain aluminum sodium dihydroxycarbonate [$AlNa(OH)_2CO_3$].

All of these antacid substances can react with the hydrochloric acid present in the stomach.

Alka-Seltzer, another commercial antacid contains calcium dihydrogen phosphate [$Ca(H_2PO_4)_2$], sodium bicarbonate ($NaHCO_3$), citric acid, and aspirin. When placed in water, the bicarbonate ions react with the acidic components to produce carbon dioxide gas (CO_2), which provides the "fizz" or effervescence. The ionic reaction is

Inorganic Chemistry **194**

$$H^+ + HCO_3^- \longrightarrow CO_2\uparrow + H_2O$$

(The prefix *bi* is sometimes used to indicate hydrogen in a compound. Sodium bicarbonate is also known as sodium hydrogen carbonate.) Sodium bicarbonate, $NaHCO_3$, may also be used to remove excess stomach acidity. However, continued use of this latter substance may interfere with the normal digestive processes taking place in the stomach. In addition, the continued use of $NaHCO_3$ adds a considerable amount of sodium ions to the body.

Strong acids will attack clothing. Vegetable fibers such as cotton and linen, animal fibers such as wool and silk, and synthetic fibers are rapidly destroyed by strong acids. All these effects are actually due to the hydrogen ions present in the acids.

Strong acids (acids with a high hydrogen ion concentration) also have an effect on tissues. Concentrated nitric acid (HNO_3) and concentrated sulfuric acid (H_2SO_4) are extremely corrosive to the skin, therefore, great care must be exercised in handling them. The yellowing of the skin by nitric acid is a test that is specific for protein (see page 363). If a strong acid is spilled on the skin, a serious burn may result. The area should be washed copiously with water. Then it should be treated with sodium bicarbonate to neutralize any remaining acid. Dilute acids are not as corrosive to the tissues. A few may even be used internally in the body.

Drugs are absorbed from the gastrointestinal tract more rapidly when they are nonionized. If a weakly acidic drug is swallowed, it will remain nonionized in the stomach because of the low pH (high acid content) of the stomach. Since the drug is nonionized, it will be absorbed rapidly. Conversely, a weakly basic drug will be highly ionized in the stomach and thus will be poorly absorbed there.

Aspirin, acetylsalicylic acid (see page 280), is over 90 percent nonionized at a pH of 2 whereas it is about 1 percent nonionized at a pH of 7. Thus we should expect aspirin to be absorbed rapidly from the stomach where the pH is near 2 and more slowly from the small intestines where the pH is above 7.

Uses of Acids   Acids such as hydrochloric acid (HCl, commercially known as muriatic acid), are used industrially and in laboratory work in large amounts. Several acids are also used medically; among these are hydrochloric, nitric, hypochlorous, boric, acetylsalicylic, and ascorbic acids.

Hydrochloric acid, normally found in the gastric juices, is necessary for the proper digestion of proteins in the stomach. Patients who have a lower than normal amount of hydrochloric acid in the stomach, a condition called hypoacidity, are given dilute hydrochloric acid orally before meals to overcome this deficiency.

Nitric acid (HNO_3) is used to test for the presence of albumin in urine because it will coagulate protein. Nitric acid has been used to remove warts, but dichloroacetic acid (bichloracetic acid) and trichloroacetic acid are now commonly used for this purpose.

Acids and Bases   **195**

Hypochlorous acid (HClO) is used as a disinfectant for floors and walls in the hospital.

Boric acid (H_3BO_3) has had extensive use as a germicide. Although boric acid has been used in eyewashes, its use in solutions or as a powder on extensive inflamed surfaces or in body cavities is now practically obsolete. Containers of boric acid should have a label reading "poison."

Acetylsalicylic acid (aspirin) is widely used as an analgesic* and as an antipyretic.* Aspirin is frequently taken by people with a cold to relieve headache, muscle pain, and fever. However, the aspirin does not remove the source of infection nor effect a cure. Aspirin also may interfere with the normal clotting of the blood and may cause bleeding in the stomach of some individuals (see page 280).

Ascorbic acid (vitamin C) is normally found in citrus fruits and is used in the prevention and treatment of scurvy.

Bases Bases may be defined as substances that yield hydroxide (OH^-) ions in a water solution. That is, bases increase the hydroxide ion concentration in water. If we write the ionization reactions (see Chapter 12) of the bases sodium hydroxide and potassium hydroxide, we have

$$NaOH \longrightarrow Na^+ + OH^-$$

$$KOH \longrightarrow K^+ + OH^-$$

A more general definition of a base is that of Bronsted: **a base is a substance that accepts protons.** According to this definition, substances that yield hydroxide ions in solution are bases, as are substances that yield bicarbonate ions, because these ions are then free to combine with or accept protons (hydrogen ions) as indicated in the following reactions:

$$OH^- + H^+ \longrightarrow H_2O$$

$$\underset{\text{base}}{HCO_3^-} + \underset{\text{proton}}{H^+} \longrightarrow H_2CO_3$$

Strong bases are highly ionized and have a great attraction for protons. Weak bases are slightly ionized and have a weak attraction for protons. Ammonia (NH_3) is a base according to the Bronsted definition because it accepts a proton from water or acids.

$$NH_3 + H_2O \longrightarrow NH_4^+ + OH^-$$

C_2H_5OH (ethyl alcohol) is not a base because it does not accept a proton; it does not ionize in water.

Table 13–3 indicates several commonly used bases. Note that they consist of a metal ion ionically bonded to an OH^- ion. The only exception to this rule is the base ammonium hydroxide, NH_4OH, in which the ammonium ion, NH_4^+, is considered to act as a metal ion. Bases are produced when metallic oxides are dissolved in water, for example

$$\underset{\substack{\text{metal} \\ \text{oxide}}}{CaO} + \underset{\text{water}}{H_2O} \longrightarrow \underset{\substack{\text{calcium hydroxide,} \\ \text{a base}}}{Ca(OH)_2}$$

Inorganic Chemistry   **196**

TABLE 13-3. Commonly Used Bases

Name	Formula
Sodium hydroxide	NaOH
Ammonium hydroxide	NH_4OH
Potassium hydroxide	KOH
Calcium hydroxide	$Ca(OH)_2$
Magnesium hydroxide	$Mg(OH)_2$

(handwritten margin notes: "strong" pointing to the first group, "weak" and "medium" pointing to the lower entries)

Properties of Bases Solutions of bases have a slippery, soapy feeling and a biting, bitter taste. Like acids, bases also react with indicators. Bases turn red litmus blue, turn methyl orange from red to yellow, and turn phenolphthalein from colorless to red.

Bases neutralize acids to form water and a salt, for example

$$\underset{\text{base}}{Ca(OH)_2} + \underset{\text{acid}}{H_2SO_2} \longrightarrow \underset{\text{water}}{2H_2O} + \underset{\text{salt}}{CaSO_4}$$

Strong bases react with certain metals to produce hydrogen gas, for example

$$\underset{\text{aluminum}}{2Al} + \underset{\substack{\text{sodium hydroxide,}\\ \text{a strong base}}}{6NaOH} + \underset{\text{water}}{6H_2O} \longrightarrow \underset{\text{hydrogen}}{3H_2\uparrow} + \underset{\substack{\text{sodium aluminate,}\\ \text{a soluble compound}}}{2Na_3Al(OH)_6}$$

Thus a strong base such as lye (NaOH) should never be used or stored in an aluminum container because it will rapidly react with and dissolve the container.

Strong bases have a high hydroxide ion concentration. They have a corrosive effect on tissues because of their ability to react with proteins and fats. If a strong base is spilled on the skin, a serious burn may result. The procedure in this case is to apply copious amounts of water followed by treatment with a weak acid such as acetic acid to neutralize any base that might be left.

Strong laundry soaps are quite basic and should not be used for washing woolen clothing because the hydroxide ion will attack the fibers and cause them to shrink. Particular care must be taken not to use strong soap on diapers because, if it is not thoroughly removed, the basic soap may cause severe sores on the tender skin of a baby.

Uses of Bases Sodium hydroxide (NaOH), commonly known as lye, is used to remove fats and grease from clogged drains. It is quite caustic and care must be exercised in handling this substance. Sodium hydroxide is also used in the conversion of fat to soap (see page 328).

Calcium hydroxide solution [$Ca(OH)_2$], commonly known as lime water, is used to overcome excess acidity in the stomach. It is also used medicinally as an antidote for oxalic acid poisoning because it reacts with the oxalic acid to form an insoluble compound, calcium oxalate.

Magnesium hydroxide [$Mg(OH)_2$] is commonly known as milk of magnesia. In dilute solutions it is used as an antacid for the stomach. In the form of a suspension of magnesium hydroxide in water, it is used as a laxative.

Acids and Bases   **197**

Spirits of ammonia, which contains ammonium hydroxide (NH_4OH) and ammonium carbonate [$(NH_4)_2CO_3$], is used as a heart and respiratory stimulant. Ammonium hydroxide, also known as household ammonia, is used as a water softener for washing clothes.

Acid-Base Titration

When an acid reacts with a base, a salt and water are produced. This reaction may be carried out in the laboratory by a process called **titration** (see Figure 13–1). In this process, a buret is filled with an acid of known concentration. A buret is a cylindrical glass tube with graduated markings, so that the exact volume of liquid withdrawn can be easily determined. A flask placed below the buret contains a measured volume of a base of unknown concentration. An indicator is added to the flask. The indicator is one that will change in color when the acid has reacted with all of the base present. This is called the *endpoint,* or equivalence point of the titration.

The acid is added drop by drop to the flask until the indicator just begins to change color. The concentration of the base (or acid if the buret contains a base and the flask an acid) can be determined by using the following formula.

$$\text{Volume}_{acid} \times \text{Normality}_{acid} = \text{Volume}_{base} \times \text{Normality}_{base}$$

buret

graduated markings

volume is read before and after the addition.

solution of known concentration

stopcock

know volume of substance being titrated

FIGURE 13–1. Titration of acid with base.

Inorganic Chemistry

EXAMPLE 13-1. 27.8 ml of 0.1 N HCl solution reacts with 20.0 ml of NaOH solution. What is the concentration of the NaOH solution?

Using the above formula

$$27.8 \text{ ml} \times 0.1 \, N = 20.0 \text{ ml} \times X$$

$$X = 0.139 \, N \, \text{NaOH}$$

EXAMPLE 13-2. 35.2 ml 0.15 N KOH reacts with 40.0 ml of H_2SO_4 solution. What is the normality of the acid?

$$35.2 \text{ ml} \times 0.15 \, N = 40.0 \text{ ml} \times X$$

$$X = 0.132 \, N \, H_2SO_4$$

Ionization of Water

Even though pure water does not conduct electricity, very exact measurements show that a very slight amount of ionization does take place. The reaction is

$$H_2O \rightleftharpoons H^+ + OH^-$$

At 25°C, only one water molecule out of 10 million ionizes (dissociates). The concentration of hydrogen ions in pure water is 10^{-7} M, as is the hydroxide ion concentration. Since the hydrogen and hydroxide ion concentrations are equal, pure water is neutral.

The equilibrium constant for water (page 93) can be written as

$$K_{eq} = \frac{[H^+][OH^-]}{[H_2O]}$$

where the [ ] indicates concentration in moles per liter. However, the concentration of water remains constant, so that the equilibrium constant may be rewritten as

$$K_{eq} \times [H_2O] = [H^+][OH^-] = K_w$$

where K_w, the ion product of water, is itself the product of two constants, K_{eq} and $[H_2O]$.

At equilibrium at 25°C, pure water contains 10^{-7} M H$^+$ and 10^{-7} M OH$^-$, so

$$K_w = [H^+][OH^-] = (10^{-7}) \times (10^{-7}) = 10^{-14}$$

Since $[H^+][OH^-]$ always equals 10^{-14}, if $[H^+]$ increases, the $[OH^-]$ must decrease, and vice versa. A solution in which the $[H^+]$ is greater than the $[OH^-]$ is acidic; a solution in which the $[H^+]$ is less than the $[OH^-]$ is basic. For example, in 0.01 M HCl, $[H^+]$ is 10^{-2}. Therefore, since $[H^+][OH^-] = 10^{-14}$, $(10^{-2})[OH^-] = 10^{-14}$ and $[OH^-] = 10^{-12}$. The solution is acidic because the $[H^+]$ is greater than $[OH^-]$; likewise, in a 0.1 M NaOH solution, $[OH^-] = 10^{-1}$, so $[H^+] = 10^{-13}$. The solution is basic since $[H^+]$ is less than $[OH^-]$.

pH

A few drops of concentrated hydrochloric acid in water produce a dilute acid solution. A few more drops produce another solution, still dilute but a

Acids and Bases

little stronger than the previous one. If a piece of blue litmus paper is placed in either of these two solutions it will turn red, indicating that the solution is acidic. However, it will not tell which one is more strongly acidic. Likewise if a piece of red litmus paper turns blue when placed in a solution, it merely indicates that the solution is basic or alkaline. It does not tell how strongly basic. The term pH is used to indicate the exact strength of an acid or a base. The pH indicates the hydrogen ion concentration in a solution.

Mathematically, pH may be defined as the negative logarithm of the hydrogen ion concentration, or

$$pH = -\log[H^+]$$

A logarithm is an exponent. Therefore, the logarithm (log) of 10^{-2} is -2 and the log 10^{-12} is -12.

Thus, a solution that has $[H^+] = 10^{-4}$ has a pH of 4; that is,

$$pH = -\log[H^+] = -\log 10^{-4} = -(-4) = 4$$

A pH of 7 indicates a neutral solution because $[H^+] = [OH^-]$. pH values below 7 indicate an acidic solution: pHs between 5 and 7 indicate a weakly acidic solution; values between 2 and 5, a moderately acidic solution; and pHs between 0 and 2, a strongly acidic solution.

Likewise, pHs above 7 indicate a basic solution: pH values between 7 and 9 indicate a weakly basic solution; those between 9 and 12, a moderately basic solution; and pHs between 12 and 14, a strongly basic solution. This is summarized in Table 13-4.

The pHs of some common body fluids and some household substances are listed in Table 13-5. From these values it can be seen that blood is a slightly basic liquid, the gastric juices strongly acidic, bile weakly basic, and urine and saliva both weakly acidic or weakly basic. The pH of pure water is 7.0.

A difference of 1 in pH value represents a tenfold difference in strength. That is, an acid of pH 4.5 is ten times as strong as one of pH 5.5. Likewise, a base of pH 10.7 is ten times as strong as one of pH 9.7, and 100 times as strong (10×10) as one of pH 8.7. Therefore, a small change in pH indicates a definite change in acid or base strength.

To measure pH in a laboratory, a pH meter (Figure 13-2) may be used. This instrument is standardized by placing the electrodes into a solution of

TABLE 13-4. pH Values[a]

pH	0	1	2	3	4	5	6	7	8	9	10	11	12	13	14
Strength of acid (H^+ in mol/L)	10^0	10^{-1}	10^{-2}	10^{-3}	10^{-4}	10^{-5}	10^{-6}	10^{-7}	10^{-8}	10^{-9}	10^{-10}	10^{-11}	10^{-12}	10^{-13}	10^{-14}
Strength of base (OH^- in mol/L)	10^{-14}	10^{-13}	10^{-12}	10^{-11}	10^{-10}	10^{-9}	10^{-8}	10^{-7}	10^{-6}	10^{-5}	10^{-4}	10^{-3}	10^{-2}	10^{-1}	10^0

strong acid ← → moderate acid ← → weak acid → neutral ← weak base ← → moderate base ← → strong base

[a] See Appendix A for an explanation of the use of negative exponential numbers in scientific notation.

TABLE 13-5. pH Values of Body Fluids and Household Substances

Fluid	pH Range	Substance	pH Range
Blood	7.35–7.45	Black coffee	4.8–5.2
Gastric juices	1.6–1.8	Eggs	7.6–8.0
Bile	7.8–8.6	Lemons	2.8–3.4
Urine	5.5–7.5	Milk	6.3–6.6
Saliva	6.2–7.4	Tap water	6.5–8.0

FIGURE 13-2. Digital pH meter. (Courtesy of Corning Glass Works, Corning, NY.)

Acids and Bases

known pH to see that it is functioning and recording properly. Then the electrodes are placed in a solution of unknown pH and the pH is determined by reading the value on the pH meter. A quicker but less accurate method is to touch a drop of the liquid to a specially prepared piece of indicator paper and then determine the pH by comparison with a pH color scale.

Summary

Acids are compounds that yield hydrogen ions or protons in solution. The general properties of acids are sour taste, effect on colors of indicators, reaction with metal oxides and hydroxides (neutralization), reaction with metals to yield hydrogen gas, reaction with carbonates and bicarbonates to produce carbon dioxide gas, effect on clothing, and effect on tissues.

Antacids are used to neutralize excess acidity in the stomach.

Acids and bases are used industrially, pharmaceutically, and in the hospital and laboratory.

Bases are compounds yielding hydroxide (OH^-) ions in solution. Bases are also compounds that accept protons. Bases have a slippery, soapy feeling; they affect the colors of indicators, neutralize acids, react with certain metals to produce hydrogen, and affect tissue and clothing.

Titration is a method for determining the strength of an unknown acid (or base) by using a buret containing a base (or acid) and an indicator.

The ion product of water, K_w, $= [H^+][OH^-] = 10^{-14}$.

The pH of a solution indicates numerically the acid (or base) strength of a solution in terms of its hydrogen ion concentration. A pH of 7 indicates a neutral solution; a pH below 7, an acid solution; a pH above 7, a basic solution.

Questions and Problems

A

1. Define (a) acid; (b) base; (c) neutralization; (d) pH.
2. List the general properties of acids.
3. List the general properties of bases.
4. What effect does an acid have on litmus paper?
5. What effect does a base have on litmus paper?
6. Will aluminum replace the hydrogen from an acid? Explain.
7. Why are acids usually stored in a container made of glass rather than metal?
8. What substances might be used to lower the acidity of the contents of the stomach?
9. What treatment should be given if a strong acid is accidentally spilled on the skin?
10. Name four acids used in the hospital and give one medical use for each.
11. Name three bases used in the hospital and give one medical use for each.
12. How may pH be measured?
13. What is the pH of blood? of urine? of saliva?
14. Indicate whether each of the substances in question 13 is acidic, basic, or neutral?

B

15. Compare the general and Bronsted definitions of an acid and of a base.
16. Explain how antacids work.
17. Compare the ionization of strong and weak acids and strong and weak bases.
18. Discuss the absorption of aspirin from the gastrointestinal system in terms of pH.
19. Why is KOH a base and C_2H_5OH not a base?

20. If a solution has a [H$^+$] of 10^{-3}, what is the [OH$^-$]? What is the pH? Is the solution acidic or basic?
21. According to Table 13–5, the pH of water is 6.5 to 8.0. Why isn't the pH 7.0?
22. Why do lemons have such a low pH?
23. 29.7 ml of what strength HNO$_3$ will 38.6 ml of 0.25 N KOH react with?
24. 31.8 ml of what strength NaOH will 46.5 ml of 0.40 N H$_2$SO$_4$ react with?
25. How many milliliters of 0.15 N Ca(OH)$_2$ will 29.5 ml of 0.10 N HCl react with?

References

DICKSON, T. R. *Introduction to Chemistry,* 4th ed. John Wiley & Sons, Inc., New York, 1983, Chapter 12.

EBBING, DARRELL D. *General Chemistry.* Houghton Mifflin Company, Boston, 1984, Chapters 17, 18.

MCQUARRIE, DONALD A. and PETER A. ROCK. *General Chemistry.* W. H. Freeman and Company, New York, 1984, Chapters 17, 18.

MILLER, FRANCIS MARION. *Chemistry, Structure and Dynamics.* McGraw-Hill Book Company, New York, 1984, Chapter 16.

MORTIMER, CHARLES E. *Chemistry,* 5th ed. Wadsworth Publishing Co., Belmont, Calif., 1983, Chapter 14.

PETRUCCI, RALPH H. and ROBERT E. WISMER. *General Chemistry with Qualitative Analysis.* Macmillan Publishing Company, New York, 1983, Chapter 17.

SACKHEIM, GEORGE I. *Chemical Calculations,* 12th ed., Series B. Stipes Publishing Co., Champaign, Ill., 1983, Chapter 20.

STOKER, H. STEPHEN. *Introduction to Chemical Principles.* Macmillan Publishing Company, New York, 1983, Chapter 14.

14 Salts

CHAPTER
OUTLINE

Solubility of Salts
Reactions of Salts
   Hydrolysis
   Reaction with Metals

Reaction with Other Salts
Reaction with Acids and Bases
Uses of Salts
Buffer Solutions

Acids have one ion in common, the hydrogen ion (H^+). Consider the dissociation of the following salts

$$NaCl \longrightarrow Na^+ + Cl^-$$

$$K_2SO_4 \longrightarrow 2K^+ + SO_4^{2-}$$

$$Mg(NO_3)_2 \longrightarrow Mg^{2+} + 2NO_3^-$$

Salts have no common ion. Salts in solution yield a positive ion and a negative ion.

Salts are formed by the reaction of an acid and a base, for example

acid		*base*		*salt*		*water*
HCl	+	KOH	$\longrightarrow$	KCl	+	H_2O
H_2SO_4	+	$Mg(OH)_2$	$\longrightarrow$	$MgSO_4$	+	$2H_2O$
$2HNO_3$	+	$Zn(OH)_2$	$\longrightarrow$	$Zn(NO_3)_2$	+	$2H_2O$

Recall that the reaction of an acid with a base is called neutralization.

Solubility of Salts

Some salts are quite soluble in water. Others are classified as slightly soluble or insoluble. Table 14–1 indicates the solubility of most common salts, and

TABLE 14-1. Solubility of Common Salts and Bases

Soluble	Insoluble
Sodium salts	Carbonates (except sodium, potassium, ammonium)
Potassium salts	
Ammonium salts	Phosphates (except sodium, potassium, ammonium)
Acetates	
Nitrates	
Chlorides (except silver, lead, and mercury +1)	Sulfides (except sodium, potassium, ammonium)
Sulfates (except calcium, barium, and lead)	Hydroxides (except sodium, potassium, ammonium)

TABLE 14-2. Water Solubility of Some Salts

Name of Salt	Formula	Solubility
Sodium chloride	NaCl	Soluble
Silver chloride	AgCl	Insoluble
Sodium sulfate	Na_2SO_4	Soluble
Zinc nitrate	$Zn(NO_3)_2$	Soluble
Barium sulfate	$BaSO_4$	Insoluble
Calcium phosphate	$Ca_3(PO_4)_2$	Insoluble
Magnesium carbonate	$MgCO_3$	Insoluble

Table 14–2 indicates the solubilities in water of various salts as predicted by using Table 14–1.

Reactions of Salts

Hydrolysis

Hydrolysis is the reaction of a compound with the hydrogen ion or the hydroxide ion derived from water. Ions derived from a weak acid or base hydrolyze (react with water) to form the corresponding acid or base. Ions derived from a strong acid or base do not hydrolyze. For simplicity we will assume that the acids and bases listed in Table 14–3 are strong and that all other commonly used acids and bases are weak. (For a discussion of strong and weak acids and bases see page 188).

TABLE 14-3. Strong Acids and Bases in Common Use

	Strong Acids			Strong Bases	
HCl	Hydrochloric acid		NaOH	Sodium hydroxide	
HNO_3	Nitric acid		KOH	Potassium hydroxide	
H_2SO_4	Sulfuric acid		$Ca(OH)_2$	Calcium hydroxide	

Since salts are produced by the reaction of an acid with a base, salts must contain parts of each. The positive ion of a salt is derived from a base, and the negative ion of a salt is derived from an acid.

Let us consider the hydrolysis of a salt such as sodium cyanide (NaCN). We first write the formula of the salt in ionic form, sodium ion (Na^+) and cyanide ion (CN^-). Directly below these ions we write the ionized formula for water, with the OH^- ion below the positive ion of the salt and the H^+ ion below the negative ion of the salt, or

$$Na^+ \quad | \quad CN^- \qquad (14\text{--}1)$$
$$OH^- \quad | \quad H^+$$

The sodium ion is derived from one of the strong bases (NaOH) and does not hydrolyze. The CN^- ion is not derived from one of the strong acids and does hydrolyze. Reading upward on the right side of the line in setup (14–1), we have the essentially nonionized compound HCN. Thus the products of hydrolysis of NaCN are the two ions on the left side of the line—Na^+ and OH^-—and the nonionized compound on the right side of the line—HCN. The hydrolysis reaction for NaCN may be written as

$$Na^+ + CN^- + H_2O \rightleftharpoons Na^+ + OH^- + HCN$$

Salts

Since the hydrolysis reaction produces OH^- ions, the solution will be basic. This is what we should expect from the hydrolysis of NaCN, which is derived from a strong base and a weak acid.

Now consider the hydrolysis of NH_4Cl. If we write this compound in ionic form, with water in its ionized form below it, and place the OH^- ion below the positive ion of the salt and the H^+ ion of the water below the negative ion of the salt, we have setup (14–2)

$$\begin{array}{c|c} NH_4^+ & Cl^- \\ OH^- & H^+ \end{array} \qquad\qquad (14\text{–}2)$$

The NH_4^+ ion is not derived from one of the strong bases and does hydrolyze. The nonionized compound formed, as indicated by reading down on the left side of the line, is NH_4OH. The Cl^- ion is derived from one of the strong acids and does not hydrolyze. The right side of the line in (14–2) indicates the ions remaining in solution—Cl^- and H^+. Thus the hydrolysis reaction is

$$NH_4^+ + Cl^- + H_2O \rightleftharpoons NH_4OH + H^+ + Cl^-$$

The resulting solution will be acidic because of the presence of hydrogen ions. This is what should be expected, since the compound NH_4Cl is derived from a weak base and a strong acid.

Reaction with Metals Some metals react with salt solutions to form another salt and a different metal. Refer to the activity series of metals (page 193) and recall that any metal can replace a metal ion below it in the activity series. Thus zinc can replace the copper from the copper sulfate solution because the zinc is higher in the activity series than copper. This is an example of a single replacement reaction

$$Zn + CuSO_4 \longrightarrow ZnSO_4 + Cu$$

Reaction with Other Salts Two different salts in solution may react by double displacement. Consider reactions (14–3) and (14–4)

$$K_2SO_4 + Ba(NO_3)_2 \longrightarrow 2KNO_3 + BaSO_4\downarrow \qquad (14\text{–}3)$$

$$K_2SO_4 + Zn(NO_3)_2 \longrightarrow \text{no reaction} \qquad (14\text{–}4)$$

Why does reaction (14–3) proceed whereas (14–4) does not? Look at the solubility rules (page 204). Note that one of the products formed in reaction (14–3), $BaSO_4$, is insoluble in water. Therefore reaction (14–3) will proceed. In reaction (14–4), the products, if formed, would be $ZnSO_4$ and KNO_3. Both of these salts are soluble and ionized, therefore, no reaction will take place. **In order for a reaction to take place between solutions of two salts, at least one of the products must be insoluble in water, a weak electrolyte, or a nonionized compound.**

Reaction with Acids and Bases Salts react with acids or bases to form other salts and other acids and bases. These reactions will proceed if one of the products is insoluble in water or is an insoluble gas.

Inorganic Chemistry

$$CaCO_3 + 2HCl \longrightarrow CaCl_2 + H_2O + CO_2\uparrow \text{ (a gas is formed)}$$

$$AlCl_3 + 3NaOH \longrightarrow 3NaCl + Al(OH)_3\downarrow \text{ (a precipitate is formed)}$$

Uses of Salts   Salts are necessary for the proper growth and metabolism of the body. Iron salts are necessary for the formation of hemoglobin; iodine salts for the proper functioning of the thyroid gland; calcium and phosphorus salts for the formation of bones and teeth; sodium and potassium salts help regulate the acid-base balance of the body. Salts regulate the irritability of nerve and muscle cells and the beating of the heart. Salts help maintain the proper osmotic pressure of the cells.

Many salts have specific uses. Barium sulfate ($BaSO_4$) is used for X-ray work. Even though barium compounds are poisonous, barium sulfate is insoluble in body fluids and so has no effect on the body. Barium sulfate is opaque to X rays and, when swallowed, it can be used to outline the gastro-intestinal (GI) system for X-ray photographs (see Figure 14–1).

Table 14–4 lists some common salts and their specific uses in medicine.

FIGURE 14–1. X ray of the stomach. (Courtesy of Dr. Leonard Berlin, Director of Radiology, Skokie Valley Community Hospital, Skokie, IL.)

Table 14-4. Common Salts and Their Uses

Classification	Formula	Chemical Name	Common Name
Antacid			
	$CaCO_3$	Calcium carbonate	Precipitated chalk
	$NaHCO_3$	Sodium bicarbonate	Baking soda
Cathartic			
	Na_2SO_4	Sodium sulfate	Glaubers salt
	$MgSO_4$	Magnesium sulfate	Epsom salt
	$MgCO_3$	Magnesium carbonate	—
	—	Magnesium citrate	Citrate of magnesia
	$KNaC_4H_4O_6 \cdot 4H_2O$	Potassium sodium tartrate	Rochelle salt
Diuretic			
	NH_4Cl	Ammonium chloride	Sal ammoniac
Expectorant			
	NH_4Cl	Ammonium chloride	Sal ammoniac
	KI	Potassium iodide	—
Germicide			
	$AgNO_3$	Silver nitrate	Lunar caustic
Miscellaneous Uses			
X-ray work	$BaSO_4$	Barium sulfate	Barium
Caries reduction	NaF	Sodium fluoride	—
	SnF_2	Stannous fluoride	—
For casts	$(CaSO_4)_2 \cdot H_2O$	Calcium sulfate hydrate	Plaster of Paris
Treatment of anemia	$FeSO_4$	Ferrous sulfate	—
Decrease of blood clotting time	$CaCl_2$	Calcium chloride	—
Physiologic saline solution used for irrigation and as IV replacement fluid	$NaCl$	Sodium chloride	Table salt
Thyroid treatment	KI	Potassium iodide	—
	NaI	Sodium iodide	—
Prevent clotting of stored blood	$Na_3C_6H_5O_7$	Sodium citrate	—

Buffer Solutions

The pH of pure water (a neutral solution) is 7.0. If an acid is added to water, the pH goes down. How far below 7.0 it goes depends on how much acid and how strong an acid is added. When a base is added to pure water, the pH rises above 7.0.

However, when small amounts of acid or base are added to a buffer solution, the pH does not change appreciably. A buffer solution is defined as a solution that will resist changes in pH upon the addition of small amounts of either acid or base.

Buffer solutions, or buffers, are found in all body fluids and are responsible for helping maintain the proper pH of those fluids. The normal pH

Inorganic Chemistry

range of the blood is 7.35 to 7.45. Even a slight change in pH can cause a very definite pathologic condition. When the pH falls below 7.35, the condition is known as acidosis. Alkalosis is the condition under which the pH of the blood rises above 7.45 (see page 462).

What does a buffer solution consist of and how does it work? A buffer system consists of a weak acid and a salt of a weak acid or a weak base and its salt. There are several buffer systems in the blood. One of these consists of carbonic acid (H_2CO_3), a weak acid, and sodium bicarbonate ($NaHCO_3$), the salt of a weak acid.

Suppose that an acid such as hydrochloric acid (HCl) enters the bloodstream. The HCl reacts with the $NaHCO_3$ part of the buffer according to the reaction

$$HCl + NaHCO_3 \longrightarrow NaCl + H_2CO_3$$

The NaCl produced is neutral; it does not hydrolyze (see page 205). The H_2CO_3 produced is part of the original buffer system and is only slightly ionized. In the body, acids (hydrogen ions) are produced by various metabolic processes. When these acids enter the bloodstream, they are removed by this reaction or a similar reaction with other buffers.

A base such as sodium hydroxide (NaOH) would react with the carbonic acid part of the buffer

$$NaOH + H_2CO_3 \longrightarrow H_2O + NaHCO_3$$

forming water, a harmless neutral normal metabolite, and sodium bicarbonate, part of the original buffer. Thus, when either acid or base is added to the buffer, something neutral (NaCl or water) is formed plus more of the buffer system (H_2CO_3 or $NaHCO_3$). Therefore, the pH of the blood should not change because the buffer system has reduced the number of free hydrogen or hydroxide ions.

In addition to the carbonate buffer system there are also phosphate buffers and several organic buffer systems. These will be discussed in Chapter 30.

If there is an overproduction of acid in the tissues and if these acids cannot be excreted rapidly enough, a condition known as acidosis results during which the buffers are unable to handle the excess acid. Acidosis may occur in certain diseases, such as diabetes mellitus and during starvation (see page 462).

Prolonged vomiting may result in alkalosis because of the continued loss of the acid contents of the stomach.

Summary Salts are formed by the reaction of an acid with a base. Salts yield ions other than hydrogen or hydroxide.

Some salts are soluble and others are insoluble in water. The solubility of most common salts can be determined from the solubility rules.

Hydrolysis is a double displacement reaction in which water is a reactant.

Salts react with some metals to yield other salts and other metals. Salts may react with other salts by a double displacement reaction. Salts may react with acids or bases to form other salts and other acids or bases.

Salts serve a definite purpose in the various metabolic processes of the body.

Buffer solutions do not change in pH upon the addition of small amounts of acid or base. Buffer solutions help maintain the proper pH of the body fluids.

Questions and Problems

A

1. Define (a) salt; (b) hydrolysis; (c) buffer solution.
2. Name five soluble salts.
3. Name ten insoluble salts.
4. Indicate whether the hydrolysis of the following salts will produce an acidic, a basic, or a neutral solution: (a) sodium carbonate; (b) magnesium chloride; (c) ammonium nitrate; (d) lead nitrate; (e) potassium sulfate.
5. Give an example of the reaction of a salt with a metal.
6. Give an example of the reaction of a salt with another salt.
7. Give an example of the reaction of a salt with an acid.
8. Give an example of the reaction of a salt with a base.
9. Name ten salts commonly used in the hospital and indicate what each is used for.
10. What is acidosis? alkalosis?
11. Explain how a buffer solution works.

B

12. Why do ions derived from weak acids or bases hydrolyze whereas those from strong acids or bases do not?
13. Why are buffer solutions important in the body?
14. Is silver chloride soluble in water? Will it hydrolyze in water?
15. When the following compounds are placed in water, will the resulting solution have a pH of 7? above 7? below 7?
    (a) KCl   (b) NaClO   (c) NH_4NO_3

References   CHISOLM, J. J., JR. Lead poisoning. *Scientific American,* **224:**15–23 (Feb. 1971).

DEEVEY, E. S., JR. The mineral cycle. *Scientific American,* **223:**148–158 (Sept. 1970).

HOYLE, G. How is muscle turned on and off? *Scientific American,* **222:**85–93 (April 1970).

STOKER, H. STEPHEN. *Introduction to Chemical Principles.* Macmillan Publishing Company, New York, 1983, Chapter 14.

UNIT II

Organic Chemistry

15 Introduction to Organic Chemistry

CHAPTER
OUTLINE

Importance of Organic Chemistry
   Comparison of Organic and Inorganic
    Compounds
Bonding
Structural Formulas
Isomers

Three-Dimensional Arrangement of the
   Bonds in the Carbon Atom
Bonding Ability of Carbon
Carbon Compounds with Other
   Elements

In the eighteenth century it was believed that a "vital force" was needed to make the compounds produced by living cells. These compounds were said to be organic compounds. However, this belief was overthrown by a German chemist, Fredrick Wöhler, in 1828. He prepared urea, a compound normally found in the blood and urine, by heating a solution of ammonium cyanate, an inorganic compound.

$$NH_4CNO \xrightarrow{\text{heat}} NH_2-\overset{\displaystyle \overset{O}{\|}}{C}-NH_2$$

ammonium cyanate   urea

After Wöhler's work many other organic compounds were produced in the laboratory. This led to the subdivision of chemistry into two parts—inorganic and organic. **Organic chemistry** was defined as the chemistry of carbon compounds. Why have one category for the element carbon and place all other elements in the other category? The answer is that although there are tens of thousands of inorganic compounds known today, *millions* of organic compounds are known.

Importance of Organic Chemistry

Organic chemistry is important in that it is the chemistry associated with all living matter in both plants and animals. Carbohydrates, fats, proteins, vitamins, hormones, enzymes, and many drugs are organic compounds. Wool, silk, cotton, linen, and such synthetic fibers as nylon, rayon, and dacron contain organic compounds. So do perfumes, dyes, flavors, soaps, detergents, plastics, gasolines, and oils.

Comparison of Organic and Inorganic Compounds

Organic compounds differ from inorganic compounds in many ways. The most important of these are listed below.

1. Most organic compounds are flammable. Most inorganic compounds are nonflammable.
2. Most organic compounds have low melting points. Most inorganic compounds have high melting points.
3. Most organic compounds have a low boiling point. Most inorganic compounds have a high boiling point point.
4. Most organic compounds are soluble in nonpolar liquids. Most inorganic compounds are insoluble in nonpolar liquids.
5. Most organic compounds are insoluble in water. Many inorganic compounds are soluble in water.
6. Organic compounds are held together by covalent bonds. Many inorganic compounds contain ionic bonds.
7. Organic reactions usually take place between molecules. Inorganic reactions usually take place between ions.
8. Organic compounds generally contain many atoms. Inorganic compounds usually contain relatively few atoms.
9. Organic compounds have a complex structure. Inorganic compounds have a simpler structure.

Bonding

Organic compounds—compounds of carbon—are held together by covalent bonds. Recall that covalent bonds are formed by sharing electrons. In organic chemistry the term **bond** is used to designate a shared pair of electrons. Thus, the statement is made that carbon forms four bonds; it has an oxidation number of -4. Bonds are usually represented by a short, straight line connecting the atoms.

Each carbon atom in the following compounds forms four bonds.

| four single bonds to carbon | double bond between carbons | triple bond between carbons |

Likewise, since the oxygen atom has an oxidation number of -2, it forms two bonds, as shown in the following compounds.

two single bonds to oxygen   double bond to oxygen

Nitrogen, with an oxidation number of -3, forms three bonds.

| triple bond to nitrogen | three single bonds to nitrogen | one single and one double bond to nitrogen |

Note that in all the preceding examples hydrogen, with an oxidation number of $+1$, forms only one bond. The halogen (fluorine, chlorine, bromine, and iodine), all with an oxidation number of -1, also form only one bond.

Structural Formulas

As will be seen later, organic compounds are often written using a structural rather than a molecular formula. What is the difference between a structural formula and a molecular formula? And why use the former and not the latter?

Consider an organic compound with a molecular formula C_2H_6O. In inorganic chemistry a formula of this type designates a specific compound. However, in organic chemistry this is not always true; the same formula may designate more than one compound. Let us see how this is possible.

If the carbons, hydrogens, and oxygens in C_2H_6O are arranged in such a manner that each carbon atom has four bonds attached to it, each hydrogen atom has one bond, and the oxygen has two bonds, there will be two possible structures, both having the formula C_2H_6O.

These two structural formulas are

$$
\begin{array}{ccccc}
 & \text{H} & \text{H} & & \text{H} & & \text{H}\\
 & | & | & & | & & |\\
\text{H}-\text{C}-\text{C}-\text{O}-\text{H} & \text{and} & \text{H}-\text{C}-\text{O}-\text{C}-\text{H}\\
 & | & | & & | & & |\\
 & \text{H} & \text{H} & & \text{H} & & \text{H}
\end{array} \qquad (15\text{-}1)
$$

Each compound contains two carbons, six hydrogens, and one oxygen so that each satisfies all of the bond requirements. These two compounds have different structures, different properties, and actually represent different compounds. They are isomers of each other. The first compound is called ethyl alcohol, the second dimethyl ether. This difference in the structure of compounds having the same molecular formula illustrates the importance of using structural rather than molecular formulas for organic compounds.

In diagram (15-1) the lines represent bonds or shared electrons. If the same structures were written using electron dots, they would be

$$
\begin{array}{ccccc}
\text{H} & \text{H} & & \text{H} & \text{H}\\
\text{H}:\ddot{\text{C}}:\ddot{\text{C}}:\ddot{\text{O}}:\text{H} & \text{and} & \text{H}:\ddot{\text{C}}:\ddot{\text{O}}:\ddot{\text{C}}:\text{H}\\
\text{H} & \text{H} & & \text{H} & \text{H}
\end{array}
$$

It is simpler to write a structural formula using the "bond" notation.

Isomers

Isomers are defined as compounds having the same molecular formula but different structural formulas. Thus, the compound C_2H_6O has two isomers. The compound C_6H_{14} has five isomers, as illustrated in Figure 15–1. $C_6H_{12}O_6$ is usually called glucose. Actually this molecular formula represents 16 different compounds or isomers, each of which is a different sugar (see page 307).

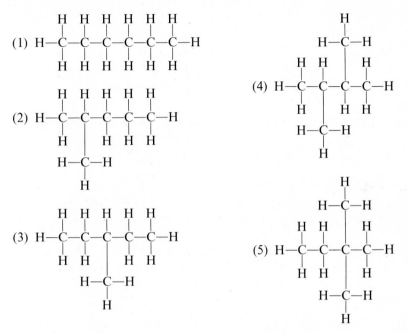

FIGURE 15–1. Isomers of C_6H_{14}.

Three-Dimensional Arrangement of the Bonds in the Carbon Atom

It should be realized that the compounds represented by structural formulas are three dimensional and not planar. For example, each carbon atom has four bonds attached to it. If these bonds are symmetrically arranged, the structure, in a planar representation, is as follows:

$$-\overset{|}{\underset{|}{C}}-$$

What does it actually look like in three dimensions? The four bonds of the carbon atom are arranged in a tetrahedral* shape. The carbon atom lies at the center of the tetrahedron; the angle between the bonds is 109.5°. Therefore the compound CH_4, methane, may be represented as shown in Figure 15–2.

Bonding Ability of Carbon

What is unique about the element carbon that it forms so many compounds? The other elements form relatively few compounds. The answer is that the carbon atom has the ability to bond other carbon atoms to itself to form very large and complex molecules. Carbon atoms may join together to form con-

Introduction to Organic Chemistry

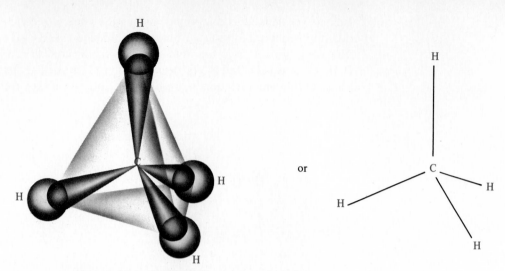

FIGURE 15-2. Tetrahedral structure of methane, CH$_4$.

tinuous or branched chains of carbon atoms. Compounds of this type are called **aliphatic compounds** (Figure 15-3a). Carbon compounds may also bond together in the shape of rings to form **cyclic** (also called **aromatic**) compounds (Figure 15-3b). A third type of organic compounds are the **heterocyclic compounds**, which also have a ring structure. However, this ring

FIGURE 15-3. Types of carbon compounds.

structure contains some element other than carbon in the ring (Figure 15-3c). In this particular case the other element is nitrogen.

Carbon Compounds with Other Elements

Carbon also forms compounds with other elements besides hydrogen and oxygen. If a chlorine atom is bonded to a carbon atom, the compound chloromethane or methyl chloride is formed.

Examples of carbon bonded to oxygen and nitrogen are indicated on page 216.

Summary

Organic chemistry is defined as the chemistry of carbon compounds. Most organic compounds differ from inorganic compounds as follows: they are combustible; they have lower melting points; they are insoluble in water; reaction takes place between molecules rather than between ions; the molecules contain many atoms; the molecules have a complex structure.

In organic chemistry the term *bond* is used rather than oxidation number. A bond is indicated by a short line and represents a pair of shared electrons. The carbon atom always has four bonds associated with it; the oxygen atom, two; the hydrogen atom, one.

Structural formulas are used for organic compounds rather than molecular formulas because the same molecular formula may represent more than one structural formula.

Isomers are compounds having the same molecular formula but different structural formulas.

The four single bonds of the carbon atom are arranged in three dimensions in a tetrahedral structure with the carbon atom at the center and each bond pointing to a corner.

Organic compounds may be divided into three categories: aliphatic compounds, aromatic compounds, and heterocyclic compounds. Heterocyclic compounds contain elements other than carbon in the ring.

Carbon also forms compounds with other elements besides hydrogen and oxygen.

Questions and Problems

A

1. What was Wöhler's best known contribution to organic chemistry?
2. Compare the properties of organic and inorganic compounds.
3. What is a "bond" in an organic compound?
4. How are the bonds arranged around the carbon atom in methane?
5. Why are structural formulas rather than molecular formulas used for organic compounds?
6. What are isomers? Do all organic compounds have isomers?
7. The compound C_5H_{12} has three isomers. Draw their structures.
8. What are the three major types of organic compounds?

B

9. Phosphorus is in group VA of the periodic chart. How many bonds should be attached to a phosphorus atom?

10. How many bonds should be attached to sulfur? bromine?
11. What is the tetrahedral angle?
12. Is it possible for a heterocyclic compound to contain oxygen in the ring? hydrogen?

References BAUM, STUART J. *Introduction to Organic and Biological Chemistry,* 3rd ed. Macmillan Publishing Company, New York, 1982, Chapter 1.

MORRISON, ROBERT T. and ROBERT N. BOYD. *Organic Chemistry,* 4th ed. Allyn and Bacon, Inc., Boston, 1983, Chapter 1.

ZIMMERMAN, HENRY and ISAAK ZIMMERMAN. *Elements of Organic Chemistry,* 2nd ed. Macmillan Publishing Company, New York, 1983, Chapter 1.

16 Hydrocarbons

CHAPTER
OUTLINE

Alkanes
   General Formula
   Alkyl Groups
Naming Hydrocarbons
Cycloalkanes
Haloalkanes
Alkenes
Alkynes

Saturated and Unsaturated Hydrocarbons
   Reactions of Saturated Hydrocarbons
   Reactions of Unsaturated Hydrocarbons
Sources of Hydrocarbons
Uses of Hydrocarbons
   Polymers

Alkanes

As the name implies, **hydrocarbons** are compounds that contain carbon and hydrogen only.

Consider the hydrocarbon of only one carbon atom. Since a carbon atom must have four bonds, four hydrogen atoms may be attached to that carbon atom. The hydrocarbon thus formed is called **methane** and has the structural formula shown in Figure 16-1.

If two carbon atoms are bonded together, six hydrogen atoms may be joined to them. This hydrocarbon is called **ethane.** The molecular formula is C_2H_6, and the structure is shown in Figure 16-2.

The hydrocarbon of three carbon atoms needs eight hydrogens to satisfy all the bonds. This compound, C_3H_8, is called **propane** (see Figure 16-3).

These compounds are called **alkanes,** and they are said to be **saturated;** that is, they have single covalent bonds between carbon atoms.

FIGURE 16-1. Methane.

FIGURE 16-2. Ethane.

Table 16–1 lists several hydrocarbons. Note that the names of all alkanes end in **-ane.** The names of the first four compounds are not systematic; they were named before a system of nomenclature was devised. Beginning with the hydrocarbon containing five carbon atoms, however, the names follow a definite pattern. The name **pentane** was derived from the prefix **penta-,** meaning five; pentane contains five carbon atoms. The name **hexane** is derived from the prefix **hexa-,** which means six; and so on through the series.

Structural formulas may be condensed, as indicated in Table 16–1.

or

FIGURE 16-3. Propane.

Organic Chemistry

222

TABLE 16-1. Alkanes

Number of Carbon Atoms	Name	Molecular Formula	Structural Formula	Condensed Structural Formula
1	Methane	CH_4	(structure)	CH_4
2	Ethane	C_2H_6	(structure)	CH_3-CH_3 or CH_3CH_3
3	Propane	C_3H_8	(structure)	$CH_3-CH_2-CH_3$ or $CH_3CH_2CH_3$
4	Butane	C_4H_{10}	(structure) and (structure)	$CH_3-CH_2-CH_2-CH_3$ or $CH_3(CH_2)_2CH_3$ $CH_3-CH-CH_3$ with CH_3 or $CH_3CH(CH_3)CH_3$
5	Pentane	C_5H_{12}	3 isomers[a]	
6	Hexane	C_6H_{14}	5 isomers	
7	Heptane	C_7H_{16}	9 isomers	
8	Octane	C_8H_{18}	18 isomers	
9	Nonane	C_9H_{20}	35 isomers	
10	Decane	$C_{10}H_{22}$	75 isomers	

[a] The number of isomers increases rapidly as the compound contains more carbon atoms. $C_{40}H_{82}$ has 62,491,178,805,831 possible isomers.

General Formula   The general formula for alkanes is

$$C_nH_{2n+2}$$

where n represents the number of carbon atoms. That is, if a compound contains n carbon atoms, the number of hydrogen atoms is twice n plus two more.

Butane contains four carbon atoms. The number of hydrogens should be $(2 \times 4) + 2$ or 10, which agrees with the molecular formula for butane

Hydrocarbons   **223**

listed in Table 16–1. Likewise, octane has eight carbon atoms and so should have $(2 \times 8) + 2$ or 18 hydrogen atoms, which it does.

Continuing with a larger number of carbon atoms, the alkane containing 16 carbon atoms would have $(2 \times 16) + 2$ or 34 hydrogen atoms, giving it the formula $C_{16}H_{34}$.

Alkyl Groups

When a hydrogen atom is removed from an alkane, an alkyl group is formed. The names of the alkyl groups are obtained by changing the ending of the name from *-ane* to *-yl*. The alkyl group of one carbon atom formed from the alkane methane is called the methyl group. The alkyl group of two carbon atoms formed from ethane is called the ethyl group. The alkyl group of three carbon atoms formed from propane is called propyl (see Table 16–2).

TABLE 16–2. Simple Alkyl Groups

Name of Alkyl Group	Condensed Structural Formula
Methyl	$CH_3—$
Ethyl	$CH_3—CH_2—$ *or* $C_2H_5—$
Propyl	$CH_3—CH_2—CH_2—$ *or* $C_3H_7—$
Butyl	$CH_3—CH_2—CH_2—CH_2—$ *or* $C_4H_9—$

The compound CH_3Cl, or

is made up of a methyl group ($CH_3—$) attached to a chlorine atom. It is called methyl chloride. The compound C_2H_5I consists of an ethyl group ($C_2H_5—$) bonded to an iodine. It is called ethyl iodide.

$$H—\overset{\displaystyle H}{\underset{\displaystyle H}{C}}—\overset{\displaystyle H}{\underset{\displaystyle H}{C}}—I$$

Naming Hydrocarbons

An international system of nomenclature for organic compounds has been devised and is recognized and used by chemists all over the world. This system was devised and approved by the International Union of Pure and Applied Chemistry and is frequently designated by the initials IUPAC. The rules of the IUPAC system are

1. Pick out the longest continuous chain of carbon atoms.
2. Identify that chain as an alkane.
3. Pick out the alkyl groups attached to that chain.
4. Number the carbons in the chain, starting at whichever end of the

chain will give the smallest numbers to the carbons to which the alkyl groups are attached. Continue the numbering of this carbon chain in the same direction from one end to the other.

5. List the numbers and the names of the alkyl groups in alphabetical order.

6. Use commas between numbers and a dash between a number and a letter.

EXAMPLE 16-1. Name the following compound:

$$CH_3-CH-CH_2-CH_2-CH_2-CH_3$$
$$|$$
$$CH_3$$

The longest chain contains six carbon atoms; therefore, this compound is a *hexane*. To identify the alkyl group attached to the chain and also to identify the chain itself, it is sometimes easier to draw a box around the chain. Then whatever is attached to the chain, the alkyl groups, will be outside the box and can be easily noticed. Thus the compound can be written with the six-carbon chain inside the box.

$$\boxed{CH_3-CH-CH_2-CH_2-CH_2-CH_3}$$
$$|$$
$$CH_3$$

Attached to the chain (sticking out of the box) is an alkyl group of one carbon atom, the CH_3- or methyl group. Thus, this compound is a methylhexane.

The next step calls for numbering the carbons in the chain. They can be numbered in either direction, from left to right or from right to left. It should be observed that the methyl group is on the second carbon atom from the left end or on the fifth carbon atom from the right end. The rule states that the numbering should be such that the carbon to which the alkyl group is attached has the smallest number. Therefore the correct name of this compound is 2-methylhexane, which indicates that there is a methyl group on the second carbon from the end in a chain consisting of six carbon atoms. If the methyl group had been pointing upward instead of down, the compound would still be the same and so would the name. ■

EXAMPLE 16-2. Name the following compound:

$$CH_3$$
$$|$$
$$CH_3-CH_2-CH-CH-CH_3$$
$$|$$
$$CH_3$$

2,3 dimethyl pentane

The longest chain contains five carbon atoms. This compound is a *pentane*. There are two methyl groups attached to the chain, one on the second carbon and one on the third carbon. This time the numbering is from right to left in order to obtain the lowest numbers for the alkyl groups.

Hydrocarbons

$$\underset{\text{5}\quad\text{4}\quad\text{3}\quad\text{2}\quad\text{1}}{CH_3-CH_2-CH-CH-CH_3}$$

with CH_3 above carbon 2 and CH_3 below carbon 3.

This compound is called 2,3-dimethylpentane, where the prefix *di-* indicates that there are two identical groups. Dimethyl means two methyl groups and the numbers tell us on which carbon atoms they are located.

Whenever an alkyl group appears more than once in a compound, a prefix is used to designate how many of these alkyl groups are present in that compound. The most commonly used prefixes are

> **di-** which means two
> **tri-** which means three
> **tetra-** which means four
> **penta-** which means five

EXAMPLE 16-3. Name the following compound:

We first draw a box around the longest chain. This chain contains eight carbon atoms so the compound is an *octane*.

Attached to the chain are three methyl groups and one ethyl group. The chain should be numbered from left to right in order to obtain alkyl groups of the lowest numbers. There are methyl groups on carbons numbered 2, 3, and 6 and an ethyl group on carbon number 5 of the eight carbon chain.

The correct name of this compound is 5-ethyl-2,3,6-trimethyloctane. Note that the alkyl groups are named in alphabetical order. Also note that the prefix *tri-* is used to indicate three alkyl groups of the same type.

EXAMPLE 16-4. Name the following compound:

First draw a box around the longest chain. Note that this chain contains seven carbon atoms so that this compound is a *heptane*.

Attached to the chain are three methyl groups at carbons numbered 2, 4, and 5. Thus the name of this compound is 2,4,5-trimethylheptane. Recall rule number 1 (page 224), which says "pick out the longest continuous chain of carbon atoms." If you had picked a chain of six carbon atoms (straight across) this would not have been the longest continuous chain of carbon atoms. ∎

Many simple hydrocarbons and hydrocarbon derivatives have common names that were in use before the IUPAC* system was adopted. Many of these names are still in use although IUPAC naming is preferred. Table 16–3 indicates the IUPAC name and the common name for the three isomers of pentane, C_5H_{12}. Note that the prefix *n* (for normal) indicates a straight chain compound.

TABLE 16–3. Names of Simple Hydrocarbons

Structure	IUPAC Name	Common Name
CH_3—CH_2—CH_2—CH_2—CH_3	*n*-pentane	*n*-pentane
CH_3—CH—CH_2—CH_3 　　　｜ 　　　CH_3	2-methylbutane	isopentane
CH_3 　　　｜ CH_3—C—CH_3 　　　｜ 　　　CH_3	2,2-dimethylpropane	neopentane

Cycloalkanes　Alkanes also exist in the shape of a ring. Such structures are called cycloalkanes. They are named by placing the prefix **cyclo** before the name of the corresponding straight chain alkane. Thus, the cyclic alkane of three carbons is called **cyclopropane**. Its structure is

$$\begin{array}{c} CH_2 \\ \diagup \quad \diagdown \\ H_2C \text{——} CH_2 \end{array}$$

Cyclopropane is used medicinally as a general anesthetic. Both induction and recovery time are short. Muscular relaxation is greater than with nitrous oxide but less than with ether. As with ether the danger of explosion is great, so care must be taken in its use. Note that cyclopropane is a saturated hydrocarbon since it contains only single bonds.

The structures of cycloalkanes may also be abbreviated by using a geometric shape in which each line represents a bond between carbon atoms and each corner a carbon atom and its hydrogens. The following structures represent cyclopropane and cyclobutane, respectively.

cyclopropane   cyclobutane

When alkyl groups are attached to a cycloalkane, the compound is numbered in such a manner as to give the groups the lowest numbers. When only one group is attached to a cycloalkane, the number 1 is understood and not written.

1,3-dimethylcyclohexane   methylcyclopropane

For an additional method of naming cycloalkanes, see page 301.

Haloalkanes Alkanes may have one or more halogen* atoms replacing hydrogens. Such compounds are called haloalkanes. The simplest chloroalkane is

chloromethane
(methyl chloride)

The IUPAC name is given first followed by the common name in parentheses.

Further substitution of chlorines for hydrogen leads to

dichloromethane   trichloromethane   tetrachloromethane
(methylene chloride) (chloroform)   (carbon tetrachloride)

Similar compounds can be formed with bromine and iodine. $CHCl_3$ is called chloroform. Likewise, $CHBr_3$ is called bromoform, and CHI_3 is called iodoform.

chloroform   bromoform   iodoform

Since there is only one carbon atom, no numbers are necessary.

Table 16–4 indicates the IUPAC and the common names of simple haloalkanes.

A hydrocarbon derivative used as an anesthetic is halothane, 2-bromo-2-chloro-1,1,1-trifluoroethane. (Note that the groups attached to the carbons are named in alphabetical order.)

Its main advantage over other anesthetics formerly used is that it is non-flammable and nonirritating to the respiratory passages. Halothane is usually used in conjunction with nitrous oxide (see page 128) and with muscle relaxants to provide general anesthesia for surgery of all types, but it can also be administered alone.

A similar compound, chloral hydrate, induces sleep and prevents convulsions. A combination of ethyl alcohol and chloral hydrate is known as a "Mickey Finn" or "knock-out drops."

chloral hydrate

TABLE 16–4. IUPAC and Common Names of Some Haloalkanes

Structure	IUPAC Name	Common Name
$CH_3-CH_2-CH_2-CH_2Br$	1-bromobutane	*n*-bromobutane
$CH_3-CH_2-\underset{\underset{Br}{\vert}}{CH}-CH_3$	2-bromobutane	*sec*-bromobutane[a]
$CH_3-\underset{\underset{CH_3}{\vert}}{CH}-CH_2Br$	1-bromo-2-methylpropane	isobutylbromide
$CH_3-\overset{\overset{CH_3}{\vert}}{\underset{\underset{Br}{\vert}}{C}}-CH_3$	2-bromo-2-methylpropane	*tert*-bromopropane[a]

[a] Where *sec* stands for secondary and *tert* for tertiary.

Hydrocarbons

In veterinary medicine, chloral hydrate is used as a narcotic and anesthetic for cattle, horses, and poultry.

Other widely used haloalkanes include ethyl chloride, a fast-acting topically applied local anesthetic; Freon-12, used in aerosol containers and in refrigeration and air conditioning units (see page 114); Teflon and polyvinyl chloride (PVC), which are polymers. Teflon is used as a coating material for cooking utensils and PVC is use in making plastic containers. Their structures are as follows:

ethyl chloride   Freon-12

Teflon   polyvinyl chloride

Alkenes

Alkanes have a single bond between the carbon atoms. Alkenes have a double bond (two bonds) between two of the carbon atoms.

$$C=C$$

Consider two carbon atoms connected by a double bond. Since this double bond uses four electrons from both carbons, a total of only four hydrogen atoms will satisfy all of the remaining bonds. Recall that a single bond represents a pair of shared electrons; a double bond represents two pairs of shared electrons.

This compound thus becomes

and has the molecular formula of C_2H_4. It is called **ethene.**

When three carbon atoms are arranged in a chain with a double bond between two of the carbon atoms, $C=C-C$, how many hydrogen atoms must be connected to these carbon atoms in order to satisfy all of the bond requirements? The answer is six, so that the structure becomes

$$
\begin{array}{cccc}
 & H & H & H \\
 & | & | & | \\
H- & C= & C- & C-H \\
 & & & | \\
 & & & H
\end{array}
$$

where the molecular formula is C_3H_6. The name of this compound is **propene.**

Note that the names of these compounds end in **-ene.** This is true of all

Organic Chemistry

alkenes. It should be noted also that the names of these compounds are similar to the alkanes except for the ending, which is *-ene* instead of *-ane*.

Compare the structures of ethane (C_2H_6) and ethene (C_2H_4).

ethane   ethene

The three-carbon alkane is propane, and the three-carbon alkene is propene. Likewise the four-carbon alkane is called butane while the corresponding alkene is called butene. The names and formulas of some of the alkenes are listed in Table 16–5.

The general formula for alkenes is

$$C_nH_{2n}$$

There are twice as many hydrogen atoms as carbon atoms in every alkene. Thus octene has 8 carbon atoms and 16 hydrogen atoms, and the formula of an alkene of 15 carbon atoms would be $C_{15}H_{30}$.

Consider the two isomers of butene listed in Table 16–5. The first is called 1-butene, indicating that the double bond is between carbons 1 and 2. The second compound is called 2-butene, indicating that the double bond lies between carbons 2 and 3. Note that the double bond is always given the lowest number, even if other groups are present.

The following examples illustrate the naming of alkenes containing other groups.

3-methyl-1-butene

cyclobutene

(1 is understood, so it is assumed that the double bond is between carbon atoms 1 and 2)

The following cycloalkene is numbered to show the double bond having the number 1 (understood) and the methyl group having the lowest number. If the numbering had been in the other direction, then the methyl group would have a larger number.

3-methylcyclopentene

The vinyl group has the structure

TABLE 16-5. Some Simple Alkenes

No. of Carbon Atoms	Name	Molecular Formula	Structural Formula	Condensed Structural Formula
2	Ethene	C_2H_4	$H-C=C-H$ (with H's)	$CH_2=CH_2$
3	Propene	C_3H_6	(structural formula)	$CH_3-CH=CH_2$
4	Butene	C_4H_8	(structural formula) _or_ (structural formula)	$CH_2=CH-CH_2-CH_3$ _or_ $CH_3-CH=CH-CH_3$
5	Pentene	C_5H_{10}	(structural formula) _or_ 5 other isomers	$CH_2=CH-CH_2-CH_2-CH_3$
6	Hexene	C_6H_{12}	(structural formula) _or_ 14 other isomers	$CH_2=CH-CH_2-CH_2-CH_2-CH_3$
7	Heptene	C_7H_{14}	30 isomers	
8	Octene	C_8H_{16}	66 isomers	

Vinyl chloride is used in the manufacture of such consumer products as floor tile, raincoats, phonograph records, fabrics, and furniture coverings. However, evidence has shown that several workers exposed to vinyl chloride during their work have died from a very rare form of liver cancer. In addition, exposure to vinyl chloride is suspected as being responsible for certain types of birth defects.

The structure of vinyl chloride is

$$\begin{array}{cc} H & H \\ | & | \\ H-C & = C - Cl \end{array}$$

Alkynes Consider two carbon atoms connected by a triple bond.

$$C \equiv C$$

How many hydrogen atoms must be connected to these two carbon atoms in order to satisfy all the bond requirements? The answer is two, so that the molecular formula of this compound is C_2H_2. This compound is called **ethyne**. Its structure is

$$H-C \equiv C-H \qquad (H : C :: C : H)$$

Ethyne is commonly called acetylene. However, this name is not preferred because the ending *-ene* denotes a double bond, whereas this compound actually has a triple bond between the carbon atoms.

If three carbon atoms are placed in a chain with a triple bond between two of these carbon atoms

$$C \equiv C - C$$

only four hydrogen atoms can be placed around these carbons in order to satisfy all the bonds. The compound then becomes

with the molecular formula C_3H_4. This compound is called **propyne**.

These two compounds, ethyne and propyne, are alkynes. They have a triple bond between two of the carbon atoms. All their names end in **-yne**. The general formula for alkynes is

$$C_nH_{2n-2}$$

Thus hexyne, which has six carbon atoms, has the formula $C_6H_{(2 \times 6)-2}$ or C_6H_{10}. Likewise, octyne has the molecular formula C_8H_{14}.

Alkynes are relatively rare compounds and do not normally occur in the human body.

As with alkenes, alkynes are named with the triple bond having the smallest number.

Hydrocarbons

TABLE 16-6. Hydrocarbons

No. of Carbon Atoms	Alkanes	Alkenes	Alkynes
1	Methane CH_4	—	—
2	Ethane C_2H_6	Ethene C_2H_4	Ethyne C_2H_2
3	Propane C_3H_8	Propene C_3H_6	Propyne C_3H_4
4	Butane C_4H_{10}	Butene C_4H_8	Butyne C_4H_6
General formula	C_nH_{2n+2}	C_nH_{2n}	C_nH_{2n-2}

$$HC\equiv C-CH_2-CH_2-CH_3 \qquad CH_3-C\equiv C-CH_2-CH_3 \qquad CH_3-C\equiv C-\underset{\underset{CH_3}{|}}{CH}-CH_2-CH_3$$

1-pentyne   2-pentyne   4-methyl-2-hexyne

It should be noted that there can be no hydrocarbon with four bonds between the carbon atoms because then there would be no bonds available for any hydrogen atoms. (Recall that hydrocarbons must contain both carbon and hydrogen.)

A summary of the names and formulas of some hydrocarbons can be found in Table 16-6.

Saturated and Unsaturated Hydrocarbons

Saturated hydrocarbons are those that have only single bonds between the carbon atoms. Alkanes are saturated compounds.

Unsaturated hydrocarbons contain at least one double bond or triple bond. Both alkenes and alkynes are unsaturated compounds.

Reactions of Saturated Hydrocarbons

Saturated hydrocarbons react by a process known as substitution. When ethane reacts with chlorine, Cl_2 or $Cl-Cl$, one of the chlorine atoms substitutes for one of the hydrogen atoms in the saturated compound.

$$H-\overset{\overset{H}{|}}{\underset{\underset{H}{|}}{C}}-\overset{\overset{H}{|}}{\underset{\underset{H}{|}}{C}}-H + Cl-Cl \xrightarrow{\text{light or heat}} H-\overset{\overset{H}{|}}{\underset{\underset{H}{|}}{C}}-\overset{\overset{H}{|}}{\underset{\underset{H}{|}}{C}}-Cl + HCl$$

ethane   + chlorine ⟶ chloroethane   + hydrogen
              (ethyl chloride)   chloride

Further chlorination may substitute additional chlorines for hydrogens.

Alkanes may be oxidized to yield carbon dioxide, water, and energy as indicated in the following reactions.

$$CH_4 + 2O_2 \longrightarrow CO_2 + 2H_2O + energy$$
methane

Organic Chemistry

$$2CH_3-\underset{\underset{\displaystyle CH_3}{|}}{\overset{\overset{\displaystyle CH_3}{|}}{C}}-CH_2-\underset{\overset{\displaystyle CH_3}{|}}{CH}-CH_3 + 25O_2 \longrightarrow 16CO_2 + 18H_2O + energy$$

2,2,4-trimethylpentane
(isooctane)

Incomplete oxidation (combustion) of alkanes yields carbon monoxide in place of carbon dioxide. The equation for the incomplete oxidation of methane is

$$2CH_4 + 3O_2 \longrightarrow 2CO + 4H_2O + energy$$

Incomplete combustion of isooctane, a major component of gasoline, also yields carbon monoxide. This carbon monoxide is released into the air and becomes a deadly pollutant. Carbon monoxide is poisonous because it combines with hemoglobin and prevents that compound from carrying oxygen to the cells (see pages 461, 462).

Reactions of Unsaturated Hydrocarbons

When ethene reacts with hydrogen (H_2) it reacts by a process known as addition. That is, the hydrogen atoms add to the double bond, making a single bond out of it. Chlorine (Cl_2) reacts similarly with propene.

ethene   + hydrogen ⟶   ethane

propene   + chlorine ⟶   1,2-dichloropropane

Like alkenes, alkynes undergo addition reactions. Ethyne (acetylene) reacts with chlorine by a process of addition to form a single bond between the carbon atoms.

$$H-C\equiv C-H + 2Cl-Cl \longrightarrow \quad H-\underset{\underset{\displaystyle Cl}{|}}{\overset{\overset{\displaystyle Cl}{|}}{C}}-\underset{\underset{\displaystyle Cl}{|}}{\overset{\overset{\displaystyle Cl}{|}}{C}}-H$$

ethyne   +   chlorine ⟶   1,1,2,2-tetrachloroethane

In general the addition reaction takes place more rapidly and under milder conditions than the substitution reaction. Note that in these examples an unsaturated reactant has been changed into a saturated product. A practical application of this will be discussed in the hydrogenation of fats and oils (see page 328).

Hydrocarbons   **235**

Sources of Hydrocarbons

The chief sources of hydrocarbons are petroleum and natural gas. Petroleum is a very complex mixture of solid, liquid, and gaseous hydrocarbons plus a few compounds of other elements. Natural gas is primarily a mixture of alkanes of one to four carbon atoms. In general, alkanes are gaseous if the compounds contain between 1 and 4 carbon atoms, liquid if they contain between 5 and 16 carbon atoms, and solid if they contain over 16 carbon atoms. The various hydrocarbons present in petroleum are isolated by a process known as fractional distillation.

One of the chief products of the fractional distillation of petroleum is gasoline. One measure of the quality of a gasoline is *octane number*. The octane number of a gasoline refers to how smoothly it burns. A high octane gasoline delivers power smoothly to the pistons. A low octane fuel burns too rapidly and causes the engine to "knock." Isooctane, 2,2,4-trimethylpentane, which has excellent combustion properties, was arbitrarily assigned an octane rating of 100. Normal heptane, *n*-heptane (C_7H_{16}), which causes considerable engine knocking, was assigned an octane rating of 0. Mixtures of these two compounds were burned in test engines to establish an "octane scale." That is, if a sample of gasoline has the same amount of knock as a 87 percent isooctane–13 percent heptane mixture, then that gasoline has an octane rating of 87.

$$CH_3-\underset{\underset{CH_3}{|}}{\overset{\overset{CH_3}{|}}{C}}-CH_2-\underset{\overset{CH_3}{|}}{CH}-CH_3 \qquad CH_3-CH_2-CH_3-CH_2-CH_2-CH_2-CH_3$$

isooctane *n*-heptane

A common additive to gasolines was tetraethyl lead, $Pb(C_2H_5)_4$. This substance reduced knocking and increased octane ratings of gasolines. However, it caused large amounts of lead compounds to be discharged into the air, with resulting hazards to human health. For that reason, unleaded fuels are now in common use.

Uses of Hydrocarbons

Methane is used for heating and cooking purposes both in the laboratory and in the home. Mineral oil is a mixture of saturated hydrocarbons and is used extensively in the hospital for lubricating purposes and also as a laxative. Rubber is also a hydrocarbon. Ethene (ethylene) and propene (propylene) have been used extensively to make plastics called polyethylene and polypropylene, respectively. Ethylene has been used as an anesthetic, but its popularity has declined since the introduction of neuromuscular blocking drugs. Acetylene has been employed by European surgeons as an anesthetic; however, the main use of acetylene (ethyne) in North America is for welding.

Polymers

When many small molecules are joined together to form a much larger molecule, the process is called **polymerization.** The product is called a polymer. Naturally occurring polymers include starch, cellulose, rubber, and protein. Synthetic polymers include plastics and man-made fibers such as

Organic Chemistry

Figure 16-4. Plastic container in use for an intravenous infusion. (Courtesy of American Hospital Supply Corporation, Evanston, IL.)

nylon, rayon, and dacron (see page 244). Medical uses of polymers include synthetic heart valves and blood vessels, surgical mesh, disposable syringes, and drug containers (see Figure 16-4).

The equation that follows indicates the formation of polyethylene from ethene (ethylene). Note that an initiator is required. This substance starts the reaction, which continues until a long chain is obtained. The number of units of ethylene joined together varies between 100 and 1000.

$$CH_2{=}CH_2 \xrightarrow[\text{initiator}]{\text{heat, pressure}} -(CH_2{-}CH_2){-}(CH_2{-}CH_2){-} \text{ etc. } \text{ or } (-CH_2{-}CH_2{-})_n$$

ethene
(ethylene)   polyethylene

If the starting material is propene (propylene), then the polymer produced is called polypropylene. If styrene is the starting material, polystyrene is produced. Likewise, polyvinyl chloride (PVC) is produced from vinyl chloride.

Summary   Hydrocarbons are organic compounds that contain the elements carbon and hydrogen only. The simplest hydrocarbon, the hydrocarbon containing only one carbon atom, is methane (CH_4). The hydrocarbon of two carbon atoms is called ethane; that of three carbon atoms, propane. These compounds are called alkanes. The general formula for alkanes is C_nH_{2n+2} where n is the number of carbon atoms. The

Hydrocarbons   **237**

names of all alkanes end in *-ane*. Beginning with pentane, the prefixes indicate the number of carbon atoms present.

When an alkane loses a hydrogen atom, it forms an alkyl group whose name ends in *-yl*. The alkyl group of one carbon atom, derived from methane, is called the methyl group (CH_3-). The alkyl group of two carbon atoms, derived from ethane, is called the ethyl group (C_2H_5-).

To identify and name a hydrocarbon compound, pick out the longest continuous chain of carbon atoms and name that chain. Then pick out the alkyl groups attached to that chain. Number the carbons, starting at whichever end of the chain will give alkyl groups with the smallest numbers. List the numbers and names of the alkyl groups, using prefixes to designate alkyl groups occurring more than once.

Alkanes that occur in the shape of a ring are called cycloalkanes.

Haloalkanes have one or more hydrogens of an alkane replaced by a halogen.

Alkenes have a double bond between two of the carbon atoms. The names of all alkenes end in *-ene*. The general formula for alkenes is C_nH_{2n}.

Alkynes have a triple bond between two of the carbon atoms and have the general formula C_nH_{2n-2}. The names of all alkynes end in *-yne*.

A saturated hydrocarbon has only single bonds between the carbon atoms. An unsaturated hydrocarbon has double or triple bonds between its carbon atoms. Saturated hydrocarbons react by a process known as substitution. Unsaturated hydrocarbons react by a process known as addition. The addition reaction is usually much more rapid than the substitution reaction.

The chief sources of hydrocarbons are petroleum and natural gas.

Polymers consist of many small molecules joined together. Examples are polyethylene and polypropylene.

Questions and Problems

A

1. Name the following compounds:
   (a) Alkane of five carbon atoms; of two carbon atoms.
   (b) Alkyne of four carbon atoms; of three carbon atoms.
   (c) Alkene of eight carbon atoms; of two carbon atoms.

2. Classify the following hydrocarbons as alkanes, alkenes, or alkynes.
   (a) C_3H_6 (b) C_9H_{20} (c) $C_{14}H_{26}$
   (d) C_3H_8 (e) $C_{22}H_{44}$ (f) $C_{45}H_{88}$
   (g) C_5H_8 (h) C_5H_{10}

3. What is an alkyl group? Name and draw the structure of the alkyl group derived from ethane.

4. Name the following compounds

   (a) $CH_3-CH_2-\underset{\underset{CH_3}{|}}{CH}-CH_2-CH_3$

   (b) $CH_3-\underset{\underset{CH_3}{|}}{CH}-\overset{\overset{CH_3}{|}}{CH}-CH_2-CH_2-CH_3$

   (c) $CH_3-\underset{\underset{CH_3}{|}}{CH}-CH_2-\underset{\underset{CH_3}{|}}{CH}-CH_2-\overset{\overset{CH_3}{|}}{CH}-CH_2-CH_3$

5. What does the term saturated refer to in hydrocarbons?

Organic Chemistry

6. What does the term unsaturated mean in terms of hydrocarbons?
7. How do saturated hydrocarbons react? Give an example of such a reaction.
8. How do unsaturated hydrocarbons react? Give an example of such a reaction.
9. What are the chief sources of hydrocarbons?
10. List several uses of hydrocarbons.

B 11. What is the IUPAC name for isooctane? Write the equation for its complete oxidation.
12. Draw the structures for (a) ethylcyclobutane, (b) 1,3-dichlorocyclobutane, (c) cyclopentane.
13. Draw structures for (a) 2-chloropropane, (b) *n*-pentane, (c) 2-iodo-2-methylbutane, (d) 1,3-dichloropropane.
14. What does the prefix *sec* refer to? Give an example.
15. Name the following compounds:

16. Compare complete and incomplete combustion of alkanes.
17. How are polymers formed? Give examples of uses of three different polymers.
18. Discuss the advantages and the disadvantages of the use of unleaded gasoline versus "ethyl" gas.

References   BAUM, STUART J. *Introduction to Organic and Biological Chemistry,* 3rd ed. Macmillan Publishing Company, New York, 1982, Chapters 2, 3, 5.

MORRISON, ROBERT T. and ROBERT N. BOYD. *Organic Chemistry,* 4th ed. Allyn and Bacon, Inc., Boston, 1983, Chapters 2, 3, 7, 8, 13.

SOLOMONS, T. W. GRAHAM. *Organic Chemistry,* 3rd ed. John Wiley & Sons, New York, 1984, Chapters 1–6.

ZIMMERMAN, HENRY and ISAAK ZIMMERMAN. *Elements of Organic Chemistry,* 2nd ed. Macmillan Publishing Company, New York, 1983, Chapters 2, 3, 4.

17 Alcohols and Ethers

CHAPTER
OUTLINE

Alcohols
  Uses
  Types
  Reactions

Thiols
Ethers
  Ether as an Anesthetic

Alcohols

A functional group is a particular arrangement of a few atoms that imparts certain characteristic properties to an organic molecule. Alcohols are derivatives of hydrocarbons in which one or more of the hydrogen atoms has been replaced by a hydroxyl (—OH) functional group. Other functional groups, which will be discussed in Chapter 18, are those of aldehydes, ketones, esters, acids, amines, and amides (see Appendix B).

In the IUPAC system, alcohols are named according to the longest continuous chain of carbon atoms. The ending **ane** is changed to **ol,** to indicate the functional group.

In the common system, alcohols are named by taking the name of the alkyl group and adding the word "alcohol."

Examples of the names of alcohols in these two systems are

$$CH_3-OH \qquad CH_3-CH_2-OH \qquad CH_3-\overset{\displaystyle |}{\underset{\displaystyle OH}{C}}H-CH_3$$

methanol	ethanol	2-propanol
(methyl alcohol)	(ethyl alcohol)	(isopropyl alcohol)

Although the IUPAC system is preferred by chemists, medical personnel usually refer to alcohols by their common names. We will do so in the following sections.

The general formula for an alcohol is **ROH,** where the R signifies an alkyl group attached to an —OH functional group.

Alcohols contain an —OH group that does not ionize. Because alcohols do not ionize, their reactions are much slower than those of inorganic bases, which contain a hydroxide ion (OH^-). Solutions of alcohols are nonelectrolytes; they are not bases. However, alcohols do react with acids to form a compound called an ester, which will be discussed in Chapter 18.

METHYL ALCOHOL

Methyl alcohol (methanol), CH_3OH, is commonly known as wood alcohol. It is used as a solvent in many industrial reactions. Methyl alcohol should never be applied directly to the body nor should the vapors be inhaled because this substance can be absorbed both through the skin and through the respiratory tract. Ingestion of as little as 15 ml of methyl alcohol can cause blindness and 30 ml can cause death.

Methyl alcohol can be prepared from the distillation of wood. It is prepared commercially from carbon monoxide.

$$CO + 2H_2 \xrightarrow[\text{heat}]{\text{Pt catalyst}} CH_3OH$$

ETHYL ALCOHOL

Ethyl alcohol (ethanol), CH_3CH_2OH, is known commonly as grain alcohol. In the hospital the word *alcohol* means ethyl alcohol.

One important property of ethyl alcohol is its ability to denature protein (see page 362). Because of this property, ethyl alcohol is widely used as an antiseptic. As an antiseptic, 70 percent alcohol is preferred to a stronger solution. It would seem that if 70 percent alcohol is a good antiseptic then 100 percent alcohol would be even better; however, the reverse is true. The 70 percent alcohol is actually a better antiseptic than the 100 percent alcohol.

Pure alcohol coagulates protein on contact. Suppose that pure alcohol is poured over a single-celled organism. The alcohol would penetrate the cell wall of that organism in all directions, coagulating the protein just inside of the cell wall, as shown in Figure 17–1. This ring of coagulated protein would then prevent the alcohol from penetrating farther into the cell so that no more coagulation would take place. At this time the cell would become dormant, but not dead. Under the proper conditions the organism can again begin to function. If 70 percent alcohol is poured over a single-celled organism, the diluted alcohol also coagulates the protein, but at a slower rate, so that it penetrates all the way through the cell before coagulation takes place.

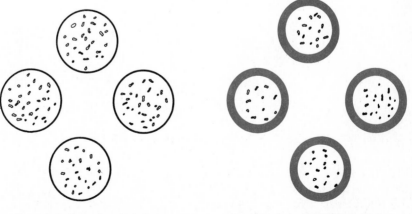

FIGURE 17–1. Effect of 100 percent alcohol on bacteria.

Bacteria before using alcohol

Bacteria after using 100% alcohol. Note that only outer layer is coagulated.

Alcohol and Ethers

Then all the cell proteins are coagulated and the organism dies (see Figure 17-2).

Alcohol (ethyl) may also be used for sponge baths to reduce the fever of a patient. When alcohol is placed on the skin it evaporates rapidly. In order to evaporate, alcohol requires heat. This heat comes from the patient's skin. Thus an alcohol sponge bath will remove heat from the patient's skin and so lower the body temperature. A water sponge bath will do the same thing, but water evaporates more slowly than alcohol and the heat removal is slower. However, water sponge baths are in common use in many hospitals because they are cheaper. Since alcohol is flammable it cannot be used in a room where oxygen is in use.

Alcohol is used as a solvent for many substances. Alcohol solutions are called tinctures. Tincture of iodine consists of iodine dissolved in alcohol.

Ethyl alcohol is also used as a beverage. The concentration of alcohol in alcoholic beverages is expressed as a "proof." The proof is twice the percentage of alcohol in the solution. Thus a beverage marked "100 proof" contains 50 percent alcohol. Alcohol slows reaction time so that driving under the influence of alcohol can be very dangerous. Alcohol is not a stimulant. It actually depresses the nervous system and can remove the normal inhibitions of a person. Excessive use of alcohol may cause the destruction of the liver, a condition known as cirrhosis.

Alcohol has a high tax rate because of its use as a beverage. For use in industry, substances are added to make the alcohol unfit for drinking. Such an alcohol is called **denatured.** It is not fit to drink but is still useful for industrial purposes. Common denaturants are wood alcohol, formaldehyde, and gasoline.

Alcohol (ethyl) can be prepared from the fermentation of blackstrap molasses, the residue that results from the purification of cane sugar. The prin-

FIGURE 17-2. Effect of 70 percent alcohol on bacteria.

Bacteria before using alcohol

Bacteria after using 70% alcohol. Note that bacterial protein is coagulated all the way through.

Organic Chemistry

ciple constituent of molasses is sucrose, $C_{12}H_{22}O_{11}$. The fermentation reaction is brought about by the enzymes present in yeast.

$$C_{12}H_{22}O_{11} + H_2O \xrightarrow{\text{enzymes}} 4C_2H_5OH + 4CO_2$$
sucrose   ethyl alcohol

The starches present in grains can be converted into sugar by malt. The sugar thus produced can be fermented, under the influence of the enzymes in yeast to yield ethyl alcohol. Hence the name grain alcohol.

Ethyl alcohol may also be prepared synthetically from ethene.

$$CH_2{=}CH_2 + H_2O \xrightarrow{\text{catalyst}} C_2H_5OH$$
ethene   ethyl alcohol

ISOPROPYL ALCOHOL   Isopropyl alcohol has the structural formula

isopropyl alcohol

The IUPAC name for this compound is 2-propanol, indicating that the —OH functional group is on the second carbon of a three-carbon chain. Isopropyl alcohol is toxic and should not be taken internally. Since it is not absorbed through the skin, it is commonly used as rubbing alcohol and as an astringent.*

GLYCEROL   Glycerol (sometimes called glycerin) is a trihydric or trihydroxy alcohol; it contains three —OH groups. Recall that an alcohol must contain at least one —OH group. A monohydric or monohydroxy alcohol contains one —OH group, a dihydric alcohol two. The structural formula for glycerol is

glycerol

The IUPAC name for glycerol is 1,2,3-propanetriol, since there is an —OH functional group on each carbon atom of the three-carbon chain.

Glycerol is an important alcohol in terms of body chemistry, especially as a constituent of fats (see Chapter 22). It is a byproduct of the manufacture of soap (see page 328), and is used in the preparation of cosmetics and hand lotions and also in suppositories. Glycerol is used in the laboratory as a lubricant for rubber tubing and stoppers. When treated with nitric acid, glycerin forms nitroglycerin, an explosive. Medicinally, nitroglycerin is used as a heart stimulant. It causes a dilation of the coronary arteries, thus increasing the supply of blood to the heart muscles.

ETHYLENE GLYCOL   The term glycol refers to compounds with two —OH functional groups. The structure of ethylene glycol is

$$CH_2—CH_2$$
$$\quad|\qquad|$$
$$OH\quad OH$$

Ethylene glycol is used in preparations to moisten the skin. It is also used as a permanent antifreeze in car radiators and as a raw material in the manufacture of the polymer Dacron. The IUPAC name for ethylene glycol is 1,2-ethanediol.

OTHER ALCOHOLS   Menthol is an example of a cyclic alcohol. It has a cooling, refreshing feeling when rubbed on the skin and so is a frequently used ingredient in cosmetics and shaving lotions. Menthol is used in cough drops and nasal sprays.

menthol

Other alcohols of biological importance are cholesterol, retinol (vitamin A), and tocopherol (vitamin E). These will be discussed later in appropriate chapters.

Types   A primary alcohol (**1°**) is one that contains an —OH functional group attached to a carbon that has one or no carbon atoms attached to it. All the

PRIMARY ALCOHOLS   structures in diagram (17–1) are primary alcohols.

(17–1)

Methyl alcohol (methanol) is an example of a primary alcohol in which the —OH functional group is attached to a carbon atom with no other carbons attached to it. Ethyl alcohol (ethanol) and propyl alcohol (propanol) are examples of primary alcohols in which the —OH functional group is attached to a carbon atom with one carbon atom attached to it. Note that in a primary alcohol the functional group (—OH) is at the end of the chain.

SECONDARY ALCOHOLS   A secondary alcohol (**2°**) is one in which the —OH is attached to a carbon atom having two other carbon atoms attached to it.

Organic Chemistry   **244**

$$CH_3-\underset{\underset{\textstyle OH}{|}}{CH}-CH_3$$

isopropyl alcohol, 2-propanol

Isopropyl alcohol is an example of a secondary alcohol. Note that in a secondary alcohol the functional group is not at the end of the chain.

TERTIARY ALCOHOLS   A tertiary alcohol (3°) is one in which the —OH is attached to a carbon atom having three carbon atoms attached to it.

$$CH_3-\underset{\underset{\textstyle OH}{|}}{\overset{\overset{\textstyle CH_3}{|}}{C}}-CH_3$$

2-methyl-2-propanol,
commonly known as
tertiary butyl alcohol

Reactions   In the presence of a dehydrating agent, such as H_2SO_4, alcohols may be dehydrated to form alkenes.

DEHYDRATION

ethanol   ethene

2-pentanol   1-pentene   2-pentene

FORMATION OF ETHERS   As will be shown in the next section, alcohols may also react in the presence of H_2SO_4 to form ethers.

OXIDATION   Primary alcohols may be oxidized to form aldehydes and then further oxidized to form acids and eventually CO_2 and H_2O. These reactions will be discussed in the next chapter. Some of these oxidation products are responsible for the toxicity of various alcohols.

$$\underset{\text{primary alcohol}}{ROH} \xrightarrow{\text{oxidation}} \underset{\text{aldehyde}}{RCHO} \xrightarrow{\text{oxidation}} \underset{\text{acid}}{RCOOH}$$

Secondary alcohols may be oxidized to yield ketones (see next chapter).

$$\underset{\text{secondary alcohol}}{ROH} \xrightarrow{\text{oxidation}} \underset{\text{ketone}}{RCOR}$$

Tertiary alcohols cannot be oxidized under ordinary conditions. Alcohols also react with organic acids to yield compounds called esters (see page 259).

Alcohol and Ethers   **245**

Thiols Thiols are sulfur analogs of alcohols and contain an —SH functional group in place of an —OH group. The IUPAC names of thiols are formed by adding the ending *-thiol* to the name of the parent hydrocarbon. The common name of thiols is formed by first naming the alkyl group and then adding the word mercaptan.

$$CH_3—SH \qquad\qquad CH_3—\underset{\underset{\textstyle SH}{|}}{CH}—CH_3$$

methanethiol   2-propanethiol
(methyl mercaptan) (isopropyl mercaptan)

Many thiols are found in nature and they have a disagreeable odor. When an onion is cut, 1-propanethiol is released; garlic owes its odor to the presence of thiols; and thiols are responsible for the odor given off by skunks. Since natural gas used for heating and cooking is odorless, thiols are added so that a gas leak may be easily detected.

Thiols may be prepared by heating alkyl halides with sodium hydrogen sulfide, NaHS.

$$CH_3—CH_2—CH_2—Cl + NaHS \longrightarrow CH_3—CH_2—CH_2—SH + NaCl$$

Thiols are easily oxidized to disulfides.

$$\underset{\text{a thiol}}{R—CH_2—SH} + O_2 \longrightarrow \underset{\text{a disulfide}}{R—CH_2—S—S—CH_2—R}$$

An example of such an oxidation is in the conversion of cysteine to cystine, a reaction that takes place when hair is given a "permanent" (see page 138).

$$2H—\underset{\underset{\textstyle NH_2}{|}}{\overset{\overset{\textstyle COOH}{|}}{C}}—CH_2—SH \underset{\text{reduction}}{\overset{\text{oxidation}}{\rightleftharpoons}} H—\underset{\underset{\textstyle NH_2}{|}}{\overset{\overset{\textstyle COOH}{|}}{C}}—CH_2—S—S—CH_2—\underset{\underset{\textstyle NH_2}{|}}{\overset{\overset{\textstyle COOH}{|}}{C}}—H$$

cysteine   cystine

Disulfide bonds are also involved in the formation of some proteins (see page 357).

Thiols (also called sulfhydryls) are also important in enzymes involved in carbohydrate metabolism.

Ethers An ether is formed during the dehydration of an alcohol. In this reaction the sulfuric acid may be considered as a dehydrating agent that removes water from two molecules of alcohol. Consider the following reaction, where R indicates an alkyl group and hence ROH indicates an alcohol.

$$\underset{\text{alcohol}}{R—OH} + \underset{\text{alcohol}}{HO—R} \overset{H_2SO_4}{\longrightarrow} \underset{\text{ether}}{R—O—R} + H_2O$$

This equation indicates that two molecules of alcohol (with the second molecular formula written backward) react in the presence of sulfuric acid to form water and an ether. When methyl alcohol is reacted with sulfuric acid, methyl ether (also called dimethyl ether) is formed.

$$CH_3-OH + HO-CH_3 \xrightarrow{H_2SO_4} CH_3-O-CH_3 + H_2O$$

methyl   methyl   methyl ether
alcohol   alcohol   (dimethyl ether)

When ethyl alcohol is treated with sulfuric acid, ethyl ether (also called diethyl ether) is formed.

$$CH_3-CH_2-OH + HO-CH_2-CH_3 \xrightarrow{H_2SO_4} CH_3-CH_2-O-CH_2-CH_3 + H_2O$$

ethyl alcohol   ethyl alcohol   ethyl ether
(diethyl ether)

The ether is named for the alcohol from which it is made: ethyl ether from ethyl alcohol and methyl ether from methyl alcohol. The general formula for an ether is **ROR.**

Under the IUPAC system, the $-OCH_3$ group is called methoxy and the $-OCH_2CH_3$ group is called ethoxy. Thus, methyl ether, CH_3-O-CH_3, is called methoxymethane and $CH_3-CH_2-O-CH_2-CH_3$, ethyl ether, is called ethoxyethane.

If two different alcohols are reacted, a mixed ether is formed. Mixed ethers are named as alkoxy derivatives of hydrocarbons with the shorter chain being named as the alkoxy group and the longer chain as the alkane.

Under the common system, mixed ethers are named by listing the alkyl groups followed by the word ether.

$$CH_3-O-CH_2-CH_3 \qquad CH_3-O-\underset{\underset{CH_3}{|}}{CH}-CH_3$$

methoxyethane   2-methoxypropane
(methyl ethyl ether)   (methyl isopropyl ether)

Recall from the previous section that alcohols react with H_2SO_4 to form alkenes. Here it is indicated that alcohols react with H_2SO_4 to form ethers. What causes two different reactions to take place? When alcohols react with H_2SO_4 at a temperature of 140°C, ethers are formed. At temperatures above 150°C, alkenes are formed.

Ethers have a low boiling point because the molecules do not form hydrogen bonds (see page 144). Ethers are good solvents because they are inert—they do not react with the solute. Ethyl ether is frequently used to extract organic material from naturally occurring substances. The low boiling point of the ether allows it to be easily removed and recovered. However, ethyl ether is very flammable and must be used with care. Ethers that remain in a laboratory for a long period of time may contain organic peroxides that are extremely explosive. Care must be taken that ethers are not allowed to stand undisturbed for a long period of time.

Ether As an   Ethyl ether, commonly known as ether, has been used quite extensively as a
Anesthetic   general anesthetic. It is very easy to administer, is an excellent muscular relaxant, and has very little effect upon the rate of respiration, blood pres-

sure, or pulse rate. However, the disadvantages of ether outweigh its advantages. It is very flammable, it is irritating to the membranes of the respiratory tract; and it has an aftereffect of nausea. Today ether is infrequently employed as a general anesthetic except in laboratory work. It has been replaced by such nonflammable anesthetics as nitrous oxide (see page 128) and halothane (see page 229).

Methoxyflurane, 2,2-dichloro-1,1-difluoroethylmethyl ether, has also been used as a general anesthetic, but its use has been discontinued in several hospitals because of its effects on renal function.

methoxyflurane

Divinyl ether has been used as a surgical anesthetic but is now obsolete for this purpose. The structure of divinyl ether is

divinyl ether

Summary   Alcohols are derivatives of hydrocarbons with one or more of the hydrogen atoms replaced by an —OH group. The —OH (hydroxyl) group is a functional group that imparts to alcohol its particular properties.

The general formula for an alcohol is ROH, where the R represents an alkyl group attached to the —OH group.

Alcohols do not ionize; they are not bases; their reactions are slower than those of inorganic hydroxides.

The simplest alcohol is methyl alcohol, CH_3OH, also known as methanol. This alcohol is poisonous and should never be used internally or externally.

Ethyl alcohol, C_2H_5OH, is also known as ethanol. It is used as a disinfectant because it has the property of coagulating protein. It may also be used for sponge baths to reduce body temperature. Solutions of medications in alcohol are called tinctures.

Isopropyl alcohol is used primarily as rubbing alcohol. It is toxic and should never be used internally.

Glycerol or glycerin is a trihydric alcohol; it has three —OH groups in its molecule. Glycerol is a constituent of fats.

Alcohols may be divided into three categories: primary, where the —OH group is attached to a carbon atom having one or no carbon atoms attached to it; secondary, where the —OH group is attached to a carbon atom having two carbon atoms attached to it; and tertiary, where the —OH is attached to a carbon atom having three carbon atoms attached to it.

Thiols are sulfur analog of alcohols and contain a —SH group.

Ethers are produced by the dehydration of an alcohol. Ethers are named according to the alcohol or alcohols from which they were produced.

Ethyl ether has been used as a general anesthetic. It is an excellent muscular relaxant and has little effect on the rate of respiration or pulse rate. However, ether is irritating to the membranes of the respiratory tract, it may cause nausea, and it is very flammable. It has been replaced by nonflammable, nonirritating anesthetics such as halothane and nitrous oxide.

Questions and Problems

A

1. What is the general formula for an alcohol?
2. Indicate several general properties of alcohols.
3. Draw the structure of (a) methyl alcohol; (b) ethyl alcohol; (c) isopropyl alcohol; (d) propyl alcohol; (e) glycerin. Give the IUPAC name for each.
4. Why should methyl alcohol never be used medicinally?
5. Explain why 70 percent alcohol is a better disinfectant than 100 percent alcohol.
6. Why is alcohol frequently used for sponge baths?
7. Why may water be substituted for alcohol in a sponge bath?
8. What is a tincture?
9. What is denatured alcohol? Where is it used?
10. What does the word "proof" mean in terms of alcohol?
11. How may alcohol be prepared commercially?
12. What is a common use for isopropyl alcohol?
13. Why is glycerol important in the body?
14. What is nitroglycerin used for in the body? How may it be prepared?
15. List the three types of alcohols and give an example of each.
16. How may an ether be prepared? What reagents are needed?
17. Write the equation for the formation of ethyl ether from ethyl alcohol.
18. What is a mixed ether? How may it be prepared?
19. List disadvantages of ether as a general anesthetic.

B

20. What is a functional group?
21. How is methyl alcohol produced commercially? ethyl alcohol?
22. Why does the dehydration of 2-pentanol produce two different products?
23. Complete the following reactions:

$$CH_3CH_2CH_2CH_2OH \xrightarrow[\text{low temp}]{H_2SO_4}$$

$$CH_3CH_2CH_2CH_2OH \xrightarrow[\text{high temp}]{H_2SO_4}$$

24. Name the following compounds according to both the IUPAC system and the common system.

(a) CH_3—O—CH_2CH_3

(b) CH_3CH_2—O—$CH_2CH_2CH_3$

(c) CH_3CH_2—O—$\underset{\underset{CH_3}{|}}{C}HCH_2CH_3$

(d) CH_3—O—CH_3

(e) CH_3—CH_2—SH

(f)

References

MORRISON, ROBERT T. and ROBERT N. BOYD. *Organic Chemistry,* 4th ed. Allyn and Bacon, Inc., Boston, 1983, Chapters 10, 11, 12.

SOLOMONS, T. W. GRAHAM. *Organic Chemistry,* 3rd ed. John Wiley & Sons, New York, 1984, Chapter 15.

ZIMMERMAN, HENRY and ISAAK ZIMMERMAN. *Elements of Organic Chemistry,* 2nd ed. Macmillan Publishing Company, New York, 1983, Chapters 7, 9.

18 Other Organic Compounds

CHAPTER
OUTLINE

Aldehydes
   Oxidation of a Primary Alcohol
   Uses of Aldehydes
   Test for Aldehydes
   Reactions of Aldehydes
Ketones
   Oxidation of a Secondary Alcohol
   Reactions of Ketones
Hemiacetals and Hemiketals
Organic Acids
   Oxidation of an Aldehyde

Properties and Reactions of Organic
   Acids
   Medically Important Organic Acids
Esters
   Thioesters
   Phosphate Esters
Amines
   Amino Acids
Amides

The oxidation of primary, secondary, and tertiary alcohols gives different types of products. If we consider oxidation as the removal of hydrogens (see page 132), then the oxidation of an alcohol may be said to involve the removal of one hydrogen from the —OH group of the alcohol and of a second hydrogen from the carbon atom to which the —OH group is attached. The oxidation of a primary alcohol may be written as

$$\underset{\text{primary alcohol}}{R-\overset{\displaystyle H}{\underset{\displaystyle H}{C}}-OH} + [O] \longrightarrow \underset{\text{aldehyde}}{R-\overset{\displaystyle H}{C}=O} + H_2O$$

The oxidation of an alcohol involves the use of some oxidizing agent such as $KMnO_4$, $K_2Cr_2O_7$, or CuO. However, for the sake of simplicity the oxidizing agent in the preceding and in the following reactions is simply listed as [O], which stands for any substance that will yield the oxygen needed for the reaction.

Aldehydes

Oxidation of a Primary Alcohol

Recall that a primary alcohol has the —OH functional group bonded to a carbon with one or no other carbon atom attached to it. The following equation indicates the oxidation of methyl alcohol, CH_3OH, a primary alcohol.

methyl alcohol   formaldehyde

Observe that, during the oxidation, one H was removed from the —OH group and another H from the carbon to which the —OH group was attached (the only carbon in this compound). Water is one product of this reaction; the other product is a new kind of compound called an aldehyde. In this example, the product is called formaldehyde. The formula for formaldehyde may also be written as HCHO.

The following reaction indicates the oxidation of ethyl alcohol (also a primary alcohol).

ethyl alcohol   acetaldehyde

The oxidation of ethyl alcohol, a primary alcohol, yields acetaldehyde, whose formula may also be written as CH_3CHO. In general,

$$\text{primary alcohol} \xrightarrow{\text{oxidation}} \text{aldehyde}$$

Aldehydes all have the —**CHO** group at the end of the chain. The general formula for an aldehyde is **RCHO,** which indicates that some alkyl group (R) is attached to a —CHO group at the end of the molecule.

The colored part of the following —CHO is called a **carbonyl group.** This group is also present in other types of compounds, as will be discussed in the following sections.

As we have seen, the oxidation of methyl alcohol, a primary alcohol of one carbon atom, yields an aldehyde of one carbon atom, HCHO, formaldehyde. The oxidation of ethyl alcohol, a primary alcohol of two carbon atoms, yields an aldehyde of two carbon atoms, CH_3CHO, acetaldehyde. Note that the term *aldehyde* comes from the words *al*cohol *dehyd*rogenation.

The IUPAC names for all aldehydes end in **al.** To name an aldehyde according to the IUPAC system, take the name of the longest chain containing the aldehyde group, drop the ending *e* and replace it with the ending *al.* Thus, the following aldehyde, which contains four carbons, is called butanal.

$$CH_3—CH_2—CH_2—CHO$$

The aldehyde group is always at the end of the chain, at carbon 1, with that number being understood and not written, as indicated in the following compound.

Other Organic Compounds   **251**

$$CH_3-\underset{\underset{\displaystyle Cl}{|}}{CH}-CH_2-CH_2-CHO$$

4-chloropentanal

Table 18–1 compares the IUPAC and common names for some simple aldehydes.

TABLE 18–1. Comparison of the Names of Some Aldehydes

Condensed Structural Formula	IUPAC Name	Common Name
HCHO	Methanal	Formaldehyde
CH_3CHO	Ethanal	Acetaldehyde
CH_3-CH_2-CHO	Propanal	Propionaldehyde
$CH_3-\underset{\underset{\displaystyle CH_3}{|}}{CH}-CHO$	2-Methylpropanal	Isobutyraldehyde

Uses of Aldehydes   Formaldehyde is a colorless gas with a very sharp odor. It is used in the laboratory as a water solution containing about 40 percent formaldehyde. The 40 percent solution, commonly known as formalin, is an effective germicide for the disinfection of excreta, rooms, and clothing. Formalin hardens protein, making it very insoluble in water. It is used in embalming fluids and also as a preservative for biologic specimens. Formaldehyde solutions should not be used directly on the patient or even in the room with the patient because of irritating fumes.

Formaldehyde and its oxidation product, formic acid, are primarily responsible for the systemic toxicity of methyl alcohol.

Glutaraldehyde is superior to formaldehyde as a sterilizing agent and is gradually replacing it. Glutaraldehyde is microcidal against all microorganisms, including spores and viruses. Glutaraldehyde does not have the disagreeable odor that formaldehyde does and it is less irritating to the eyes and skin.

Paraldehyde is formed by the polymerization (joining) of three molecules of acetaldehyde. Paraldehyde depresses the central nervous system. It is used as an hypnotic—a sleep producer. Paraldehyde is also used in the treatment of alcoholism (see following paragraph). In therapeutic dosages it is nontoxic; it does not depress heart action or respiration. Its disadvantages are its disagreeable taste and its unpleasant odor.

glutaraldehyde   glyceraldehyde (2,3-dihydroxypropanal)   paraldehyde

Organic Chemistry   **252**

Acetaldehyde (ethanal) is responsible for many of the unpleasant side effects of ethyl alcohol consumption. The drug Antabuse, used to treat alcoholics, functions by increasing the concentration of acetaldehyde in the body.

Another aldehyde, glyceraldehyde, is an important component in the metabolism of carbohydrates (see page 402).

Test for Aldehydes   In general aldehydes are good reducing agents. Laboratory tests for the presence of aldehydes are based on their ability to reduce copper (II) or cupric ions to form copper (I) or cuprous oxide. When an aldehyde is heated with Benedict's or Fehling's solution or treated with a Clinitest tablet (all of which contain Cu^{2+} complex ion) a red precipitate of copper (I) or cuprous oxide (Cu_2O) is formed. This is actually the test for glucose (sugar) in urine since glucose is an aldehyde (see page 309).

Another laboratory test for the presence of an aldehyde involves the use of Tollen's reagent, which contains an Ag^+ complex ion. In this test, the presence of an aldehyde causes the formation of a bright, shiny mirror on the inside of the test tube. Hence the name "silver mirror test" (see page 310).

Reactions of Aldehydes

OXIDATION   Aldehydes can be oxidized to form acids, a type of reaction that will be discussed later in this chapter.

$$RCHO + [O] \longrightarrow RCOOH$$
aldehyde   acid

Note that this type of oxidation involves the addition of an oxygen (see page 132).

Aldehydes can be oxidized by $Cu(OH)_2$, according to the following reaction.

$$RCHO + Cu(OH)_2 \longrightarrow RCOOH + Cu_2O\downarrow + H_2O$$

This is the basis of the test for an aldehyde that was discussed in the previous section.

REDUCTION   Aldehydes may be reduced to the corresponding primary alcohols.

$$RCHO + [H] \longrightarrow RCH_2OH$$
aldehyde   primary alcohol

This is the reverse of the reaction whereby a primary alcohol was oxidized to yield an aldehyde.

Ketones

Oxidation of a Secondary Alcohol   Recall that a secondary alcohol is one in which the —OH group is bonded to a carbon atom having two carbon atoms attached to it. Isopropyl alcohol is an example of a secondary alcohol.

$$CH_3-\underset{\underset{OH}{|}}{\overset{\overset{H}{|}}{C}}-CH_3$$

isopropyl alcohol, 2-propanol

The oxidation of isopropyl alcohol is indicated by the following equation

isopropyl alcohol,
2-propanol

acetone
propanone

As before, the oxygen atom from the oxidizing agent reacts with the H from the —OH group and with the H attached to the same carbon as the —OH group, forming water and a new class of compounds called ketones.

The oxidation of a secondary alcohol yields a ketone, of the general formula **RCOR**. That is, a ketone has two alkyl groups attached to a $>C=O$ or a **carbonyl group.** This carbonyl group is present in both aldehydes and ketones. However, the carbonyl group is at the end of the chain in an aldehyde and not at the end in a ketone.

aldehyde   ketone

In the IUPAC system, the names of ketones end in **-one.** To name a ketone according to this system, take the name of the longest alkane containing the carbonyl group, drop the ending *e*, and add *one*. Thus, the following compound is called butanone.

$$CH_3-\underset{\underset{O}{\|}}{C}-CH_2-CH_3$$

butanone

In the common system for naming ketones, each alkyl group attached to the carbonyl group is named and the word ketone is added afterward. Thus the name of the preceding compound, according to the common system, is methyl ethyl ketone, since there is a methyl group attached to one end of the carbonyl group and an ethyl group attached to the other end.

Table 18–2 gives both common and IUPAC names of several ketones.

Acetone (propanone) is the simplest ketone. Acetone is a good solvent for fats and oils. It is also frequently used in fingernail polish and in polish remover. Acetone is normally present in small amounts in the blood and urine. In diabetes mellitus it is present in larger amounts in the blood and urine and even in the expired air. Dihydroxyacetone is an intermediate in carbohydrate metabolism.

$$HO-CH_2-\underset{\underset{O}{\|}}{\overset{\overset{O}{\|}}{C}}-CH_2-OH$$

dihydroxyacetone

TABLE 18-2. Names of Some Simple Ketones

Structure	IUPAC	Common Name
$CH_3-\overset{\overset{\displaystyle }{\|}}{\underset{\underset{\displaystyle O}{}}{C}}-CH_3$	Propanone	Dimethyl ketone (commonly known as acetone)
$CH_3-\overset{\|}{\underset{O}{C}}-CH_2-CH_3$	Butanone	Methyl ethyl ketone
$CH_3-\overset{\|}{\underset{O}{C}}-CH_2-CH_2-CH_3$	2-Pentanone	Methyl propyl ketone
$CH_3-CH_2-\overset{\|}{\underset{O}{C}}-CH_2-CH_3$	3-Pentanone	Diethyl ketone

Reactions of Ketones

What happens when a ketone is oxidized? Consider the formula for a ketone, acetone

$$CH_3-\overset{\|}{\underset{O}{C}}-CH_3$$

acetone

There are no hydrogen atoms on the carbon atom of the carbonyl group. Therefore, ketones are not easily oxidized. They are normally unreactive. Ketones give a negative test with such reducing agents as Benedict's solution or Clinitest tablets. Recall that aldehydes give a positive test with these reagents.

The test for acetone and ketone bodies makes use of the reaction between sodium nitroprusside and ketones or ketone bodies to produce a lavender color.

Hemiacetals and Hemiketals

The reaction of an aldehyde or a ketone with an alcohol yields compounds known as hemiacetals* or hemiketals,* respectively.

These types of compounds are important in discussing the structures of monosaccharides (see page 306).

If a hemiacetal or hemiketal reacts with a second molecule of alcohol, an acetal* or ketal,* respectively, is formed. These structures are important in disaccharides and polysaccharides (pages 312–313, 317–318).

Organic Acids

Oxidation of an Aldehyde

The oxidation of a primary alcohol yields an aldehyde. Aldehydes in turn can be easily oxidized. When an aldehyde is oxidized, the reaction is

$$\underset{\text{acetaldehyde}}{CH_3\overset{\displaystyle H}{\underset{}{C}}=O} + [O] \longrightarrow \underset{\text{acetic acid}}{CH_3\overset{\displaystyle OH}{\underset{}{C}}=O} \qquad (\text{also written as } CH_3COOH)$$

The resulting compound is acidic because it yields hydrogen ions in solution. (Note that this reaction involved oxidation because of a gain in oxygen—see page 132).

The functional group of an organic acid is —**COOH,** so that the oxidation of an aldehyde to an acid may be written functionally as

$$\underset{\text{aldehyde}}{R\text{—CHO}} \xrightarrow{[O]} \underset{\text{acid}}{R\text{—COOH}}$$

The oxidation of methyl alcohol, a primary alcohol, to an aldehyde and then to an acid is illustrated in the following equations

Primary alcohols may also be oxidized directly to acids.

The IUPAC names for acids end in **-oic acid.** To name an acid according to the IUPAC system, take the longest alkane containing the acid group, drop the ending *e* and add *oic acid*. Thus, formula 18–1 shows ethanoic acid.

$$CH_3-\overset{\displaystyle O}{\underset{\displaystyle \|}{C}}-OH$$

(18–1)

ethanoic acid

The common names of acids are derived from the names of the aldehyde from which they may be prepared. Thus formula (18–1), derived from acetaldehyde, is called acetic acid.

The general formula for an acid is **RCOOH.** All organic acids contain at least one —COOH group. This group is called the **carboxyl group** and it is this group that yields hydrogen ions.

Table 18–3 gives the common and IUPAC names of several common acids.

TABLE 18-3. Names of Common Acids

Formula	IUPAC Name	Common Name
HCOOH	Methanoic acid	Formic acid
CH_3COOH	Ethanoic acid	Acetic acid
CH_3CH_2COOH	Propanoic acid	Propionic acid
$CH_3CH_2CH_2COOH$	Butanoic acid	Butyric acid

Properties and Reactions of Organic Acids

Most organic acids are relatively weak acids since they ionize only slightly in water.

$$CH_3COOH \rightleftharpoons H^+ + CH_3COO^-$$

acetic acid   hydrogen ion   acetate ion

Organic acids react with bases to form salts and water. The general formula for the reaction of an organic acid with a base to form a salt and water may be written as follows:

$$RCOOH + NaOH \rightleftharpoons RCOONa + H_2O$$

organic acid   base   organic salt   water

$$CH_3COOH + NaOH \rightleftharpoons CH_3COONa + H_2O$$

acetic acid   sodium hydroxide   sodium acetate (a salt)   water

Organic acids containing few carbon atoms are soluble in water. As the length of the carbon chain increases, the solubility in water decreases.

Organic acids also react with alcohols to form a class of compounds called esters, which will be dealt with later in this chapter.

Medically Important Organic Acids

Formic acid, HCOOH, is a colorless liquid with a sharp irritating odor. Formic acid is found in the sting of bees and ants and causes the characteristic pain and swelling when it is injected into the tissues. It is one of the strongest organic acids.

Acetic acid, CH_3COOH, is one of the components of vinegar, where it is usually found as a 4 to 5 percent solution. Anhydrous acetic acid freezes at 17°C and then looks like a chunk of ice. For this reason it is called *glacial acetic acid*. Acetic acid can be made by the oxidation of ethyl alcohol. The

acetyl group, $CH_3C—$, derived from acetic acid, is very important in metabolic reactions.

Citric acid is found in citrus fruits. Its formula indicates that it is an alcohol as well as an acid. Citric acid contains one alcohol (—OH) group and three acid (—COOH) groups. It is an example of a tricarboxylic acid.

citric acid

Magnesium citrate, a salt of citric acid, is used as a cathartic (a medication for stimulating the evacuation of bowels). Sodium citrate, another salt of citric acid, is used as a blood anticoagulant. (It removes Ca^{2+} from the blood.)

Lactic acid is found in sour milk. It is formed from the fermentation of milk sugar, lactose. Its formula is

lactic acid

Lactic acid is also both an acid and an alcohol. It is formed whenever the body produces energy anaerobically (see page 400).

Oxalic acid is another one of the strong, naturally occurring organic acids. Its formula is

oxalic acid

Oxalic acid is used to remove stains, particularly rust and potassium permanganate stains, from clothing. It is poisonous when taken internally. Oxalate salts also prevent clotting by removing Ca^{2+} from the blood. However, oxalate can only be used for blood samples that are to be analyzed in the laboratory because these salts are poisonous and cannot be added directly to the bloodstream.

Pyruvic acid is produced during the anaerobic oxidation of glucose (see page 405). It is a keto acid.

pyruvic acid

In muscle, pyruvic acid is reduced to lactic acid. In the tissues, pyruvic acid is changed to acetyl coenzyme A, which then enters the citric acid cycle (page 405).

Tartaric acid is another one of the organic acids that is both an acid and an alcohol. Its formula is written as

tartaric acid

Tartaric acid is found in several fruits, particularly grapes. Potassium hydrogen tartrate, an acid salt called cream of tartar, is used in making baking powders. Rochelle salts, or potassium sodium tartrate, is used as a mild cathartic. Antimony potassium tartrate, known as tartar emetic, is used in the treatment of schistosomiasis (a disease caused by a type of parasitic flatworm), but its use is inadvisable in the presence of severe hepatic, renal, or cardiac insufficiency.

Stearic acid is a solid greaselike acid that is insoluble in water. It is an example of a fatty acid. Its formula is $C_{17}H_{35}COOH$. The sodium salt of stearic acid, sodium stearate, is a commonly used soap.

$$C_{17}H_{35}COOH + NaOH \longrightarrow C_{17}H_{35}COONa + H_2O$$

stearic acid   sodium stearate

Esters Esters are produced by the reaction of an organic acid with an alcohol and have the general formula

$$RCOOR' \quad \text{or} \quad R\overset{\displaystyle O}{\overset{\|}{C}}OR'$$

The general reaction of an alcohol with an acid is illustrated by the following equation (where R and R' may be the same or different alkyl groups).

$$RCOOH + R'OH \rightleftharpoons RCOOR' + H_2O$$

acid   alcohol   ester   water

Note that the reaction is written with a double arrow, indicating that it is an equilibrium reaction; that is, the reverse reaction also takes place. Thus,

Other Organic Compounds

TABLE 18-4. Names of Several Common Esters

Ester	Acid Part
$H-\overset{O}{\underset{\|\|}{C}}-O-CH_2-CH_3$	$H-\overset{O}{\underset{\|\|}{C}}-OH$
$CH_3-\overset{O}{\underset{\|\|}{C}}-O-CH_3$	$CH_3-\overset{O}{\underset{\|\|}{C}}-OH$
$CH_3-CH_2-\overset{O}{\underset{\|\|}{C}}-O-CH_2-CH_3$	$CH_3-CH_2-\overset{O}{\underset{\|\|}{C}}-OH$
$CH_3-CH_2-CH_2-\overset{O}{\underset{\|\|}{C}}-CH_2-CH_2-CH_3$	$CH_3-CH_2-CH_2-\overset{O}{\underset{\|\|}{C}}-OH$

esters hydrolize to form organic acids and alcohols. Esters do not readily ionize in water solution.

When an organic acid reacts with an alcohol, the name of the ester is determined as follows:

IUPAC Name

1. Write the name of the alkyl group of the alcohol
2. Write the name of the acid minus the ending *-ic*
3. Add the ending *-ate* to the name of the acid

Common Name

1. Write the name of the alcohol
2. Write the name of the acid minus the ending *-ic*
3. Add the ending *-ate* to the name of the acid

An example is given in reaction (18–2).

$$CH_3-\overset{O}{\underset{\|\|}{C}}-OH + HOCH_3 \rightleftharpoons CH_3-\overset{O}{\underset{\|\|}{C}}-OCH_3 + H_2O \quad (18-2)$$

ethanoic acid (acetic acid)   methanol (methyl alcohol)   methyl ethanoate (methyl acetate)

Consider reaction 18–3 between ethyl alcohol and formic acid.

$$H-\overset{O}{\underset{\|\|}{C}}-OH + HO-CH_2-CH_3 \rightleftharpoons H-\overset{O}{\underset{\|\|}{C}}-O-CH_2-CH_3 + H_2O \quad (18-3)$$

formic acid   ethyl alcohol   ethyl formate

In reactions (18–2) and (18–3), the acid loses the —OH group and the alcohol an —H. This may be indicated in diagram (18–4) of the structure of an ester.

$$R-\overset{O}{\underset{\|\|}{C}}\!\!\mid\!\!O\!-\!R' \quad (18-4)$$

acid part | alcohol part

Organic Chemistry

TABLE 18-4. (*Continued*)

Alcohol Part	IUPAC Name	Common Name
CH_3—CH_2OH	Ethyl methanoate	Ethyl formate
CH_3OH	Methyl ethanoate	Methyl acetate
CH_3—CH_2OH	Ethyl propanoate	Ethyl propionate
CH_3—CH_2—CH_2—OH	Propyl butanoate	Propyl butyrate

Table 18–4 shows the derivation and compares the common and IUPAC names of several common esters.

Esters are important as solvents, perfumes, and flavoring agents. Table 18–5 indicates some of the esters used in preparing synthetic flavors. Many esters are also used medicinally (see Table 18–6).

The hydrolysis of esters takes place in the body when fats and oil are digested. The reaction, in general, is

$$RCOOR' + H_2O \xrightarrow{\text{enzymes}} RCOOH + R'OH$$

This type of reaction will be discussed in Chapter 22.

TABLE 18-5. Esters and Synthetic Flavors

Ester	Flavor
Amyl acetate	Banana
Ethyl butyrate	Pineapple
Amyl butyrate	Apricot
Isoamyl acetate	Pear
Octyl acetate	Orange

TABLE 18-6. Some Medical Uses of Esters

Esters	Use
Ethyl aminobenzoate (benzocaine)	Local anesthetic
Glyceryl trinitrate (nitroglycerin)	Used to dilate coronary arteries and lower blood pressure
Methyl salicylate (oil of wintergreen)	Used as a flavoring agent and also as a counterirritant in many liniments
Phenyl mercuric acetate	Used to disinfect instruments and as an antiseptic on cutaneous and mucosal surfaces

Other Organic Compounds

Thioesters Thioesters have the general formula

$$\text{R}\text{—}\overset{\displaystyle O}{\overset{\displaystyle \|}{\text{C}}}\text{—S—R}'$$

where the prefix *thio* indicates the presence of a sulfur atom (see page 246). Many thioesters are found in biologic systems. The most important of these is acetyl coenzyme A, abbreviated acetyl CoA. Acetyl CoA is a key compound in metabolic reactions in the body. Acetyl coenzyme A is involved in the formation of fats (page 417), ketone bodies (page 419), and amino acids.

The structure of acetyl CoA is abbreviated as

$$\text{CH}_3\text{—}\overset{\displaystyle O}{\overset{\displaystyle \|}{\text{C}}}\text{—S—CoA}$$

The complete structure of acetyl CoA is given on page 375.

Phosphate Esters When an organic compound containing an —OH group reacts with phosphoric acid (H_3PO_4), phosphate esters are formed. Phosphate esters serve many important functions in the body. They are present in

Adenosine triphosphate (ATP), adenosine diphosphate (ADP), and adenosine monophosphate (AMP), the body's energy compounds.

Cyclic adenosine monophosphate (*c*-AMP), a chemical messenger that regulates cellular enzymes.

Deoxyribonucleic acid (DNA) and ribonucleic acid (RNA), the hereditary material of the cell.

Phospholipids, which are found in cell membranes and also in all tissue, particularly brain, liver, and spinal.

Phosphorylases, enzymes involved in the adding of phosphate groups to carbohydrates.

These uses of phosphate esters will be discussed later in appropriate chapters.

Amines Amines are organic compounds derived from ammonia. There are three classes of amines: primary, secondary, and tertiary. Note that in relation to amines, the terms primary, secondary, and tertiary refer directly to the number of hydrogen atoms of ammonia that have been replaced by alkyl groups. In the case of alcohols, the terms primary, secondary, and tertiary refer to the number of carbon atoms attached to the carbon having the —OH group on it.

Primary amines are those in which one of the hydrogen atoms of ammonia (NH_3) has been replaced by an alkyl group. Primary amines have the general formula RNH_2.

Secondary amines are those in which two of the hydrogen atoms of the ammonia have been replaced by alkyl groups. Secondary amines have the general formula R_2NH.

Tertiary amines are those in which all three hydrogen atoms of the ammonia have been replaced by alkyl groups. Tertiary amines have the general formula R_3N.

The common system names amines by placing the name of the alkyl group before the word amine. If two or three identical alkyl groups are present, the prefixes di- or tri- are used, as indicated in Table 18–7. The common system is used primarily for simple compounds. For more complex compounds, the IUPAC system is used. With this system, the prefix **amino** is used to denote the presence of an —NH_2 group.

The following compounds illustrate the IUPAC names for some amino compounds (common names in parentheses)

2-aminopropane   2-aminoethanoic acid
(isopropyl amine)   (aminoacetic acid)

Among the amines that are found in the body or are used medicinally are

TABLE 18–7. Some Common Amines

Name	Formula	Example

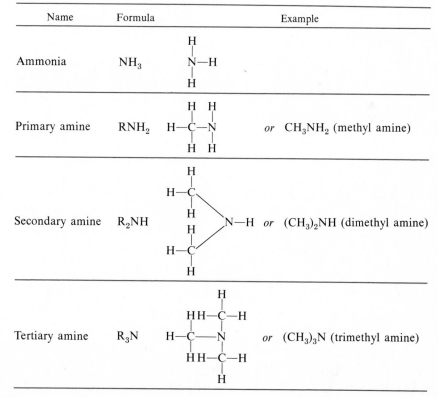

histamines (page 431), barbiturates (pages 289–290), psychedelics (page 291), amphetamines (page 290), and nucleic acids (page 526).

Amines produced during the decay of once-living matter include putrescine and cadaverine (page 431).

$$\underset{\substack{|\\ NH_2}}{CH_2}-CH_2-CH_2-\underset{\substack{|\\ NH_2}}{CH_2} \qquad \underset{\substack{|\\ NH_2}}{CH_2}-CH_2-CH_2-CH_2-\underset{\substack{|\\ NH_2}}{CH_2}$$

putrescine
1,4-diaminobutane   cadaverine
1,5-diaminopentane

When amines react with an acid such as hydrochloric acid, ammonium salts are produced. These ammonium salts are frequently named by placing the word hydrochloride after the name of the amine. Examples are thiamine hydrochloride (vitamin B_1) and procaine hydrochloride (Novocain, a local anesthetic). The hydrochlorides are administered rather than the amines themselves because they are more soluble in water.

Amines in general are basic compounds. They react with inorganic acids to form salts. Recall that one definition of a base is "a substance that accepts protons (H^+) (see page 133). Compare the following reactions of ammonia and amines with HCl, the reaction of a base with an acid to form a salt.

$$NH_3 + HCl \longrightarrow NH_4^+ + Cl^-$$
$$RNH_2 + HCl \longrightarrow RNH_3^+ + Cl^-$$
$$R_2NH + HCl \longrightarrow R_2NH_2^+ + Cl^-$$
$$R_3N + HCl \longrightarrow R_3NH^+ + Cl^-$$

Quaternary ammonium salts are formed by the action of tertiary amines with organic halogen compounds. An example of this type of reaction is that between trimethyl amine and methyl iodide. Tetramethyl ammonium iodide is formed.

trimethyl   methyl   tetramethyl
amine   iodide   ammonium
iodide

Some quaternary ammonium salts have both a detergent action and antibacterial activity. They are used medicinally as antiseptics. Benzalkonium chloride (zephiran chloride) is used in 0.1 percent solution for storage of sterilized instruments. A 0.01 to 0.02 percent solution is applied as a wet dressing to denuded areas. A 0.005 percent solution is used for irrigations of the bladder and the urethra.

Amino Acids Amino acids are organic acids that contain an amine group. Examples of amino acids are

glycine, an
α-amino acid

an α-amino
acid

a β-amino
acid

Note that Greek letters are used to designate the position of the amino group in the chain. The carbon atom next to the acid group, the —COOH group, is called the alpha (α) carbon. Then next in order comes the beta (β), the gamma (γ), and the delta (δ) carbon atoms.

Amino acids contain an acid group, —COOH, which naturally is acidic. Amino acids also contain an —NH₂ group, which is basic (see page 264). Thus, amino acids exhibit both acidic and basic properties; amino acids can react with either acids or bases. Compounds that can act as, or react with, either acids or bases are called **amphoteric compounds.**

α-Amino acids are the building blocks of proteins. That is, proteins are polymers of α-amino acids (see Chapter 23).

Amides   Organic acids can react with ammonia or with amines to form a class of compounds called amides. Amides have a bond between the carbonyl group (—C=O) and the nitrogen.

$$R-\overset{\overset{O}{\parallel}}{C}-OH + H-\overset{\overset{H}{|}}{N}-H \xrightarrow{\text{heat}} R-\overset{\overset{O}{\parallel}}{C}-NH_2 + H_2O$$

acid   ammonia   amide

Amides are named as follows:

IUPAC system

1. Drop ending *-oic* and the word acid from the name of the acid
2. Add *amide*

Common System

1. Drop ending *-ic* and the word acid from the name of the acid
2. Add *amide*

For example,

ethanoic acid   ammonia   ethanamide
(acetic acid)   (ammonia)   (acetamide)

If an organic acid reacts with a primary or secondary amine, a substituted amide is formed.

acid   primary   a substituted
                  amine   amide

$$H-\overset{\overset{\displaystyle O}{\|}}{C}-OH + H-\overset{\displaystyle H}{\underset{}{N}}-CH_2-CH_3 \longrightarrow H-\overset{\overset{\displaystyle O}{\|}}{C}-\overset{\displaystyle H}{\underset{}{N}}-CH_2-CH_3 + H_2O$$

methanoic acid   ethyl amine   N-ethylmethanamide
(formic acid)   (ethyl amine)   (N-ethylformamide)

$$CH_3-\overset{\overset{\displaystyle O}{\|}}{C}-OH + H-\overset{\displaystyle CH_3}{\underset{}{N}}-CH_3 \longrightarrow CH_3-\overset{\overset{\displaystyle O}{\|}}{C}-\overset{\displaystyle CH_3}{\underset{}{N}}-CH_3 + H_2O$$

ethanoic acid   dimethyl amine   N,N-dimethylethanamide
(acetic acid)   (dimethyl amine)   (N,N-dimethylacetamide)

Alkyl groups attached to the nitrogen are indicated by the letter N.

If two amino acids combine with the acid part of one reacting with the amine part of the other, the following type of reaction may occur.

$$R-\underset{\underset{\displaystyle NH_2}{|}}{CH}-\overset{\overset{\displaystyle O}{\|}}{C}-OH + H-\overset{\displaystyle H}{\underset{\underset{\displaystyle R}{|}}{N}}-CH-COOH$$

amino acid   amino acid

$$R-\underset{\underset{\displaystyle NH_2}{|}}{CH}-\overset{\overset{\displaystyle O}{\|}}{C}-\overset{\displaystyle H}{\underset{\underset{\displaystyle R}{|}}{N}}-CH-COOH + H_2O$$

a peptide

These two amino acids are said to be linked by a peptide (amide) bond. Compounds of this type will be discussed in Chapter 23.

Niacin, one of the B vitamins, is administered as an amide, niacinamide. Urea, one of the metabolic products of protein metabolism, may be considered as the diamide of carbonic acid.

$$HO-\overset{\overset{\displaystyle O}{\|}}{C}-OH \qquad H_2N-\overset{\overset{\displaystyle O}{\|}}{C}-NH_2$$

carbonic acid   urea

Summary   During the oxidation of an alcohol, the oxygen atom reacts with the H from the —OH group and with a hydrogen attached to the same carbon that has the —OH group.

The oxidation of a primary alcohol yields an aldehyde. Aldehydes contain the —CHO group and have the general formula RCHO. The aldehyde of one carbon atom is known as formaldehyde or methanal; that of two carbon atoms, as acetaldehyde or ethanal. A water solution of formaldehyde, known as formalin, is commonly used as a germicide. Paraldehyde, formed by polymerizing molecules of acetaldehyde, depresses the central nervous system.

Aldehydes are good reducing agents. When an aldehyde is heated with $Cu(OH)_2$, a red precipitate of Cu_2O is formed.

The oxidation of a secondary alcohol yields a ketone. A ketone may not be further oxidized without decomposing it. Likewise, tertiary alcohols are not easily oxidized.

The oxidation of an aldehyde yields an acid. The general formula for an acid is RCOOH. The —COOH group, called the carboxyl group, furnishes hydrogen ions and so causes the acidic properties. Organic acids react with bases to form organic salts.

Formic acid, HCOOH, is found in the sting of bees. Acetic acid, CH_3COOH, is one of the components of vinegar. Citric acid is found in citrus fruits, lactic acid in milk.

When an organic acid reacts with an alcohol, a compound called an ester is produced. Esters have the general formula RCOOR′. Esters are named according to the alcohol and the acid from which they were made.

Amines are organic compounds in which an alkyl group has replaced one or more of the hydrogen atoms of ammonia, NH_3. Amines are basic compounds and readily form salts.

Amino acids are organic acids that contain an amine group. α-Amino acids are the building blocks of protein.

Amides are formed by the reaction of an organic acid with ammonia or with an amine. Amino acids are held together by peptide (amide) bonds.

Questions and Problems

A

1. Write the equation for the oxidation of methyl alcohol. What product is formed?
2. Write the equation for the formation of acetaldehyde from ethyl alcohol.
3. What is the general formula for an aldehyde?
4. What does the suffix -al indicate?
5. What does the suffix -one indicate?
6. Indicate some uses for formaldehyde.
7. What is paraldehyde? What is it used for?
8. Describe the test for aldehydes.
9. Write the reaction for the oxidation of isopropyl alcohol.
10. The oxidation of a primary alcohol yields what type of compound?
11. The oxidation of a secondary alcohol yields what type of product?
12. Describe the oxidation of a tertiary alcohol; of a ketone.
13. Write the equation for the oxidation of formaldehyde and name the product.
14. Write the equation for the oxidation of acetaldehyde and name the product.
15. What is the general formula for an acid?
16. Write the equation for the reaction between formic acid and potassium hydroxide.
17. Name several organic acids and indicate where each can be found.
18. What is an ester? Indicate its general formula.
19. Write the equation for the reaction between formic acid and ethyl alcohol. Name the product.
20. Name and give the medical use of two esters.
21. What is an amine? Compare the structures of primary, secondary, and tertiary amines.
22. How do the terms *primary, secondary,* and *tertiary* for amines compare with the usage of these same terms for alcohols?
23. What is an amino acid? What properties does it have?
24. For what purposes does the body use amino acids?
25. Why are amino acids amphoteric?
26. What is the type structure for an amide?
27. Write the reaction when formic acid and ammonia are heated. What is the name of the product?
28. What is a peptide bond? Where is it found?
29. Why is urea called a diamide?

Other Organic Compounds 267

B **30.** In what type of compounds is a carbonyl group present?

31. Name the following compounds according to the IUPAC system.

(a) $CH_3-CH-CH_2-C=O$ with H above the C and Cl below the first CH

(b) $Cl-C-C-OH$ with Cl and O above, Cl below

(c) $CH_3-CH-CH_2-C=O$ with CH_3 below the first CH and H below the C

(d) $CH_3-C-CH-CH_3$ with CH_3 above and O below the C

(e) $CH_3-CH-C-OH$ with O above the C and NH_2 below the CH

(f) $CH_3-CH_2-C-CH-CH_2-CH_3$ with O above the C and CH_3 below the CH

(g) $H-C-N-CH_2-CH_3$ with O above the C and H below the N

32. Reduction of an aldehyde yields what type of compound? reduction of a ketone?

33. Why do aldehydes give a positive test with Clinitest whereas ketones give a negative test?

34. What is a hemiacetal? an acetal? Why are they important in the body?

35. What is a hemiketal? a ketal? Why are they important in the body?

36. Why does the removal of calcium ions from the blood prevent clotting?

References   BAUM, STUART J. *Introduction to Organic and Biological Chemistry,* 3rd ed. Macmillan Publishing Company, New York, 1982, Chapters 7, 8, 9.

MORRISON, ROBERT T. and ROBERT N. BOYD. *Organic Chemistry,* 4th ed. Allyn and Bacon, Inc., Boston, 1983, Chapters 18, 19, 20, 22, 23.

SOLOMONS, T. W. GRAHAM. *Organic Chemistry,* 3rd ed. John Wiley & Sons, New York, 1984, Chapters 16–19.

ZIMMERMAN, HENRY and ISAAK ZIMMERMAN. *Elements of Organic Chemistry,* 2nd ed. Macmillan Publishing Company, New York, 1983, Chapters 10, 14.

19 Aromatic Compounds

CHAPTER
OUTLINE

Benzene
   Structure
   Properties
   Halogen Derivatives
   Other Derivatives
Other Aromatic Compounds
   Phenols

Phenol Derivatives
Aldehydes
Ketones
Acids
Amines
Amides

The term *aromatic* originally referred to certain compounds that had a pleasant odor and similar chemical and physical properties. Further studies of these compounds showed that they all had a ring-shaped structure. However, many compounds have a pleasant odor and do not have this ring-shaped structure. The term **aromatic** is now usually used to designate compounds whose bonding has features in common with that of benzene.

Benzene

Structure

Benzene has the formula C_6H_6. Since there is one hydrogen atom for every carbon atom, we might expect benzene to have several double bonds in order to fulfill the bonding requirements for carbon, thus making it unsaturated and predictably very reactive. On the contrary, however, benzene is quite stable. The structure for the benzene molecule was first deduced by Kekulé in 1865. He stated that the six carbon atoms were arranged in a ring with alternate single and double bonds, each carbon atom having one hydrogen atom attached to it. Kekulé also suggested that the position of the double and single bonds could change, producing two structures that represent benzene.

resonance structures of benzene

269

The actual structure of benzene is intermediate between these two Kekulé structures. This is indicated by the double-headed arrow. The two Kekulé structures are called **resonance*** structures. The electron-cloud picture (Figure 19–1) of the benzene molecule shows two continuous doughnut-shaped electron clouds, one above and the other below the plane of the atoms.

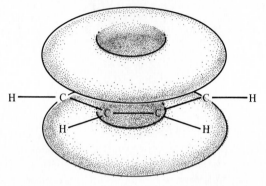

FIGURE 19-1. Electron-cloud picture of benzene.

The benzene structure is the basis of many thousands of organic compounds. The chemist has devised an abbreviated version of the benzene formula.

Abbreviated resonance structures for benzene found in other texts are

In all these representations it is assumed that a hydrogen atom is present on each carbon or at each corner unless otherwise indicated.

If one of the hydrogen atoms is replaced by a methyl group, CH_3—, it is indicated as follows

Properties Benzene is a colorless liquid with a distinct gasolinelike odor. It is insoluble in water but soluble in alcohol and ether. Benzene is toxic when taken internally. Contact with the skin is harmful, and continued inhalation of benzene vapors decreases red and white blood cell count. Benzene is now considered to be mildly carcinogenic and care must be taken with its use. For this reason, the use of benzene in laboratory experiments by students has, or should be, discontinued. Also, benzene, commonly known as naphtha, has been banned as an ingredient in consumer products.

Halogen Derivatives Although benzene has three double bonds, it does not easily undergo addition reactions as do alkenes. Instead, like alkanes, benzene usually undergoes substitution reactions. This difference is due to resonance in the benzene structure.

When benzene is treated with chlorine, chlorobenzene is produced.

The structure of chlorobenzene indicates that one of the hydrogen atoms in the benzene ring has been replaced by a chlorine atom. Since all six carbon atoms and all six hydrogen atoms are equivalent in the benzene ring, there is only one possible *mono*substitution product. That is, all of the structures shown in diagram (19–1) are identical—they represent the same compound, chlorobenzene.

(19–1)

However, when two of the hydrogen atoms in the benzene ring are replaced more than one possible *di*substitution product is possible. One of the disubstitution products obtained upon the reaction of chlorine with chlorobenzene is indicated as follows.

For the IUPAC name, the benzene ring is numbered from 1 to 6. The numbers must be such that the substituents attached to the ring have the lowest possible numbers, as shown in structure (19–2). The name of this compound is 1,2-dichlorobenzene, which indicates two chlorines on a benzene ring in positions 1 and 2.

(19–2)

Actually, when chlorine reacts with chlorobenzene, three different disubstitution products (isomers) are obtained. Their structures and names are indicated in (19–3).

Aromatic Compounds   **271**

1,2-dichlorobenzene   1,3-dichlorobenzene   1,4-dichlorobenzene

(19–3)

If the disubstitution products on the benzene ring are different, the same system of naming may be used. Consider the compound

It may be numbered with either the bromine atom at position 1 and the chlorine atom at position 2 or vice versa, as shown in (19–4).

(19–4)

Thus the compound may be named either 1-bromo-2-chlorobenzene or 1-chloro-2-bromobenzene. The preferred name lists the substituents in alphabetical order, but frequently the pharmaceutical companies use several different systems for naming their drugs.

The common system for naming disubstituted benzene compounds is based upon the use of prefixes rather than numbers to designate positions in the benzene ring. The prefix **ortho** indicates substances on the benzene ring in positions next to each other. The compound shown in (19–5) is called *ortho*-dichlorobenzene, or simply *o*-dichlorobenzene.

(19–5)

The compound shown in (19–6) may be called either *o*-chlorobromobenzene or *o*-bromochlorobenzene; the alphabetic sequence is preferred.

(19–6)

When substituents on the benzene ring are separated by one carbon atom (in positions 1 and 3), the prefix used is **meta.** The compound shown in (19–7) is called *meta*-dichlorobenzene or *m*-dichlorobenzene.

(19–7)

Organic Chemistry

And structure (19-8) is called *m*-bromochlorobenzene.

(19–8)

When two substituents on the benzene ring are separated by two carbon atoms (in positions 1 and 4) the prefix used is **para**. The compound indicated in (19–9) is called *para*-dichlorobenzene or *p*-dichlorobenzene. It is a modern version of mothballs.

(19–9)

The structure of *p*-bromochlorobenzene is shown in (19–10).

(19–10)

Other Derivatives

TOLUENE

The methyl derivative of benzene is commonly called toluene. Its IUPAC name is methylbenzene. Its structure is

Toluene is a colorless liquid with a benzenelike odor. It is insoluble in water and soluble in alcohol and ether. Toluene is used as a preservative for urine specimens and in the preparation of dyes and explosives. Toluene is one ingredient in airplane glue. When "sniffed," it can produce blurred vision, a lack of coordination, and may even cause a fatality. Toluene, however, is much less toxic than benzene and now is frequently being substituted for benzene.

A derivative of toluene, trinitrotoluene (TNT) is a powerful explosive. Its structure is

XYLENE   Xylene is a dimethylbenzene. Again, with two substitutions on the benzene ring, there are three possible structures of xylene.

o-xylene   m-xylene   p-xylene

Xylenes are good solvents for oils and are used in cleaning lenses in microscopes.

NAPHTHALENE   Naphthalene, $C_{10}H_8$, is an aromatic compound containing two benzene rings. These two rings are attached to each other in such a manner that they share two carbon atoms.

or

Naphthalene is a white crystalline solid obtained from coal tar. Napthalene crystals are frequently used in the home under the name mothballs. Functional groups may be attached to naphthalene in either of two positions, called alpha (α) and beta (β). These positions in α- and β-naphthol are

alpha-naphthol   beta-naphthol
or α-naphthol   or β-naphthol

Note that naphthalene has four alpha positions and also four beta positions.

ANTHRACENE AND   Anthracene and phenanthrene are aromatic compounds containing three
PHENANTHRENE   benzene rings joined together. Their structures are

Organic Chemistry   **274**

anthracene   phenanthrene

Anthracene is used commercially in the manufacture of dyes. Phenanthrene is an isomer of anthracene. It also contains three benzene rings but in a different structural arrangement. Phenanthrene has the basic structure of many biologically and medically important compounds. Among these are the male and female sex hormones, vitamin D, cholesterol, bile acids, and some alkaloids.

OTHER POLYCYLIC AROMATIC COMPOUNDS

When coal or wood is burned, compounds containing several benzene rings are obtained. Such compounds are carcinogenic (cancer producing). One of the most active of this group of carcinogens is benzpyrene. In the seventeenth century chimney sweeps in England were the first known to develop cancer from such compounds, which are also found in the "tar" of cigarettes. Industrial nations emit large amounts of benzpyrene into the air. This dangerous substance is also found in well-done charbroiled meats and smoked fish.

benzpyrene

Other Aromatic Compounds

Phenols

When an —OH group is attached to a benzene ring, a class of compounds known as phenols is formed. Generally, phenols are like alcohols but have been placed in a class by themselves because phenols are weak acids, and alcohols are not.

phenol

Phenol reacts with aqueous sodium hydroxide solution to form a water-soluble salt, sodium phenoxide. Alcohols such as ethanol and cyclohexanol do not react with basic solutions.

phenol   sodium phenoxide

Aromatic Compounds

$$CH_3CH_2OH + NaOH \longrightarrow \text{no reaction}$$

ethanol

+ NaOH ⟶ no reaction

cyclohexanol

Pure phenol is a white crystalline solid with a low melting point, 41°C. However, on exposure to light and air phenol turns reddish. Phenol is poisonous if taken internally, and externally it causes deep burns and blisters on the skin. If phenol should accidentally be spilled on the skin, it should be removed as quickly as possible with 50 percent alcohol, glycerin, sodium bicarbonate solution, or water.

Phenol was the original Lister antiseptic* and is still used as a disinfectant for surgical instruments and utensils, clothing and bed linens, floors, toilets, and sinks. Phenol is used commercially in the manufacture of dyes and plastics.

Phenol is the standard of reference for germicidal activity of disinfectants; that is, their activity is compared to that of phenol. If a 1 percent solution of a germicide kills organisms in the same time that a 5 percent solution of phenol does, then that germicide is said to have a **phenol coefficient** of 5.

Phenol Derivatives   The methyl derivatives of phenol are called cresols. There are three different cresols—*ortho, meta,* and *para.*

o-cresol   m-cresol   p-cresol

Commonly, cresol is a mixture of all three of these isomers. Cresol is a better antiseptic than phenol and also is less toxic. One commonly used disinfectant, lysol, is a mixture of the three cresols in water with soap added as an emulsifying agent. Even though cresols are less toxic than phenol, they are still poisonous and should be used for external purposes only.

Resorcinol is *m*-dihydroxybenzene. It is also an antiseptic but is not as good as phenol. Its structure is

resorcinol

A resorcinol derivative, hexylresorcinol, is a much better antiseptic and germicide. It is commonly used in mouthwashes. Its structure is

hexylresorcinol

Hexachlorophene has marked antibacterial activity. Its phenol coefficient is 125. Its activity is retained in the presence of soaps so that soaps containing hexachlorophene are used for surgical scrubs and also by food handlers and dentists. Hexachlorophene has also been employed in deodorants and cleansing creams, but its use for all these purposes has largely been discontinued because of the possibility of adverse effects on brain tissue, particularly in premature infants. The structure of hexachlorophene is

hexachlorophene

Two compounds commonly found in foods (listed as food preservatives) are BHA (butylated hydroxyanisole) and BHT (butylated hydroxytoluene).

Hydroquinone is 1,4-dihydroxybenzene. Hydroquinone is easily oxidized to quinone. Quinone, in turn, is easily reduced to hydroquinone.

hydroquinone   quinone

Hydroquinone and quinones are important in the respiratory system. One such compound, ubiquinone, is also known as coenzyme Q (see page 377).

ubiquinone (coenzyme Q)

reduced form   oxidized form

Aldehydes   Aromatic aldehydes have a general formula **ArCHO**, where Ar stands for an aromatic ring. The simplest aromatic aldehyde is benzaldehyde, which consists of an aldehyde group attached to a benzene ring. Benzaldehyde is prepared by the mild oxidation of toluene, as shown in equation (19–11). Note that the side chain, the methyl group, is more susceptible to oxidation than the fairly stable benzene ring.

toluene   benzaldehyde

$$(19\text{--}11)$$

Benzaldehyde is a colorless oily liquid with an almondlike odor. It is used in the preparation of flavoring agents, perfumes, drugs, and dyes.

Vanillin occurs in vanilla beans and gives the particular taste and odor to vanilla extract. It also has an aldehyde structure. Cinnamic aldehyde (cinnamaldehyde) is present in oil of cinnamon, an oil found in cinnamon bark. Both vanillin and cinnamic aldehyde may be prepared synthetically, and both are used as flavoring agents.

vanillin   cinnamic aldehyde

Ketones   Aromatic ketones have the general formula **ArCOAr'** or **ArCOR**. The simplest aromatic ketone is acetophenone.

acetophenone

Acetophenone has been used as a hypnotic but has been supplanted for this purpose of newer and safer drugs.

Chloracetophenone is a lacrimator* and is used as a tear gas.

chloracetophenone

Among the aromatic ketones in the body are the sex hormones estrone, progesterone, testosterone, and androsterone (see pages 520–522).

Acids   Aromatic acids have the —COOH group just as aliphatic acids. Aromatic acids are represented by the general formula **ArCOOH.** The simplest aromatic acid is benzoic acid, which consists of a —COOH attached to a benzene ring. Benzoic acid can be produced by the oxidation of toluene.

toluene   benzoic acid

Benzoic acid is a white crystalline compound slightly soluble in cold water and more soluble in hot water. It is used medicinally as an antifungal agent. The sodium salt of benzoic acid, sodium benzoate, is used as a preservative.

Salicylic acid is both an alcohol and an acid, as can be seen from its structure.

salicylic acid

Salicylic acid is a white crystalline compound with properties similar to those of benzoic acid. It is used in the treatment of fungal infections and also for the removal of warts and corns.

Commonly used compounds of salicylic acid are the salt sodium salicylate and the ester methyl salicylate.

sodium salicylate   methyl salicylate

Sodium salicylate is used as an antipyretic (to reduce fever) and also to relieve pain of arthritis, bursitis, and headache. Methyl salicylate is a liquid with a pleasant odor, that of wintergreen. It is used topically to relieve pain in muscles and joints.

The acetyl derivative of salicylic acid (the acetyl group is CH_3CO-) is acetylsalicylic acid, more commonly known as aspirin.

acetylsalicylic acid (aspirin)

Aspirin is used as an analgesic,* as an antipyretic,* and for the treatment of colds, headaches, minor aches, and pains. Aspirin is also used in the treatment of rheumatic fever. Over 50 tons of aspirin are used daily in the United States. Aspirin is contraindicated after surgery because it interferes with the normal clotting of the blood and can induce hemorrhaging. Aspirin can cause bleeding of the stomach and, therefore, should not be taken on an "empty" stomach. About 1 person in 10,000 is allergic to aspirin.

The action of aspirin is related directly to that of the prostaglandins (see page 339). Aspirin stimulates respiration directly and overdoses can cause serious acid-base balance disturbances.

Recent evidence appears to indicate that aspirin can prevent blood clots from forming by interfering with the action of the blood platelets. Evidence has also shown that aspirin seems to help prevent heart attacks. While aspirin can prevent sickling of red blood cells (see page 538) in test tubes, clinical evidence of this effect on humans is far from complete.

Acetaminophen (Tylenol) has been used as a substitute for aspirin because it does not cause gastrointestinal bleeding and does not affect blood clotting. However, overdoses can lead to hepatic damage, as can be the case with aspirin itself. Also, it is not very anti-inflammatory.

acetaminophen (Tylenol)

Amines The simplest aromatic amine is aniline, which consists of an amine group attached to the benzene ring. It is prepared by the reduction of nitrobenzene.

nitrobenzene   aniline

Aniline is used commercially in the preparation of many dyes and drugs. When aniline is reacted with acetic acid, acetanilide is produced.

aniline   acetic acid   acetanilide

Acetanilide has been used as an antipyretic and as an analgesic. A related compound, phenacetin, has also been used for similar purposes, but its use has largely been discontinued because of liver and kidney toxicity.

phenacetin

When aniline is heated with concentrated sulfuric acid, it forms *p*-aminobenzenesulfonic acid, commonly known as sulfanilic acid.

sulfanilic acid

In 1936 a derivative of sulfanilic acid, sulfanilamide, was discovered to have definite therapeutic effects against such diseases as pneumonia, diarrhea, and streptococcal infections. However, further investigation showed that sulfanilamide had several disadvantages. It caused nausea, dizziness, anemia, and other toxic reactions in the body. Pharmaceutical chemists then

Aromatic Compounds   **281**

developed a group of related sulfanilamide compounds with equal or better therapeutic value and with greatly decreased toxic effects. These were called "the sulfa drugs."

All of the sulfa drugs contain the *p*-aminobenzenesulfonamide group, which gives them their characteristic properties.

p-aminobenzenesulfonamide group

Examples of some sulfa drugs follow.

sulfanilamide

sulfapyridine

sulfadiazine

sulfacetamide

sulfamethoxazole

Since 1935, when the antibacterial action of Prontosil was discovered by Domagk, over 5000 sulfonamide (sulfa-type) compounds have been prepared and tested. Of these only a few have clinical use. The different groups attached to the parent substance determine the potency and toxicity. Most of the sulfa drugs are white crystalline substances that are insoluble in water. Their sodium compounds, however, are readily soluble.

The sulfa drugs are classified as bacteriostatic* and not bactericidal.* They appear to weaken or inhibit the growth of susceptible bacteria and make them more vulnerable to the action of phagocytes in the bloodstream of the host.

It is believed that the sulfa drugs interfere and compete with the use of *p*-aminobenzoic acid (PABA) for the formation of folic acid by bacteria. Note the similarity of structures of sulfa drugs and PABA (see page 382).

p-Aminobenzoic acid is also used in suntan lotions to prevent the dangerous ultraviolet rays from reaching the skin.

sulfanilamide, a sulfa drug   PABA

Amides   The simplest aromatic amide is benzamide, which is formed by the reaction of benzoic acid with ammonia.

benzoic acid   ammonia   benzamide

Aromatic amides have the general formula $ArCONH_2$. The amide of niacin, niacinamide, is one of the B vitamins (see page 491).

niacin   niacinamide

Summary

Benzene (C_6H_6) is a symmetrical six-sided ring compound with a hydrogen at each corner. One or more of the hydrogen atoms of benzene may be replaced by a halogen yielding halogen derivatives.

There is only one monosubstitution product of benzene because all six positions on the ring are equivalent.

There are three possible disubstitution products of benzene. These compounds may be named numerically. If both the substituents are chlorine, the disubstitution products are 1,2-dichlorobenzene, 1,3-dichlorobenzene, and 1,4-dichlorobenzene.

Prefixes are also used to designate positions on the benzene ring. The prefix *ortho* corresponds to positions 1,2; *meta-* to 1,3; and *para-* to 1,4.

Naphthalene contains two benzene rings joined together. Anthracene and phenanthrene contain three benzene rings joined together.

The simplest ring alcohol is phenol, a benzene ring with an —OH group attached. Phenol is used as a disinfectant of surgical instruments.

Cresols are methyl derivatives of phenol. Cresol is a better antiseptic than phenol and is also less toxic.

Benzoic acid consists of a benzene ring with a carboxyl (—COOH) group attached. Benzoic acid may be produced by the oxidation of toluene.

Acetylsalicylic acid, commonly known as aspirin, is an analgesic, an antipyretic, and is used in the treatment of colds, headaches, minor aches, and pains. Aspirin is contraindicated after surgery.

Aniline consists of an amine group attached to a benzene ring. Aniline is the basic compound for many dyes and drugs. Among these are the sulfa drugs.

Questions and Problems

A

1. Indicate the resonance structures for benzene.
2. What is the abbreviation for the structure of benzene?
3. What effects does benzene vapor have on the body?
4. Draw the structure of chlorobenzene.
5. Why is there only one monosubstitution product for benzene?
6. Why are there three and only three disubstitution products for benzene?
7. Draw the structures for the following compounds: (a) 1,3-dibromobenzene; (b) 1,4-diiodobenzene; (c) 1-chloro-2-iodobenzene.
8. Name the following compounds numerically:

9. Name the compounds in question 8 using the prefix system.
10. Draw the structure of each of the following compounds: (a) *o*-dichlorobenzene; (b) *m*-bromochlorobenzene; (c) *p*-xylene.
11. Draw the structure of toluene and indicate one medical use for it.
12. What are xylenes used for?
13. Draw the structure of naphthalene; of α-naphthol.
14. Why does naphthalene have only two possible monosubstitution products?
15. Draw the structures of phenanthrene and anthracene. Why is the phenanthrene structure important biologically?
16. Draw the structure of phenol. For what is this compound used?
17. What are cresols? How many cresols are there? For what are they used?
18. Draw the structures of resorcinol and hexylresorcinol.
19. How can benzaldehyde be prepared? Write the equation.
20. What kind of compound is acetophenone?
21. How can benzoic acid be prepared? Write the equation.
22. Write the formula for sodium benzoate. What is it used for?
23. What is methyl salicylate used for? sodium salicylate?
24. Draw the structure of aspirin. What is its chemical name?
25. List several uses for aspirin.
26. Why is the use of aspirin after surgery contraindicated?
27. How can acetanilide be prepared?
28. Draw the structure of sulfanilic acid. Of what medical importance is this compound?
29. To what do sulfa drugs owe their activity?
30. What is the general structure for the following types of aromatic compounds: acids, aldehydes, amines, amides?
31. Write the reaction between benzoic acid and ammonia; between benzoic acid and methyl amine.

B

32. Compare the structures of cyclohexane and cyclohexene; of cyclohexene and benzene.
33. How do the compounds in question 32 react with halogens?

Organic Chemistry

34. Are anthracene and phenanthrene isomers? anthracene and naphthalene? Explain.
35. Benzpyrene contains how many rings? Where is it found? Why is it a dangerous compound?
36. Many germicides have a phenol coefficient of 500 or over. What does this mean?
37. Why are BHA and BHT added to foods?
38. Compare the use of R and Ar in "general formulas."
39. Name several aromatic ketones of biologic importance.
40. Why is niacinamide an important biologic compound? What does it do?

References   BAUM, STUART J. *Introduction to Organic and Biological Chemistry,* 3rd ed. Macmillan Publishing Company, New York, 1982, Chapter 4.

MORRISON, ROBERT T. and ROBERT N. BOYD. *Organic Chemistry,* 4th ed. Allyn and Bacon, Inc., Boston, 1983, Chapters 14, 24.

SOLOMONS, T. W. GRAHAM. *Organic Chemistry,* 3rd ed. John Wiley & Sons, New York, 1984, Chapter 12.

ZIMMERMAN, HENRY and ISAAK ZIMMERMAN. *Elements of Organic Chemistry,* 2nd ed. Macmillan Publishing Company, New York, 1983, Chapter 5.

20 Heterocyclic Compounds

CHAPTER
OUTLINE

Some Common Heterocyclic Com-
  pounds
Psychoactive Drugs
  Narcotic Analgesics—Opiates
  Sedative Hypnotics—Barbiturates

Stimulants—Amphetamines
Psychedelics
Other Heterocyclic Compounds
  Alkaloids

Heterocyclic compounds are ring compounds that contain some element other than carbon in the ring. The elements most commonly found in the ring other than carbon are nitrogen, sulfur, and oxygen. Heterocyclics are primarily five- and six-membered rings, sometimes joined to one another.

Some Common Heterocyclic Compounds

A few of the common heterocyclic rings in structural and abbreviated form follow; also indicated are the biologically and medically important compounds based on these structures. The compound after which the group is named is given in color.

Five-membered rings

pyrrole

hemoglobin
chlorophyll
bilirubin
(in bile)
vitamin B_{12}

thiazole

penicillins
thiamine
(vitamin B_1)

Six-membered rings

pyridine

niacin (a B-complex
vitamin)
vitamin B_6
NAD (a coenzyme)
sulfapyridine
nicotine⎫ alkaloids
coniine⎭

pyrimidine

nucleoprotein
barbiturates

purine

caffeine
dramamine
theobromine
theophylline
nucleic acids
ATP, ADP,
AMP, c-AMP
coenzyme A

The DNA (deoxyribonucleic acid) structure, which is the basis of genetic information in the cell, contains four heterocyclic rings; two of these have a purine base and two have a pyrimidine base. The purines are adenine and guanine; the pyrimidines are cytosine and thymine. The cell messenger, ribonucleic acid (RNA) (see Chapter 33), contains the pyrimidine uracil in place of thymine. The structures of these important heterocyclics are

adenine

guanine

cytosine

uracil

thymine

One important class of derivatives of pyrrole is called the porphyrins. Porphyrins are formed by joining four pyrrole rings by means of —CH— bridges. The simplest porphyrin, called porphin is shown structurally below.

Porphyrins bind metal ions in the space between the four nitrogens. Examples of porphyrins of biologic importance are hemoglobin, myoglobin, and the cytochromes (all of which bind iron), chlorophyll (which binds magnesium), vitamin B_{12} (which binds cobalt), and cytochrome oxidase (which binds copper).

Heterocyclic Compounds

porphin

Psychoactive Drugs

Psychoactive drugs affect the central nervous system. There are several categories of psychoactive drugs, depending upon their action and the responses they elicit. Among them are the narcotic analgesics, sedative hypnotics,* stimulants, and psychedelics.* A selected example of each category will be discussed in the following sections. Most of these drugs are heterocyclic compounds containing one or more nitrogen atoms in their rings.

Narcotic Analgesics—Opiates

Opiates are morphine narcotics that are obtained from the opium poppy. The dried unripened pod of this plant is the source of opium, which is a complex mixture of many narcotics. Among them are morphine, codeine, and papaverine. Heroin can be prepared from morphine by a process called acetylation. Synthetic opiates, compounds with morphinelike properties, include meperidine (Demerol) and methadone.

The opiates depress the central nervous system. The principal effects are analgesia, sedation, drowsiness, lethargy, and euphoria.* The major reason for the abuse of opiates is the relief of apprehension and elevation of mood. However, as time passes, the euphoria wears off and the user becomes apathetic and suddenly falls asleep. Opiates depress the respiratory center, and death from an overdose results from respiratory failure.

Morphine is used as an analgesic for the relief of postoperative pain, for cardiac pain, and for conditions for which other narcotics are ineffective. However, the chief disadvantage of the continued use of morphine is that it leads to addiction.

Codeine (methylmorphine) depresses the cough center of the brain and so is used in cough medicines. It is also used in the management of pain.

Papaverine, another opiate, is an antispasmodic;* it is a nonspecific smooth muscle relaxant. The drug has been used to dilate blood vessels but is now practically obsolete.

One of the most commonly abused opiates is heroin, which is a bitter-tasting, water-soluble compound. Heroin is two and one half times as powerful as morphine and has a correspondingly greater possibility of addiction. Its use in the United States has been outlawed except for research purposes. A user of heroin develops a dependence on the drug and also builds up a tolerance to it. As the tolerance develops, increased amounts of heroin are required, so that the addict may be using an amount that would be fatal to a nonuser.

Rapid intravenous injection of heroin produces a warm flushing of the skin and a sensation in the lower abdomen described by addicts as a "thrill." Morphine behaves similarly. Actually, heroin is converted into morphine by the body.

If an addict is without the drug for 10 to 12 hr, the following symptoms appear: vomiting, diarrhea, tremors, pains, restlessness, and mental disturbances. A pregnant heroin addict can pass the dependency on to the child, who must then spend the first few days of life withdrawing from the drug. If not treated properly, the infant may die within a week.

Heroin and other opiates reduce aggression and sexual drive and, therefore, are unlikely to induce crime. However, many individuals commit crimes to pay for their habit.

The currently preferred treatment for heroin addiction is the use of methadone. Methadone is itself an addictive narcotic, but it does not induce euphoria. It eliminates the desire for heroin and also reduces the withdrawal symptoms that normally accompany abstention from heroin. The amount of methadone used is gradually reduced as withdrawal symptoms lessen.

Substitutes for the opiates have been developed for the treatment of intense pain, chronic coughing, or chronic diarrhea. Opiate antagonists counteract overdoses. Naloxone is the best known of these. When given intravenously, it will remove the effect of an opiate within 1 to 2 min.

Brompton's cocktail, a mixture of morphine and cocaine in alcohol, is given orally to relieve the pain of terminal cancer. The original Brompton cocktail, developed in England, contained heroin as a narcotic analgesic, cocaine as a central nervous system stimulant, and alcohol as a flavor enhancer. Syrup and chloroform water were added to improve the mixtures taste and texture.

Sedative Hypnotics— Barbiturates The barbiturates are a class of synthetic drugs that have sedative and hypnotic (sleep-producing) properties when administered in therapeutic dosages. The structure of a barbiturate is

Table 20–1 indicates some of the barbiturates that can be prepared by varying the constituents R_1 and R_2.

In general, the more rapid the onset of action of a barbiturate, the shorter the duration of its physiologic effect. Phenobarbital is a long-acting barbiturate (10 to 12 hr), whereas secobarbital (Seconal) and pentobarbital (Nembutal) are short-acting drugs (3 to 4 hr).

Heterocyclic Compounds　　　　　　　　　　　　　　　　　　　**289**

TABLE 20-1. Composition and Names of Some Barbiturates

Name	R$_1$	R$_2$	Trade Name
Phenobarbital	ethyl, C$_2$H$_5$—	phenyl, C$_6$H$_5$—	Luminal
Pentobarbital	ethyl, C$_2$H$_5$—	1-methylbutyl, CH$_3$CH$_2$CH$_2$CH(CH$_3$)—	Nembutal
Secobarbital	allyl, CH$_2$=CHCH$_2$—	1-methylbutyl, CH$_3$CH$_2$CH$_2$CH(CH$_3$)—	Seconal

Phenobarbital is used as an anticonvulsant agent in the treatment of epilepsy by potentiation of inhibitory pathways in the nervous system.

In general, barbiturates depress the central nervous system. A person who takes repeated doses of barbiturates develops a tolerance for the drug and soon requires many times the original amount to produce the desired effect. Small amounts of barbiturates produce the symptoms of chronic alcoholism—the user is sociable, relaxed, and good humored, but his or her ability to react and alertness are decreased. Large amounts of the drug result in blurred speech, confusion, mental sluggishness, and loss of emotional control and may induce a coma.

Barbiturates are a definite hazard to the user in that, even though the tolerance builds up with increased use, the lethal dose remains about the same, thus reducing an addict's margin of safety.

In the United States the names of all barbiturates end in *-al*, even though the compounds are ketones rather than aldehydes. In the British Commonwealth, the ending *-one* is used.

Stimulants— Amphetamines

The amphetamines, known as "pep pills" or uppers, are one type of the synthetic drugs that stimulate the central nervous system. These drugs are useful in the treatment of such conditions as narcolepsy (an overwhelming compulsion to sleep) and mild depression. Their use for obesity is no longer recommended since the reduction in appetite induced by amphetamines is temporary. Frequent misusers of amphetamines are overtired truckdrivers and business persons, students cramming for exams, and athletes who need a "pick up" before a game. Prolonged use or misuse leads to serious effects because the amphetamines tend to concentrate in the brain and cerebrospinal fluid. A tolerance to the drug develops rapidly, and increasing amounts lead to long periods of sleeplessness, loss of weight, and severe paranoia.*

The amphetamine Benzedrine was synthesized to simulate the action of epinephrine (adrenaline) (see page 513). Note the similarity of their structures.

Drug users refer to Benzedrine as "bennies" and dextroamphetamine as "dexies." Amphetamine and methamphetamine, used intravenously, are known as "speed."

Organic Chemistry

amphetamine
(Benzedrine)

epinephrine
(adrenaline)

Psychedelics   The psychedelic drugs produce "visions." Among these drugs are the **halucinogens,** drugs that stimulate sensory perceptions, and the **psychomimetics,** drugs that seem to mimic psychoses.

The "psychedelic state" includes several major effects. There is a heightened awareness of sensory input. The individual has an enhanced sense of clarity but a reduced control over what is experienced. One part of the individual seems to be observing what the other part is seeing and doing. The environment may be perceived as harmonious and beautiful with interplays of light and color in minute detail. Colors may be heard and sounds may be seen. There is a loss of boundary between the real and the unreal.

The most abused of these drugs are the hallucinogens, such as LSD (lysergic acid diethylamide), mescaline (3,4,5-trimethoxyphenylethylamine), and STP (2,5-dimethoxy-4-methylamphetamine) (the initials STP in drug culture refer to serenity, tranquility, and peace).

The structures of LSD, mescaline, and STP are as follows.

LSD

mescaline

STP

Of all the hallucinogens, LSD ("acid") is the most powerful. An average "trip" dose of LSD is 0.1 mg. To obtain the same effect from STP requires 5 mg, and from mescaline 400 mg. Certain susceptible individuals feel the psychologic effects of LSD in doses as low as 20 to 25 mcg (0.020 to 0.025 mg). The effects on the central nervous system begin within 1 hr and may last 8 to 12 hr.

In addition to the hallucinogenic effects, LSD causes dilation of the pupils of the eyes, an increased blood pressure, tachycardia,* nausea, and increased body temperature.

Heterocyclic Compounds

It is believed that LSD exerts its effect by interfering with serotonin, a hormone found in the brain, which plays an important part in the thought process. Note the similarity in structure between LSD (above) and serotinin.

serotonin

LSD has been used by psychiatrists and psychologists in the treatment of psychoneuroses* and social delinquency. It has also been used for the treatment of terminal cancer patients because it lessens their pain and awareness.

Cannabis, also known as marijuana, hashish, "pot," "grass," or "Mary Jane," is obtained from the flowery tops of hemp plants. In the Middle East and North Africa the dried resinous extract of the tops is called hashish and charas in the Far East. In the United States the term *marijuana* (or *marihuana*) is used to describe any part of the plant that induces psychic changes in humans.

Marijuana acts on both the central nervous system and the cardiovascular system. When it is smoked, the effects can be felt within a few minutes. If eaten with food, the effects are delayed about an hour. The physiologic effects include a voracious appetite, nausea, bloodshot eyes, increased pulse rate, dry mouth and throat, and dilation of the pupils. In addition, there is a sense of euphoria, intensified visual images, a keener sense of hearing, and a distortion of space and time.

Large doses of marijuana can induce hallucinations, delusions, and paranoiac feelings. Anxiety may replace euphoria.

Marijuana is not a narcotic in that it is not a derivative of opium or synthetic substitutes, but it is so labeled by law.

Other Heterocyclic Compounds

Although many of the biologically active heterocyclic compounds contain nitrogen in the ring, other elements may also be present. For example, both thiamine and biotin, which are B vitamins, contain sulfur in the ring. Glucose has an oxygen in its ring structure.

thiamine   biotin   glucose

Alkaloids   One particular group of heterocyclic amines contains compounds called alkaloids. They are found chiefly in plants and usually have a marked physiologic effect on the body. Examples of alkaloids, in addition to morphine, codeine, heroin, and LSD follow.

CAFFEINE   Caffeine occurs in coffee and tea. It stimulates the central nervous system and also acts as a diuretic.* Caffeine is used for various headache remedies in conjunction with analgesic drugs.

COCAINE   Obtained from the leaves of a coca shrub in South America, cocaine is administered medicinally in the form of a hydrochloride. Because it blocks nerve conduction, cocaine is widely used as a local anesthetic. However, it has largely been supplanted by synthetic drugs, which are less habit forming and less toxic.

NICOTINE   Found in tobacco leaves, nicotine is one of the few alkaloids soluble in water. It has no therapeutic use but is used as an insecticide. Nicotine is found in the body after cigarette smoking. It increases the blood pressure and pulse rate and constricts the blood vessels.

QUININE   Obtained from the bark of the cinchona tree in South America, quinine was formerly used primarily in the treatment of malaria. It has been replaced by less toxic and more effective synthetic antimalarial drugs. Quinine has been used as an antipyretic and analgesic for muscular pain and headaches.

Quinine acts on skeletal muscle by three different mechanisms: (1) it increases the refractory* period by direct action on the muscle fiber; (2) it decreases the excitability of the motor end plate: and (3) it affects the distribution of calcium within the muscle fiber.

EPHEDRINE   Obtained from twigs of a Chinese plant, ma-huang, ephedrine is used to elevate blood pressure during spinal anesthesia. It is used in the treatment of asthma, coughs, and colds. It is also used as a nasal decongestant.

RESERPINE   Obtained from the shrub of *Rauwolfia serpentina,* in India and the Malay peninsula, reserpine has been used for the treatment of hypertension but has some adverse side-effects.* It is also used as a sedative and as a relaxant.

Summary

Heterocyclics are compounds containing some element other than carbon in the ring, the most common being nitrogen, sulfur, and oxygen. Heterocyclics are usually five- or six-membered rings sometimes joined together.

The parent compounds of some of the more important heterocyclic compounds are pyrrole, a five-membered ring with a nitrogen in it; pyridine, a six-membered ring containing a nitrogen; pyrimidine, a six-membered ring containing two nitrogens; and purine, a six-membered ring containing two nitrogens joined to a five-membered ring containing two nitrogens.

The purines and the pyrimidines are the parent compounds for the base of the nucleic acids DNA and RNA.

Psychoactive drugs affect the central nervous system. Among the categories of psychoactive drugs are narcotic analgesics, sedative hypnotics, stimulants, and psychedelics.

The following heterocyclics are but a few of the many used medically: caffeine, as a stimulant; cocaine, as a local anesthetic; ephedrine, as a nasal decongestant; reserpine, for treatment of hypertension.

1. Define the term *heterocyclic*.
2. Which heterocyclic bases are used in the DNA and RNA molecules?
3. What are opiates?
4. Name two naturally occurring opiates; one semisynthetic opiate; two synthetic opiates.
5. What are the effects of opiates on the body?
6. For what purposes is morphine used? What is its chief disadvantage?
7. What is codeine used for? How is it related structurally to morphine?
8. What are the dangers of use of heroin? What are the symptoms of heroin withdrawal?
9. How is heroin addiction treated?
10. What properties do barbiturates have? How do they differ structurally?
11. What is one use for phenobarbital?
12. Why is there greater danger of a fatal overdose with barbiturates than with opiates?
13. What is narcolepsy? How is it treated?
14. Who are frequent misusers of amphetamines?
15. What are the effects of the use of psychedelic drugs?
16. What is the most powerful psychedelic drug?
17. What is believed to be the method of action of LSD?
18. Cannabis is known by what other names? What are the effects of small amounts of cannabis? large amounts?

19. Name one compound containing an oxygen in the ring; one with both a sulfur and a nitrogen.
20. Why are there warnings about the use of reserpine?
21. How does a hallucinogenic drug differ from a psychomimetic drug?
22. What effects does nicotine have on the human body?

References

GOODMAN, L. S. and A. GILMAN (eds). *The Pharmacological Basis of Therapeutics,* 7th ed. Macmillan Publishing Company, New York, 1985, Chapter 16.

MORRISON, R. T. and R. N. BOYD. *Organic Chemistry,* 4th ed. Allyn and Bacon, Inc., Boston, 1983, Chapter 35.

SOLOMONS, T. W. GRAHAM. *Organic Chemistry,* 3rd ed. John Wiley & Sons, New York, 1984, pages 878 and 888.

VAN DYKE, CRAIG and ROBERT BYCK, Cocaine. *Scientific American,* **246:**128–41 (March 1982).

UNIT III

Biochemistry

Biochemistry is the study of life itself—

The interrelationships of the metabolism of carbohydrates, fats, and proteins

The need for enzymes, vitamins, and hormones in various body processes

The formation and excretion of waste products

The properties and functions of the body's fluids, including blood and urine

The cause and cure of certain pathologic conditions

The study of human reproduction and its molecular basis as evidenced by the study of DNA

21 Carbohydrates

CHAPTER OUTLINE

Classification
Origin
    Oxygen–Carbon Dioxide Cycle in Nature
Optical Activity
    Structural Isomers
    Functional Isomers
    Geometric Isomers
    Optical Isomers
Monosaccharides
    Trioses
    Tetroses
    Pentoses
    Hexoses
    Reactions of the Hexoses
Disaccharides

Structure
Reducing Properties
Fermentation
Sucrose
Maltose
Lactose
Sweetness of Sugars
Polysaccharides
    Starch
    Cellulose
    Glycogen
    Dextrin
    Heparin
    Dextran
    Structure of the Polysaccharides

Carbohydrates (which contain the elements carbon, hydrogen, and oxygen) are a class of organic compounds that includes sugars, starches, and cellulose. Originally all known carbohydrates were considered to be hydrates of carbon because they contain hydrogen and oxygen in the ratio of two to one just as in water. The formula for glucose, $C_6H_{12}O_6$, was written as $C_6(H_2O)_6$. Likewise sucrose, $C_{12}H_{22}O_{11}$, was written as $C_{12}(H_2O)_{11}$. However, later investigation showed that rhamnose, another carbohydrate, has the formula $C_6H_{12}O_5$. It did not fit the general formula for a hydrate of carbon yet it was a carbohydrate. Also, such compounds as acetic acid ($C_2H_4O_2$) and pyrogallol ($C_6H_6O_3$) did fit such a system but were not carbohydrates.

Carbohydrates are now defined as polyhydroxyaldehydes or polyhydroxyketones or substances that yield these compounds on hydrolysis. **Polyhydroxy** means "containing several alcohol groups." Thus simple carbohydrates are alcohols and also are either aldehydes of ketones (they contain a carbonyl group, $>C=O$; see Chapter 18).

Classification   Carbohydrates are divided into three major categories: monosaccharides, disaccharides, and polysaccharides.

Monosaccharides (*mono-* means one) are simple sugars. They cannot be changed into simpler sugars upon hydrolysis (reaction with water).

Disaccharides (*di-* means two) are double sugars. On hydrolysis, they yield two simple sugars.

$$\text{disaccharides} \xrightarrow{\text{hydrolysis}} \text{2 monosaccharides}$$

Polysaccharides (*poly-* means many) are complex sugars. On hydrolysis, they yield many simple sugars.

$$\text{polysaccharides} \xrightarrow{\text{hydrolysis}} \text{many simple sugars}$$

Monosaccharides, or simple sugars, are called either **aldoses** or **ketoses,** depending upon whether they contain an aldehyde (—CHO) or a ketone ($>$C$=$O) group. Aldoses and ketoses are further classified according to the number of carbon atoms they contain. An aldopentose is a five-carbon simple sugar containing an aldehyde group. A ketohexose is a six-carbon simple sugar containing a ketone group.

Although there are simple sugars with three carbon atoms (trioses), four carbon atoms (tetroses), and five carbon atoms (pentoses), the hexoses (six-carbon simple sugars) are the most common in terms of the human body because they are the body's main energy-producing compounds.

Polysaccharides are sometimes called hexosans or pentosans, depending upon the type of monosaccharide they yield on hydrolysis. That is, hexosans on hydrolysis yield hexoses and pentosans yield pentoses.

Origin Plants pick up carbon dioxide from the air and water from the soil and combine them to form carbohydrates in a process called **photosynthesis.** Enzymes, chlorophyll, and sunlight are necessary. The overall reaction is represented in equation (21–1).

$$6CO_2 + 6H_2O \xrightarrow[\substack{\text{chlorophyll} \\ \text{enzymes}}]{\text{sunlight}} \underset{\text{sugar}}{C_6H_{12}O_6} + 6O_2\uparrow \qquad (21\text{–}1)$$

However, it should be understood that even though reaction (21–1) appears simple, it is very complex, with many intermediate steps between the original reactants and the final products.

During photosynthesis oxygen is given off into the air, thus renewing our vital supply of this element.

The carbohydrate produced in reaction (21–1), $C_6H_{12}O_6$, is a monosaccharide. Plant cells also have the ability to combine two molecules of a monosaccharide into one of a disaccharide, as indicated in (21–2).

$$\underset{\text{monosaccharide}}{2C_6H_{12}O_6} \longrightarrow \underset{\text{disaccharide}}{C_{12}H_{22}O_{11}} + H_2O \qquad (21\text{–}2)$$

Reaction (21–2) is the reverse of hydrolysis—water is removed when two molecules of a monosaccharide combine.

Plant (and animal) cells can also combine many molecules of monosaccharide into large polysaccharide molecules. The *n* in equation (21–3) represents a number larger than 2:

Carbohydrates **299**

$$nC_6H_{12}O_6 \longrightarrow (C_6H_{10}O_5)_n + nH_2O \qquad (21\text{-}3)$$

monosaccharide   polysaccharide

This is an example of a polymerization reaction (see page 236).

Polysaccharides occur in plants as cellulose in the stalks and stems and as starches in the roots and seeds. Monosaccharides and disaccharides are generally found in plants in their fruits.

Plants as well as animals are able to convert carbohydrates into fats and proteins.

Oxygen–Carbon Dioxide Cycle in Nature

Although plants have the ability to pick up carbon dioxide from the air and water from the ground to form carbohydrates, animals are unable to do this and must rely on plants for their carbohydrates.

Animals oxidize carbohydrates in their bodies to yield carbon dioxide, water, and energy:

$$C_6H_{12}O_6 + 6O_2 \longrightarrow 6CO_2 + 6H_2O + energy$$

Again, this reaction is not as simple as it appears; many steps are involved between the reactants and the products, and many different enzymes are required.

It should be noted that this overall reaction during metabolism is the reverse of that taking place during photosynthesis. Both reactions can be summarized by equation (21-4).

$$energy + 6CO_2 + 6H_2O \underset{\substack{animal \\ metabolism}}{\overset{\substack{plant \\ photosynthesis}}{\rightleftharpoons}} C_6H_{12}O_6 + 6O_2 \qquad (21\text{-}4)$$

Thus, there is a cycle in nature. During photosynthesis, plants pick up carbon dioxide from the air and give off oxygen; both plants and animals pick up oxygen from the air and give off carbon dioxide.

During photosynthesis, the energy from the sun is needed for the reaction (that is, the reaction is endothermic*). During metabolism of these carbohydrates in animals, this same amount of energy is liberated (the reaction is exothermic*). Thus, all the energy from the burning of carbohydrates by animals comes originally from the sun. Plants store solar energy in carbohydrates, and this energy is utilized by all living organisms during the metabolic process. It has been estimated that only about 1 percent of the total solar energy falling on plants is converted into useful stored energy.

Optical Activity

In Chapters 15 and 16 the topic of isomers was mentioned. However, isomers may be subdivided into four classifications: structural, functional, geometric, and optical.

Structural Isomers

Structural isomers are compounds with the same molecular formula, same functional groups, but different structural formulas. Examples are propyl alcohol and isopropyl alcohol, o-dichlorobenzene and m-dichlorobenzene, and 2-methylhexane and 3-methylhexane.

Biochemistry

CH₃—CH₂—CH₂OH   CH₃—CH—CH₃

$$CH_3-CH_2-CH_2OH \qquad CH_3-\underset{\underset{\displaystyle OH}{|}}{CH}-CH_3$$

propyl alcohol   isopropyl alcohol

o-dichlorobenzene

m-dichlorobenzene

$$CH_3\underset{\underset{\displaystyle CH_3}{|}}{CH}CH_2CH_2CH_2CH_3 \qquad CH_3CH_2\underset{\underset{\displaystyle CH_3}{|}}{CH}CH_2CH_2CH_3$$

2-methylhexane   3-methylhexane

Functional Isomers

Functional isomers are compounds having the same molecular formula but different functional groups. Examples are ethyl alcohol and dimethyl ether, and propanoic acid and 2-hydroxypropanal.

$$CH_3CH_2OH \qquad CH_3OCH_3$$

ethyl alcohol   dimethyl ether

$$CH_3CH_2COOH \qquad CH_3\underset{\underset{\displaystyle OH}{|}}{CH}CHO$$

propanoic acid   2-hydroxypropanal

Geometric Isomers

Geometric isomers are compounds with the same molecular formula but different structural formulas owing to a restricted rotation because of either a double bond or a ring system.

If two carbon atoms are connected by a double bond, those two carbon atoms and the four groups attached to them all lie in a single plane. There are two possible isomeric structures, one having similar groups on the same "side" of the double bond and one having similar groups on opposite "sides" of the double bond. An example of geometric isomerism is

cis-1,2-dichloroethene   trans-1,2-dichloroethene

The prefix **cis-** means on the same side and **trans-** means across or on opposite sides.

If two groups attached to one of the doubly bonded carbon atoms are identical, only one structure is possible. The two groups attached to each carbon must be different for geometric isomerism to occur.

Cis-trans isomerism is also possible for ring structures. In cyclopropane, the three carbon atoms all lie in one plane. Substituents on adjacent carbons

Carbohydrates   301

may both be on the same side of the plane (*cis*) or on opposite sides of the plane (*trans*), such as

cis-1,2-dimethylcyclopropane   trans-1,2-dimethylcyclopropane

Cis-trans isomerism occurs in fatty acids (see Chapter 22) and is very important in the rhodopsin–vitamin A cycle (see page 482).

An example of a biologically active geometric isomer in *trans*-diethylstilbestrol (DES). This compound was formerly used during pregnancy but its use has been discontinued because of its carcinogenic effects. The *cis*-isomer is biologically inactive.

trans-diethylstilbestrol

Optical Isomers   Optical isomers are compounds with the same molecular formula but with structures that are the mirror image of one another. Such isomers rotate the plane of polarized light equally but in opposite directions. Let us see what this means and why.

Polarized light vibrates in one plane only as opposed to ordinary light, which vibrates in all planes. When polarized light is passed through a solution of an optically active substance, the plane of polarized light is rotated (see Figure 21–1).

What causes such a rotation of the plane of polarized light? According to the theory of van't Hoff, such an effect upon the plane of polarized light is due to the presence of one (or more) **asymmetric**† carbon atoms. An asymmetric carbon atom is one having four different groups attached to it.

The simplest carbohydrate is glyceraldehyde, whose structural formula is

glyceraldehyde

---

† Some texts use the word **chiral** in place of asymmetric. An asymmetric carbon is also called a chiral center. Molecules that are not superimposable on their mirror images are said to be chiral and are optically active.

Biochemistry   **302**

FIGURE 21-1. Schematic representation of the production of polarized light and its rotation by an optically active substance.

Glyceraldehyde has an aldehyde group at one end of the molecule, a primary alcohol at the other end, and a secondary alcohol in the middle. The central carbon atom in glyceraldehyde is asymmetric (chiral)—it has four different groups attached to it. They are

$$\text{—CHO} \qquad \text{—OH} \qquad \text{—CH}_2\text{OH} \qquad \text{—H}$$

This compound can exist in two optically active forms. The two structures are mirror images of one another (see Figure 21-2); they are *not* superimposable. Your right and left hands are mirror images; they are not superimposable. You wear a right and a left shoe; they too are mirror images and are not superimposable.

The Fischer projection formula is a two-dimensional representation of the mirror-image structures. In this system, the two isomers of glyceraldehyde are represented as

D-glyceraldehyde   L-glyceraldehyde

The horizontal lines indicate bonds extending forward from the paper, and the vertical lines indicate bonds extending backward from the paper. Com-

FIGURE 21-2. Ball-and-stick models of the two forms of glyceraldehyde. (Reproduced from S. J. Baum and C. W. Scaife: *Chemistry: A Life Science Approach,* 2nd ed. Macmillan Publishing Co., New York, 1980.)

Carbohydrates

303

pare these two diagrams with those in Figure 21–2. The Fischer projection formulas are *always* written with the aldehyde (or ketone) group—the most highly oxidized—at the top. Thus, in the above Fischer formulas, the —H and —OH groups project forward from the paper and the —CHO and —CH$_2$OH groups project backward from the paper.

Fischer called the glyceraldehyde with the —OH group on the right side of the asymmetric carbon atom D-glyceraldehyde. Likewise, the one with the —OH group on the left side of the asymmetric carbon he called L-glyceraldehyde.

Glyceraldehyde is considered the parent compound from which more complex sugars may be derived. Those whose terminal structure (the primary alcohol and the asymmetric carbon) is similar to that of D-glyceraldehyde belong to the D series; those whose terminal end is similar to that of L-glyceraldehyde belong to the L series. Note in Figure 21–3 that D-erythrose and D-threose have structures similar to that of D-glyceraldehyde. The corresponding L structures are also similar. D and L refer to structure only, *not* to the direction of rotation of polarized light.

Figure 21–3 illustrates the D family of aldoses. The colored areas indicate the D conformation. A table of the mirror images of these aldoses would represent the L forms.

The number of optical isomers depends upon the number of asymmetric carbon atoms present in a compound and may be calculated by using the formula 2^n where n is the number of asymmetric carbons. Thus, glyceraldehyde, which has one asymmetric carbon, has 2^1 or 2 optical isomers, as was shown. Glucose, which will be discussed later in this chapter, has four asymmetric carbons and so has 2^4 or 16 optical isomers. Of these 16 isomers, 8 belong to the D series and 8 to the L series (one set of 8 is the mirror image of the other set).

Optical activity is of great importance in the body because many enzymes will interact with only one particular optical isomer. In the human body, the D series is the primary configuration for carbohydrates whereas the L series is the primary one for proteins.

Monosaccharides

Trioses

A triose is a three-carbon simple sugar. Trioses are formed during the metabolic breakdown of hexoses in muscle metabolism.

An example of a triose is glyceraldehyde (glycerose), whose optical isomers are shown on page 303.

Tetroses

Tetroses are four-carbon sugars. One tetrose, erythrose, is an intermediate in the hexose-monophosphate shunt for the oxidation of glucose (see page 405).

Pentoses

Pentoses are five-carbon sugar molecules. The most important of these are ribose and deoxyribose, which are found in nucleic acids. Ribose forms part of ribonucleic acid (RNA), and deoxyribose forms part of deoxyribonucleic acid (DNA). Both DNA and RNA are components of every cell nucleus and

FIGURE 21-3. D family of aldoses.

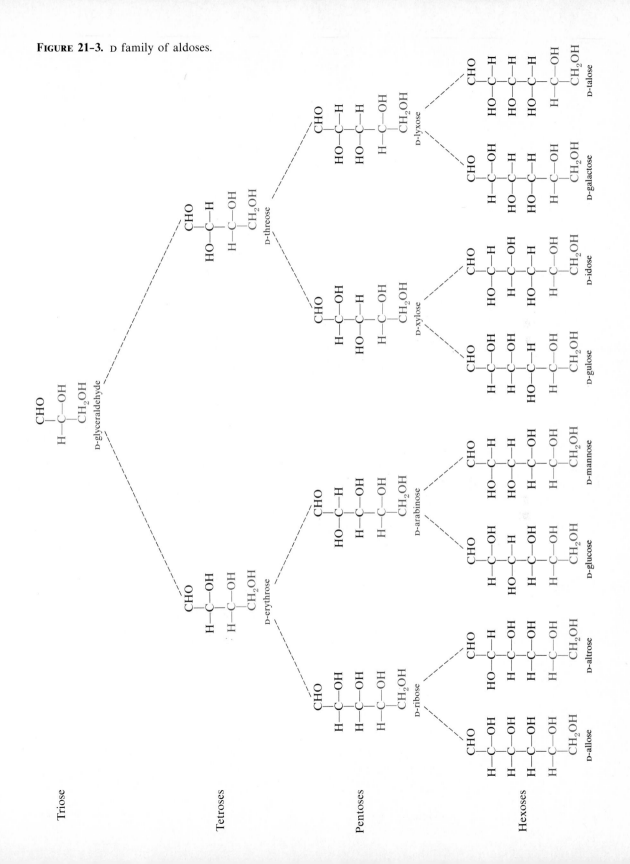

cytoplasm. The prefix *de* means without, so deoxy means without oxygen. Note that deoxyribose has one less oxygen atom than does ribose.

$$(21\text{-}1)$$

D-ribose   D-deoxyribose

Structures 21–1, the Fischer projection representations for the pentoses, are called open-chain structures. However, the predominant form for pentoses is a ring structure. Recall that aldehydes react with alcohols to form hemiacetals (page 255). In the case of ribose, the aldehyde can react with the alcohol at carbon 4 to form two different compounds.

ribose   α-ribose   β-ribose

Another representation for the hemiacetal (ring) structure of ribose, and other monosaccharides, is called the Haworth projection (equation 21–2). In projection (21–2) the ring, consisting of carbons at each corner and an oxygen where indicated, is considered to be in a plane perpendicular to the paper. The shaded line in the ring indicates the section closest to you; the lighter line that part of the ring farther from you. The —H and —OH groups are above and below that plane. The Fischer and Haworth projections are related as follows:

1. The groups on the right side of the Fischer projection are written below the plane in the Haworth projection. Those on the left side are written above the plane.
2. One exception to rule 1 occurs at carbon 4 in pentoses and at carbon 5 in hexoses because of the nature of the reaction occurring there. At these carbons rule 1 is reversed.
3. At carbon 1 the α form is indicated by the —OH being written below the plane; the β form has the —OH above the plane.

Other pentoses are ribulose, which is formed in the metabolic breakdown of glucose; lyxose, which is found in heart muscle; arabinose, which is found in gum arabic and the gum of the cherry tree; and xylose, which is obtained from the hydrolysis of wood gums.

ribose   α-ribose   β-ribose   (21-2)

Hexoses

The hexoses, the six-carbon sugars, are the most common of all the carbohydrates. Of the several hexoses, the most important as far as the human body is concerned are *glucose, fructose,* and *galactose.* All three of these hexoses have the same molecular formula, $C_6H_{12}O_6$, but different structural formulas; they are isomers.

GLUCOSE

Glucose, $C_6H_{12}O_6$, is an aldohexose and may be represented structurally as

D-glucose   α-D-glucose†   β-D-glucose†

Fischer projection   Haworth projection

Note that glucose contains four asymmetric carbon atoms (numbers 2, 3, 4, 5) and so has 2^4 or 16 optical isomers.

Medically, when the word glucose is mentioned, the D isomer is meant because that is the biologically active isomer. Likewise, for the other hexoses, the D isomer is commonly called by name only, without the prefix D.

Glucose is known commonly as dextrose or grape sugar. It is a white crystalline solid, soluble in water and insoluble in most organic liquids. It is found, along with fructose, in many fruit juices. It may be prepared by the hydrolysis of sucrose, a disaccharide, or by the hydrolysis of starch, a polysaccharide.

Glucose is the most important of all the monosaccharides. It is normally found in the bloodstream and in the tissue fluids. As will be discussed in Chapter 26 (Carbohydrate Metabolism), glucose requires no digestion and

† The chemical name for these ring compounds are α-D-glucopyranose and β-D-glucopyranose, respectively, but this system of naming is of interest primarily to organic chemists.

can be given intravenously to patients who are unable to take food by mouth (see Figure 21-4).

Glucose is found in the urine of patients suffering from diabetes mellitus and is an indication of this disease. The presence of glucose in the urine is called glycosuria. Glucose may also show up in the urine during extreme excitement (emotional glycosuria), after ingestion of large amounts of sugar (alimentary glycosuria), or because of other factors that will be discussed in the chapter on carbohydrate metabolism.

GALACTOSE   Galactose, an isomer of glucose, is also an aldohexose. The structures of galactose are

d-galactose   α-d-galactose   β-d-galactose

Glucose and galactose differ from each other only in the configuration of the H and OH about a single carbon atom. Two sugars that differ only in the configuration about a single carbon atom is called **epimers.** D-Galactose is converted to D-glucose in the liver by a specific enzyme called an epimerase. Galactose is present in some glycoproteins and glycolipids (see page 338).

Galactosemia, a severe inherited disease, results in the inability of infants to metabolize galactose because of a deficiency of either the enzyme galactose 1-phosphate uridyl transferase or the enzyme galactokinase. The galactose concentration increases in the blood and urine (galactosuria).

Biochemistry   **308**

FRUCTOSE   Fructose is a ketohexose. Its molecular formula, like that of glucose and galactose, is $C_6H_{12}O_6$. It, too, may be represented as a straight-chain or a ring compound (see structures 21–3). The ring structure is predominant. Note that the ring structure represents a hemiketal (see page 255).

α-D-fructose β-D-fructose   (21–3)

Reactions of the ***Hexoses***   Fructose is often called levulose or fruit sugar. It occurs naturally in fruit juices and honey. It may be prepared by the hydrolysis of sucrose, a disaccharide, and also by the hydrolysis of inulin, a polysaccharide found in Jerusalem artichokes. Fructose is the most soluble sugar and also the sweetest of all sugars, being approximately twice as sweet as glucose.

REDUCTION

Fructosemia, fructose intolerance, is an inherited disease due to a deficiency of the enzyme fructose 1-phosphate aldolase. An infant suffering from this disease experiences hypoglycemia, vomiting, and severe malnutrition. Such a condition is treated by placing the infant on a low fructose diet.

Hexoses, which are either aldoses or ketoses, show reducing properties. This reducing property is the basis of the test for sugar in the urine and in the blood. When a reducing agent is treated with an oxidizing agent such as Cu^{2+} complex ion,† a red-orange precipitate of copper (I) oxide, Cu_2O, is formed. The unbalanced equation for the reaction of an aldehyde with copper (II) complex ion may be written as follows

$$\text{aldehyde} + \underset{\substack{\text{deep blue}\\\text{solution}}}{Cu^{2+}} \xrightarrow[\text{NaOH}]{\text{heat}} \text{acid} + \underset{\substack{\text{red-orange}\\\text{precipitate}}}{Cu_2O\downarrow} + \text{water}$$

† Fehling's solution is an alkaline solution of Cu^{2+} ions complexed with tartrate; Benedict's solution is an alkaline solution of Cu^{2+} ions complexed with citrate.

Carbohydrates   **309**

In this reaction the aldehyde is oxidized to the corresponding acid. When glucose is treated with Cu^{2+} complex ion and the mixture is heated, the reaction is

<table>
<tr><td>D-glucose</td><td>copper II
complex ion
(deep blue color)</td><td>copper (I)
oxide
(red-orange
precipitate)</td><td>D-gluconic acid</td></tr>
</table>

Laboratory tests for the presence of glucose in urine use Benedict's solution or Fehling's solution, both of which contain copper (II) complex ion. Clinitest tablets, which also contain a copper (II) complex, give a rapid quantitative measurement of the concentration of glucose present. If the blue liquid turns green, a trace of sugar (glucose) is present. This is frequently recorded as +. A yellow color, indicated by + +, indicates up to 0.5 percent sugar; an orange color, + + +, 0.5 to 1.5 percent; and a red color, + + + +, over 1.5 percent sugar.

Glucose does not normally appear in the urine for any extended period of time. Its presistent presence usually indicates something is wrong with the metabolism of carbohydrates—such as diabetes mellitus.

Another laboratory test for the presence of a reducing sugar uses Tollen's reagent, which contains Ag^+ complex ion. In this reaction glucose is oxidized to gluconic acid as before and the silver complex ion is reduced to free silver, which appears as a bright shiny mirror on the inside of the test tube.

$$\text{glucose} + \underset{\substack{\text{Tollen's}\\\text{reagent}}}{Ag^+} \xrightarrow[\text{NH}_4\text{OH}]{\text{heat}} \text{gluconic acid} + \underset{\text{silver mirror}}{Ag\downarrow} + \text{water}$$

FERMENTATION   Glucose ferments in the presence of yeast, forming ethyl alcohol and carbon dioxide. This reaction will not readily occur in the absence of yeast. Yeast contains enzymes that catalyze this particular reaction.

$$\underset{\text{glucose}}{C_6H_{12}O_6} \xrightarrow{\text{enzymes}} \underset{\text{ethyl alcohol}}{2C_2H_5OH} + 2CO_2'$$

Fructose will also ferment; galactose will not readily ferment. Pentoses do not ferment in the presence of yeast.

OXIDATION   An aldose contains an aldehyde group as well as several —OH groups. If the aldehyde end of the molecule is oxidized, the product is named an **-onic**

Biochemistry   **310**

acid. When the aldehyde end of glucose is oxidized, the product is called gluconic acid (see page 310). When the aldehyde end of galactose is oxidized, the product is called galactonic acid. If the alcohol at the end opposite the aldehyde (the other end of the molecule) is oxidized, the product is called a **-uronic acid.** The oxidation of the alcohol end of glucose yields glucuronic acid. Glucuronic acid is a minor product of glucose metabolism. It is also part of the heparin molecule (see page 317).

glucose   glucuronic acid

Likwise, if the alcohol end of galactose is oxidized, galacturonic acid is formed.

If both ends of the glucose molecule are oxidized at the same time, the product is called saccharic acid.

glucose   saccharic acid

REDUCTION   The aldohexoses may be reduced to alcohols. When glucose is reduced, sorbitol is formed. Sorbitol accumulation in the eye is a major factor in the formation of cataracts due to diabetes.

glucose   sorbitol

Reduction of galactose yields dulcitol and reduction of fructose yields a mixture of mannitol and sorbitol.

Carbohydrates   **311**

Disaccharides   There are three common disaccharides—sucrose, maltose, and lactose—all of which are isomers with the molecular formula $C_{12}H_{22}O_{11}$. On hydrolysis these disaccharides yield two monosaccharides. The general reaction may be written as follows

$$C_{12}H_{22}O_{11} + H_2O \xrightarrow{\text{hydrolysis}} C_6H_{12}O_6 + C_6H_{12}O_6$$

a disaccharide		a monosaccharide	+	a monosaccharide
sucrose	$\longrightarrow$	glucose	+	fructose
maltose	$\longrightarrow$	glucose	+	glucose
lactose	$\longrightarrow$	glucose	+	galactose

The disaccharides, just like the monosaccharides, are white, crystalline, sweet solids. Sucrose is very soluble in water; maltose is fairly soluble; and lactose is only slightly soluble. The disaccharides are also optically active; they rotate the plane of polarized light. However, even though they are soluble in water, they are too large to pass through cell membranes.

Structure   Disaccharides are formed by the combination of two monosaccharides. In the last section we noted that monosaccharides were either hemiacetals or hemiketals. If a hemiacetal or hemiketal (a monosaccharide) combines with an alcohol (another monosaccharide) an acetal or a ketal will be formed (see page 256). Such a bond between the two monosaccharides is called a **glycosidic linkage.***

Consider the combination of a molecule of α-glucose with a molecule of β-glucose, as shown in equation (21–5). The products of such a reaction are β-maltose and water.

The linkage in β-maltose is between carbon 1 of one glucose and carbon 4 of the other glucose. Such a linkage is called an α-1,4 linkage; α-maltose has an —OH on carbon 1 of the second glucose molecule below the plane rather than above. Both α- and β-maltose exist, but the predominant form is the β.

If a molecule of β-glucose combines with another molecule of β-glucose, cellobiose, a compound with a β-1,4 glucosidic linkage, is formed.

Biochemistry   **312**

Enzymes are specific in the type of glycosidic linkage (α or β) whose hydrolysis they can catalyze. For example, maltase (page 379) catalyzes the hydrolysis of maltose, which contains an α glycosidic linkage. It does not catalyze the hydrolysis of cellobiose, which contains a β glycosidic linkage.

Conversely, an enzyme that catalyzes the hydrolysis of β glycosidic linkages catalyzes the hydrolysis of cellobiose. Such β glycosidic linkage hydrolysis enzymes are not found in the human digestive system. That is why humans cannot digest cellulose and cellobiose, both of which have β-glycosidic linkages.

Consider reaction (21–6) of a molecule of α-glucose with a molecule of β-fructose. The products of such a reaction are sucrose and water.

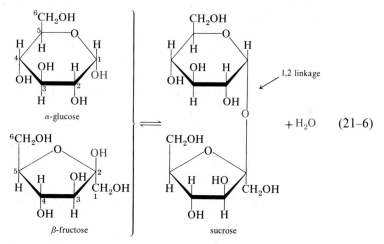

$$+ H_2O \qquad (21\text{–}6)$$

The linkage in sucrose is an α-1,2 glycosidic linkage because it occurs between carbon 1 of the glucose molecule and carbon 2 of the fructose. There is only one form of sucrose; α and β forms do not exist.

If a molecule of β-galactose reacts with a molecule of glucose (α or β), the products are water and lactose (α or β). The linkage is β-1,4.

Reducing Properties   In maltose, the aldehyde groups are at carbon 1 in each of the original glucose molecules. Since the linkage is 1,4, one free aldehyde group remains. Therefore, maltose acts as a reducing sugar (see page 253).

In sucrose, the glucose part had the aldehyde at carbon 1 and the fructose part had the ketone group at carbon 2. Since the linkage is 1,2, neither group is free. Therefore, sucrose is not a reducing sugar.

Lactose, which has a 1,4 linkage, acts as a reducing sugar because both of the original aldehyde groups were on carbon 1 and one of them is free to react.

Fermentation   Sucrose and maltose will ferment when yeast is added because yeast contains the enzymes sucrase and maltase; lactose will not ferment when yeast is added because yeast does not contain lactase. The identity of a disaccharide can be deduced on the basis of its fermentation reaction and its reducing properties.

Suppose that a test tube contains a disaccharide, $C_{12}H_{22}O_{11}$. It is sucrose, lactose, or maltose? The identity can be determined by the following method.

1. Mix the unknown disaccharide with alkaline Cu^{2+} complex and warm gently. If there is no reaction, the disaccharide must be sucrose. In this case, no further test is necessary to prove the identity of the disaccharide.
2. If the unknown disaccharide gives a positive test with alkaline Cu^{2+} complex, it must be either maltose or lactose. In this case, another sample of the disaccharide is mixed with yeast and allowed to stand to observe whether fermentation takes place or not. If the disaccharide does ferment, then it must be maltose. If it does not ferment, then it must be lactose.

The same two laboratory tests may be performed in reverse order with the same results.

1. Mix the unknown disaccharide with yeast and allow to stand, to observe whether fermentation takes place. If no fermentation is observed, the disaccharide is lactose, and no further test is necessary.
2. If fermentation does occur, the disaccharide is either sucrose or maltose. In this case take another sample of the unknown disaccharide, mix with alkaline Cu^{2+} complex, and warm gently. If the color remains blue, the unknown disaccharide must be sucrose. If the unknown gives a positive test with alkaline Cu^{2+} complex, it must be maltose.

Sucrose   Sucrose is the sugar used ordinarily in the home. It is also known as cane sugar. Sucrose is produced commercially from sugar cane and sugar beets. It also occurs in sorghum, pineapple, and carrot roots.

When sucrose is hydrolyzed, it forms a mixture of glucose and fructose. This 50:50 mixture of glucose and fructose is called **invert sugar**. Honey contains a high percentage of invert sugar.

Biochemistry   **314**

Maltose   Maltose, commonly known as malt sugar, is present in germinating grain. It is produced commercially by the hydrolysis of starch.

Lactose   Lactose, commonly known as milk sugar, is present in milk. It differs from the preceding sugars in that it has an animal origin. Certain bacteria cause lactose to ferment, forming lactic acid. When this reaction occurs, the milk is said to be sour. Lactose is used in high-calcium diets and in infant foods. Lactose can be used for increasing calorie intake without adding much sweetness. Lactose is found in the urine of pregnant women and, since it is a reducing sugar, it gives a positive test with Cu^{2+} complex ions.

Sweetness of Sugars   When we speak of sugar, we think of a substance with a sweet taste. However, some sugars are sweeter than others. If we arbitrarily assign a sweetness of 100 to sucrose, then the sweetest sugar of all is fructose, as shown in Table 21–1. Because of its great sweetness, fructose is commonly used in the manufacture of candies. It is also used in diet foods because it takes much less carbohydrate to give a desired sweetness.

Noncarbohydrate sweetners include saccharin and aspartame. Cyclamates, which were formerly used in the United States, are still in use in Canada.

TABLE 21–1. Relative Sweetness of Sugars and Other Compounds

Fructose	173
Galactose	32
Glucose	74
Lactose	16
Maltose	32
Sucrose	100
Aspartame	20,000
Cyclamate	3,000
Saccharin	30,000

Polysaccharides   Polysaccharides are polymers of monosaccharides. Complete hydrolysis of polysaccharides produces many molecules of monosaccharides. The polysaccharides differ from monosaccharides and disaccharides in many ways, as is indicated in Table 21–2.

Polysaccharides can be formed from pentoses (five-carbon sugars) or from hexoses (six-carbon sugars). Polysaccharides formed from pentoses are called **pentosans.** Those formed from hexoses are called **hexosans** (or sometimes **glucosans**).

The hexosans (or glucosans) are the most important in terms of physiology. The hexosans have the general formula $(C_6H_{10}O_5)_x$ where x is some

Carbohydrates   **315**

TABLE 21-2. Comparison of Polysaccharides with Monosaccharides and Disaccharides

Property	Monosaccharides and Disaccharides	Polysaccharides
Molecular weight	Low	Very high
Taste	Sweet	Tasteless
Solubility in water	Soluble	Insoluble
Size of particles	Pass through a membrane[a]	Do not pass through a membrane
Test with Cu^{2+} complex ions (an oxidizing agent)	Positive (except for sucrose)	Negative

[a] Only monosaccharides.

large number. Some of the common hexosans are starch, cellulose, glycogen, and dextrin. All are made up of only glucose molecules.

Starch Plants store their foods in the form of starch granules. Starch is actually a mixture of the polysaccharides amylopectin and amylose. Amylopectin is a branched polysaccharide present in starch to a large extent (80 to 85 percent). It is usually present in the covering of the starch granules. Amylose is a nonbranched polysaccharide present in starch to an extent of 15 to 20 percent.

Starch is insoluble in water. When starch is placed in boiling water, the granules rupture forming a paste that gels on cooling. When a small amount of starch is added to a large amount of boiling water, a colloidal dispersion of starch in water is formed.

Starch gives a characteristic deep blue color with iodine. This test is used to detect the presence of starch because it is conclusive even when only a small amount of starch is present. That is, if iodine is added to an unknown and a blue color is produced, starch is present. This text may also be used to check for the presence of iodine. If starch is added to an unknown and a blue color is produced, iodine must be present.

When starch is hydrolyzed, it forms dextrins (amylodextrin, erythrodextrin, achroodextrin), then maltose, and finally glucose. Erythrodextrins turn red in the presence of iodine. Both maltose and glucose produce no color in the presence of iodine. Thus, it is possible to follow the hydrolysis of the starch by observing the changing colors when iodine is added.

$$\text{starch} \longrightarrow \text{erythrodextrins} \longrightarrow \text{maltose} \longrightarrow \text{glucose}$$
| blue | red | colorless | colorless |

Cellulose Wood, cotton, and paper are composed primarily of cellulose. Cellulose is the supporting and structural substance of plants. Like starch, cellulose is a polysaccharide composed of many glucose units. It is not affected by any of the enzymes present in the human digestive system and so cannot be digested. However, it does serve a purpose when eaten with other foods: it gives bulk to the feces and prevents constipation.

Cellulose does not dissolve in water nor in most ordinary solvents. It gives no color test with iodine and gives a negative test with Cu^{2+} complex ions.

Cotton is nearly pure cellulose. When cotton fibers are treated with a strong solution of sodium hydroxide, then stretched and dried, the fibers take on a high luster. Such cotton is called *mercerized* cotton.

Cellulose is also used to make rayon. In this process, purified wood pulp (nearly pure cellulose) is converted into a viscous liquid called viscose by treatment with sodium hydroxide and carbon disulfide. When the viscose is forced through small openings in a block suspended in an acid solution, the cellulose is regenerated into fibers that can then be formed into threads.

Glycogen
Glycogen is present in the body and is stored in the liver and the muscles, where it serves as a reserve supply of carbohydrate. Glycogen has an animal origin, as opposed to the plant origin of starch.

Glycogen forms a colloidal dispersion in water and gives a red color with iodine. It gives no test with alkaline Cu^{2+} complex. Glycogen is formed in the body cells from molecules of glucose. This process is called **glycogenesis** (see page 398). When glycogen is hydrolyzed into glucose, the process is called **glycogenolysis.**

$$\text{glucose} \underset{\text{glycogenolysis}}{\overset{\text{glycogenesis}}{\rightleftharpoons}} \text{glycogen}$$

Dextrin
Dextrin is produced during the hydrolysis of starch. Dextrin is an intermediate between starch and maltose. It forms sticky colloidal suspensions with water and is used in the preparation of adhesives. The glue on the back of postage stamps is a dextrin. Dextrin is also used when starch digestion may be a problem as with infants and elderly persons.

Heparin
Heparin is a polysaccharide used as a blood anticoagulant. It accelerates the inactivation of thrombin and other blood-clotting agents (see page 459). The structure of heparin consists of repeating units of glucuronic acid and glucosamine with some sulfate groups on the amino and hydroxyl groups. Heparin is the strongest organic acid present in the body.

heparin

Dextran
Dextran (not the same as dextrin) is a polysaccharide produced by certain bacteria when they are grown on sucrose. There are various types of dextrans, differing in chain length and degree of branching. Medically, dextrans are used as blood extenders to hold water in the bloodstream and

Carbohydrates

help prevent drops in blood volume and blood pressure. Dextrans growing on the surfaces of teeth are an important component of dental plaque.

Structure of the Polysaccharides The ring structures of some of the polysaccharides are indicated in (21–7).

$x = 100$ to 400

(note α-1,4 linkages)

amylose

(21–7)

(note α-1,4 and 1,6 linkages)

amylopectin

$x =$ about 15, $y = 8$ or 9 for amylopectin

$x =$ about 6, $y = 3$ for glycogen

cellulose   (β-1,4 linkages)

Summary Carbohydrates are polyhydroxyaldehydes or polyhydroxyketones or substances that yield these compounds on hydrolysis. Carbohydrates are divided into three categories: monosaccharides, disaccharides, and polysaccharides—based upon hydrolytic possibilities.

There are four types of isomers: structural, functional, geometric, and optical. Structural isomers have the same molecular formula, same functional groups, but different structural formulas. Functional isomers have the same molecular formula but different functional groups. Geometric isomers have the same molecular formula but different structural formulas owing to a restricted rotation because of either a double bond or a ring system. Optical isomers have the same molecular formula but have structural formulas that are mirror images of each other.

Carbohydrates are formed in plants by a process called photosynthesis. Plant cells take carbon dioxide from the air and water from the ground and combine them in the presence of sunlight and chlorophyll to produce monosaccharides, at the same time giving off oxygen into the air. Plant cells also have the ability to convert the monosaccharides thus formed into disaccharides and polysaccharides. When carbohydrates are burned in the body, carbon dioxide and water are formed, thus returning these substances for reuse by plants.

Monosaccharides, or simple sugars, are either aldoses or ketoses, depending upon whether they contain an aldehyde or a ketone group. The six-carbon monosaccharides, the hexoses, are the most common in terms of the human body.

The most important hexoses in terms of the human body are glucose, fructose, and galactose. These compounds are isomers with the molecular formula $C_6H_{12}O_6$.

Glucose is an aldohexose whose structure may be represented as a linear or ring-shaped molecule. Glucose is commonly known as dextrose or grape sugar. It is the most important of all monosaccharides and is normally found in the blood stream and in the tissue fluids.

Galactose is also an aldohexose. It occurs in nature as one of the constituents of lactose.

Fructose, a ketohexose, is commonly known as levulose or fruit sugar. Fructose is the sweetest of all sugars. It occurs in nature as one of the constituents of sucrose and is found free in fruit juices and in honey.

The hexoses are either aldehydes or ketones and can act as reducing agents. When a hexose is treated with alkaline Cu^{2+} complex (Fehling's solution, Benedict's solution, or Clinitest), a red-orange precipitate of Cu_2O is formed. This reaction is the basis for the test for sugar (hexoses) in the urine. Hexoses will also reduce Tollen's reagent (Ag^+ complex) to free silver.

Hexoses will ferment in the presence of enzymes found in yeast.

When the aldehyde end of a monosaccharide is oxidized, an -*onic* acid is formed.

When the alcohol end of a monosaccharide is oxidized, an -*uronic* acid is formed.

The three common disaccharides—sucrose, maltose, and lactose—are isomers with the molecular formula $C_{12}H_{22}O_{11}$. On hydrolysis a disaccharide yields two monosaccharides.

Of the three disaccharides only maltose and lactose show reducing properties with alkaline Cu^{2+} complex ions. Sucrose is not a reducing sugar.

Sucrose and maltose will ferment with yeast owing to the presence of the enzymes sucrase and maltase. Lactose will not ferment with yeast because of the absence of the enzyme lactase.

Polysaccharides are polymers of monosaccharides and yield monosaccharides upon hydrolysis.

Polysaccharides have a high molecular weight, are insoluble in water, are tasteless, and give negative tests for reducing sugars. These properties are the opposite of those for monosaccharides and disaccharides.

Three common polysaccharides are starch, cellulose, and glycogen. Plants store their food as starch; plants use cellulose as supporting and as structural parts; animals use glycogen as a reserve supply of carbohydrate.

Questions and Problems

A

1. What is a carbohydrate?
2. What are aldoses? aldopentoses? ketohexoses?
3. What are structural isomers? Give an example.
4. What are geometric isomers? Give an example.
5. What are functional isomers? Give an example.
6. What are optical isomers? Give an example.
7. Draw the structure for (a) *cis*-1,2-dibromocyclopentane, (b) *trans*-1,2-dibromopropene.
8. What is meant by the term *asymmetric carbon atom?* Give an example.

Carbohydrates **319**

9. How can the number of asymmetric carbon atoms be used to predict the number of optical isomers?
10. If a compound has three asymmetric carbons, how many optical isomers are possible?
11. What is the difference between ordinary light and polarized light?
12. What effect does a solution of an optical isomer have on the plane of polarized light?
13. What do the letters D and L refer to in terms of optical isomers?
14. What are epimers? Give an example.
15. Is the D or the L form the predominant one in terms of carbohydrates that the body uses?
16. What is the reference compound for the configurations of carbohydrates?
17. What is a hexosan? a pentosan?
18. What are the three types of carbohydrates?
19. How are carbohydrates formed in nature? Are they formed directly as polysaccharides?
20. Are animals able to synthesize carbohydrates from raw materials? Explain.
21. What are trioses? pentoses? hexoses?
22. Name the three important hexoses and draw their linear structural formulas.
23. How do the three important hexoses differ in molecular formula? in structure?
24. Why can glucose be given intravenously whereas sucrose cannot?
25. Where is glucose normally found in nature?
26. Where are fructose and galactose normally found in nature?
27. Where is glucose found in the body?
28. How do the hexoses affect alkaline Cu^{2+} complex ions? What use is made of this reaction?
29. What are the trade names given to alkaline Cu^{2+} complex ions used in testing for hexoses?
30. What is Tollen's reagent? What is it used for?
31. Do all hexoses ferment in the presence of yeast? Why or why not?
32. What product is formed when the aldehyde end of glucose is oxidized?
33. What product is formed when the alcohol end of glucose is oxidized?
34. What product is formed when both ends of glucose are oxidized?
35. What product is formed when the aldehyde end of glucose is reduced?
36. Do all three disaccharides act as reducing agents? Why?
37. Do all three disaccharides ferment in the presence of yeast? Why?
38. Explain how you could identify a disaccharide on the basis of its reducing action and its fermentation.
39. Compare the ring structures of the three disaccharides and use these structures to explain their reaction to alkaline Cu^{2+} complex.
40. Where is sucrose found in nature?
41. Where is maltose found in nature?
42. Where is lactose found in nature?
43. Compare the properties of the polysaccharides with those of monosaccharides and disaccharides.
44. What is starch?
45. What is the test for the presence of starch? of iodine?
46. What products are formed when starch is slowly hydrolyzed? How may the presence of these products be detected?
47. For what purpose do plants use cellulose?
48. What is mercerized cotton?

Biochemistry   **320**

49. For what purpose does the body use glycogen?

50. What is glycogenesis? glycogenolysis?

51. What are dextrins? How are they used commercially?

52. What type of liquid mixture does starch form in boiling water?

B **53.** What is a hemiacetal? Draw the hemiacetal structure for α-D-glucose.

54. What is a hemiketal? Draw the hemiketal structure for α-D-fructose.

55. What is a Fischer projection? How does it indicate three-dimensional structure?

56. What is a Haworth projection? How does it indicate three-dimensional structure?

57. Draw the Fischer and Haworth projections for D-galactose.

58. What does the representation $+ + + +$ indicate in regards to the use of Clinitest tablets?

59. What is a glycosidic linkage?

60. What type of glycosidic linkage is present in maltose? sucrose? lactose?

61. Why are alpha and beta forms of maltose possible?

62. Why can't the body's enzymes digest cellulose?

References BAUM, STUART J. *Introduction to Organic and Biological Chemistry,* 3rd ed. Macmillan Publishing Company, New York, 1983, Chapters 11, 12.

MARTIN, D. W., P. A. MAYES, and V. W. RODWELL. *Harper's Review of Biochemistry,* 19th ed. Lange Medical Publications, Los Altos, Calif., 1983, Chapter 12.

MORRISON, ROBERT T. and ROBERT N. BOYD. *Organic Chemistry,* 4th ed. Allyn and Bacon, Inc., Boston, 1983, Chapters 28, 29.

RAWN, J. DAVID. *Biochemistry.* Harper & Row, New York, 1983, Chapter 8.

SOLOMONS, T. W. GRAHAM. *Organic Chemistry,* 3rd ed. John Wiley & Sons, New York, 1984, Chapter 21.

ZIMMERMAN, HENRY and ISAAK ZIMMERMAN. *Elements of Organic Chemistry,* 2nd ed. Macmillan Publishing Company, New York, 1983, Chapters 6, 11, 12.

22 Lipids

CHAPTER OUTLINE

General Properties
Fatty Acids
Classification
  Simple Lipids
  Compound Lipids
  Derived Lipids
Fats and Oils
  Structure
  Iodine Number
  Use of Fats in the Body
  Physical Properties
  Chemical Reactions
Soaps
  Cleansing Action

Detergents
Waxes
Phospholipids
  Cell Membranes
  Phosphoglycerides
  Phosphospingosides
Glycolipids
Eicosanoids
  The Prostaglandins
  Prostacyclin and Thromboxanes
  Leukotrienes
Steroids

General Properties

A second group of organic compounds that serve as food for the body is called lipids. Lipids have the following general properties.

1. Insoluble in water.
2. Soluble in organic solvents such as alcohol, ether, acetone, and carbon tetrachloride.
3. Contain carbon, hydrogen, and oxygen; sometimes contain nitrogen and phosphorus.
4. Yield fatty acids on hydrolysis or combine with fatty acids to form an ester.
5. Take part in plant and animal metabolism.

Fatty Acids

Both simple and compound lipids yield fatty acids on hydrolysis. Fatty acids are straight-chain organic acids. The fatty acids that are found in natural fats usually contain an even number of carbon atoms. Fatty acids may be one of two types: saturated and unsaturated. Saturated fatty acids contain only single bonds between carbon atoms. Unsaturated fatty acids contain one or more double bonds between carbon atoms.

Table 22–1 lists some of the common fatty acids and indicates where they are found in nature. Note that they all contain an even number of carbon atoms.

322

TABLE 22-1. Common Fatty Acids

Name	Formula		Source
		Saturated Fatty Acids	
Butyric	C_3H_7COOH		Butter fat
Caproic	$C_5H_{11}COOH$		Butter fat
Caprylic	$C_7H_{15}COOH$		Coconut oil
Capric	$C_9H_{19}COOH$		Palm oil
Lauric	$C_{11}H_{23}COOH$		Laurel
Myristic	$C_{13}H_{27}COOH$		Nutmeg oil, coconut oil
Palmitic	$C_{15}H_{31}COOH$		Palm oil, lard, cottonseed oil
Stearic	$C_{17}H_{35}COOH$		Plant and animal fats such as lard, peanut oil
Arachidic	$C_{19}H_{39}COOH$		Peanut oil
		Unsaturated Fatty Acids	
Oleic	$C_{17}H_{33}COOH$	(contains 1 double bond)	Olive oil
Linoleic	$C_{17}H_{31}COOH$	(contains 2 double bonds)	Linseed oil
Linolenic	$C_{17}H_{29}COOH$	(contains 3 double bonds)	Linseed oil
Arachidonic	$C_{19}H_{31}COOH$	(contains 4 double bonds)	Animal tissues, corn oil, linseed oil

Unsaturated fatty acids have lower melting points than the corresponding saturated fatty acids, and the greater the degree of unsaturation, the lower the melting point. The 18-carbon saturated fatty acid, stearic acid, melts at 70°C. The 18-carbon fatty acid with one double bond, oleic acid, melts at 13°C. The 18-carbon fatty acid with two double bonds, linoleic acid, melts at −5°C; and the 18-carbon fatty acid with three double bonds, linolenic acid, melts at −10°C.

Linoleic acid is called the **essential fatty acid**—it is essential for the complete nutrition of the human body. It cannot be synthesized in the body and must be supplied from food we eat. Arachidonic and linolenic acids, which were formerly also designated as essential fatty acids, can be synthesized in the body from linoleic acid. Linoleic acid is found in large concentrations in oils such as corn, cottonseed, peanut, and soybean but *not* in coconut or olive oils. One of the functions of essential fatty acids is in the synthesis of the prostaglandins (see page 339).

The absence of essential fatty acids from the diet of an infant causes loss of weight and also eczema.* Such conditions may be cured by administering corn oil or linseed oil. Commercial boiled linseed oil should never be used for this purpose because it can contain litharge, a lead compound that is poisonous to the body.

The percentages of fatty acids in corn oil, linseed oil, butter, and lard are listed in Table 22-2. The percentages listed in Table 22-2 are given as averages since the percentage composition of a fat or oil can vary considerably because of weather conditions or the type of food eaten by the animal, or both.

In addition to these straight-chain fatty acids, there are also cyclic fatty acids. An example of this is chaulmoogric acid, whose formula is

Lipids

chaulmoogric acid

Chaulmoogric acid occurs in chaulmoogra oil and has been used in the treatment of leprosy, although it has been supplanted in this use by newer and more effective drugs.

TABLE 22–2. Average Percentage of Fatty Acids in Fats and Oils

		Saturated				Unsaturated			
		Myristic Acid	Palmitic Acid	Stearic Acid	Other Acids	Oleic Acid	Linoleic Acid	Other Acids	Iodine Number
Vegetable oils	cotton- seed oil	0–3	17–23	1–3	—	23–44	34–55	0–1	103–115
	corn oil	0–2	8–10	1–4	—	36–50	34–56	0–3	116–130
Animal fats	butter	8–13	25–32	8–13	4–11	22–29	3	3–9	26–45
	lard	1	25–30	12–16	—	41–51	3–8	5–8	46–66

Oleic acid, $C_{17}H_{33}COOH$, occurs in nature as the *cis* configuration (see page 301), as do most naturally occurring unsaturated fatty acids. The *trans* form is called elaidic acid.

oleic acid (*cis* form)

elaidic acid (*trans* form)

Classification   Lipids are divided into three main categories: simple, compound, and derived.

Simple Lipids   Simple lipids are esters of fatty acids. The hydrolysis of a simple lipid may be expressed as

$$\text{simple lipid} + H_2O \xrightarrow{\text{hydrolysis}} \text{fatty acid(s)} + \text{alcohol}$$

If the hydrolysis of a simple lipid yields three fatty acids and *glycerol,* the simple lipid is called a *fat* or *oil.*

Biochemistry

If the hydrolysis of a simple lipid yields a fatty acid and a high-molecular-weight monohydric alcohol, the simple lipid is called a *wax*.

Compound Lipids

Compound lipids on hydrolysis yield a fatty acid(s), an alcohol, and some other type of compound. In this category are phospholipids and glycolipids (also called cerebrosides because they are found in the cerebrum of the brain). These compound lipids undergo hydrolysis as follows

phospholipids + H_2O $\xrightarrow{\text{hydrolysis}}$
    fatty acid + alcohol + phosphoric acid + a nitrogen compound

glycolipids + H_2O $\xrightarrow{\text{hydrolysis}}$ fatty acid + a carbohydrate + sphingosine
    (a nitrogen-containing alcohol)

Derived Lipids

Derived lipids are compounds produced when simple and compound lipids undergo hydrolysis. Derived lipids include such substances as fatty acids, glycerol, other alcohols, sterols, which are solid alcohols having a high molecular weight, fatty aldehydes, and ketone bodies (see page 418).

Fats and Oils

Structure

Fats are esters formed by the combination of a fatty acid with one particular alcohol, glycerol. If one molecule of glycerol reacts with one molecule of stearic acid (a fatty acid), glyceryl monostearate is formed.

stearic acid   glycerol   glyceryl monostearate

The product of this reaction may react with a second molecule and then with a third molecule of stearic acid.

Glyceryl tristearate (also called tristearin) is formed by the reaction of one molecule of glycerol with three molecules of stearic acid. Since stearic acid is a saturated fatty acid, the product is a fat. As the degree of unsaturation of the fatty acids increases, the melting point decreases (see page 323). Fats with a melting point below room temperature are called oils.

glyceryl distearate

$$C_{17}H_{35}COO—\overset{\displaystyle H}{\underset{\displaystyle H}{C}}—H-$$
$$C_{17}H_{35}COO—\overset{\displaystyle }{\underset{\displaystyle }{C}}—H$$
$$C_{17}H_{35}COOH + HO—\overset{\displaystyle }{\underset{\displaystyle H}{C}}—H$$

glyceryl tristearate,
a fat

The glycerol molecule contains three —OH groups and so combines with three fatty acid molecules. However, these fatty acid molecules do not have to be the same. Fats and oils can contain three different fatty acid molecules, either saturated, unsaturated, or some combination of these.

An example of a mixed triglyceride† formed from the reaction of glycerol with three different fatty acid molecules follows. The fatty acids are oleic, stearic, and linoleic.

$$CH_3CH_2CH_2CH_2CH_2CH_2CH_2CH_2CH=CHCH_2CH_2CH_2CH_2CH_2CH_2CH_2COO—\overset{\displaystyle H}{C}—H$$
(from oleic acid—one double bond)

$$CH_3CH_2CH_2CH_2CH_2CH_2CH_2CH_2CH_2CH_2CH_2CH_2CH_2CH_2CH_2CH_2CH_2COO—C—H$$
(from stearic acid—saturated—no double bonds)

$$CH_3CH_2CH_2CH_2CH_2CH=CHCH_2CH=CHCH_2CH_2CH_2CH_2CH_2CH_2COO—\underset{\displaystyle H}{C}—H$$
(from linoleic acid—two double bonds)
a mixed triglyceride

Oleic acid has a *cis* configuration around its double bond; linoleic acid has a *cis-cis* configuration.

The preceding formula for a mixed triglyceride may be written in condensed form as shown in structure (22–1).

$$CH_3(CH_2)_7CH=CH(CH_2)_7COO—\overset{\displaystyle H}{C}—H$$
$$CH_3(CH_2)_{16}COO—C—H \qquad (22–1)$$
$$CH_3(CH_2)_4CH=CHCH_2CH=CH(CH_2)_7COO—\underset{\displaystyle H}{C}—H$$

or simply as

$$C_{17}H_{33}COO—\overset{\displaystyle H}{C}—H$$
$$C_{17}H_{35}COO—C—H \qquad (22–2)$$
$$C_{17}H_{31}COO—\underset{\displaystyle H}{C}—H$$

† According to the International Union of Pure and Applied Chemistry (IUPAC) and the International Union of Biochemistry (IUB), monoglycerides are to be designated as monoacylglycerols, diglycerides as diacylglycerols, and triglycerides as triacylglycerols. Throughout this text, these systems may be used interchangeably.

Biochemistry

A more correct representation of the triglyceride structure (22–2) is

indicating the L-configuration of most naturally occurring triglycerides, but for simplicity we will use structure (22–2).

Iodine Number

Unsaturated fats and oils will readily combine with iodine, whereas saturated fats and oils will not do so very readily. The more unsaturated the fat or oil, the more iodine it will react with.

The iodine number of a fat or oil is the number of grams of iodine that will react with the double bonds present in 100 g of that fat or oil. The higher the iodine number, the greater the degree of unsaturation of the fat or oil. The iodine numbers of some fats and oils are listed in Table 22–2.

In general, animal fats have a lower iodine number than do vegetable oils. This indicates that vegetable oils are more unsaturated. This increasing unsaturation is also accompanied by a change of state—animal fats are solid; vegetable oils are liquid. Fats have an iodine number below 70, whereas oils have iodine numbers above 70.

Animal and vegetable oils should not be confused with mineral oil, which is a mixture of saturated hydrocarbons, or with essential oils, which are volatile aromatic liquids used as flavors and perfumes.

Use of Fats in the Body

Fats serve as a fuel in the body, producing more energy per gram than either carbohydrate or protein. Metabolism of fat produces 9 kcal/g, whereas the metabolism of either carbohydrate or protein produces 4 kcal/g.

Fats also serve as a reserve supply of food and energy for the body. If a 70-kg person stored energy in the form of carbohydrate rather than fat, that person would weigh an additional 55 kg. Fat is stored in the adipose tissue and serves as a protector for the vital organs. That is, fats surround the vital organs to keep them in place and also act as shock absorbers. Fats in the outer layers of the body act as heat insulators, helping to keep the body warm in cold weather. Fats act as electrical insulators and allow rapid propagation of nerve impulses. The fat content of nerve tissue is particularly high. Fats are a constituent of lipoproteins, which are found in cell membranes and in the mitochondria and also serve as a means of transporting lipids in the bloodstream.

Physical Properties

Pure fats and oils are generally white or yellow solids and liquids, respectively. Pure fats and oils are also odorless and tasteless. However, over a period of time fats become rancid; they develop an unpleasant odor and taste.

Lipids

Fats and oils are insoluble in water but are soluble in such organic liquids as benzene, acetone, and ether. Fats do not diffuse through a membrane. Fats are lighter than water and have a greasy feeling. Fats and oils form a temporary emulsion when shaken with water. The emulsion may be made permanent by the addition of an emulsifying agent such as soap. Fats and oils must be emulsified by bile in the body before they can be digested.

Chemical Reactions

HYDROLYSIS

When fats are treated with enzymes, acids, or bases, they hydrolyze to form fatty acids and glycerol. When tripalmitin (glyceryl tripalmitate) is hydrolyzed, it forms palmitic acid and glycerol and requires three molecules of water. Recall that in the formation of a fat, water is a product.

tripalmitin   palmitic acid   glycerol

When fats are hydrolyzed to fatty acids and glycerol, the glycerol separates from the fatty acids and can be drawn off and purified. Glycerol is used both medicinally and industrially.

SAPONIFICATION

Saponification is the heating of a fat with a strong base such as sodium hydroxide to produce glycerol and the salt of a fatty acid.

$$C_{17}H_{35}COO-CH_2$$
$$C_{17}H_{35}COO-CH + 3NaOH \xrightarrow{heat} 3C_{17}H_{35}COONa + glycerol$$
$$C_{17}H_{35}COO-CH_2$$

tristearin   sodium stearate,   glycerol
                          a soap

The sodium salt (or potassium salt) of a fatty acid is called a soap. Reactions and properties of soaps will be discussed later in this chapter.

HYDROGENATION

Fats and oils are similar compounds except that oils are more unsaturated; that is, oils contain many double bonds. These double bonds may be changed to single bonds upon the addition of hydrogen. Vegetable oils may be converted to fats by the addition of hydrogen in the presence of a catalyst. This process is called hydrogenation. Hydrogenation is used to produce the so-called vegetable shortenings used in the home. Oleomargarine is prepared by the hydrogenation of certain fats and oils with the addition of flavoring and coloring agents, plus vitamins A and D. Compounds that give butter its characteristic flavor are sometimes added.

Biochemistry   **328**

triolein, an oil
(contains double bonds)

tristearin, a fat
(contains single bonds)

In actual practice, vegetable oils are not completely hydrogenated. Enough hydrogen is added to produce a solid at room temperature. If the oil were completely hydrogenated, the solid fat would be hard and brittle and unsuitable for cooking purposes.

As should be expected, hydrogenation lowers the iodine number to a value within the range of fats.

ACROLEIN TEST The acrolein test, which is a test for the presence of glycerol, is sometimes used as a test for fats and oils, since all fats and oils contain glycerol.

When glycerol is heated to a high temperature, especially in the presence of a dehydrating agent such as potassium bisulfate ($KHSO_4$), a product called acrolein results.

glycerol   acrolein

This substance is easily recognized by its strong, pungent odor. When fats or oils are heated to a high temperature or are burned, the disagreeable odor is that of acrolein.

RANCIDITY Fats develop an unpleasant odor and taste when allowed to stand at room temperature for a short period of time. That is, they become rancid. Rancidity is due to two types of reactions—hydrolysis and oxidation.

Oxygen present in the air can oxidize some unsaturated parts of fats and oils. If this oxidation reaction produces short-chain acids or aldehydes, the fat turns rancid, as evidenced by a disagreeable odor and taste. Since oxidation, as well as hydrolysis, takes place more rapidly at higher temperatures, fats and foods containing a high percentage of fats should be stored in a cool place. Oxidation of fats, especially in hydrogenated vegetable compounds, can be inhibited by the addition of antioxidants, substances that prevent oxidation. Two naturally occurring antioxidants are vitamine C and vitamin E.

When butter is allowed to stand at room temperature, hydrolysis takes place between the fats and the water present in the butter. The products of

Lipids   **329**

this hydrolysis are fatty acids and glycerol. One of the fatty acids produced, butyric acid, has the disagreeable odor that causes one to say that the butter is rancid. The catalysts necessary for the hydrolysis reaction are produced by the action of microorganisms present in the air acting on the butter. At room temperature this reaction proceeds rapidly so that the butter soon turns rancid. This effect may be overcome by keeping the butter refrigerated and covered.

Soaps

Soaps are produced by the saponification of fats. Soaps are salts of fatty acids. When the saponifying agent used is sodium hydroxide, a sodium soap is produced. Sodium soaps are bar soaps. When the saponifying agent used is potassium hydroxide, a potassium soap is produced. Potassium soaps are soft or liquid soaps.

Soaps may also be produced by the reaction of a fatty acid with an inorganic base, although this method is much too expensive to be of commercial value.

$$C_{17}H_{35}COOH + NaOH \longrightarrow C_{17}H_{35}COONa + H_2O$$

stearic acid	sodium hydroxide	sodium stearate, a soap

Various substances may be added to soaps to give them a pleasant color and odor. Floating soaps contain air bubbles. Germicidal soaps contain a germicide. Scouring soaps contain some abrasive. Tincture of green soap is a solution of a potassium soap in alcohol.

Calcium and magnesium ions present in hard water react with soap to form insoluble calcium and magnesium soaps.

$$2Na\ soap + Ca^{2+} \longrightarrow Ca\ soap{\downarrow} + 2Na^+$$

$$2Na\ soap + Mg^{2+} \longrightarrow Mg\ soap{\downarrow} + 2Na^+$$

The soap "precipitate" is mostly organic and floats to the top rather than sinking to the bottom as most precipitates. This precipitated soap is seen as "the ring around the bathtub." More soap is required to produce a lather in hard water than in soft water (see page 152).

Zinc stearate is an insoluble soap used as a dusting powder for infants. It has antiseptic properties but is irritating to mucous membranes. Zinc undecylenate is used in the treatment of athlete's foot.

Children who suffer from celiac disease cannot absorb fatty acids from the small intestine. The unabsorbed fatty acids combine with calcium ions to form insoluble calcium compounds, or soaps. These calcium compounds are eliminated from the body, and the body will become deficient in calcium unless additional amounts of this necessary element are given to the child.

Cleansing Action

Soaps are cleansing agents. Consider a soap molecule such as sodium stearate.

$$CH_3—CH_2—CH_2—CH_2—CH_2—CH_2—CH_2—CH_2—CH_2—$$
$$CH_2—CH_2—CH_2—CH_2—CH_2—CH_2—CH_2—CH_2—COONa$$

The long-chain aliphatic part is nonpolar whereas the carboxylate part is polar. A simplified representation of a soap molecule is ○— where the line represents the nonpolar part and the circle the polar part.

In general, nonpolar compounds dissolve in nonpolar liquids and polar compounds dissolve in polar liquids (see page 160). If soap is added to a mixture of water and oil and then shaken rapidly, the nonpolar end of the soap molecule will dissolve in the oil, a nonpolar liquid. At the same time, the polar end of the soap molecule will dissolve in the water, a polar liquid. The nonpolar end of the soap molecule is said to be **hydrophobic,*** water repelling. The polar end is **hydrophillic,*** water soluble. The carboxylate end of the soap molecule, which is in the water, ionizes into sodium ions, which are free to move about. This may be represented as follows:

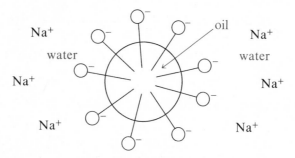

Structures such as this are called micelles.

Note that the oil drop has a negative charge because of the negative ends of the soap molecules sticking out into the water. This negatively charged oil drop will repel all other oil drops, which will have acquired a like charge. That is, the oil will have become emulsified with the soap acting as the emulsifying agent.

This is the manner in which soap cleanses, since most dirt is held on skin and clothing by a thin layer of grease or oil. Mechanical washing causes the oil or grease to break up into small drops. The soap then emulsifies that oil or grease, which can then be easily washed away. Soap also acts as a surfactant (page 167); it lowers the surface tension of the water, making emulsification easier.

Soap has little effect as an antibacterial agent. Nurses and surgeons in the operating room scrub for at least 10 min to remove most of the debris, such as keratin and natural fats, from the skin. A germicidal soap, one that contains a germ-killing compound, usually is used.

Detergents   Detergents (syndets) are synthetic compounds used as cleansing agents. They work like soaps but are free of several of the disadvantages that soaps have.

Detergents work as well in hard water as they do in soft water. That is, calcium and magnesium salts of detergents are soluble and do not precipitate out of solution (as do calcium and magnesium soaps). Recall that soaps do not work as well in hard water because insoluble calcium and magnesium salts precipitate out of solution. Detergents are generally neutral compounds compared to soaps, which are usually alkaline or basic substances. Therefore, detergents may be used on silks and woolens but soaps may not. Detergents are used in washing clothes and also as cleansing agents in toothpastes and toothpowders.

Detergents are sodium salts of long-chain alcohol sulfates. For example, sodium lauryl sulfate may be prepared by treating lauryl alcohol, a 12-carbon alcohol, with sulfuric acid and then neutralizing with sodium hydroxide. The reactions are

$$\underset{\text{lauryl alcohol}}{C_{11}H_{23}CH_2OH} + H_2SO_4 \longrightarrow \underset{\text{lauryl hydrogen sulfate}}{C_{11}H_{23}CH_2OSO_3H} + H_2O$$

$$\underset{\substack{\text{lauryl hydrogen} \\ \text{sulfate}}}{C_{11}H_{23}CH_2OSO_3H} + NaOH \longrightarrow \underset{\substack{\text{sodium lauryl sulfate,} \\ \text{a detergent}}}{C_{11}H_{23}CH_2OSO_3Na} + H_2O$$

Note that the detergent, like a soap, has a nonpolar part and a polar part.

Detergents containing straight chains are **biodegradable** and do not cause water pollution, whereas those containing branched chains are nonbiodegradable and cause pollution.

Waxes A wax is a compound produced by the reaction of a fatty acid with a high-molecular-weight monohydric alcohol such as myricyl alcohol ($C_{30}H_{61}OH$) and ceryl alcohol ($C_{26}H_{53}OH$). Carnauba wax is largely $C_{25}H_{51}COOC_{30}H_{61}$, an ester of myricyl alcohol. Beeswax is largely $C_{15}H_{31}COOC_{30}H_{61}$, also an ester of myricyl alcohol.

Note that waxes are primarily esters of long-chain fatty acids with an even number of carbon atoms and long-chain alcohols, also with an even number of carbon atoms. The number of carbon atoms is usually 26 to 34. The alcohol may also be a steroid such as lanosterol. The wax thus produced, lanolin, is widely used in cosmetics and ointments.

Waxes are insoluble in water, nonreactive, and flexible; hence, waxes make excellent protective coatings. Excessive loss of water through the feathers of birds, through the fur of animals, and through the leaves of plants is prevented by the presence of waxes.

Some of the common waxes are listed in Table 22–3.

TABLE 22–3. Common Waxes

Name	Source	Use
Beeswax	Honeycomb of bee	Polishes and pharmaceutical products
Spermaceti	Sperm whale	Cosmetics and candles
Carnauba	Carnauba palm	Floor waxes and polishes
Lanolin	Wool	Skin ointments

Paraffin wax is different from these waxes because it is merely a mixture of hydrocarbons and is not an ester.

Phospholipids   Phospholipids are phosphate esters and may be divided into two categories—phosphoglycerides and phosphosphingosides—depending on whether the alcohol is glycerol or sphingosine. As indicated on page 325, phospholipids also contain a nitrogen compound. Phospholipids are found in all tissues in the human body, particularly in brain, liver, and spinal tissue.

  Phospholipids also occur in the membranes of all cells. Their peculiar properties are responsible for passage of various substances into and out of the cells.

  Consider a phosphoglyceride whose structure may be represented as

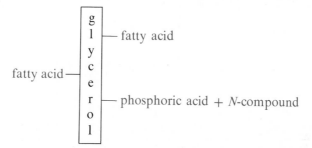

  At carbons 1 and 2 of the glycerol there are esters of fatty acids. At carbon 3 there is a phosphate group, which in turn is bonded to a nitrogen compound. There are many different phosphoglycerides, depending upon the types of fatty acids bonded to the glycerol and also on the identity of the nitrogen compound bonded to the phosphate group. Most phosphoglycerides have a saturated fatty acid connected at carbon 1 and an unsaturated fatty acid at carbon 2.

  The phosphate group and the nitrogen compound are polar substances whereas the fatty acid molecules are nonpolar.

  The fatty acid chains are *hydrophobic**—they point away from water. The other end of the molecule, the one containing the nitrogen compound and phosphoric acid, is *hydrophilic** and dissolves in water. Molecules of this type, with a hydrophobic (nonpolar) and a hydrophilic (polar) end, are said to be **amphipathic.***

Cell Membranes   Cell membranes serve two important functions: (1) a mechanical support to separate the contents of a cell from its external environment and (2) a structural support for certain proteins that serve to transport ions and polar molecules across the membrane. Some of these proteins act as "gates" and "pumps" to move certain materials through the membrane but exclude others. Other membrane proteins act as "receptor sites" by which molecules outside the cell can send messages inside the cell. An example of such a protein is the hormone insulin, which regulates the metabolism of glucose in certain cells but does not cross membranes itself. Instead, the insulin reacts with the specific receptor protein on the outer surface of the membrane, and that receptor protein in turn communicates the specific message to the inside of the cell.

Lipids   **333**

Cell membranes are composed, on the average, of 40 to 50 percent lipids and 50 to 60 percent protein. However, these percentages vary considerably even among the cells of the same individual, as shown in the following table.

Percentages of Lipids in Certain Membranes	
Myelin	82
Red blood cells	48
Mitochondria, outer membrane	48
Mitochondria, inner membrane	24

In addition, membranes also contain cholesterol and a small amount of carbohydrate.

The cell membrane is relatively fluid, as it must be in order to account for the flexibility of the cell and its deformation without disruption of structure.

How do lipids form a membrane and where do the proteins fit into that membrane? Recall that phospholipids have a polar end and a nonpolar end. In the following diagram, the long lines represent the nonpolar (hydrophobic) end, the fatty acid chains, whereas the circles represent the polar (hydrophillic) end, the end that dissolves in water. Such amphipathic molecules can form a bilayer, as shown below.

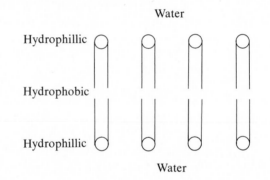

Such a simple model is not satisfactory for cell membranes because this type of bilayer would be highly impermeable to ions and most polar molecules, which cannot pass through the center of such a system. The current theory of cell membranes involves a phospholipid bilayer in which are embedded proteins, as shown in Figure 22-1.

In this type of membrane, called the fluid-mosaic model, some proteins are embedded in the surface of the membrane, others are embedded in the center, and still others provide channels all the way through in order to transport polar molecules and ions through the membrane. The proteins are believed to be mobile and to move through the bilayer as well as across its surface.

Phosphoglycerides One category of phospholipid is the phosphoglycerides, whose general structure is shown below. Phosphoglycerides may in turn be subdivided into

FIGURE 22-1. Fluid mosaic model of plasma membrane structure.

several types, depending upon the nitrogen compound present. Among these are the lecithins and the cephalins.

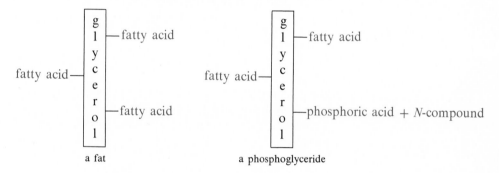

<table>
<tr><td>glycerol</td><td>—fatty acid</td></tr>
</table>

fatty acid—[glycerol]—fatty acid
—fatty acid

a fat

fatty acid—[glycerol]—fatty acid
—phosphoric acid + *N*-compound

a phosphoglyceride

LECITHINS   Lecithins, now called phosphatidylcholines, are compounds that are particularly important in the metabolism of fats by the liver. In lecithins, the nitrogen compound is choline, an alcohol. Choline is an example of a quaternary ammonium compound (see page 264).

$$\text{HOCH}_2\text{—CH}_2\text{—}\overset{+}{\text{N}}\text{—(CH}_3)_3 \qquad \text{OH}^-$$
choline

A typical formula for a lecithin (phosphatidylcholine) is shown on the following page.

In most lecithins, the fatty acid at carbon 1 of the glycerol is saturated whereas the fatty acid at carbon 2 is unsaturated. The carbon marked with an asterisk is asymmetric, indicating optical activity. Naturally occurring lecithins have the L form (see page 300).

Lecithins are insoluble in water but are good emulsifying agents. They are also good sources of phosphoric acid, which is needed for the synthesis of

Lipids   **335**

new tissue. Lecithin is abundant in egg yolk and soybeans. It is used commercially as an emulsifying agent in dairy products and in the manufacture of mayonnaise.

Fats are partly converted to lecithins in the body and are transported as lecithins from one part of the body to another. Lecithins are widely distributed in all cells and have both metabolic and structural functions in membranes.

Dipalmityl lecithin (lecithin where the two fatty acids are palmitic acid) is a very good surface active agent (see page 168). It prevents adherence of the inner surfaces of the lungs.

Removal of one molecule of fatty acid from lecithin produces lysolecithin. The removal of this molecule of fatty acid is catalyzed by the enzyme lecithinase A, which is found in the venom of poisonous snakes. The venom is poisonous because it produces lysolecithin, which in turn causes hemolysis—the destruction of the red blood cells.

CEPHALINS   Cephalins are similar to lecithins except that another nitrogen compound, ethanolamine, is present instead of choline. The newer names for this compound is phosphatidylethanolamine.

$$HO—CH_2—CH_2—NH_2$$
ethanolamine

a cephalin

Cephalins are important in the clotting of the blood and also are sources of phosphoric acid for the formation of new tissue.

Similar compounds, phosphatidylserine and phosphatidylinositol, are abundant in brain tissue. In these compounds, serine and inositol, respectively, occur in place of choline or ethanolamine in the preceding diagrams.

$$HO-CH_2-\overset{\overset{\displaystyle NH_2}{|}}{CH}-COOH$$

serine

inositol

PLASMALOGENS   Plasmalogens structurally resemble lecithin and cephalin but they have an unsaturated ether at carbon 1 instead of an ester. The fatty acid at carbon 2 of the glycerol is usually unsaturated. Plasmalogens constitute up to 10 percent of the phospholipids found in membranes of brain and muscle cells. The structure of a plasmalogen is

Phosphosphingosides   Phosposphingosides, also called sphingolipids, differ from phosphoglycerides in that they contain the alcohol sphingosine in place of glycerol. One particular type of sphingolipid, called sphingomyelin, is present in large amounts in brain and nerve tissue. The general formula for a sphingolipid and the structural formula for sphingomyelin are given below.

In Niemann-Pick disease, a disease of infancy or early childhood, sphingomyelins accumulate in the brain, liver, and spleen. The accumulation of the sphingomyelins causes mental retardation and early death. It is caused by the lack of a specific enzyme, sphingomyelinase.

a sphingolipid

Lipids

sphingomyelin

Note that the fatty acid in sphingomyelin is bonded to an $-NH_2$ group rather than to an $-OH$ group as in phosphoglycerides.

Glycolipids   Glycolipids are similar to sphingomyelins except that they contain a carbohydrate, often galactose, in place of the choline and phosphoric acid. The general structure for a glycolipid is

As in sphingomyelins, the fatty acid is bonded to an $-NH_2$ group on the sphingosine molecule.

Glycolipids produce no phosphoric acid on hydrolysis because they do not contain this compound. Glycolipids are also called cerebrosides because they are found in large amounts in the brain tissue.

Among the glycolipids are kerasin, cerebron, nervon, oxynervon, and the gangliosides. These compounds differ primarily in the identity of the fatty acid attached to the sphingosine.

In Gaucher's disease glycolipids accumulate in the brain and cause severe mental retardation and death by age 3. Juvenile and adult forms of this disease are characterized by enlarged spleen and kidneys, hemorrhaging, mild anemia, and fragile bones. This disease is caused by the lack of a specific enzyme, β-glucosidase.

In the absence of a particular enzyme, hexosaminidase A, glycolipids accumulate in the tissues of the brain and eyes. This effect, called Tay–Sachs disease, is usually fatal to infants before they reach age 2.

Eicosanoids

The eicosanoids are a biologically active group of compounds derived from arachidonic acid. They are extremely potent compounds with a variety of actions, as will be discussed in the following paragraphs. Among the eicosanoids are the prostaglandins, the thromboxanes, prostacyclin, and the leukotrienes.

The Prostaglandins

The prostaglandins consist of 20-carbon unsaturated fatty acids containing a five-membered ring and two side chains. One side chain has seven carbon atoms and ends with an acid group (COOH). The other chain contains eight carbon atoms with an —OH group on the third carbon from the ring (see structure given). The E series of prostaglandins has, in addition to four asymmetric carbon atoms, a *trans* configuration.

Prostaglandins are derived from arachidonic acid, which is formed from the essential fatty acid linoleic acid. The structures of arachidonic acid and prostaglandin E_1 (PGE_1) are

arachidonic acid

prostaglandin E_1(PGE_1)

The abbreviation PGE_1 refers to prostaglandin E with one double bond. Likewise, PGE_2 refers to prostaglandin E with two double bonds.

Prostaglandins have been isolated from most mammalian tissues, including male and female reproductive systems, liver, kidneys, pancreas, heart, lungs, brain, and intestines. The richest source of prostaglandins is human seminal fluid.

Prostaglandins have a wide range of physiologic effects. They seem to be involved in the body's natural defenses against all forms of change including those induced by chemical, mechanical, physiologic, and pathologic stimuli. Aspirin and other anti-inflammatory drugs appear to partially operate by inhibiting prostaglandin synthesis. Prostaglandins are involved at the cellular level in regulating many body functions, including gastric acid secretion, contraction and relaxation of smooth muscles, inflammation and vascular permeability, body temperature, and blood platelet aggregation. Prostaglandins stimulate steroid production by the adrenal glands and also stimulate the release of insulin from the pancreas. Prostaglandins markedly stimulate the movement of calcium ions from bone. Excessive production of prostaglandins by malignant tissue may provide a partial answer for the hypercalcemia* and osteolysis* observed in patients afflicted with such a condition.

Prostaglandins have also been used clinically to induce abortion or to induce labor in a term pregnancy, to treat hypertension, to relieve bronchial asthma, and to heal peptic ulcers.

Prostaglandins increase cyclic adenosine monophosphate (c-AMP) (see page 503) in blood platelets, thyroid, corpus luteum, adenohypophysis, and lungs but decrease c-AMP in adipose tissue.

Prostaglindin E_1 (PGE$_1$) is now used to strengthen babies born with cyanotic congenital heart disease, "blue babies," to prepare them for corrective surgery. Another use of prostaglandins is in animal husbandry, particularly in the management of breeding farm animals.

Prostacyclin and Thromboxanes

Prostacyclin is so-called because it contains a second five-membered ring in addition to the ring found in prostaglandins. Thromboxanes have a cyclopentane ring interrupted by an oxygen atom. The structures of prostacyclin and thromboxane B$_2$ (TXB$_2$) are

prostacyclin   TXB$_2$

Prostacyclin is a potent inhibitor of platelet aggregation and is a powerful vasodilator.

Thromboxanes have an effect opposite to that of prostacyclin. They are potent aggregators of blood platelets and have a profound contractive effect on a variety of smooth muscles.

Thromboxanes function in conjunction with prostacyclin in maintaining a healthy vascular system. Both substances exert their influence by regulating the production of c-AMP with the thromboxanes acting as inhibitors and prostacyclin as a stimulator of c-AMP production.

Leukotrienes

Leukotrienes are another group of eicosanoids derived from arachidonic acid. The *tri* refers to three alternate sets of double bonds in the molecule. One of this group, leukotriene C, is involved in the body's allergic responses. It constricts air passages to the bronchi during an asthma attack. The structure of leukotriene C is

Biochemistry   **340**

Steroids

Steroids are high-molecular-weight tetracyclic (four-ring) compounds. Those containing one or more —OH groups and no C=O groups are called sterols. The most common sterol is cholesterol, which is found in animal fats but not in plant fats. Cholesterol is found in all animal tissues, particularly in brain and nervous tissue, in the bloodstream, and as gallstones. Cholesterol aids in the absorption of fatty acids from the small intestine. Several theories have been proposed relating cholesterol to coronary malfunction, but no definite evidence has yet been found linking the two together.

Most of the body's cholesterol is derived or synthesized from other substances, such as carbohydrates and proteins as well as from fats.

Atherosclerosis, a form of arteriosclerosis, results from the deposition of excess lipids, primarily triglycerides and cholesterol, from the bloodstream. Of these two, cholesterol poses a greater threat to the well-being of a person, although excess triglycerides also present a significant risk. One way of combating heart disease and atherosclerosis is to reduce the concentration of lipids in the bloodstream—either by reducing lipid intake or by the use of antihyperlipidemic drugs, those that tend to reduce blood lipid levels. It has been found that certain unsaturated fish and vegetable oils, when substituted for saturated fats, lower the serum cholesterol level.

Another substance, Mevinolin, isolated from the fungus *Asperigillus terreus,* inhibits the synthesis of cholesterol and may be helpful in the prevent of atherosclerosis.

Ergosterol is a sterol similar to cholesterol. When ergosterol is irradiated (exposed to radiation) with ultraviolet light, one of the products formed is calciferol (vitamin D_2, see page 483).

Other steroids include bile salts, the sex hormones, and the hormones of the adrenal cortex. The similarities of the structure of some of these steroids are indicated in the following structures.

cholesterol

estradiol

testosterone

ergosterol

Summary   Lipids yield fatty acids on hydrolysis or combine with fatty acids to form esters. Lipids are insoluble in water but are soluble in organic solvents such as ether, acetone, and carbon tetrachloride.

Lipids may be classified into three types: simple, compound, and derived. Simple lipids are esters of fatty acids. A simple lipid that yields fatty acids and glycerol upon hydrolysis is called a fat or oil. A simple lipid that, on hydrolysis, yields fatty acids and a high-molecular-weight alcohol is called a wax.

Compound lipids yield fatty acids, alcohol, and some other type of compound on hydrolysis.

Derived lipids are compounds produced when simple or compound lipids undergo hydrolysis. Fatty acids are straight-chain organic acids. Those found in nature usually contain an even number of carbon atoms. Saturated fatty acids have only single bonds between carbon atoms. Unsaturated fatty acids have one or more double bonds in the molecule and occur in nature in the *cis* form.

The essential fatty acid, so-called because it is necessary in the diet, is linoleic acid.

Unsaturated fats and oils react with iodine, whereas saturated ones do not. The iodine number of a fat or oil is the number of grams of iodine that will react with (the double bonds present in) 100 g of that fat or oil.

Fats serve as fuel for the body—1 g of fat produces 9 kcal as compared to only 4 kcal/g of carbohydrate. Fats protect nerve endings and also act as insulators to keep the body warm in cold weather.

Fats and oils are odorless and tasteless when pure. They are insoluble in water but are soluble in organic solvents. Fats and oils must be emulsified before being digested.

When fats are hydrolyzed, they form fatty acids and glycerol. When fats are saponified, they form salts of fatty acids (soaps) and glycerol.

When oils are hydrogenated, the double bonds are changed to single bonds and the (liquid) oil becomes a (solid) fat.

When fats or oils are heated to a high temperature, especially in the presence of

Biochemistry

a dehydrating agent, a product known as acrolein is produced. The odor of burning fat or oil is due to the presence of acrolein.

When fats are allowed to stand at room temperature, they become rancid because of hydrolysis and oxidation. Keeping fats cool prevents their becoming rancid.

Soaps are salts of fatty acids—sodium soaps are solid or bar soaps and potassium soaps are soft or liquid soaps.

Calcium and magnesium soaps are insoluble in water and are formed when sodium or potassium soaps are used in hard water. The precipitated calcium and magnesium soaps are seen as the "ring around the bathtub."

Detergents are similar to soaps in their cleansing properties. However, detergents do not precipitate in hard water because their calcium and magnesium compounds are soluble.

A wax is a compound produced by the reaction of a fatty acid with a high-molecular-weight monohydric alcohol.

Phospholipids contain fatty acids, an alcohol, a nitrogen compound, and phosphoric acid. Two types of phospholipids are phosphoglycerides and phosphosphingosides.

Phosphoglycerides include phosphatidylcholines (lecithin) and phosphatidylethanolamine (cephalin). Lecithins are important in the metabolism of fats by the liver and also are a source of phosphoric acid, which is needed for the formation of new tissue. Cephalins are important in clotting of the blood and also are a source of phosphoric acid for the formation of new tissue.

Sphingomyelins are an example of phosphosphingosides and are present in large amounts in brain and nerve tissue.

Glycolipids, also called cerebrosides, are found in large amounts in brain tissue.

Phospholipids are found in all cell membranes as bilayers and are responsible for the passage of various substances into and out of the cells.

The eicosanoids are a biologically active group of compounds derived from arachidonic acid. Among the eicosanoids are the prostaglandins, the thromboxanes, prostacyclin, and leukotrienes.

Steroids are high-molecular-weight, four-ring compounds. Those containing —OH groups are called sterols. The most common sterol in the body is chholesterol. Other steroids are vitamin D, bile salts, sex hormones, and hormones of the adrenal cortex.

Questions and Problems

A

1. State the general properties of lipids.
2. What are simple lipids?
3. What is the difference between a fat and a wax? a fat and an oil?
4. What is a compound lipid? Give examples of several.
5. What is a derived lipid? Give examples of several.
6. What is a fatty acid?
7. What is the difference between a saturated and an unsaturated fatty acid?
8. What is unusual about the number of carbon atoms in naturally occurring fatty acids?
9. What is an essential fatty acids? Why is it important?
10. Why should commercial boiled linseed oil never be used to overcome a deficiency of the essential fatty acid?
11. What fatty acid has been used in the treatment of leprosy?
12. What is the iodine number of a fat or oil? What determines this number?
13. Which have higher iodine numbers, animal or vegetable fats?

14. Draw the structure of glyceryl tripalmitate.
15. Draw the structure of the fat formed from the reaction of glycerol with palmitic, stearic, and oleic acids.
16. What is the function of fat in the body?
17. What are the general physical properties of fats and oils?
18. What products are formed when a fat is hydrolyzed?
19. What products are formed when a fat is saponified?
20. How can an unsaturated oil be changed to a saturated fat? Is the fat thus formed completely saturated? Why?
21. What is the test for the presence of a fat or oil?
22. What causes rancidity in a fat or oil?
23. Compare soaps with detergents on the basis of structure.
24. Compare soaps with detergents on the basis of their reaction with hard water.
25. What causes a soap to float?
26. What is a germicidal soap? How is it made?
27. Why do surgeons scrub so vigorously before surgery?
28. What causes celiac disease?
29. What is a phospholipid?
30. What are the types of phospholids?
31. What is a lysolecithin? What effect does it have on the body? How is it produced?
32. Compare the structures of the phosphoglycerides.
33. How do phospholipds help control the passage of materials into or out of cells?
34. What is meant by the term *amphipathic*?
35. What causes atherosclerosis? What can be done to prevent it?
36. What causes Niemann–Pick disease? Tay–Sachs disease? Gaucher's disease?
37. What is the most common sterol in the body?
38. Give the names of several steroids. Where is each found?
39. Why does the elimination of cholesterol-containing foods in the diet have little effect on the body's cholesterol? What can be done to reduce serum cholesterol?

B 40. Compare the structures of oleic and elaidic acids.
41. Explain the cleansing action of soap.
42. What do the terms *hydrophobic* and *hydrophillic* mean?
43. What are biodegradable detergents?
44. Why are waxes important biologically?
45. What effect do prostaglandins have on Ca^{2+} concentration?
46. What are prostacyclins? For what purpose are they used?
47. How does the fluid-mosaic model account for the movement of polar substances through a membrane?
48. What does the abbreviation PGF_2 indicate?
49. How do prostacyclin and thromboxanes affect the production of *c*-AMP?
50. From what compound are the eicosanoids derived? What are the main types of eicosanoids?

References   BAUM, STUART J. *Introduction to Organic and Biological Chemistry,* 3rd ed. Macmillan Publishing Company, New York, 1982, Chapter 13.
CAPALDI, R. A. A dynamic model of cell membranes. *Scientific American,* **230**:26–33 (March 1974).
CULLITUN, B. J. Prostaglandins—something for everyone. *Science News,* **98**:306–307 (Oct. 10, 1970).

Biochemistry   **344**

GREEN, D. E. Synthesis of fat. *Scientific American,* **202**:46–51 (Feb. 1960).

KEYNES, R.D. Ion channels in the nerve-cell membrane. *Scientific American,* **240**:126–135 (March 1979).

LODISH, H. F. and J. E. ROTHMAN. The assembly of cell membranes. *Scientific American,* **240**:48–63 (Jan. 1979).

MARTIN, D. W., P. A. MAYES, and V. W. RODWELL. *Harper's Review of Biochemistry,* 19th ed. Lange Medical Publications, Los Altos, Calif., 1983, Chapter 16.

MORRISON, ROBERT T. and ROBERT N. BOYD. *Organic Chemistry,* 4th ed. Allyn and Bacon, Inc., Boston, 1983, Chapter 27.

RAWN, J. DAVID. *Biochemistry.* Harper & Row, New York, 1983, Chapter 11.

SOLOMONS, T. W. GRAHAM. *Organic Chemistry,* 3rd ed. John Wiley & Sons, New York, 1984, Chapter 22.

UNWIN, NIGEL. The structure of proteins in biological membranes. *Scientific American* **250**:78–94 (Feb. 1984).

ZIMMERMAN, HENRY and ISAAK ZIMMERMAN. *Elements of Organic Chemistry,* 2nd ed. Macmillan Publishing Company, New York, 1983, Chapter 13.

23 Proteins

CHAPTER
OUTLINE

Sources
Functions
Molecular Weight
Amino Acids
   Composition
   Amphoteric Nature
Dipeptides
Structure
Percentage Composition
Classification
   Classification According to Composi-
   tion
   Classification According to Function
   Classification According to Shape
Properties

Colloidal Nature
Denaturation
Reagents or Conditions that Cause
   Denaturation
Color Tests
   Xanthoproteic Test
   Biuret Test
   Millon's Test
   Hopkins–Cole Test
   Ninhydrin Test
Chromatography
   Column Chromatography
   Paper Chromatography
   Thin-Layer Chromatography
   Gas-Liquid Chromatography

Other than water, proteins are the chief constituents of all cells of the body. Proteins are much more complex than either carbohydrates or fats. All proteins contain the elements carbon, hydrogen, oxygen, and nitrogen. Most proteins also contain sulfur; some contain phosphorus; and a few, such as hemoglobin, contain some other element.

Sources   Plants synthesize proteins from inorganic substances present in the air and in the soil. Animals cannot synthesize proteins from such materials. Animals must obtain proteins from plants or from other animals, who, in turn, have obtained them from plants.

Animals excrete waste materials containing many nitrogen compounds. These nitrogen compounds along with decaying animal and plant matter are converted into soluble nitrogen compounds by soil bacteria. Plants in turn use these soluble nitrogen compounds to manufacture more protein, thus completing the cycle in nature. A simplified version of the nitrogen cycle is shown in Figure 23–1.

Functions   The word **protein** is derived from the Greek word *proteios,* which means "of first importance." Proteins function in the body in the building of new cells, the maintenance of existing cells, and the replacement of old cells. Thus,

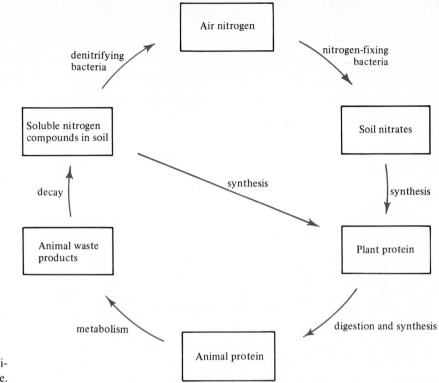

Figure 23-1. The nitrogen cycle.

proteins are the most important type of compound in the body. Proteins are also a valuable source of energy in the body. The oxidation of 1 g protein yields 4 kcal—just as does the oxidation of 1 g carbohydrate.

Proteins are involved in the regulation of metabolic processes (hormones), in the catalysis of biochemical reactions (enzymes), in the transportation of oxygen (hemoglobin), in the body's defense against infection (antibodies), in the transmission of impulses (nerves), in muscular activity (contraction), and in genetic regulation (DNA). Proteins are components of skin, hair, and nails as well as connecting and supporting tissue.

Molecular Weight

Proteins have very high molecular weights. A comparison of the molecular weight of proteins with carbohydrates and fats can be seen in Table 23-1.

Amino Acids

Proteins are polymers built up from simple units called amino acids. Hydrolysis of proteins yields amino acids. There are 20 known amino acids that can be produced by the hydrolysis of protein.† All these amino acids, except

† γ-Aminobutyric acid (GABA) is an amino acid that is not incorporated into protein. It is manufactured almost exclusively in the brain and spinal cord and functions as an inhibitory transmitter. A specific deficiency of GABA in the brain occurs in Huntington's chorea,* an inherited neurological syndrome* characterized by uncontrollable body movements.

Type of Compound	Molecular Weight
Inorganic compounds	
Water	18
Sodium chloride	58.5
Plaster of paris	290
Organic compounds	
Benzene	78
Ethyl alcohol	46
Carbohydrates	
Glucose	180
Sucrose	342
Lipids	
Tristearin	891
Cholesterol	384
Proteins	
Insulin	12,000–48,000[a]
Lactalbumin	17,500
Hemoglobin	68,000
Serum globulin	180,000
Fibrinogen	450,000
Thyroglobin	630,000
Hemocyanin	9,000,000
Tobacco mosaic virus	59,000,000

[a] Even though the minimum calculated molecular weight of
human insulin is 5734 (see structure page 355), insulin exists in
several different polymeric forms depending upon pH, temperature, and concentration.

glycine, which has no asymmetric carbon, have the L configuration. Compare structures 23–1 of the L-amino acid with L-glyceraldehyde.

Composition   Amino acids are organic acids having an amine ($-NH_2$) group attached to
a chain containing an acid group. Although the amine group can be any-
where on the chain, amino acids found in nature usually have the amine
group on the alpha (α) carbon—that is, the carbon atom next to the acid
group. The second carbon from the acid group is the beta (β) carbon. Then
come the gamma (γ) and the delta (δ) carbons, respectively.

α-Amino acids may be represented by the following general formula
where R can be many different radicals.

$$
\begin{array}{cc}
\text{COOH} & \text{CHO} \\
| & | \\
\text{H}_2\text{N}-\text{C}-\text{H} & \text{HO}-\text{C}-\text{H} \\
| & | \\
\text{R} & \text{CH}_2\text{OH} \\
\text{L-amino acid} & \text{L-glyceraldehyde}
\end{array}
\qquad (23\text{–}1)
$$

Certain microorganisms can prepare D-amino acids, which are used as
antibiotics.

Biochemistry   **348**

Amino acids can be divided into two groups, polar and nonpolar, depending upon the polarity of the R group attached to the alpha carbon. If the R group is primarily hydrocarbon, which is nonpolar, then the amino acid will not dissolve in a polar liquid such as water. Thus, amino acids containing a nonpolar R group will be insoluble in water. Exceptions to this are glycine and alanine.

An R group that is polar, such as —OH, —SH, —NH_2, or —COOH, produces an amino acid that is polar. Such amino acids are soluble in water. Table 23–2 lists the polar and nonpolar amino acids.

TABLE 23-2. Nonpolar and Polar Amino Acids

Structure	Name	IUPAC Abbreviation	Isoelectric Point
	Nonpolar		
COOH | H_2N—C—H | CH_3	Alanine	Ala	6.00
COOH | H_2N—C—H | CH / \\ CH_3 CH_2—CH_3	Isoleucine	Ile	6.02
COOH | H_2N—C—H | CH_2 | CH / \\ H_3C CH_3	Leucine	Leu	5.98
COOH | H_2N—C—H | CH_2 | CH_2 | S | CH_3	Methionine	Met	5.74
COOH | H_2N—C—H | CH_2 | ⬡	Phenylalanine	Phe	5.48

TABLE 23-2. Nonpolar and Polar Amino acids (*Continued*)

Structure	Name	IUPAC Abbreviation	Isoelectric Point
Nonpolar (*Continued*)			
	Proline	Pro	6.30
	Tryptophan	Trp	5.89
	Valine	Val	5.96
Polar			
	Arginine	Arg	10.76
	Aspartic acid	Asp	2.97
	Asparagine	Asn	5.41

TABLE 23-2. Nonpolar and Polar Amino acids (*Continued*)

Structure	Name	IUPAC Abbreviation	Isoelectric Point
	Polar (*Continued*)		

Structure	Name	IUPAC Abbreviation	Isoelectric Point
H_2N—C—H with COOH, CH$_2$, SH	Cysteine	Cys	5.07
H_2N—C—H with COOH, CH$_2$, CH$_2$, COOH	Glutamic acid[a]	Glu	3.22
H_2N—C—H with COOH, CH$_2$, CH$_2$, O=C—NH$_2$	Glutamine	Gln	5.65
H_2N—C—H with COOH, H	Glycine	Gly	5.97
H_2N—C—H with COOH, CH$_2$, imidazole ring	Histidine	His	7.59
H_2N—C—H with COOH, CH$_2$—CH$_2$—CH$_2$—CH$_2$—NH$_2$	Lysine	Lys	9.74

TABLE 23-2. Nonpolar and Polar Amino acids (*Continued*)

Structure	Name	IUPAC Abbreviation	Isoelectric Point
	Polar (*Continued*)		

$$
\begin{array}{c}
\text{COOH} \\
| \\
\text{H}_2\text{N}-\text{C}-\text{H} \\
| \\
\text{CH}_2\text{OH}
\end{array}
$$

Serine — Ser — 5.68

$$
\begin{array}{c}
\text{COOH} \\
| \\
\text{H}_2\text{N}-\text{C}-\text{H} \\
| \\
\text{H}-\text{C}-\text{OH} \\
| \\
\text{CH}_3
\end{array}
$$

Threonine — Thr — 5.60

$$
\begin{array}{c}
\text{COOH} \\
| \\
\text{H}_2\text{N}-\text{C}-\text{H} \\
| \\
\text{CH}_2
\end{array}
$$

Tyrosine — Tyr — 5.66

ᵃ Monosodium glutamate (MSG), a salt of glutamic acid, is widely used as a flavor enhancer and seasoning in restaurants and also in food processing. Persons sensitive to this substance develop "Chinese restaurant syndrome," characterized by nausea, headache, and a tightness in facial and neck muscles.

The body can synthesize some, but not all, of the amino acids that it needs. Those that it cannot synthesize must be supplied from food consumed. These are called the nutritionally **essential amino acids** and are listed in Table 23–3 along with the daily requirements per kilogram of body weight.

Amphoteric Nature   Amino acids contain a —COOH group, which is acidic, and an —NH$_2$ group, which is basic (see page 262). In solution, the carboxyl group can donate a hydrogen ion to the amino group, forming a dipolar ion, called a **zwitterion.**

$$
\begin{array}{ccc}
\text{R}-\text{CH}-\text{COOH} & \longrightarrow & \text{R}-\text{CH}-\text{COO}^- \\
| & & | \\
\text{NH}_2 & & \text{NH}_3^+
\end{array}
$$

amino acid   zwitterion form of an amino acid

Amino acids are amphoteric compounds; that is, they can react with either acids or bases. When an amino acid is placed in a basic solution, it forms a negatively charged ion that will be attracted toward a positively

Biochemistry

TABLE 23-3. Essential Amino Acids and
Their Daily Requirement in
Milligrams per Kilogram
of Body Weight

	Adult	Infant
Isoleucine	14	83
Leucine	17	135
Lysine	14	99
Methionine	15	58
Phenylalanine	19	141
Threonine	9	68
Tryptophan	4	21
Valine	13	92
Arginine (can be synthesized by the body but too slowly to be of practical use)		
Histidine (required primarily during childhood)		33

charged electrode. In an acid solution, the amino acid forms a positively charged ion that will be attracted toward a negatively charged electrode.

$$R-CH-COOH \underset{H^+}{\rightleftharpoons} R-CH-COO^- \xrightarrow{OH^-} R-CH-COO^-$$
$$\quad\ |\qquad\qquad\qquad\quad |\qquad\qquad\qquad\qquad |$$
$$\quad NH_3^+\qquad\qquad\qquad NH_3^+\qquad\qquad\qquad\ NH_2$$

positively charged ion   zwitterion   negatively charged ion
(in acid solution)   (in basic solution)

Since amino acids are amphoteric,* proteins, which are made up of amino acids, are also amphoteric. This amphoteric nature of proteins accounts for their ability to act as buffers in the blood; they can react with either acids or bases to prevent an excess of either.

At a certain pH (that is, a certain hydrogen ion concentration) amino acids will not migrate toward either the positive or the negative electrode. At this pH amino acids will be neutral; there will be an equal number of positive and negative ions. This point is called the **isoelectric point*** (see Table 23-2).

Proteins, which are composed of amino acids, also have an isoelectric point, which is different for each protein. At their isoelectric point proteins have a minimum solubility, a minimum viscosity, and also a minimum osmotic pressure. At a pH above the isoelectric point, a protein has more negative than positive charges. At a pH below the isoelectric point a protein has more positive than negative charges. The isoelectric points of a few proteins are listed in Table 23-4.

Dipeptides Proteins consist of many amino acids joined together by what is called a **peptide linkage** or a **peptide bond** (see page 266). Suppose that a glycine

TABLE 23-4. Isoelectric Points of Some Proteins

Protein	Isoelectric Point (pH)
Egg albumin	4.7
Casein	4.6
Hemoglobin	6.7
Insulin	5.3
Serum globulin in blood	5.4
Fibrinogen in blood	5.6

molecule reacts with an alanine molecule. This reaction may occur in two different ways. That is, the amine part of the glycine may react with the acid part of the alanine (equation 23–2), or the acid part of the glycine may react with the amine part of the alanine (equation 23–3). Both of these reactions are illustrated.

$$CH_3-CH-\overset{\overset{\textstyle O}{\|}}{C}-OH + H-NH-CH_2-COOH \longrightarrow$$

NH₂ region: alanine

glycine

peptide bond

$$CH_3-CH-\overset{\overset{\textstyle O}{\|}}{C}-NH-CH_2-COOH + H_2O \qquad (23-2)$$

alanyl-glycine (Ala-Gly)

$$NH_2-CH_2-\overset{\overset{\textstyle O}{\|}}{C}-OH + HNH-CH-COOH \longrightarrow$$

glycine   alanine (CH₃)

peptide bond

$$NH_2-CH_2-\overset{\overset{\textstyle O}{\|}}{C}-NH-CH-COOH + H_2O \qquad (23-3)$$

glycyl-alanine (Gly-Ala)

When two amino acids combine, the product is called a **dipeptide**. When three amino acids combine, the product is called a **tripeptide**. When four or more amino acids join together, the product is called a **polypeptide**. For just two amino acids, glycine and alanine, two different combinations have already been indicated—glycyl-alanine and alanyl-glycine, where the first member of each group acts as the one furnishing the OH from the acid group. For three different amino acids—such as glycine, alanine, and valine—there are six possible combinations (or tripeptide linkages).

Biochemistry   **354**

1. Glycyl-alanyl-valine
   (Gly-Ala-Val)
2. Glycyl-valyl-alanine
   (Gly-Val-Ala)
3. Alanyl-glycyl-valine
   (Ala-Gly-Val)

4. Alanyl-valyl-glycine
   (Ala-Val-Gly)
5. Valyl-glycyl-alanine
   (Val-Gly-Ala)
6. Valyl-alanyl-glycine
   (Val-Ala-Gly)

By convention, peptides are written with the —NH$_2$ end (the *N*-terminal) at the left and the —COOH (the *C*-terminal) at the right.

Proteins contain a large number of peptide linkages, and the number of possible combinations of the many amino acids in the formation of a protein is beyond all comprehension. Insulin (see Figure 23–2) illustrates the peptide linkages. It has an A chain, containing 21 amino acids, and a B chain, which contains 30 amino acids. Note that both chains are connected by two disulfide bridges (see page 357).

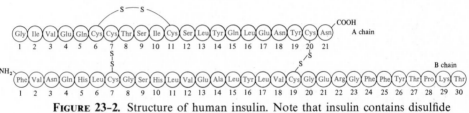

Figure 23–2. Structure of human insulin. Note that insulin contains disulfide bridges between Cys groups. Breaking these disulfide bridges inactivates insulin.

Structure

When a protein is hydrolyzed (by acids, bases, or certain enzymes), it breaks down into smaller and smaller units, eventually forming amino acids. Likewise, when amino acids combine (under the influence of certain enzymes), they first form dipeptides, then tripeptides, then polypeptides, and so on, until they eventually form a protein.

$$\text{protein} \underset{H_2O}{\rightleftharpoons} \text{proteoses} \underset{H_2O}{\rightleftharpoons} \text{peptones} \underset{H_2O}{\rightleftharpoons} \text{polypeptides} \underset{H_2O}{\rightleftharpoons}$$

$$\text{tripeptides} \underset{H_2O}{\rightleftharpoons} \text{dipeptides} \underset{H_2O}{\rightleftharpoons} \text{amino acids}$$

Proteins have a three-dimensional structure that can be considered as being composed of simpler structures.

The **primary structure** of a protein refers to the number and sequence of the amino acids in the protein. These amino acids are held together by peptide bonds. The primary structure of human insulin is indicated in Figure 23–2.

A slight change in the amino acid sequence can change the entire protein (see normal hemoglobin and sickle cell hemoglobin, page 538).

The **secondary structure** of a protein refers to the regular recurring arrangement of the amino acid chain. One such arrangement, called the α-helix, occurs when the amino acids form a coil or spiral. The coil consists of

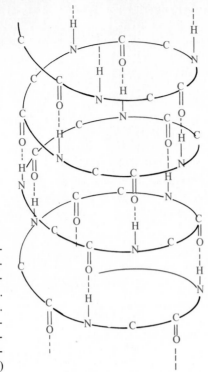

loops of amino acids held together by hydrogen bonds [between the —H of the —NH_2 of one amino acid and the O of the C=O of the acid part of another amino acid (see Figure 23–3)]. Each turn of the helix contains an average of 3.6 amino acids. Such a structure is both flexible and elastic. Hair and wool are examples of protein in such a helical structure.

When the amino acids are coiled, they may form either a right- or left-handed spiral. However, since α-amino acids in protein are all of the L-configuration, the coils always are right handed.

A second type of secondary structure, the β-pleated sheet (also called the pleated sheet) consists of parallel strands of polypeptides held together by hydrogen bonds. Such a structure (Figure 23–4) is flexible but not elastic.

FIGURE 23-4. A β-pleated structure formed by hydrogen bonds between two polypeptide chains.

Biochemistry 356

FIGURE 23-5. Tertiary structure of a protein. Note that the coiled helix represents the secondary structure, which in turn is made up of the various amino acids in the sequence specified by the primary structure.

Silk has such a pleated sheet structure. It is strong, but resistant to stretching. This type of structure is less common than the α-helix.

The **tertiary structure** of a protein refers to the specific folding and bending of the coils into specific layers or fibers (see Figure 23-5). It is the tertiary structure that gives proteins their specific biologic activity (see enzymes, page 373). Tertiary structures are stabilized by several different types of bonds as indicated in Figure 23-6. (a) There are salt bridges, which are formed between positively and negatively charged groups within the protein molecule. Examples of such groups are the carboxyl and amino side chains found in glutamic acid, lysine, arginine, and aspartic acid. (b) Hydrogen bonds can form between different segments of the coil. (c) Disulfide bonds can form between cysteine groups in different parts of the coil. (d) Hydrophobic bonds can be formed. In general, nonpolar amino acids are folded on

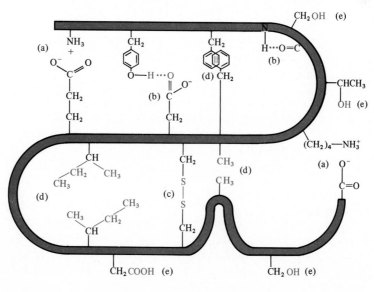

FIGURE 23-6. Various types of bonds that stabilize the tertiary structure of a protein.

Proteins

357

FIGURE 23–7. Quaternary structure of hemoglobin.

the "inside" of the protein and polar amino acids are on the "outside," where they can react with water molecules to form polar group interactions (also hydrogen bonds) (e).

Some proteins have a **quaternary structure,** which occurs when several protein units, each with its own primary, secondary, and tertiary structure, combine to form a more complex unit. An example of a protein with a quaternary structure is hemoglobin (Figure 23–7). It consists of two identical alpha chains (light colored) and two identical beta chains (dark colored). Each chain enfolds a heme (iron-containing) group. The oxygen-binding site is marked O_2.

Percentage Composition

The average percentage of nitrogen present in protein is 16 percent; that is, about one sixth of protein is nitrogen. Because protein is the major food that contains nitrogen, the chemist can determine the amount of protein present in a food substance by determining the amount of nitrogen present. This amount is about one sixth of the amount of protein present. Therefore, the amount of protein in the food can be calculated by multiplying the weight of nitrogen by six and converting this to a percentage of the total. For example, suppose that a 100-g sample of food yielded 4 g nitrogen upon chemical analysis. Since the amount of nitrogen in protein is one sixth of the total amount of protein present, the amount of protein present is 6×4 g, or 24 g. Then the percentage of protein present in the original 100-g sample is 24 percent.

Classification

Proteins are divided into three categories; simple, conjugated, and derived. On hydrolysis, simple proteins yield only amino acids or derivatives of amino acids. On hydrolysis, conjugated proteins yield amino acids plus some other type of compound. Conjugated protein consists of a simple protein combined with a nonprotein compound. Derived proteins are produced by the action of chemical, enzymatic, and physical forces on the other two classes of protein. Derived proteins include proteoses, peptones, polypeptides, tripeptides, and dipeptides.

Proteins may be classified according to their composition, according to their function, or according to their shape.

Classification According to Composition

Simple proteins are classified according to their solubility in various solvents and also as to whether they are coagulated by heat (see Table 23-5). Conjugated proteins are classified according to the nature of the nonprotein portion of the molecule (see Table 23-6).

GLYCOPROTEINS

Glycoproteins are proteins containing carbohydrates in varying amounts. Glycoproteins have molecular weights from 15,000 to over 1 million. The carbohydrates present in glycoproteins include the hexoses mannose and galactose, the pentoses arabinose and xylose, and sialic acids, which are derivatives of neuraminic acid.

TABLE 23-5. Properties of Simple Proteins

Type of Simple Protein	Solubility	Coagulated by Heat	Examples
Albumins	Soluble in water, precipitated by saturated salt solution	Yes	Egg albumin; serum albumin; lactalbumin
Globulins	Soluble in dilute salt solution, insoluble in water and moderately concentrated salt solution	Yes	Serum globulin; lactoglobulin; vegetable globulin
Albuminoids	Insoluble in all neutral solvents and in dilute acid and alkali	No	Keratin in hair, nails; feathers; collagen
Histones	Soluble in water and very dilute acid; insoluble in very dilute NH_4OH	No	Nucleohistone in thymus gland; globin in hemoglobin

TABLE 23-6. Conjugated Proteins

Type	Nonprotein Portion of the Combination	Examples
Nucleoproteins	Nucleic acid	Chromosomes
Glycoproteins	Carbohydrates	Mucin in saliva
Phosphoproteins	Phosphate	Casein in milk
Chromoproteins	Chromophore group (color-producing group)	Hemoglobin, hemocyanin, flavoproteins, cytochrome
Lipoproteins	Lipids	Fibrin in blood
Metalloproteins	Metals	Ceruloplasmin (containing Cu) and siderophilin (containing Fe) in blood plasma

Proteins

neuraminic acid (sialic acids have an R—C=O group
in place of the H marked with the asterisk)

Glucose is not found in glycoproteins with the exception of collagen.

Glycoproteins are present in most organisms including animals, plants, bacteria, viruses, and fungi. Human cell membranes contain about 5 percent carbohydrate present as glycoproteins and glycolipids. Glycophorin is a glycoprotein found in the membranes of human erythrocytes.*

In addition to their functions in membranes, glycoproteins serve in the following ways: as structural proteins (collagen); as lubricants (mucin and mucous secretions); as transportation molecules for vitamins, lipids, minerals, and trace elements; as immunoglobulins such as interferon; as hormones such as thyrotropin (TSH); as enzymes such as the hydrolases and nuclases; as hormone receptor sites; and for the specification of human blood types.

LIPOPROTEINS   Lipoproteins are part of cell membranes. Thromboplastin, a lipoprotein, is released into the bloodstream by injured tissue (see page 459).

The blood transports fats (which are insoluble in water) in the form of lipoproteins, which consist of cholesterol, esters, and phospholipids bonded to protein. Lipoproteins are classified into four types, as indicated in Table 23–7.

The low-density lipoproteins and the high-density lipoproteins contain a higher percentage of cholesterol than chylomicrons and very low density lipoproteins. Cholesterol, in the form of HDL, reduces the risk of developing coronary heart disease. However, cholesterol in the form of LDL increases the risk. It has been found that atherosclerosis* and coronary heart disease are associated with high serum levels of low-density lipoproteins.

Long distance runners and other athletes usually have an increased amount of high-density lipoproteins.

TABLE 23–7. Lipoproteins

Type	Density (g/ml)	Cholesterol (%)	Lipids (%)
Chylomicrons	less than 0.96	1	98–99
Very low density lipoproteins (VLDL)	0.96–1.006	8	90–93
Low-density lipoproteins (LDL)	1.006–1.063	9–10	79–89
High-density lipoproteins (HDL)	1.063–1.21	6–10	43–67

Biochemistry   **360**

Proteins may also be classified according to their biologic function. Table 23–8 lists the various categories of proteins classified by this method.

TABLE 23–8. Proteins Classified According to Function

Type of Protein	Example	Use
Structural	Collagen	In structure of connective tissue
	Keratin	In structure of hair and nails
Contractile	Myosin, actin	In muscle contraction
Storage	Ferritin	In storage of iron needed to make hemoglobin
Transport	Hemoglobin	In carrying oxygen
	Serum albumin	In carrying fatty acids
Hormones	Insulin	In metabolism of carbohydrates
Enzymes	Pepsin	In digestion of protein
Protective	Gamma globulin	In antibody formation
	Fibrinogen	In blood clotting
Toxins	Venoms	Poisonous

**Classification
According to Shape**

Proteins may also be classified according to their shape and dimensions. **Globular proteins** consist of polypeptides folded into the shape of a "ball." They have a length to width ratio of less than 10. Globular proteins are soluble in water or form colloidal dispersions and have an active function. Proteins classified as globular are hemoglobin, albumin, and the globulins.

Fibrous proteins consist of parallel polypeptide chains that are coiled and stretched out. They have a length to width ratio greater than 10. Fibrous proteins are insoluble in water. Examples include collagen, fibrin, and myosin.

Properties

Colloidal Nature

Proteins form collidal dispersions in water. Being colloidal, protein will pass through a filter paper but not through a membrane. The inability of protein to pass through a membrane is of great importance in the body. Proteins present in the bloodstream cannot pass through the cell membranes and should remain in the bloodstream. Since proteins cannot pass through membranes, there should be no protein material present in the urine. The presence of protein in the urine indicates damage to the membranes in the kidneys—possibly nephritis.

Denaturation

Denaturation of a protein refers to the unfolding and rearrangement of the secondary and tertiary structures of a protein without breaking the peptide bonds (see Figure 23–8). A protein that is denatured loses its biologic activity. When the conditions for denaturation are mild, the protein may be restored to its original conformation by carefully reversing the conditions that caused the denaturation. This is called **reversible denaturation**. But, if the conditions that caused the denaturation are drastic, the process is irreversible; the protein will coagulate or precipitate from solution. Proteins may be denatured by a variety of agents, as indicated in the following section.

FIGURE 23–8. Reversible denaturation.

⊟ = Areas of forces (−S−S−, hydrogen bonding, ionic, etc.) stabilizing conformation

Reagents or Conditions that Cause Denaturation

ALCOHOL

SALTS OF HEAVY METALS

Alcohol coagulates (precipitates) all types of protein except prolamines. Alcohol (70 percent) is used as a disinfectant because of its ability to coagulate the protein present in bacteria (see page 241). Alcohol denatures protein by forming hydrogen bonds that compete with the naturally occurring hydrogen bonds in the protein. Such a process is not reversible.

Heavy metal salts, such as mercuric chloride (bichloride of mercury) or silver nitrate (lunar caustic), precipitate protein. These denature protein irreversibly by disrupting the salt bridges and the disulfide bonds present in the protein. They are very poisonous if taken internally because they coagulate and destroy protein present in the body. The antidote for mercuric chloride or silver nitrate when these poisons are taken internally is egg white. The heavy metal salts react with the egg white and precipitate out. (The egg white colloid has a charge opposite to that of the heavy metal ion and so attracts it.) The precipitate thus formed must be removed from the stomach by an emetic or the stomach will digest the egg white and return the poisonous material to the system.

Dilute silver nitrate solution is used as a disinfectant in the eyes of newborn infants. Stronger solutions of silver nitrate are used to cauterize fissures and destroy excessive granulation tissues.

HEAT

Gentle heating causes reversible denaturation of protein whereas vigorous heating denatures protein irreversibly by disrupting several types of bonds. Egg white, a substance containing a high percentage of protein, coagulates on heating. Heat coagulates and destroys protein present in bacteria. Hence sterilization of instruments and clothing for use in operating rooms requires the use of high temperatures. The presence of protein in the urine may be determined by heating a sample of urine, which will cause the coagulation of any protein material that might be present.

Biochemistry

Alkaloidal reagents, such as tannic acid and picric acid, form insoluble compounds with proteins. Alkaloidal reagents denature protein irreversibly by disrupting salt bridges and hydrogen bonds.

ALKALOIDAL REAGENTS

Tannic acid has been used extensively in the treatment of burns. When this substance is applied to a burn area, it causes the protein to precipitate as a tough covering, thus reducing the amount of water loss from the area. It also reduces exposure to air. Newer drugs have taken the place of tannic acid for burns, but an old-fashioned remedy still in use for emergencies involves the use of wet tea bags (which contain tannic acid).

RADIATION

Ultraviolet or X rays can cause protein to coagulate. The radiation denatures irreversibly by disrupting the hydrogen bonds and the hydrophobic bonds present in the protein. In the human body the skin absorbs and stops ultraviolet rays from the sun so that they do not reach the inner cells. Proteins in cancer cells are more susceptible to radiation than those present in normal cells, so X radiation is used to destroy cancerous tissue (see page 56).

pH

Changes in pH can disrupt hydrogen bonds and salt bridges causing irreversible denaturation. Proteins are coagulated by such strong acids as concentrated hydrochloric, sulfuric, and nitric acids. Casein is precipitated from milk as a curd when it comes in contact with the hydrochloric acid of the stomach. Heller's ring test is used to detect the presence of albumin in urine. A layer of concentrated nitric acid is carefully placed under a sample of urine in a test tube. If albumin is present, it will precipitate out as a white ring at the interface of the two liquids. If acid or base remains in contact with protein for a long period of time, the peptide bonds will break.

OXIDIZING AND REDUCING AGENTS

Oxidizing agents such as bleach and nitric acid and reducing agents such as sulfites and oxalates denature protein irreversibly by disrupting disulfide bonds (see page 357).

SALTING OUT

Most proteins are insoluble in saturated salt solutions and precipitate out unchanged. To separate a protein from a mixture of other substances, the mixture is placed in a saturated salt solution [such as $NaCl$, Na_2SO_4, or $(NH_4)_2SO_4$]. The protein precipitates out and is removed by filtration. The protein can then be purified from the remaining salt by the process of dialysis (see page 180).

Color Tests

Color tests for the presence of proteins depend on the presence of certain amino acids in that protein. It may be necessary to try several tests before deciding whether a substance is a protein or not.

Xanthoproteic Test

The word xanthoproteic means yellow protein. The test consists of adding concentrated nitric acid to a protein. The protein will then turn yellow and precipitate. Anyone who has spilled nitric acid on his or her hands will recall the yellow color produced by the reaction of the nitric acid with the protein of the skin. The xanthoproteic test works only for a protein that consists of amino acids containing a benzene ring, such as tyrosine, phenylalanine, or tryptophan.

Proteins

363

Biuret Test   If a protein suspension is made alkaline with sodium hydroxide solution and copper (II) sulfate solution is added, a violet color is produced. This test is positive for substances that contain two or more peptide linkages—that is, such substances as proteins or polypeptides. It is negative for amino acids, which do not contain a peptide linkage, or for dipeptides, which contain only one peptide linkage.

Millon's Test   Millon's reagent consists of mercury dissolved in nitric acid (forming a mixture of mercuric and mercurous nitrates). When Millon's reagent is added to a protein, a white precipitate forms. This white precipitate on heating turns brick-red. Millon's test is specific for the amino acid tyrosine.

Hopkins–Cole Test   In the Hopkins–Cole test, a protein is mixed with glyoxalic acid, CHOCOOH, and then carefully placed over a layer of concentrated sulfuric acid in a test tube. If the amino acid tryptophan is present, a purple color will appear at the area of contact of the two liquids.

Ninhydrin Test   When proteins are boiled with ninhydrin (a benzene-type compound), a blue-purple color and CO_2 are produced. This test indicates the presence of α-amino acids or peptide groups.

Chromatography

Chromatography is a method used to separate very complex mixtures of amino acids, proteins, or lipids. It may be used for very small samples or for components present in extremely low concentrations. There are several types of chromatography. Among them are column, paper, thin layer, and gas-liquid.

Column Chromatography   In column chromatography a glass tube is packed with a chemically inert material that tends to adsorb solids on its surface. A solution containing a sample is poured into the column, where it is held by packing material at the top (see Figure 23-9). A solvent in which the components of the mixture have different solubilities is poured into the column, gradually flushing the components of the mixture down the column. The component of the mixture that is most soluble (or least strongly adsorbed by the inert material) moves down the column most rapidly, whereas the component that is least soluble in the solvent (or most strongly adsorbed by the inert material) moves downward the slowest. As more solvent is added, the components move downward with greater and greater separation, until they may be collected individually.

Paper Chromatography   In paper chromatography, a piece of filter paper is used in place of the adsorbent. The paper is suspended vertically in a stoppered container. A drop of unknown is placed near the bottom of the paper and solvent is added until its level is near the unknown (see Figure 23-10). As the solvent rises through the paper by capillary action, the components of the mixture are gradually separated. Different amino acids move at different rates and can be identified by calculations of ratios of distances moved. If, after the

FIGURE 23-9. Column chromatography for a mixture of four components.

FIGURE 23-10. Paper chromatography. (Reproduced from M. E. Rafelson and J. A. Hayashi: *Basic Biochemistry,* 4th ed. Macmillan Publishing Company, New York, 1979.)

Proteins

Figure 23-11. Two-dimensional paper chromatography. (Reproduced from M. E. Rafelson and J. A. Hayashi: *Basic Biochemistry,* 4th ed. Macmillan Publishing Company, New York, 1979.)

separation of a mixture into its components, the paper is dried, turned at right angles, and then placed in another solvent, a two-dimensional chromatogram is obtained. In this method, there is a further separation of the amino acids (see Figure 23-11).

Thin-Layer Chromatography

Thin-layer chromatography is very similar to paper chromatography, except that a glass plate covered with a thin layer of adsorbent is used in place of the filter paper. The advantages of this method over paper chromatography are the rapidity of separation and the choice of adsorbents, which permits separations not possible with filter paper.

A special adaptation of thin-layer chromatography is called *zone electrophoresis.* In this method a small amount of blood serum is applied to a cellulose acetate strip and an electric current is applied. The protein bands are separated and can be visualized after staining. The results of electrophoresis are shown on page 458.

Gas-Liquid Chromatography

Gas-liquid chromatography is probably the most widely used of all chromatographic methods. In this system, a column is packed with an inert material coated with a thin layer of a high-boiling, nonvolatile liquid. A very small sample (0.001 to 0.010 ml) is injected into the top of the column. The column is heated, and an inert carrier such as helium is passed through. The mixture separates gradually as the more volatile components vaporize first. These more volatile components move faster and are carried out of the column first. As each component of the mixture is eluted from the column, a detector produces an electrical signal, which is proportional to the amount of the substance being detected. This electrical signal is used to produce a tracing of concentration versus time. Such a trace is known as a chromatogram.

Summary   Proteins are high-molecular-weight compounds containing the elements carbon, hydrogen, oxygen, and nitrogen. Some proteins also contain other elements. Proteins are the chief constituents of all cells of the body.

Animals cannot synthesize protein from raw materials. They must obtain their protein from plants or from other animals, which in turn have obtained the protein from plants.

Proteins serves to build new cells, to maintain existing cells, and to replace old cells in the body. Protein is necessary for the formation of the various enzymes and hormones in the body. The oxidation of protein yields 4 kcal/g.

Proteins are polymers of amino acids. Hydrolysis of protein yields amino acids with an amine group attached to the alpha carbon. The body can synthesize very few amino acids. Those that it needs and cannot synthesize are called essential amino acids. All the amino acids in the body, except glycine, have the L-configuration. Amino acids in which the R group is primarily hydrocarbon are nonpolar and insoluble in water. Amino acids with polar R groups are polar compounds and soluble in water.

Amino acids are amphoteric—they react with either acids or bases because they contain an acid group (—COOH) and a basic group (—NH$_2$).

When an amino acid is placed in an acid solution, it forms a positive ion and migrates toward the negative electrode. When an amino acid is placed in a basic solution it forms a negative ion and migrates toward the positive electrode. At a certain pH, the isoelectric point, the amino acid will be neutral; it will not migrate toward either electrode.

When two amino acids combine, a dipeptide is formed. When four or more amino acids combine, a polypeptide is formed. Polypeptides in turn form peptones, then proteoses, and finally protein. The hydrolysis of protein proceeds through the same types of compounds in reverse order, forming proteoses, peptones, polypeptides, dipeptides, and amino acids.

The primary structure of a protein refers to the number and sequence of the amino acids in the protein chain. The secondary structure refers to the regular recurring arrangement of the amino acid chain into a coil or a pleated sheet. The tertiary structure refers to the specific folding and bending of the coils into specific layers or fibers. The quaternary structure of a protein occurs when several protein units combine to form a more complex unit.

In general, the nitrogen content of protein is 16 percent.

Proteins may be classified according to composition, function, or shape.

Denaturation of a protein refers to the unfolding and rearrangement of the secondary and tertiary structures of a protein.

Proteins do not dissolve in water; rather they form colloidal dispersions. Proteins, being colloids, cannot pass through membranes and should not normally be present in the urine.

Proteins can be coagulated (precipitated) by means of alcohol, concentrated salt solutions, salts of heavy metals, heating, the use of alkaloidal reagents, concentrated inorganic acids, and radiation.

Proteins give certain color tests based upon the presence of certain amino acids. Among these tests are the xanthoproteic test (for benzene-ring proteins), the biuret test (for substances containing two or more peptide linkages), the Millon test (for the amino acid tyrosine), the Hopkins–Cole test (for the amino acid tryptophan), and the ninhydrin test (for α-amino acids).

Mixtures of amino acids, proteins, and lipids may be separated by chromatographic methods. Among the systems used are column, paper, thin layer, and gas-liquid chromatography.

1. All proteins contain which elements?
2. What additional elements are present in most proteins?
3. Where do plants obtain their protein?
4. Where do animals obtain their protein?
5. Describe the nitrogen cycle in nature.
6. Where did the word *protein* originate?
7. How does the energy value of protein compare with that of carbohydrate? with fat?
8. How does the molecular weight of a protein compare with that of other organic compounds?
9. What are amino acids? State the names and write the structure of three amino acids.
10. Name the essential amino acids.
11. Why are amino acids amphoteric? Why are they optically active? What configuration do they have?
12. What is meant by the term *isoelectric point* in relation to proteins?
13. What happens to the solubility of a protein at its isoelectric point?
14. What is a peptide linkage?
15. Write the reaction of glycine with valine in two different ways.
16. What is a polypeptide?
17. What amino acids are present in insulin?
18. Describe the types of structure of proteins.
19. When proteins are slowly hydrolyzed, what products are formed?
20. What percentage of protein is usually nitrogen? What use is made of this fact?
21. How are proteins classified?
22. List several different types of simple protein.
23. List several different types of conjugated protein.
24. Why should protein not normally be found in the urine?
25. Why is 70 percent alcohol a better disinfectant than 100 percent alcohol?
26. What is meant by the term *salting out* of a protein?
27. What is the antidote for $HgCl_2$ poisoning? Why must the stomach be pumped afterward?
28. What use is made of the fact that heat coagulates protein?
29. Name five color tests for protein. What reagent does each use? What is each test for?
30. Describe the separation of amino acids by column chromatography.
31. How does paper chromatography work? What is meant by the term two-dimensional paper chromatography?
32. What is thin-layer chromatography? What are its advantages over paper chromatography?
33. Describe gas-liquid chromatography.

B
34. Why are proteins important in the body?
35. Where are D-amino acids found? What function do they have?
36. Compare polar and nonpolar amino acids in terms of structure and solubility in water.
37. What is a zwitterion?

Biochemistry

38. What is an α-helix? What holds it together? Give two examples of such a structure.
39. Why are coils of proteins right handed?
40. Compare an α-helical structure with a β-pleated structure.
41. What types of bonding stabilize the tertiary structure of proteins?
42. What is a globular protein? Fibrous protein? How do they differ?
43. Give an example of a protein that performs the indicated function: storage, transportation, enzyme, hormone.
44. Compare reversible and irreversible denaturation.

References   BAUM, STUART J. *Introduction to Organic and Biological Chemistry,* 3rd ed. Macmillan Publishing Company, New York, 1982, Chapter 14.

BLOOM, FLOYD E. Neuropeptides. *Scientific American,* **245**:148–169 (Oct. 1981).

BRILL, W. J. Biological nitrogen fixation. *Scientific American,* **236**:68–81 (March 1977).

MARTIN, D. W., P. A. MAYES, and V. W. RODWELL. *Harper's Review of Biochemistry,* 19th ed. Lange Medical Publications, Los Altos, Calif., 1983, Chapters 3–5.

MORRISON, R. T. and R. N. BOYD. *Organic Chemistry,* 4th ed. Allyn and Bacon, Inc., Boston, 1983, Chapter 30.

RAUN, J. DAVID. *Biochemistry.* Harper & Row, New York, 1983, Chapters 2–4.

SOLOMONS, T. W. GRAHAM. *Organic Chemistry,* 3rd ed. John Wiley & Sons, New York, 1984, Chapter 23.

ZIMMERMAN, HENRY and ISAAK ZIMMERMAN. *Elements of Organic Chemistry,* 2nd ed. Macmillan Publishing Company, New York, 1983, Chapter 15.

24 Enzymes

CHAPTER
OUTLINE

Properties of Enzymes
   Composition
   Effects of Temperature
   pH
   Concentration
Activators and Inhibitors
Mode of Enzyme Activity
Apoenzymes and Coenzymes
   Coenzymes
Nomenclature
Classification
   Oxidoreductases
   Transferases

Hydrolases—The Hydrolytic Enzymes
Lyases
Isomerases
Ligases
Enzymes of the Kidneys
Chemotherapy
   Antibiotics
   Antimetabolites
Clinical Significance of Plasma Enzyme
   Concentrations
Isoenzymes
Allosteric Enzymes
Zymogens

Enzymes are biologic catalysts. Catalysts are substances that increase the speed of a chemical reaction. Although a catalyst influences a chemical reaction, it is not itself permanently changed nor does it cause the reaction to occur; that is, a catalyst can increase the speed of a reaction but cannot cause that reaction if it would not occur in the absence of that catalyst. Since catalysts are not used up, they may be used over and over again.

Enzymes are organic catalysts produced by living organisms. Each enzyme will affect only specific substances called **substrates.** * Enzymes provide a chemical pathway that has a lower energy of activation* than the same reaction uncatalyzed. That is, enzymes increase the rate of a reaction by lowering the energy requirements.

How do enzymes differ from catalysts and why are there thousands of enzymes present in the human body?

Enzymes are superior to catalysts in several ways:

1. They have a much greater catalytic power. Consider the reaction

$$CO_2 + H_2O \underset{}{\overset{\text{carbonic anhydrase}}{\rightleftharpoons}} H_2CO_3$$

which takes place in red blood cells (see page 461). The enzyme carbonic anhydrase increases the reaction rate over 10 million times that of the same reaction without the presence of the enzyme. In general, enzymes increase the rate of reaction from over 1 million to over

370

1 trillion times faster than a corresponding reaction without an enzyme. Few catalysts can cause such an increase in reaction rate.

2. Enzymes act on specific substrates and can distinguish between molecules that have a very similar structure. Some enzymes are specific for one particular compound and will not catalyze the reaction of closely related compounds. Other enzymes will catalyze reactions of compounds that have a common structure; that is, they can catalyze a whole series of reactions. For example, an enzyme might catalyze the reaction of D-glyceraldehyde and have no effect on the reaction of L-glyceraldehyde. That is, the enzyme is specific for one compound only. An example of an enzyme with a more general action is trypsin, which catalyzes the hydrolysis of the peptide bonds in many different proteins.

3. The activity of enzymes is closely regulated whereas that of catalysts is difficult to control. There are substances in cells that can increase or decrease the activity of an enzyme and thus control the rate of the particular reaction that that cell requires.

Properties of Enzymes

Composition

Enzymes are proteins and, as such, undergo all the reactions that proteins do. That is, enzymes may be coagulated by heat, alcohol, strong acids, and alkaloidal reagents. Many different enzymes have now been prepared in crystalline form.

Effects of Temperature

The speed of all chemical reactions is affected by temperature: the higher the temperature, the faster the rate of the reaction (see Figure 24–1). This is also true for reactions involving enzymes. However, if the temperature is

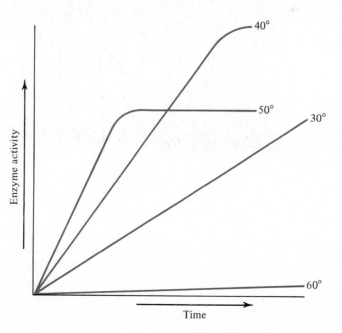

FIGURE 24-1. Effect of temperature on enzyme activity.

raised too much, the enzyme (protein) will be inactivated by denaturation and be unable to function.

The best temperature for enzyme function—the temperature at which the rate of a reaction involving an enzyme is the greatest—is called the **optimum temperature** for that particular enzyme. At higher temperatures, the enzyme will coagulate and be unable to function. At temperatures below the optimum temperature, the rate of reaction will be slower than the maximum rate.

Because many enzymes have an optimum temperature near 40°C, or close to that of body temperature, they function at maximum efficiency in the body.

pH   Each enzyme has a pH range within which it can best function (see Figure 24–2). This is called the **optimum pH range** for that particular enzyme. For example, the optimum pH of pepsin, an enzyme found in the gastric juice, is approximately 2, whereas the optimum pH of trypsin, an enzyme found in the pancreatic juice, is near 8.2. If the pH of a substrate is too far from the optimum pH required by the enzyme, that enzyme cannot function at all. However, since body fluids contain buffers, the pH usually does not vary too far from the optimum values.

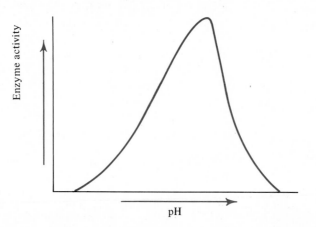

FIGURE 24–2. Effect of pH on Enzyme activity.

Concentration   As with all chemical reactions, the speed is increased with an increase in concentration of reactants. With an increased concentration of substrate, the rate of the reaction will increase until the available enzyme becomes saturated with substrate. Also with an increase in the amount of enzyme, the rate of reaction will increase, assuming an unlimited supply of substrate.

Activators and Inhibitors   Inorganic substances that tend to increase the activity of an enzyme are called **activators**. For example, the magnesium ion, Mg^{2+}, is an inorganic activator for the enzyme phosphatase, and the zinc ion, Zn^{2+}, is an activator for the enzyme carbonic anhydrase (see page 461).

Substances that tend to decrease the activity of enzymes are called **inhibitors**. Inhibitors may act by combining directly with the enzyme and so effec-

Biochemistry

tively remove it from the substrate, or they may react with the activator so that it, in turn, cannot activate the enzyme. Heat, changes in pH, strong acids, alcohol, and alkaloidal reagents all can denature protein. These are examples of **nonspecific inhibitors;** they affect all enzymes in the same manner. **Specific inhibitors** affect one single enzyme or group of enzymes. In this category are most poisonous substances, such as cyanide, CN^-, which inhibits the activity of the enzyme cytochrome oxidase (see page 407).

Cyclic AMP (*c*-AMP) acts as a chemical messenger to regulate enzyme activity within the cells that store carbohydrate and fat. Without *c*-AMP the activity of all the enzymes working at maximum speed within the cells would soon create chaos. It also appears that an inadequate supply of *c*-AMP can lead to one type of uncontrolled cell growth, which we call cancer.

Mode of Enzyme Activity

How do enzymes act? Why are they so specific toward certain substrates?

Each enzyme contains an "active site," that section of the molecule at which combination with the substrate takes place. The active site consists of different parts of the protein chain (the enzyme). These parts are brought close together by the folding and bending of the protein chain (the secondary and tertiary structures), so that the active site occupies a relatively small area. The fact that enzymes (proteins) can be denatured by heat (changed in three-dimensional configuration) indicates the importance of structural arrangement (see Figure 24–3).

It is believed that enzyme activity occurs in two steps. First, the active site of the enzyme combines with the substrate to form an enzyme-substrate complex (see Figure 24–4a). This enzyme-substrate complex then breaks up to form the products and the free enzyme that can react again. According to this theory (the lock-and-key method), the substrate must "fit" into the active site of the enzyme—hence the specificity of that enzyme. For substrates

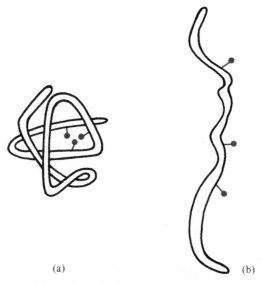

FIGURE 24–3. (a) Representation of an active site in an enzyme. **(b)** Denatured enzyme showing parts of active site no longer in close proximity.

(a)

(b)

Enzymes

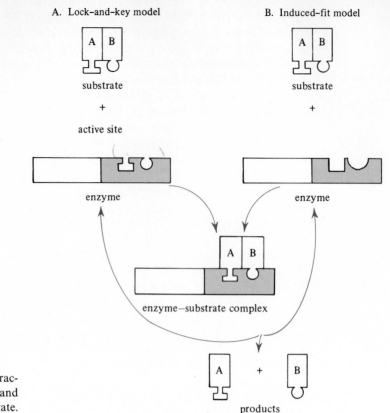

A. Lock–and–key model   B. Induced–fit model

A B

substrate

+

active site

enzyme   enzyme

A B

enzyme–substrate complex

A + B

products

FIGURE 24-4. Interaction of enzyme and substrate.

that have an optically active site, it is believed that there must be three points of attachment between the substrate and the active site of the enzyme so that only one of the two optical isomers "fits." In the body, enzymes are specific for the L-amino acids and the D-carbohydrates.

A more recent version of the activity of an enzyme suggests that the active site is not rigid as in the lock-and-key model, but flexible instead. That is, the site changes in conformation upon binding to a substrate in order to yield an enzyme-substrate fit (see Figure 24–4b).

If some other substance should fit into the active site of the enzyme, it could prevent that enzyme from reacting with the substrate. Such a substance is called a **competitive inhibitor** (see Figure 24–5).

active site

enzyme   + competitive   enzyme–inhibitor
            inhibitor   complex

FIGURE 24-5. Enzyme-inhibitor complex.

An example of a competitive inhibitor is sulfanilamide. Its structure is similar to that of *p*-aminobenzoic acid (PABA), which certain bacteria require for growth (see page 282). The "sulfa" inhibits the growth of the bacteria by competing for the active site on the enzyme.

Another type of inhibition is called **noncompetitive inhibition.** As the name implies, a noncompetitive inhibitor does not compete for the active site. Instead, it forms strong covalent bonds at another part of the enzyme, sometimes but not always near the active site, deforming the enzyme so that it cannot form an enzyme-substrate complex. Noncompetitive inhibitors do not need to have a structure similar to that of the substrate because they are not competing for the active site.

Apoenzymes and Coenzymes   It was mentioned previously that enzymes are proteins. However, some enzymes are simple proteins—they yield only amino acids on hydrolysis. Examples of such enzymes are pepsin and trypsin (page 391). Other enzymes are conjugated proteins—they contain a protein and a nonprotein part. Both parts must be present before the enzyme can function. The protein part is called the **apoenzyme*** and the nonprotein (organic) part is called the **coenzyme.***

Coenzymes   Coenzymes are not proteins and so are not inactivated by heat. Examples of coenzymes are the vitamins or compounds derived from vitamins.

The reaction involving a coenzyme may be written as follows

$$\text{coenzyme} + \text{apoenzyme} \longrightarrow \text{enzyme}$$

Coenzyme A (CoA, structure 24-1) is essential in the metabolism of carbohydrates, lipids, and proteins in the body. It also functions in certain acetyla-

(24–1)

coenzyme A

tion reactions. Hydrolysis of CoA yields pantothenic acid (a B vitamin), adenine (a purine), ribose (a sugar), phosphoric acid, and mercapto-ethanolamine (a sulfur compound).

Acetyl coenzyme A (acetyl CoA) has an acetyl group attached to the sulfur atom. Acetyl CoA functions in the oxidation of food in the Krebs cycle (see Chapter 26).

Nicotinamide is a very important constituent of two coenzymes—nicotin-amide adenine dinucleotide (NAD$^+$) and nicotinamide adenine dinucleo-tide phosphate (NADP$^+$). These coenzymes are involved in most oxidation-reduction reactions in the mitochondria. They also take part in the citric acid cycle. The structure of NAD$^+$ is indicated in formula (24–2).

When NAD$^+$ is reduced to NADH, another hydrogen atom is attached to the carbon atom indicated by an asterisk in structure (24–2). The charge on the nitrogen atom is eliminated, and the double bond between that nitrogen and the marked carbon is changed to a single bond. Recent evidence indi-cates that a defect in the enzyme responsible for the conversion of NADH to NAD$^+$, NADH dehydrogenase, may be involved in cystic fibrosis.

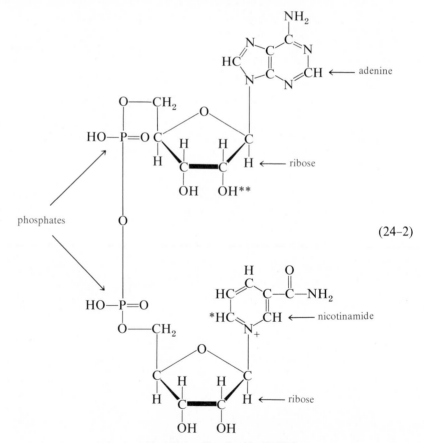

(24–2)

nicotinamide adenine dinucleotide (NAD$^+$)

In NADP$^+$, another phosphate group has been added in the position marked with a double asterisk in NAD$^+$ (structure 24-2), so that NADP$^+$ contains three phosphate groups.

Coenzyme Q is found in the mitochondria* and has a structure similar to vitamin K and vitamin E (see pages 486 and 487). The structure of coenzyme Q is

coenzyme Q

Coenzyme Q functions in electron transport and in oxidative phosphorylation.

Coenzymes frequently contain B vitamins as part of their structure. Many coenzymes involved in the metabolism of amino acids contain pyridoxine, vitamin B$_6$. Other B vitamins, such as riboflavin, pantothenic acid, nicotinamide, thiamine, and lipoic acid, are found in coenzymes involved in oxidation-reduction reactions. B vitamins such as folic acid and cobalamin (vitamin B$_{12}$) are part of different coenzymes.

Nomenclature

Formerly enzymes were given names ending in *-in,* with no relation being indicated between the enzyme and the substance it affects—the substrate. Some of the enzymes named under this system are listed in Table 24–1.

The current system for naming enzymes utilizes the name of the substrate or the type of reaction involved, with the ending *-ase.* Table 24–2 lists some enzymes and substrates named under the preferred system.

TABLE 24-1. Enzymes Named Under the Older System

Enzyme	Substrate
Rennin	Casein
Pepsin	Protein
Trypsin	Protein
Ptyalin	Carbohydrate

TABLE 24-2. Enzymes and Substrates or Reaction Types

Enzyme	Substrate or Reaction Type
Maltase	Maltose
Urease	Urea
Proteases	Proteins
Carbohydrases	Carbohydrates
Lipases	Lipids
Hydrolases	Hydrolysis reactions
Deaminases	Removing amines
Dehydrogenases	Removing hydrogens

Classification

The Commission on Enzymes of the International Union of Biochemistry has classified enzymes into six divisions. Each of these divisions can be further subdivided into several classes. The following paragraphs indicate these divisions and some of the classes. The older names of the enzymes are still in common use and are given throughout this text merely for simplicity. It is much easier to write *sucrase* than *α-glucopyrano-β-fructofurano-hydrolase.*

Oxidoreductases

Oxidoreductases are enzymes that catalyze oxidation-reduction reactions between two substrates. The enzymes that catalyze oxidation-reduction reactions in the body are important in that these reactions are responsible for the production of heat and energy. Recall that oxidation-reduction requires a transfer of electrons. Many of these enzymes are present in the mitochondria, which are the most prominent structural and functional units in animal cells, except for the nucleus (see Figure 24–6). They are sausage-shaped objects ranging in size from 0.2 to 5 μm (1 μm is one millionth of a meter). The cytoplasm of a typical cell contains from 50 to 50,000 mitochondria.

FIGURE 24-6. A typical cell.

Inside the mitochondrion is a double-layered membrane that is folded back and forth to form sacs called cristae. These cristae have a tremendous amount of surface area. On the surface of these membranes are enzyme-containing particles. Coenzymes are present in the fluid between the membranes. The mitochondria are highly organized and hold their enzymes in a definite spatial arrangement for the most efficient control of various cellular processes.

The mitochondria play an important part in oxidative phosphorylation in the citric acid cycle, which relates to carbohydrate metabolism. Mitochondria contain enzymes needed for the oxidation of fatty acids. They also are involved in the metabolism of amino acids.

Biochemistry

In addition to these functions, the mitochondria manufacture adenosine triphosphate (ATP), the main energy-supplying substance in the cell.

DEHYDROGENASES Dehydrogenases catalyze the removal of hydrogen from a substrate.

OXIDASES Oxidases activate oxygen so that it will readily combine with a substrate.

CATALASES Catalases catalyze the decomposition of hydrogen peroxide to water and oxygen.

PEROXIDASES Peroxidases also catalyze the decomposition of organic peroxides to hydrogen peroxide and water.

Transferases

Transferases are enzymes that catalyze the transfer of a functional group between two substrates. Under this category are the kinases, which aid in the transfer of phosphate groups.

Hydrolases—the Hydrolytic Enzymes

The hydrolytic enzymes catalyze the hydrolysis of carbohydrates, esters, and proteins. They are named for the substrate upon which they act. Some hydrolytic enzymes are present in the cytoplasm in organelles called lysosomes.

CARBOHYDRASES Enzymes that catalyze the hydrolysis of carbohydrates into simple sugars are called carbohydrases. The various carbohydrases are as follows:

1. **Ptyalin,** or salivary amylase, for the hydrolysis of starch to dextrins and maltose.
2. **Sucrase,** for the hydrolysis of sucrose to glucose and fructose. Sucrase occurs in the intestinal juice.
3. **Maltase,** for the hydrolysis of maltose to glucose. Maltase occurs in the intestinal juice.
4. **Lactase,** for the hydrolysis of lactose to glucose and galactose. Lactase occurs in the intestinal juice.
5. **Amylopsin,** or pancreatic amylase, for the hydrolysis of starch to dextrin and maltose. Pancreatic amylase occurs in the pancreatic juice.

ESTERASES Esterases are enzymes that catalyze the hydrolysis of esters into acids and alcohols. The various types of esterases are as follows:

1. **Gastric lipase,** for the hydrolysis of fats to fatty acids and glycerol.
2. **Steapsin,** or pancreatic lipase, for the hydrolysis of fats to fatty acids and glycerol.
3. **Phosphatases,** for the hydrolysis of phosphoric acid esters to phosphoric acid.

PROTEASES Proteases are enzymes that catalyze the hydrolysis of protein to derived protein and amino acids. These are of two types: proteinases and peptidases.

The proteinases, for the hydrolysis of proteins to peptides and amino acids, are as follows:

1. **Pepsin,** found in the gastric juice, for the hydrolysis of protein to polypeptides.
2. **Trypsin,** found in the pancreatic juice, for the hydrolysis of protein to polypeptides.

3. **Chymotrypsin,** found in the pancreatic juice, for the hydrolysis of protein to polypeptides.

The peptidases, for the hydrolysis of polypeptides to amino acids, are as follows:

1. **Aminopeptidases,** from the intestinal juices.
2. **Carboxypeptidases,** from the pancreatic juice.

NUCLEASES   Enzymes that catalyze the hydrolysis of nucleic acids are called nucleases. Examples are ribonuclease and deoxyribonuclease.

Lyases   Lyases are enzymes that catalyze the removal of groups from substrates by means other than hydrolysis, usually with the formation of double bonds. An example is fumarase, which catalyzes the change of fumaric acid to L-malic acid in the citric acid cycle (see page 408).

Isomerases   Isomerases are enzymes that catalyze the interconversion of optical, geometric, or structural isomers. One example is retinal isomerase, which catalyzes the conversion of 11-*trans*-retinal to 11-*cis*-retinal (see page 482). Another example is alanine racemase, which catalyzes the conversion of L-alanine to D-alanine.

Ligases   Ligases are enzymes that catalyze the coupling of two compounds with the breaking of pyrophosphate bonds (see page 401). One example is the enzyme that catalyzes the formation of malonyl CoA from acetyl CoA during lipogenesis (see page 420).

Enzymes of the Kidneys   If the blood pressure drops, as in the case of hemorrhaging or in hypokalemia (page 471), the kidneys secrete the enzyme renin (sometimes considered a hormone) into the bloodstream. The following reactions occur:

$$\text{angiotensinogen} \xrightarrow{\text{renin}} \text{angiotensin I} \xrightarrow[\text{enzyme}]{\text{converting}} \text{angiotensin II}$$

Angiotensin II increases the force of the heartbeat and constricts the arterioles, thus causing an increase in blood pressure. Angiotensin II brings about the contraction of smooth muscle and also triggers the release of the hormone aldosterone (page 511), which aids in the retention of water. Actually, angiotensin II is the most powerful vasoconstrictor* known. It is an octapeptide; angiotensin I is a decapeptide.

Chemotherapy   Chemotherapy is the use of chemicals to destroy infectious microorganisms and cancerous cells without damaging the host's cells. These chemicals function by inhibiting certain cellular enzyme reactions. Among the chemotherapeutic agents are the antibiotics and the antimetabolites.*

Antibiotics   Antibiotics are compounds produced by one microorganism that are toxic to another microorganism. They function by inhibiting enzymes that are essen-

Biochemistry   **380**

tial to bacterial growth. Among the most commonly used antibiotics are penicillin and tetracycline, structures (24–3).

penicillin G

tetracycline

(24–3)

Various strains of penicillin contain different groups attached to the cysteine-valine combination. Recall that both of these substances are amino acids.

The antibacterial action of penicillins is a result of their inhibition of a final stage in bacterial cell wall synthesis. In these final stages long polysaccharide chains are cross-linked together by short peptide chains. The last step in this process is the formation of a peptide bond between alanine on one peptide chain and lysine on another (see Figure 24–7). Penicillin inhibits this step, probably by irreversibly bonding to the active site of the enzyme. The similarity between alanine-alanine from the peptide chain and penicillin is shown in Figure 24–8. There is no human enzyme that uses alanine-alanine as a substrate and penicillin, therefore, does not interfere

FIGURE 24-7. The final crosslinkage of polysaccharide chains in the bacterial cell wall.

FIGURE 24-8. Comparison of the structures of alanine-alanine (D-alanyl-D-alanine) and penicillin.

alanine-alanine

penicillin

with our own enzymatic machinery. Allergic sensitivity to penicillin is due to the breakdown products of penicillin, especially to 6-aminopenicillinic acid.

Bacterial resistance to penicillin is due to the secretion of an enzyme, penicillinase, that cleaves the ring amide bond.

penicillin   penicillinic acid

This enzyme probably evolved as a detoxification mechanism since its absence does not produce any effect in the bacterial cell.

Antimetabolites

Antimetabolites are chemicals that have structures closely related to that of the substrates enzymes act on, thus inhibiting enzyme activity. One example of an antimetabolite is sulfanilamide (see page 282), whose structure is similar to that of *p*-aminobenzoic acid. Bacteria require folic acid as a coenzyme for their growth, and they synthesize it from *p*-aminobenzoic acid. Because their structure is similar to that of *p*-aminobenzoic acid, the sulfa drugs prevent the formation of folic acid and so inhibit the growth of the bacteria. This accounts for the use of sulfa drugs to fight bacterial infections.

Some chemotherapeutic agents* used in the treatment of cancer (antineoplastic agents*) are antimetabolites (mercaptopurine used in the treatment of leukemias); some are antibiotics (adriamycin used in the treatment of Hodgkin's disease); others are either alkylating agents, hormones, or natural products.

Clinical Significance of Plasma Enzyme Concentrations

The measurement of plasma enzyme levels can be of great diagnostic value. For example, the levels of glutamic pyruvic transaminase increase with infectious hepatitis; the levels of trypsin increase during acute disease of the pancreas; ceruloplasmin levels decrease during Wilson's disease (see page 474); and glutamic oxaloacetic transaminase levels rise rapidly after myocardial infarction. Many other plasma enzymes are useful in the diagnosis of different diseases (see Table 24-3).

Biochemistry

TABLE 24-3. Enzymes of Diagnostic Value

Enzyme	Possible Diagnosis
Glutamic oxaloacetic transaminase (GOT)	Infectious hepatitis, myocardial infarction
Glutamic pyruvic transaminase (GPT)	Infectious hepatitis
Trypsin	Acute pancreatic disease
Cerruloplasmin	Wilson's disease
Amylase	Liver and pancreatic disease
Acid phosphatase	Cancer of prostate
Alkaline phosphatase	Liver or bone disease
Creatine phosphokinase (CPK)	Myocardial infarction
Lactate dehydrogenase (LDH)	Myocardial infarction, leukemia
Renin	Hypertension

Isoenzymes

Isoenzymes, or isozymes, are enzymes with the same function but slightly different structural features. The reason for their existence is not known but they are made use of clinically. Lactate dehydrogenase (LDH) (see page 403), creatine kinase, and alkaline phosphatase all occur in isoenzyme form and are of diagnostic value. LDH has five forms, and Table 24–4 lists some clinically useful diagnoses based on these isoenzymes. Different tissues will contain different relative amounts of each of these isoenzymes. This difference allows a determination of tissues that have been damaged.

TABLE 24-4. Clinical Significance of Relative Amounts of LDH

Condition	Isoenzyme Pattern
Myocardial infarction	Moderate elevation of LDH_1; slight elevation of LDH_2
Acute hepatitis	Large elevation of LDH_5; moderate elevation of LDH_4
Muscular dystrophy	Elevation of LDH_1, LDH_2, LDH_3
Megaloblastic anemia	Large elevation of LDH_1
Sickle-cell anemia	Moderate elevation of LDH_1, LDH_2
Arthritis with joint effusions	Elevation of LDH_5

Allosteric Enzymes

Allosteric enzymes are key metabolic enzymes whose activity can be changed by molecules other than the substrate. It is thought that the other molecules bind to the enzyme at sites other than the active site. This binding changes the three-dimensional structure of the enzymes. Some molecules increase the catalytic rate (effectors) and some decrease it (inhibitors). This control of key enzymes is of utmost importance to ensure that biologic processes remain coordinated at all times to meet the immediate metabolic needs of the cell. The key glycolytic enzyme phosphofructokinase (see page 403) is one such allosteric enzyme.

Enzymes

Zymogens Zymogens are inactive precursors of enzymes. Most digestive and blood-clotting enzymes exist in the zymogen form until activated. In the case of digestive enzymes, this is necessary to prevent digestion of pancreatic and gastric tissue. For blood clotting, it is to avoid premature formation of blood clots.

Summary Enzymes are biologic catalysts that increase the speed of a chemical reaction but do not themselves change.

Enzymes are proteins and will undergo all the reactions of proteins. The enzymes in the body function best at about 40°C. Temperatures above or below body temperature will decrease the activity of enzymes.

Each enzyme has a certain pH at which it can best function.

An increase in the amount of enzyme will increase the rate of reaction. An increase in the amount of substrate will increase the rate of the reaction.

Inorganic compounds that increase the activity of an enzyme are called activators. Compounds that interfere with the activity of an enzyme are called inhibitors.

Enzymes contain an "active site" that binds to the substrate to form an enzyme-substrate complex. This complex yields the products and regenerates the enzyme.

Many enzymes contain two parts—a protein part and a nonprotein part. The protein part of an enzyme is called the apoenzyme.

Some enzymes require the presence of a substance called a coenzyme before they can act effectively. Coenzymes frequently contain the B vitamins or compounds derived from the B vitamins.

Under the older system of naming enzymes the substrate was not mentioned; the newer system indicates the substrate being acted upon. The names of enzymes under this system end in *-ase*.

Enzymes may be classified as oxidoreductases (enzymes that catalyze oxidation-reduction reactions between two substrates), transferases (which catalyze the transfer of a functional group between two substrates), hydrolases (which catalyze hydrolysis reactions), lyses (which catalyze the removal of groups from substrates by means other than hydrolysis), isomerases (which catalyze the interconversion of optical, geometric, or structural isomers), and ligases (which catalyze the coupling of two compounds with the breaking of pyrophosphate bonds).

Some hydrolytic enzymes are found in the lysosomes of the cytoplasm. The cytoplasm also contains mitochondria. These structural and functional units contain most of the oxidative enzymes and are deeply involved in the electron transport system of oxidation-reduction. The mitochondria also produce ATP, the cells' chief source of energy.

Chemotherapy is the use of chemicals to destroy infectious microorganisms and cancerous cells without damaging the host's cells. Among chemotherapeutic agents are antibiotics and antimetabolites.

Abnormal plasma enzyme concentrations are of clinical significance in the diagnosis of certain diseases.

Isoenzymes are enzymes with the same function but slightly different structural features.

Allosteric enzymes are key metabolic enzymes whose activity can be changed by molecules other than the substrate.

Zymogens are the precursors of enzymes.

Biochemistry

Questions and Problems

A

1. What effect do enzymes have on the speed of a reaction?
2. Most enzymes are found to be what kind of compounds?
3. What is the effect of temperature upon an enzyme?
4. What is meant by the *optimum temperature* of an enzyme?
5. What is the effect of pH upon the activity of an enzyme?
6. What is the effect of concentration of enzyme upon the rate of the reaction?
7. What is the effect of concentration of substrate upon the rate of the reaction?
8. What is an apoenzyme? a coenzyme?
9. What is CoA used for? What products does it yield upon hydrolysis?
10. Compare the newer and older systems of naming enzymes.
11. What are the general classifications of enzymes?
12. What are carbohydrases? Name three. Indicate where they are found in the body and what substrate they act upon.
13. What are esterases? Name two. Where are they found? What substrate do they act upon?
14. Name two proteases. What substrate do they act upon? What products are formed?
15. What is a nuclease?
16. Name three types of oxidation-reduction enzymes.
17. What is a transferase? an isomerase?
18. Describe the appearance of the mitochondria. What functions do they serve?
19. What is coenzyme Q? What is its function?
20. How do enzymes function? Where do they get their specificity?
21. How do enzymes distinguish between optical isomers?
22. What is a competitive inhibitor? How does it work?
23. Distinguish between specific and nonspecific inhibitors.
24. What effect does denaturing have upon the "active site" of an enzyme? Why?
25. What is chemotherapy? Give an example of two chemotherapeutic agents.

B

26. How does an antimetabolite function?
27. How can plasma enzyme concentration be used to diagnose disease?
28. Discuss enzymes in terms of activation energy.
29. Compare competitive and noncompetitive inhibitors.
30. What is renin? Where is it found? Of what diagnostic value is it?
31. Compare the lock-and-key theory of enzymes with the induced-fit theory.
32. Of what clinical use is the determination of relative amounts of LDH?
33. What are allosteric enzymes? Why are they important?
34. What are zymogens? Why are they important?

References

BAUM, STUART J. *Introduction to Organic and Biological Chemistry,* 3rd ed. Macmillan Publishing Company, New York, 1982, Chapter 14.

MARTIN, D. W., P. A. MAYES, and V. W. RODWELL. *Harper's Review of Biochemistry,* 19th ed. Lange Medical Publications, Los Altos, Calif., 1983, Chapter 6.

RAWN, J. DAVID. *Biochemistry.* Harper & Row, New York, 1983, Chapters 6, 7, 10.

25 Digestion

C H A P T E R
O U T L I N E

Salivary Digestion
Gastric Digestion
Intestinal Digestion
   Pancreatic Juice
   Intestinal Juice
   Bile
Digestion of Carbohydrates
   In the Mouth
   In the Stomach
   In the Small Intestine

Digestion of Fats
   In the Stomach
   In the Small Intestine
Digestion of Proteins
   In the Stomach
   In the Small Intestine
Absorption of Carbohydrates
Absorption of Fats
Absorption of Proteins
Formation of Feces

Most foods (carbohydrates, fats, and proteins) are composed of large molecules that are usually not soluble in water. Before these foods can be absorbed through the alimentary canal, they must be broken down into smaller soluble molecules. **Digestion** is the process by which food molecules are broken down into simpler molecules that can be absorbed into the blood through the intestinal walls.

Digestion involves the use of hydrolases—the hydrolytic enzymes. The hydrolases catalyze the hydrolysis of carbohydrates to monosaccharides, fats to fatty acids and glycerol, and proteins to amino acids.

However, not all foods require digestion. Monosaccharides are already in their simplest form and do not require digestion. Inorganic salts and vitamins also do not require digestion.

Digestion of food takes place in the mouth, the stomach, and the small intestine, each area having its own particular enzyme or enzymes that catalyze the hydrolytic reactions.

Salivary Digestion

During chewing, the food is mixed with saliva. The saliva moistens the food, so that swallowing is easier. Saliva contains approximately 99.5 percent water. The remaining 0.5 percent consists of mucin, a glycoprotein that acts as a lubricant; several inorganic salts that act as buffers; and salivary amylase, an enzyme that catalyzes the hydrolysis of starches. Saliva also acts as an excretory fluid for certain drugs, such as morphine and alcohol, and for certain inorganic ions, such as K^+, Ca^{2+}, HCO_3^-, and SCN^-. Saliva has a pH range of 5.75 to 7.0, with an optimum pH of 6.6.

Gastric Digestion

When food is swallowed, it passes down the esophagus into the stomach where it is mixed with the gastric juice. The gastric juice is secreted by glands in the walls of the stomach. When food enters the stomach, it causes the production of the hormone gastrin. Gastrin diffuses into the bloodstream, which carries it back to the stomach where it then stimulates the flow of gastric juice.

Approximately 2 to 3 L of gastric juice are secreted daily. Gastric juice is normally a clear, pale yellow liquid with a pH of 1 to 2. It contains 97 to 99 percent water and up to 0.5 percent free hydrochloric acid. It is the presence of this hydrochloric acid that causes the gastric juice to have such a low pH. In certain pathologic conditions, the acidity of the stomach may be less than normal. Such a condition is known as **hypoacidity*** and is commonly associated with stomach cancer and pernicious anemia. **Hyperacidity** is a condition in which the stomach has too high an acid concentration. It is indicative of gastric ulcers, hypertension, or gastritis (inflammation of the stomach walls).

The gastric juice contains the zymogen pepsinogen and the enzyme (gastric) lipase.

In addition to these enzymes, a substance known as the **intrinsic factor** is secreted by the parietal cells in the walls of the stomach. Vitamin B_{12} must undergo a reaction with this intrinsic factor before it can be absorbed into the bloodstream. A lack of the intrinsic factor is associated with pernicious anemia.

Intestinal Digestion

The food in the stomach is very acidic. When this acid material enters the small intestine, it stimulates the mucosa to release the hormone secretin. Secretin, in turn, stimulates the pancreas to release the pancreatic juice into the small intestine.

Three different digestive juices enter the small intestine. These digestive juices are alkaline and neutralize the acid contents coming from the stomach. The three digestive juices entering the small intestine are (1) pancreatic juice (2) intestinal juice (3) bile.

Pancreatic Juice

Pancreatic juice contains several enzymatic substances. Among these are trypsinogen, chymotrypsinogen, carboxypeptidase, pancreatic lipase, and pancreatic amylase.

Intestinal Juice

Intestinal juice contains several enzymes. Among these are aminopeptidase and dipeptidase. The intestinal juice also contains enzymes that catalyze the hydrolysis of phosphoglycerides, nucleoproteins, and organic phosphates. The intestinal mucosal cells contain the enzymes sucrase, maltase, and lactase.

Bile

Bile is produced in the liver and stored in the gallbladder. The gallbladder absorbs some of the water and other substances from the liver bile and so changes its composition slightly. When meat or fats enter the small intestine, they cause it to secrete a hormone, cholecystokinin-pancreozymin (CCK-

Digestion 387

PZ). This hormone enters the bloodstream and is carried to the gallbladder where it causes that organ to contract and empty into the duodenum through the bile duct.

Bile is a yellowish brown to green viscous liquid with a pH of 7.8 to 8.6. Because it is alkaline, it serves to neutralize the acid entering from the stomach. Primarily, bile contains bile salts, bile pigments, and cholesterol. Bile contains no digestive enzymes. Bile is the end product of cholesterol metabolism and is a primary determinant in cholesterol synthesis.

BILE SALTS Sodium glycocholate and sodium taurocholate are the two most important bile salts. They are both derived from cholic acid, a steroid similar to cholesterol in structure (see page 341).

cholic acid

Bile salts have the ability to lower surface tension and so aid in the emulsification of fats. They also increase the effectiveness of the pancreatic lipase (steapsin) in its digestive action on emulsified fats.

In addition, bile salts aid the absorption of fatty acids through the walls of the intestine. After absorption of these fatty acids, the bile salts are removed and carried back by portal circulation to the liver where they are again returned to the bile. Bile salts also help stimulate intestinal motility.

BILE PIGMENTS The average red blood cell lasts about 120 days and then is destroyed. The hemoglobin is broken down into globin and heme. The body removes the iron from the heme and reuses it. The heme, with the iron removed, becomes biliverdin. Biliverdin is reduced in the reticuloendothelial cells of the liver, spleen, and bone marrow to form bilirubin, the main bile pigment excreted into the bile by the liver. In the intestines, bilirubin is converted to urobilinogen and then to urobilin, a pigment that gives the feces its characteristic yellow-brown color. Some urobilin and urobilinogen are absorbed from the intestinal tract and appear in the urine, giving that fluid its characteristic color. These reactions may be written as follows:

hemoglobin $\longrightarrow$ heme $\longrightarrow$ biliverdin $\longrightarrow$ bilirubin $\longrightarrow$
$+$ $+$
globin iron
urobilinogen $\longrightarrow$ urobilin

As the urobilinogen and urobilin (this mixture in urine is called urochrome) are waste products, bile can be classified as an excretion as well as a secretion (see page 431).

Biochemistry   **388**

FIGURE 25-1. Granulated gallstones. (Courtesy of X-ray Department, Michael Reese Hospital and Medical Center, Chicago, IL.)

If the bile duct is blocked, the bile then goes into the bloodstream, producing jaundice. This disorder is recognizable by the yellow pigmentation of the skin. If the bile duct is blocked, no bile pigments can enter the intestine and the feces will appear clay-colored or nearly colorless.

CHOLESTEROL

The body's excess cholesterol is excreted by the liver and carried to the small intestine in the bile. Sometimes the cholesterol precipitates in the gallbladder, producing gallstones. Figure 25–1 shows gallstones present in a gallbladder.

Digestion of Carbohydrates

Digestion begins in the mouth, as chewing action reduces the size of the food particles. Thus they will have more surface area in contact with the digestive enzymes.

In the Mouth

Saliva contains salivary amylase (ptyalin), which catalyzes the hydrolysis of starch into maltose. However, this enzyme becomes inactive at a pH

Digestion   **389**

below 4 so that its activity ceases when it is mixed with the contents of the stomach, where the pH falls to about 1.5. Salivary amylase does not serve a very important function in digestion because the food does not remain in the mouth long enough for any appreciable hydrolysis to take place. Some hydrolysis of carbohydrates catalyzed by salivary amylase may take place in the stomach before the food is thoroughly mixed with the contents of the stomach, but this is of little importance because there are intestinal enzymes capable of hydrolyzing starch and maltose. The principal function of saliva is to lubricate and moisten the food so it can be easily swallowed.

In the Stomach   The stomach contains no carbohydrases, so that no digestion of carbohydrates occurs there except for that catalyzed by salivary amylase. However, the activity of salivary amylase ceases as soon as it becomes mixed with the acid contents of the stomach.

In the Small   The major digestion of carbohydrates takes place in the small intestine
Intestine   through the action of enzymes in the pancreatic and intestinal juices.
   The pancreatic juice contains the enzyme pancreatic amylase, which catalyzes the hydrolysis of starch and dextrins into maltose. The maltose thus produced is hydrolyzed to glucose through the activity of the enzyme maltase from the intestinal mucosal cells. The optimum pH of pancreatic amylase is 7.1. The intestinal mucosal cells also contain the enzymes sucrase and lactase, which catalyze the hydrolysis of sucrose and lactose, respectively.

$$(C_6H_{10}O_5)_n + H_2O \xrightarrow{\text{pancreatic amylase}} C_{12}H_{22}O_{11}$$
$$\text{starch} \qquad\qquad\qquad\qquad\qquad \text{maltose}$$

$$C_{12}H_{22}O_{11} + H_2O \xrightarrow{\text{maltase}} 2C_6H_{12}O_6$$
$$\text{maltose} \qquad\qquad\qquad\qquad \text{glucose}$$

   If a monosaccharide such as glucose is eaten, digestion is not necessary because the monosaccharide is already in its simplest form and can easily undergo absorption into the bloodstream. Many adults cannot digest milk because they lack mucosal lactase. Such adults show milk intolerance with symptoms of abdominal cramps, bloating, and diarrhea.

Digestion of Fats

As there are no lipases present in the saliva, no digestion of fats takes place in the mouth.

In the Stomach   Although gastric lipase is present in the stomach, very little digestion of fats takes place because the pH of the stomach (1 to 2) is far below the optimum pH of that enzyme (7 to 8); also, fats must be emulsified before they can be digested by lipase and there is no mechanism for emulsification of fats in the stomach. However, if emulsified fats are eaten, a small amount of hydrolysis may take place in the stomach. In infants, whose stomach pH is higher, fat hydrolysis of milk may be of some importance.

Biochemistry   **390**

In the Small Intestine In the small intestine, the pancreatic lipase catalyzes the hydrolysis of fats into fatty acids and glycerol. This action is aided by the bile, which emulsifies the fats so that they can be acted upon readily by pancreatic lipase.

$$\text{fat} + \text{water} \xrightarrow{\substack{\text{pancreatic} \\ \text{lipase}}} \text{fatty acids} + \text{glycerol}$$

Digestion of Proteins As the saliva contains no enzymes for the hydrolysis of protein there is no digestion of protein in the mouth.

In the Stomach The precursor enzyme pepsinogen is converted to pepsin when it is mixed with the hydrochloric acid of the stomach. Pepsin catalyzes the hydrolysis of protein to polypeptides.

$$\text{protein} + \text{water} \xrightarrow{\text{pepsin}} \text{polypeptides}$$

Rennin, an enzyme present in the gastric juice of calves, coagulates casein to form paracasein, which is precipitated by the calcium ions present in milk. Coagulated milk remains in the stomach longer than uncoagulated milk and so is more readily digested there. According to modern theories, rennin is not present in the gastric juice of humans.

In the Small Intestine In the small intestine, the zymogen trypsinogen from the pancreatic juice is changed into trypsin by the intestinal enzyme enterokinase. Trypsin in turn changes chymotrypsinogen, another pancreatic zymogen, into chymotrypsin. Both trypsin and chymotrypsin catalyze the hydrolysis of protein, proteoses, and peptones to polypeptides. The optimum pH of trypsin and chymotrypsin is 8 or 9.

The intestinal enzymes aminopeptidase and dipeptidase catalyze the hydrolysis of polypeptides and dipeptides into amino acids. Carboxypeptidase, an enzyme of the pancreatic juice, also catalyzes the hydrolysis of polypeptides to amino acids. Carboxypeptidase contains the element zinc.

Absorption of Carbohydrates As we have seen, the principal digestion of carbohydrates takes place in the small intestine, where the polysaccharides and disaccharides are hydrolyzed into monosaccharides—glucose, fructose, and galactose. The monosaccharides are transported through the walls of the small intestine directly into the bloodstream by diffusion and by active transport of galactose and glucose. The blood carries the monosaccharides to the liver and then into the general circulation to all parts of the body. The monosaccharides may be oxidized to furnish heat and energy. Some of the monosaccharides are converted to glycogen, a polysaccharide, and stored in the liver or the muscles, and the rest are converted to fat and stored in the adipose tissue.

Absorption of Fats The digestion of fats takes place primarily in the small intestine. The end products of digestion of fats—mono- and diglycerides, fatty acids, and glycerol—pass through the intestinal mucosa where they are reconverted into triglycerides and phosphoglycerides, which then enter the lacteals, the lymph vessels in the villi in the walls of the small intestine. From the lacteals these products pass into the thoracic duct (a main lymph vessel) and then into the bloodstream.

Bile salts are necessary for this absorption process. After the absorption of the fatty acids, the bile salts are returned to the liver to be excreted again into the bile. Fatty acids of less than 10 to 12 carbon atoms are transported through the intestinal walls directly into the bloodstream, as is any free glycerol present.

Absorption of Proteins

The end products of the hydrolysis of protein are amino acids. The L-amino acids are absorbed more rapidly than the D-isomers and pass through the capillaries of the villi directly into the bloodstream, which carries them to the tissues to be used to build or replace tissue. The amino acids may also be oxidized to furnish energy. Although the body can store carbohydrate and fat, it cannot store protein.

Formation of Feces

After the absorption of monosaccharides, glycerol, fatty acids, and amino acids, the remaining contents of the small intestine pass into the large intestine. The large intestine contains undigestible material (such as cellulose), undigested food particles, unused digestive juices, epithelial tissues from the walls of the digestive system, bile pigments, bile salts, and inorganic salts. The material passing into the large intestine is a semifluid and contains

TABLE 25-1. Summary of Digestion

Type of Digestion	Location of Digestion	Digestive Juice and Enzymes	Substrate	Product
Salivary	Mouth	Saliva		
		Salivary amylase (ptyalin)	Starch	Dextrins
Gastric	Stomach	Gastric juice		
		Pepsin	Protein	Polypeptides
		Lipase	Fats	Fatty acids + glycerol
		Hydrochloric acid	Pepsinogen	Pepsin
Intestinal	Small intestine	Intestinal juice		
		Aminopeptidase	Polypeptides	Amino acids
		Dipeptidase	Peptides	Amino acids
		Maltase	Maltose	Glucose
		Sucrase	Sucrose	Glucose + fructose
		Lactase	Lactose	Glucose + galactose
		Pancreatic juice		
		Trypsin	Protein	Polypeptides
		Chymotrypsin	Protein	Polypeptides
		Pancreatic amylase	Starch + dextrins	Maltose
		Pancreatic lipase	Fats	Fatty acids + glycerol
		Carboxypeptidase	Polypeptides	Amino acids

much water. Most of this water and some salts are reabsorbed through the walls of the large intestine, leaving behind a residue called feces. Little or no digestion takes place in the large intestine.

The conditions in the large intestine are ideal for the growth of bacteria and usually one quarter to one half of the feces consist of bacteria. The bacteria cause the fermentation of carbohydrates to produce hydrogen, carbon dioxide, and methane gases, as well as acetic, butyric, and lactic acid. The gases can cause distention and swelling of the intestinal tract, producing a feeling of discomfort. The acids may be irritating to the intestinal mucosa and cause diarrhea. Particularly in infants, the acids may cause excoriated* buttocks. Infants who have this condition are usually given a high protein-low carbohydrate diet, because the fermentation bacteria act on carbohydrates and not on protein. The bacteria also produce vitamin K.

Some of the amino acids undergo decarboxylation because of the action of intestinal bacteria to produce toxic amines called ptomaines (see page 431). For example, decarboxylation produces cadaverine from the amino acid lysine, putrescine from ornithine, and histamine from histidine. These toxic substances are reabsorbed from the large intestine, carried to the liver where they are detoxified, and then excreted in the urine.

The amino acid tryptophan undergoes a series of reactions to form the compounds indole and skatole, which are primarily responsible for the odor of the feces.

tryptophan   indole   skatole (methylindole)

Summary   Digestion is the process by which foods are broken down (hydrolyzed) into simple molecules that can then be absorbed through the intestinal walls. Digestion takes place in the mouth, the stomach, and the small intestine.

Digestion begins in the mouth. Food is mixed with saliva which moistens the food and makes swallowing easier. Saliva contains an enzyme that begins the hydrolysis of carbohydrates (starch). Saliva has a pH of 5.75 to 7.0 and contains approximately 99.5 percent water.

In the stomach the food is mixed with the gastric juices. The gastric juices contain hydrochloric acid and have a pH of 1 to 2. The gastric juice contains the zymogen pepsinogen and the enzyme gastric lipase. Upon contact with hydrochloric acid, pepsinogen is converted into pepsin, which then catalyzes the hydrolysis of protein to polypeptides. Gastric lipase is not an important enzyme because it can act only on emulsified fats and there is practically no emulsified fat present in the stomach.

The food leaving the stomach enters the small intestine where it is mixed with three digestive juices—those from the pancreas, those from the intestinal walls, and bile from the gallbladder.

Bile is produced in the liver and stored in the gallbladder. Bile is alkaline and neutralizes the acid entering the small intestine from the stomach. Bile salts lower surface tension and help emulsify fats; they aid in the absorption of fatty acids; they help stimulate intestinal motility.

Bile also contains pigments that come from the breakdown of hemoglobin. These bile pigments give the feces and the urine their characteristic color. If cholesterol crystallizes in the gallbladder, gallstones are produced.

Digestion of carbohydrates begins in the mouth. No digestion of carbohydrate takes place in the stomach except that catalyzed by salivary amylase from the saliva. Even this activity ceases when the food from the mouth reaches the low pH of the stomach. The major digestion of carbohydrates takes place in the small intestine with the acid of the enzymes pancreatic amylase, maltase, lactase, and sucrase.

No digestion of fats takes place in the mouth. No digestion of fats takes place in the stomach unless the fats are already emulsified. In that case their hydrolysis is catalyzed by gastric lipase, although to a very limited extent. Fats are emulsified in the small intestine by the action of bile and then acted on by the enzyme pancreatic lipase.

Digestion of protein begins in the stomach with the aid of pepsin. The digestion of protein continues in the small intestine with the aid of the enzymes trypsin, chymotrypsin, carboxypeptidase, aminopeptidase, and dipeptidase.

The monosaccharides produced by the digestion of carbohydrates pass through the villi of the small intestine and enter the bloodstream.

Fatty acids and glycerol, products of the digestion of fats, are converted into glycerides in the intestinal mucosa by the action of bile and pass through the lacteals into the thoracic duct and then into the bloodstream. Fatty acids of less than 10 to 12 carbon atoms pass directly into the bloodstream through the villi.

Amino acids, from the digestion of protein, pass through the villi of the small intestine into the bloodstream.

Undigested food, undigestible foods, unused digestive juices, epithelial tissues from the walls of the digestive system, bile salts, inorganic salts, and water pass from the small intestine into the large intestine. Most of the water and some salts are reabsorbed. The remaining material is excreted as feces.

Questions and Problems

A

1. Why is digestion necessary?
2. Do all foods require digestion? Why?
3. Where does digestion take place?
4. What does saliva contain? What does it do? What is its pH?
5. What is the pH of gastric juice? What causes this pH?
6. What is hypoacidity? What may cause it?
7. What is hyperacidity? What may cause it?
8. Gastric juice contains what enzymes?
9. What is the difference between pepsinogen and pepsin?
10. What converts pepsinogen into pepsin?
11. What is the function of secretion?
12. Why is gastric lipase considered an unimportant enzyme?
13. What is the intrinsic factor? What disease is associated with a lack of this substance?
14. Three different digestive juices enter the small intestine. What are they?
15. What enzymes are present in the pancreatic juice? What does each do?
16. What enzymes are present in the intestinal juice? What does each do?
17. Where is bile produced? Where is it stored?
18. What is the function of cholecystokinin-pancreozymin? Where is it produced?
19. What is the pH of bile? What does it contain?

20. What are the functions of bile salts?
21. How are bile pigments formed? Where are they excreted?
22. What is urochrome?
23. What happens when the bile duct is blocked?
24. What may cause gallstones?

B
25. Describe the digestion of carbohydrate. Where are the end products absorbed?
26. Describe the digestion of fats. Where are the end products absorbed?
27. Describe the digestion of protein. Where are the end products absorbed?
28. Describe the formation of feces.
28. What are the functions of the large intestine?
30. What may cause excoriated buttocks in infants? What may be done to overcome this effect?
31. What causes the characteristic odor of feces?
32. Where are some of the toxic putrefactive products detoxified? Where are they excreted?
33. What is enterokinase? Where does it function?

References

ALLISON, A. Lysosomes and disease. *Scientific American,* **217:**62–72 (Nov. 1967).

DAUTRY-VARSAT, ALICE and HARVEY F. LODISH. How receptors bring proteins and particles into cells. *Scientific American* **250:**52–58 (May 1984).

MARTIN, D. W., P. A. MAYES, and V. W. RODWELL. *Harper's Review of Biochemistry,* 19th ed. Lange Medical Publications, Los Altos, Calif., 1983, Chapter 38.

MOOG, FLORENCE. The lining of the small intestine. *Scientific American,* **245:**154–176 (Nov. 1981).

WURTMAN, RICHARD J. Nutrients that modify brain function. *Scientific American,* **246:**50–59 (April 1982).

26 Carbohydrate Metabolism

CHAPTER OUTLINE

Concentration of Sugar in the Blood:
  Blood Sugar Level
Source of Energy
Carbohydrate Metabolism
  Glycogenesis
  Glycogenolysis
  Glycolysis
  Other Oxidative Pathways
  The Aerobic Sequence (*Krebs Cycle*)

Gluconeogenesis
Overall Scheme of Carbohydrate Metabolism
Hormones Involved in Regulating Blood Sugar
  Insulin
  Epinephrine
  Glucagon
Glucose Tolerance Test

Concentration of Sugar in the Blood: Blood Sugar Level

The end products of carbohydrate digestion are the monosaccharides glucose, fructose, and galactose. Both fructose and galactose are converted to glucose in the liver so that the major monosaccharide remaining in the bloodstream is glucose.

The amount of glucose present in the blood will vary considerably, depending upon whether the measurements were taken $\frac{1}{2}$ hr after eating, 1 hr after eating, or during a period of fasting. The normal quantity of glucose present in 100 ml of blood taken after a period of fasting is 70 to 100 mg. This value is called the **normal fasting blood sugar.** Soon after eating a meal, the blood sugar level may rise to 120 mg per 100 ml of blood or even higher. However, the level soon drops so that after $1\frac{1}{2}$ to 2 hr the blood sugar level again returns to its normal fasting value.

During the time of fasting, even though the body is continuously using glucose for the production of heat and energy, the amount of glucose present in the blood remains fairly constant. How does the body regulate the amount of glucose present in the blood and what happens when these control mechanisms do not function properly?

When the glucose level in the blood rises, as happens after the digestion of a meal, the liver removes the excess glucose and converts it to glycogen, a polysaccharide. This process is called **glycogenesis.** This glycogen may be stored in the liver and in muscle tissue. However, only a certain amount of glycogen may be stored in the liver and muscle; the rest is changed to fat and stored as such.

Cellular uptake of glucose is greatly increased by the release of insulin (see page 411). Glucose is also removed from the blood by the normal oxidative reactions that take place continuously throughout the body.

Glucose does not normally appear in the urine except in amounts too small to be detected by Benedict's solution. However, if the blood sugar level rises above 170 to 180 mg per 100 ml of blood, the sugar "spills over" into the urine. The point at which the sugar spills over into the urine is called the **renal threshold.** The presence of glucose in the urine is called **glycosuria.**

Thus, the factors that remove excess glucose from the blood are (1) insulin secretion, (2) glycogenesis and storage as glycogen, (3) conversion to fat, (4) normal oxidation reactions in the body, and (5) excretion through the kidneys when the renal threshold is exceeded.

After a period of 2–3 hr, the liver converts glycogen back to glucose. This process is called **glycogenolysis.** Liver glycogen will be exhausted after 10 hr. The body then switches to making glucose from amino acids, this process is called **gluconeogenesis** (see Figure 26–7).

Source of Energy

Where does a muscle get its energy to contract? Where does the body get the energy necessary to synthesize protein, to send nerve impulses, to perform countless other functions?

The energy necessary for the body functions comes from certain high-energy compounds, compounds that yield a large amount of energy on hydrolysis. The key compound of this type is adenosine triphosphate (ATP). Hydrolysis of ATP to adenosine diphosphate (ADP) and inorganic phosphate liberates about 7600 cal/mol. This hydrolysis breaks one of high-energy phosphate bonds, designated by $\sim$. These two molecules—ATP and ADP—are shown in structures (26–1) and (26–2).

adenosine triphosphate (ATP)   (26–1)

This formula for ATP may be abbreviated as

(26–1a)

$$\text{(26-2)}$$

adenosine diphosphate (ADP)

This formula for ADP may be abbreviated as

$$\boxed{\text{adenosine}}-O-\overset{\overset{\displaystyle O}{\|}}{\underset{\underset{\displaystyle OH}{|}}{P}}-O\sim\overset{\overset{\displaystyle O}{\|}}{\underset{\underset{\displaystyle OH}{|}}{P}}-OH \quad \text{or} \quad A-P\sim P \qquad \text{(26-2a)}$$

However, the supply of ATP in the body is limited. There must be some mechanism of regenerating this substance so that this high-energy compound is available for continued use. How does the body change ADP back to ATP? To accomplish this, a high-energy phosphate group must be added again to the ADP. Such a process is called phosphorylation and may be indicated by the equation

$$\text{ADP} + \text{phosphate ion} + \text{fuel} \longrightarrow \text{ATP} + \text{fuel residue}$$

One of the fuels used in this reaction is glucose. The oxidation of glucose, the steps and enzymes required, the products produced, and the involvement of ADP and ATP in these processes will be discussed later in this chapter.

Carbohydrate Metabolism

The metabolism of carbohydrates in humans may be categorized as follows:

1. **Glycogenesis,** the synthesis of glycogen from glucose.
2. **Glycogenolysis,** the breakdown of glycogen to glucose.
3. **Glycolysis,** the oxidation of glucose or glycogen to pyruvic or lactic acids.
4. **Hexose monophosphate shunt,** an alternative oxidative path for glucose.
5. **Citric acid cycle and electron transport chain,** the final oxidative path to carbon dioxide and water.
6. **Gluconeogenesis,** the formation of glucose from noncarbohydrate sources.

Glycogenesis

Glycogenesis is the formation of glycogen from glucose. This process occurs primarily in the liver and the muscles. The liver may contain up to 5 percent glycogen after a high carbohydrate meal but may contain almost no glycogen after 12 hr of fasting.

The overall conversion of glucose to glycogen and vice versa may be written as

$$nC_6H_{12}O_6 \underset{\text{glycogenolysis}}{\overset{\text{glycogenesis}}{\rightleftharpoons}} (C_6H_{10}O_5)_n + nH_2O$$

$$\quad\quad \text{glucose} \quad\quad\quad\quad\quad\quad\quad\quad \text{glycogen}$$

However, the reaction is by no means as simple as this equation indicates. There are several steps involved, each one being catalyzed by its own particular enzyme.

The first step in glycogenesis involves the conversion of glucose to glucose-6-phosphate (abbreviated as glucose-6-P), a phosphate ester of glucose. ATP from the liver cells serves as a source of the phosphate group. After the loss of the phosphate group, ADP is left. The enzyme *glucokinase* is necessary to catalyze this reaction. Insulin is involved in the phosphorylation of glucose by glucokinase.

$$\text{glucose} + \text{ATP} \xrightarrow[\text{insulin}]{\text{glucokinase}} \text{glucose-6-P} + \text{ADP}$$

Glucose-6-phosphate is then rearranged so that the phosphate group moves from the number 6 position to the number 1 position, producing glucose-1-phosphate. The enzyme required for this reaction is *phosphoglucomutase:*

$$\text{glucose-6-P} \xrightarrow{\text{phosphoglucomutase}} \text{glucose-1-P}$$

Glucose-1-phosphate then reacts with uridine triphosphate (UTP) to form uridine diphosphate glucose (UDPG). (Uridine triphosphate is similar to adenosine triphosphate except that uracil takes the place of adenine.) The enzyme is *UDPG pyrophosphorylase.*

$$\text{glucose-1-P} + \text{UTP} \xrightarrow{\text{UDPG pyrophosphorylase}} \text{UDPG} + \text{pyrophosphate}$$

Then the glucose molecules in UDPG (activated glucose molecules) are joined together to form glycogen. The enzymes necessary here are *glycogen synthetase* and a branching enzyme. The former enzyme is regulated by both insulin and cyclic adenosine monophosphate (*c*-AMP). The latter enzyme aids in the formation of 1,4- and 1,6-glycosidic linkages.

$$\text{UDPG} \xrightarrow[\text{branching enzyme}]{\text{glycogen synthetase}} \text{glycogen} + \text{UDP}$$

The UDP formed in this reaction then reacts with ATP to regenerate UTP.

$$\text{UDP} + \text{ATP} \longrightarrow \text{UTP} + \text{ADP}$$

A diagram of the overall reaction is shown in Figure 26-1.

Carbohydrate Metabolism

FIGURE 26–1. Overall reaction of glycogenesis.

The figure shows the pathway:

glucose → (glucokinase (insulin); ATP → ADP) → glucose-6-P → (phosphoglucomutase) → glucose-1-P → (UDPG pyrophosphorylase; UTP → pyrophosphate) → UDPG → (branching enzyme, glycogen synthetase (insulin and cyclic-AMP)) → glycogen + UDP; with ADP → ATP branch.

Glycogenolysis

In glycogenolysis we might expect the reverse of all the reactions of glycogenesis, but it should be noted that the first reaction, that involving glucokinase, is *not* a reversible reaction.

In glycogenolysis, glycogen is converted to glucose-1-phosphate by the enzyme phosphorylase a and then to glucose-6-phosphate by the enzyme phosphoglucomutase.

Glucose-6-phosphate is then converted to glucose by the enzyme glucose-6-phosphatase, an enzyme found in the liver but not in the muscle. Therefore, muscle glycogen cannot serve as a source of blood glucose.

c-AMP (see page 504) is involved in the conversion of glycogen into glucose-6-phosphate in both the liver and the muscles. When the body is under stress, it produces hormones that are carried by the bloodstream to the liver cells, where they activate the enzyme adenyl cyclase, which in turn causes the production of *c*-AMP from ATP. *c*-AMP then activates a protein kinase, which in turn activates a phosphorylase b kinase. This phosphorylase b kinase then activates phosphorylase a, which triggers the conversion of glycogen into glucose. The same type of reaction is involved in the conversion of muscle glycogen into glucose-6-phosphate. *c*-amp also deactivates the enzyme glycogen synthetase, thereby stopping glycogenesis.

Glycogenesis and glycogenolysis may be summarized as in Figure 26–2.

Glycolysis

The breakdown of glycogen resupplies the energy used up during muscle contraction. This breakdown involves a series of steps, each catalyzed by a particular enzyme.

The breakdown of glycogen to pyruvate (pyruvic acid) and lactate (lactic acid), called the Embden–Meyerhof pathway, is the first step involved in muscle contraction. This process is also called *glycolysis* and is an anaero-

Biochemistry

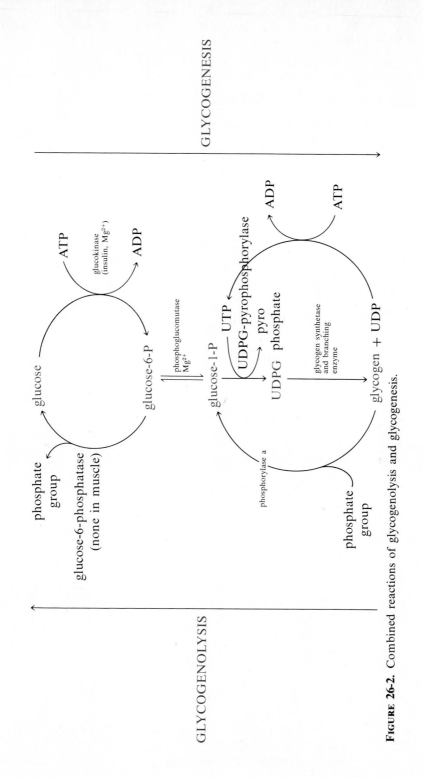

FIGURE 26-2. Combined reactions of glycogenolysis and glycogenesis.

bic* process—that is, each step takes place without oxygen. Glycolysis supplies the ATP needed for muscle contraction. Over 90 percent of the energy in the red blood cells is produced by glycolysis.

The overall reaction of glycolysis may be summarized as follows:

glucose-6-P (from glycogen or from glucose) + 3ADP $\longrightarrow$
$$2 \text{ lactic acid (or lactate)} + 3ATP$$

The ATP formed is available for muscular work. As the ATP is used, it is changed to ADP and must then be regenerated. This regeneration can be accomplished through the above pathway or by the use of another anaerobic sequence

$$\text{creatine phosphate} + ADP \longrightarrow \text{creatine} + ATP$$

The steps in glycolysis and the structural formulas of the intermediary products are given in the following chart and Figure 26–3.

Glycogen is changed to glucose-1-P by the catalytic action of the enzyme phosphorylase a. Glucose-1-P is then changed to glycose-6-P by the enzyme phosphoglucomutase. Glucose-6-P could also be formed directly from glucose with the action of ATP and the enzyme glucokinase.

Step A. Glucose-6-P is then changed to fructose 6-P by the action of the enzyme phosphoglucose isomerase.

Step B. Fructose-6-P is changed to fructose-1,6-diphosphate by the action of the enzyme phosphofructokinase. Note that during this reaction, ATP is converted to ADP.

Step C. Fructose-1,6-diphosphate is changed to the three-carbon compounds, glyceraldehyde-3-P and dihydroxyacetone-P. The enzyme involved is aldolase. Dihydroxyacetone-P is converted to glyceraldehyde-3-P by the action of the enzyme phosphotriose isomerase.

Step D. Glyceraldehyde-3-P is changed to 1,3-diphosphoglycerate by the action of the enzyme glyceraldehyde-3-P-dehydrogenase. During this reaction, nicotinamide adenine dinucleotide (NAD^+) is reduced to $NADH + H^+$.

Step E. Next, 1,3-diphosphoglycerate is changed to 3-phosphoglycerate by the action of the enzyme phosphoglycerokinase. In this reaction, two ADPs (one for each three-carbon compound) are changed to two ATPs.

Step F. Then, 3-phosphoglycerate is changed to 2-phosphoglycerate through the enzyme phosphoglyceromutase.

Step G. Next, 2-phosphoglycerate is changed to phosphoenolpyruvate through the enzyme enolase.

Step H. Phosphoenolpyruvate is changed to pyruvate through the enzyme pyruvic kinase. During this reaction, two ADPs are changed to two ATPs (one for each three-carbon compound).

Step I. Pyruvate is changed to lactate through the enzyme lactic dehydrogenase. At the same time, NADH and H^+ are changed to NAD^+.

The sequence of reactions involved in glycolysis may be summarized as shown in Figure 26–4. Three of these reactions are irreversible—the conversions of glucose to glucose-6-P, fructose-6-P to fructose-1,6-diphosphate, and phosphoenol pyruvate to pyruvate. The rate of glycolysis is primarily

Biochemistry

Figure 26-3. Glycolysis.

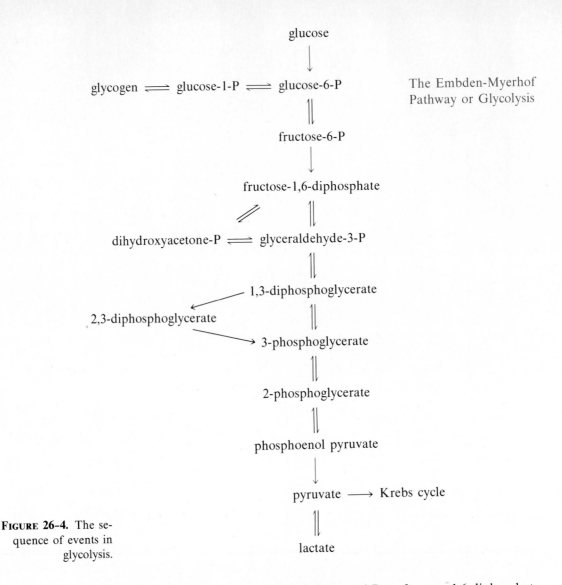

glucose

glycogen ⇌ glucose-1-P ⇌ glucose-6-P

The Embden-Myerhof
Pathway or Glycolysis

fructose-6-P

fructose-1,6-diphosphate

dihydroxyacetone-P ⇌ glyceraldehyde-3-P

1,3-diphosphoglycerate

2,3-diphosphoglycerate

3-phosphoglycerate

2-phosphoglycerate

phosphoenol pyruvate

pyruvate ⟶ Krebs cycle

lactate

FIGURE 26-4. The sequence of events in glycolysis.

controlled by the conversion of fructose-6-P to fructose-1,6-diphosphate. This conversion is stimulated by ADP and AMP and inhibited by ATP and citrate.

In addition, red blood cells have two enzymes that allow for the formation of 2,3-diphosphoglycerate (2,3-DPG) from 1,3-diphosphoglycerate. 2,3-DPG is a regulator of oxygen transport in red blood cells. When the O_2 levels in the blood drop, the 2,3-DPG levels increase so that more O_2 is delivered to the cells.

According to these reactions, muscle glycogen is changed into lactic acid (lactate). However, only about one fifth of the lactic acid thus formed is oxidized to carbon dioxide and water, resupplying the energy used up during muscle contraction. The other four fifths of the lactic acid is changed back to glycogen, reversing the above reactions. Part of the lactic acid is changed back to glycogen in the muscle. The rest of the lactic acid is carried to the liver by the bloodstream where it is converted to liver glycogen. In addition, for lactic acid to be utilized for energy, it must first be converted to pyruvic acid. Lactic acid is a metabolic dead end.

The oxidation of some of the lactic acid, the aerobic sequence, produces a large amount of energy. The oxidation of one molecule of lactic acid converts 18 molecules of ADP to ATP.

After a muscle contracts and relaxes, the net change is a partial loss of glycogen. This deficiency in glycogen can be replenished by the conversion of blood glucose to muscle glycogen (muscle glycogenesis).

This conversion of glycogen to lactic acid (lactate) and partial reconversion to glycogen, the lactic acid cycle, is shown in diagram (26–3).

Other Oxidative Pathways

The oxidation of glucose to lactic acid can also proceed through a series of reactions called the **hexose monophosphate shunt,** or the **pentose shunt.** This sequence is important because it provides the five-carbon sugars needed for the synthesis of nucleic acids and nucleotides and because it makes available NADPH, the reduced form of nicotinamide adenine dinucleotide phosphate ($NADP^+$), a coenzyme necessary for the synthesis of fatty acids.

The overall reaction may be written as follows:

$$3 \text{ glucose-6-P} + 6NADP^+ \xrightarrow{\text{enzymes}} 3CO_2 + 2 \text{ glucose-6P}$$
$$+ \text{ glyceraldehyde-3-P} + 6(NADPH + H^+)$$

The Aerobic Sequence (Krebs Cycle)

The aerobic sequence converts lactic and pyruvic acids (from anaerobic glycolysis) through a series of steps to carbon dioxide and water. This series of reactions is called the **Krebs cycle,** or **citric acid cycle** (see Figure 26–5). The citric acid cycle uses oxygen transported to the cells by hemoglobin, hence the term *aerobic*. This cycle takes place in the mitochondria (see page 378).

During the complete oxidation of one molecule of glucose, 36 high-energy phosphate bonds are produced. Four of these are formed during glycolysis. Two more are formed from the substrate level of the citric acid (Krebs) cycle, but two are used up during the phosphorylation of glucose in the glycolytic mechanism. Two high-energy phosphate bonds are formed during the Krebs cycle. The remaining come from oxidative phorphorylation. Thus, most of the energy for the body comes from oxidative phosphorylation.

Assuming 7.6 kcal per high-energy phosphate bond, the overall sum is 36×7.6 kcal or 274 kcal. Theoretically, 686 kcal should be produced from

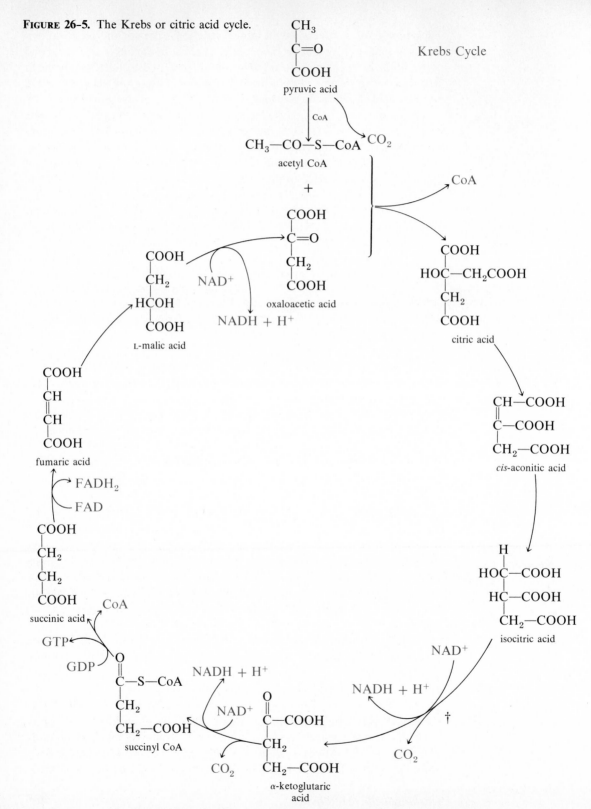

FIGURE 26-5. The Krebs or citric acid cycle.

† An enzyme-bound complex of oxalosuccinic acid occurs here as an intermediary.

1 mole of glucose; thus, the efficiency of conversion is approximately 40 percent.

The first step in the aerobic process is the formation of active acetate from pyruvic acid. This active acetate is the acetyl derivative of coenzyme A, or **acetyl CoA.** Acetyl CoA is the converting substance in the metabolism of carbohydrates, fats, and protein. Acetyl CoA becomes the "fuel" for the Krebs cycle. As will be noted, acetyl CoA reacts with oxaloacetic acid and goes through the cycle. At the end of the cycle, oxaloacetic acid is regenerated and picks up another molecule of acetyl CoA to carry it through the sequence. During the cycle, acetyl CoA is oxidized to carbon dioxide and at the same time NADH and $FADH_2$ are produced. These enter into the electron transport chain that functions on the inner membranes of the mitochondria. In the electron transport chain (also called the electron transport system), electrons are transferred from NADH through a series of steps to oxygen, with the regeneration of NAD^+ and FAD, and the formation of H_2O. The energy yielded is used for the formation of ATP (see Figure 26–6). The overall reaction in the electron transport chain is also called oxidative phosphorylation and proceeds because large amounts of NADH and $FADH_2$ are produced from the citric acid cycle and also because there is a plentiful supply of oxygen in the tissues. The overall reaction is

$$NADH + H^+ + 3P + 3ADP + \tfrac{1}{2}O_2 \longrightarrow NAD^+ + 3ATP + H_2O$$

Involved in this electron transport system are NADH, $FADH_2$, coenzyme Q, and several cytochromes, which are complexes containing heme (recall that heme is part of the hemoglobin molecule).

One of the cytochromes, cytochrome oxidase, is a complex that binds oxygen, reduces it with electrons received from other cytochromes in the electron transport system, and finally converts that oxygen to water. Note that the oxygen in this sequence (which is therefore an aerobic sequence) reacts only at the last step.

One unusual fact about cytochrome oxidase is that it contains two metals—iron and copper. This particular enzyme is mainly responsible for the introduction of oxygen into the metabolic processes of the citric acid cycle and so is considered absolutely vital to life. If the cytochrome oxidase function is blocked, as with cyanide poisoning, all cellular activity stops very quickly. It is believed that the cytochrome oxidase functions by transferring electrons from copper to iron to oxygen.

Note that another high-energy compound produced by the citric acid cycle is guanosine triphosphate (GTP). GTP is considered to be interchangeable with ATP.

Gluconeogenesis   Gluconeogenesis is the formation of glucose from noncarbohydrate substances such as amino acids and glycerol. This process takes place primarily in the liver, although a small amount also takes place in the kidneys.

Gluconeogenesis is increased in high-protein diets and decreased in high-carbohydrate diets. During starvation, gluconeogenesis supplies glucose from the amino acids of the tissue protein. In severe diabetes, gluconeo-

Krebs Cycle

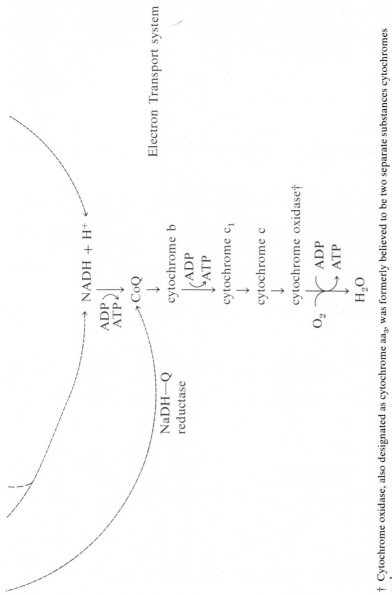

Electron Transport system

NADH + H⁺

NaDH—Q
reductase

CoQ

cytochrome b

cytochrome c₁

cytochrome c

cytochrome oxidase†

H₂O

† Cytochrome oxidase, also designated as cytochrome aa₃, was formerly believed to be two separate substances cytochromes a and a₃.

FIGURE 26–6. Oxidative phosphorylation.

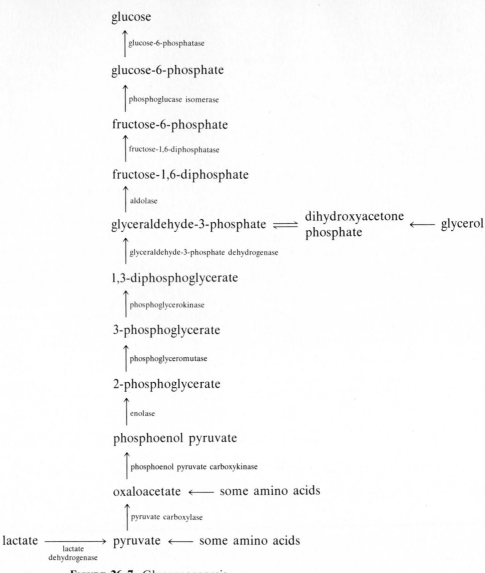

glucose

　↑ glucose-6-phosphatase

glucose-6-phosphate

　↑ phosphoglucase isomerase

fructose-6-phosphate

　↑ fructose-1,6-diphosphatase

fructose-1,6-diphosphate

　↑ aldolase

glyceraldehyde-3-phosphate ⇌ dihydroxyacetone phosphate ← glycerol

　↑ glyceraldehyde-3-phosphate dehydrogenase

1,3-diphosphoglycerate

　↑ phosphoglycerokinase

3-phosphoglycerate

　↑ phosphoglyceromutase

2-phosphoglycerate

　↑ enolase

phosphoenol pyruvate

　↑ phosphoenol pyruvate carboxykinase

oxaloacetate ← some amino acids

　↑ pyruvate carboxylase

lactate ——→ pyruvate ← some amino acids
　　　lactate
　　dehydrogenase

FIGURE 26-7. Gluconeogenesis

genesis not only from food protein but also from tissue protein may lead to emaciation. Since several reactions in glycolysis are not reversible, gluconeogenesis contains some additional reactions (see Figure 26–7).

Overall Scheme of Carbohydrate Metabolism   The interrelationship of glycogenesis, glycogenolysis, glycolysis, gluconeogenesis, the hexose monophosphate shunt, and the Krebs (citric acid) cycle, along with the metabolism of fats and proteins, is indicated in Figure 28–2 on page 432).

Hormones Involved in Regulating Blood Sugar

The liver plays a vital function in controlling the normal blood sugar level by removing sugar from and adding sugar to the blood. The activity of the liver in maintaining the normal blood sugar level is in turn controlled by several different hormones. Among these are insulin, epinephrine, and glucagon. The hormones of the anterior pituitary, the adrenal cortex, and the thyroid also have a definite effect upon carbohydrate metabolism.

Insulin

Insulin is a hormone produced by the beta cells of the islets of Langerhans in the pancreas. Insulin performs the following functions:

1. It aids in the transportation of glucose across cell membranes.
2. It accelerates the oxidation of glucose in the cells.
3. It increases the transformation of glucose to glycogen (glycogenesis) in the muscle and also in the liver. (Insulin controls the phosphorylation of glucose to glucose-6-P by means of the enzyme glucokinase; see page 399.)
4. It depresses the production of glucose (glycogenolysis) in the liver.
5. It promotes the formation of fat from glucose.

Thus, the principal function of insulin may be said to be the removal of glucose from the bloodstream and so a consequent lowering of the blood sugar level.

DIABETES MELLITUS

If the amount of insulin is decreased or eliminated (either because of decreased activity of the islets of Langerhans or by the degeneration of these cells), the blood sugar level will rise. Increased blood sugar level (hyperglycemia) leads to glycosuria (glucose in the urine) because the renal threshold is exceeded.

Also, the lack of insulin in diabetes leads to an increased oxidation of fatty acids as a source of ATP. Increased oxidation of fatty acids leads to an accumulation of acetoacetic acid, β-hydroxybutyric acid, and acetone. These substances, commonly known as ketone bodies, form faster than they can be oxidized and removed and so accumulate in the blood (and urine). A higher-than-normal concentration of these substances in the blood is known as ketosis.

The presence of ketone bodies affects the pH of the blood, since two of the three compounds are acids. If the ketone bodies accumulate and lower the pH of the blood, a condition known as acidosis exists. A decreased pH reduces the ability of hemoglobin to carry oxygen, thus, acidosis can be very serious. Prolonged acidosis first causes nausea, then depression of the central nervous system, severe dehydration, deep coma (known as diabetic coma), and finally death.

Prompt injection of insulin will alleviate the symptoms accompanying high blood sugar. Persons suffering from diabetes mellitus can lead normal lives provided that they receive insulin as needed. Since insulin is a protein, it cannot be taken orally (it would be digested as are all proteins) and so must be administered by injection.

Epinephrine   Epinephrine is a hormone secreted by the medulla* of the adrenal glands. It stimulates the formation of glucose from glycogen in the liver (glycogenolysis) (see page 399) and so has an action opposite to that of insulin. Insulin removes glucose from the bloodstream, whereas epinephrine increases the amount of glucose present in the blood.

During periods of strong emotional stress, such as anger or fright, epinephrine is secreted into the bloodstream where it promotes glycogenolysis in the liver. This increases the amount of glucose in the blood, making that glucose readily available as the body needs it to meet the emergency situation. The amount of glucose may then exceed the renal threshold (hyperglycemia) and sugar will appear in the urine. This is one example of how the presence of sugar in the urine may be due to a condition other than diabetes.

Glucagon   Glucagon is a hormone produced by the alpha cells of the pancreas. Its effects are opposite to those of insulin. Glucagon raises blood sugar levels by stimulating the activity of the enzyme phosphorylase in the liver, which changes liver glycogen to glucose. The activity of phosphorylase depends upon c-AMP. Glucagon also increases gluconeogenesis from amino acids and from lactic acid. Glucagon has no effect on phosphorylation in the muscles.

Glucose Tolerance Test   A positive Benedict's test on a urine specimen indicates that the patient *may* have diabetes mellitus. However, this test is by no means conclusive proof because the presence of sugar in the urine may be due to other conditions, such as pregnancy, emotional disturbances, large intake of fruit or fruit juices, and genetic disorders (idiopathic pentosuria, fructosuria, or galactosuria).

A patient who is suspected of being diabetic is given a glucose tolerance test. In this test, approximately 1 g of glucose is given for each kilogram of body weight after fasting for 12 hr. Then the patient's blood sugar level is checked by withdrawing blood samples at regular intervals for several hours. These samples are chemically analyzed and the concentration of sugar in the blood is plotted in relation to the time intervals. In a normal person, the blood sugar level rises from about 80 mg per 100 ml of blood to 130 mg per 100 ml of blood in about 1 hr. Then the blood sugar level gradually returns to normal after a period of about $2\frac{1}{2}$ hr. In a diabetic patient, because no insulin is being secreted, the blood sugar level rises to an even higher level than in the normal patient and remains there for a much longer period of time. Then it slowly begins to return toward its normal value.

These results may be seen in the graphs of the glucose tolerance test, as shown in Figure 26–8.

Also, in the diabetic patient, large amounts of glucose appear in the urine because of the spillover when the renal threshold is exceeded.

The glucose tolerance test is a valuable diagnostic tool because it indicates the ability of the body to utilize carbohydrate. A decreased utilization may indicate diabetes, whereas an increased utilization may indicate Addison's disease, hypopituitarism, or hyperinsulinism.

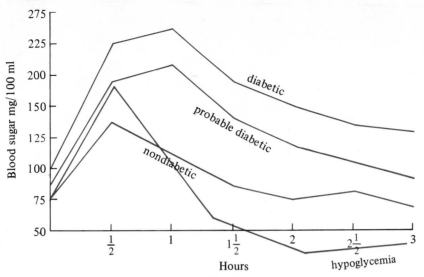

FIGURE 26-8. Criteria used for interpretation of glucose tolerance tests. (Modified from B. Pansky: *Dynamic Anatomy and Physiology*. Macmillan Publishing Co., Inc., New York, 1975.)

Venous Blood Sugar (mg per 100 ml)

	Fasting	$\frac{1}{2}$ hour	1 hour	$1\frac{1}{2}$ hours	2 hours	$2\frac{1}{2}$ hours
Normal	<100	<160	<160	–	<100–110	<100
Probable	<110–120	130–159	160–180	>135	110–120	<100–120
Diabetes	>110	>150–160	>160	>140	>120	>110
Hypoglycemia	<100	<160	<160	<70	<50	<50

Summary The end products of carbohydrate digestion are the monosaccharides. The major monosaccharide in the bloodstream is glucose. Some of the blood glucose is converted to glycogen in the liver and in the muscle. This process is called glycogenesis. Other glucose is constantly being oxidized to furnish energy for the body. If the blood sugar level rises too much, the excess spills over into the urine. The presence of glucose in the urine is known as glycosuria.

The oxidation of glucose produces energy, which is stored in high-energy compounds, especially adenosine triphosphate (ATP). Hydrolysis of ATP to adenosine diphosphate (ADP) and inorganic phosphate liberates about 7.6 kcal.

Glycogenesis—the formation of glycogen from glucose—takes place in the liver and in muscle tissue. There are many intermediate steps involved in this conversion, each being catalyzed by a specific enzyme.

Glycogenolysis—the conversion of glycogen to glucose—takes place primarily in the liver.

The breakdown of muscle glycogen to pyruvate and lactate, a process that requires no oxygen (anaerobic), is termed glycolysis. Glycolysis supplies most of the ATP needed for muscle contraction. Glycolysis proceeds through a series of steps, each catalyzed by a specific enzyme. In this process three molecules of ADP are converted to ATP, which is then available for muscular work.

About one fifth of the lactic acid formed in glycolysis is oxidized to carbon dioxide and water. The other four fifths is converted back to liver glycogen. The cycle of glucose–glycogen–lactic acid–glycogen is known as the lactic acid cycle.

The oxidation of glucose to lactic acid may also proceed through a series of reactions called the hexose monophosphate shunt or the pentose shunt. This sequence is important because it provides five-carbon sugars needed for the synthesis of nucleic acids and nucleotides and also because it makes available the reduced form of $NADP^+$, a coenzyme necessary for the synthesis of fatty acids.

The aerobic sequence for the oxidation of lactic and pyruvic acids is called the citric acid or Krebs cycle. This cycle takes place in the mitochondria.

The first step in the Krebs cycle is the formation of acetyl CoA from pyruvic acid. This acetyl CoA, also called active acetate, is the fuel for the citric acid cycle. Acetyl CoA reacts with oxaloacetic acid and then goes through a series of steps, each catalyzed by a particular enzyme. At the completion of the cycle, oxaloacetic acid is regenerated and then picks up another molecule of acetyl CoA to carry through the same cycle again. The NADH and $FADH_2$ produced in the citric acid cycle enter the electron transport chain in the mitochondria. The overall reaction, called oxidative phosphorylation, involves oxygen and produces ATP. Several different coenzymes and cytochromes are involved.

Glucose may also be formed from noncarbohydrate substances such as amino acids, fatty acids, and glycerol. Such a process is termed gluconeogenesis.

Thus carbohydrate metabolism interrelates the processes of glycogenesis, glycogenolysis, glycolysis, gluconeogenesis, and the Krebs cycle.

The liver controls the blood sugar level. This activity is governed by several hormones. Among these are insulin, epinephrine, and glucagon.

Insulin, a hormone secreted by the pancreas, accelerates oxidation of glucose in the cells, increases glycogenesis, decreases glycogenolysis, and promotes the formation of fat from glucose. Thus insulin removes glucose from the bloodstream.

Epinephrine, a hormone of the adrenal medulla, changes liver glycogen to glucose and muscle glycogen to lactic acid. Epinephrine is secreted into the bloodstream during periods of emotional stress.

Glucagon, a hormone secreted by the pancreas, has an effect opposite to that of insulin. It raises blood sugar levels.

The glucose tolerance test is given to a patient suspected of being a diabetic. He or she is fed glucose and the blood sugar level checked for several hours. In a normal person the blood sugar level rises and then gradually returns to normal after about $2\frac{1}{2}$ hr. In a diabetic the blood sugar level rises to a much higher level and remains there for a longer period of time.

Questions and Problems

A

1. Which monosaccharide is the principal one remaining in the bloodstream after passing through the liver?
2. What is meant by the term *normal fasting blood sugar?*
3. What is glycogenesis? Where does it occur?
4. What happens to excess carbohydrate that cannot be immediately utilized or converted to glycogen?
5. What is meant by the term *renal threshold?*
6. What is glycosuria?
7. How may glucose be removed from the bloodstream?
8. What types of compounds does the body use to store energy?
9. Indicate the hydrolysis reaction of ATP. How much energy is produced in this reaction?
10. Name two ways in which ADP may be converted to ATP.

Biochemistry

11. Describe the process of glycogenesis, indicating the intermediary products and enzymes necessary.
12. What is glycogenolysis?
13. Are glycogenesis and glycogenolysis reversible in both muscle and liver? Why?
14. What is glycolysis? Is it an aerobic or an anaerobic sequence?
15. Does glycolysis supply most of the body's energy?
16. Indicate the steps in glycolysis and the enzymes required at each step.
17. Is all the lactic acid formed in glycolysis oxidized to carbon dioxide and water? Explain.
18. What happens to most of the lactic acid formed during glycolysis?
19. After a muscle contracts and then relaxes, how does it replenish its glycogen?
20. Diagram and label the lactic acid cycle.
21. What is the hexose monophosphate shunt? Why is it important?
22. Explain briefly what happens in the Krebs cycle (citric acid cycle).
23. What is the function of acetyl CoA in the Krebs cycle?
24. How much energy is produced by the oxidation of glucose? What is the efficiency of conversion?
25. How does the energy produced during the Krebs cycle compare with that produced during glycolysis?

B 26. Diagram and label the Krebs cycle.
27. What is gluconeogenesis? What might increase it?
28. Show the interrelationship of glycolysis, gluconeogenesis, the Krebs cycle, glycogenesis, and glycogenolysis.
29. Why is acetyl CoA not considered to be a source of glucose?
30. What are the functions of insulin?
31. When is epinephrine secreted? What does it do?
32. Where is glucagon formed and what is its function?
33. Describe the glucose tolerance test. What is its purpose?
34. Where does the electron transport system function? Describe the steps involved.
35. What is cytochrome oxidase? What does it do? What is unusual about it? Why is it considered essential to life?

References   BAUM, S. J. *Introduction to Organic and Biological Chemistry,* 3rd ed. Macmillan Publishing Company, New York, 1982, Chapter 17.

DICKERSON, E. Cytochrome C and the evolution of energy metabolism. *Scientific American,* **242:**136–149 (March 1980).

FERNSTROM, J. D. and R. WURTMAN. Nutrition and the brain. *Scientific American,* **230:**84–91 (Feb. 1974).

FOYE, W. O. (ed.). *Principles of Medicinal Chemistry.* Lea & Febiger, Philadelphia, 1974, Chapter 23.

MARTIN, D. W., P. A. MAYES, and V. W. RODWELL. *Harper's Review of Biochemistry,* 19th ed., Lange Medical Publications, Los Altos, Calif., 1983, Chapters 17, 18.

RAWN, J. DAVID. *Biochemistry.* Harper and Row, New York, 1983, Chapters 14–17.

27 Metabolism of Fats

CHAPTER
OUTLINE

Absorption of Fat
Oxidation of Fat
   Oxidation of Glycerol
   Oxidation of Fatty Acids
   Energy Produced by Oxidation of
     Fatty Acids

Ketone (Acetone) Bodies
   Ketosis
Storage of Fat
Lipogenesis
Synthesis of Phospholipids
Cholesterol
   Synthesis

Absorption of Fat

The digestion of fats takes place primarily in the small intestines with hydrolysis yielding fatty acids and glycerol. Prior to their digestion, the fats have been emulsified by the bile salts. The products of fat digestion pass through the lacteals* of the villi* into the lymphatics* where they appear as resynthesized fats. From the lymphatics, the fats flow through the thoracic duct into the bloodstream and then to the liver. After a meal the fat content of the blood rises and remains at a high level for several hours, then gradually decreases to the fasting level.

In the liver some of the fats are changed to phospholipids, so that the blood leaving the liver contains both fats and phospholipids. These phospholipids, such as sphingomyelin and lecithin (see page 335), are necessary for the formation of nerve and brain tissue. Lecithins (phosphatidyl cholines) are also involved in the transportation of fat to the tissues. Cephalin, another phospholipid, is involved in the normal clotting of the blood. From the liver, some fat goes to the cells where it is oxidized to furnish heat and energy. The fat in excess of what the cells need is stored as adipose tissue.

Lipolysis, the hydrolysis of triacylglycerols (triglycerides) to fatty acids and glycerol, is under the control of c-AMP and various hormones. Glucagon and epinephrine stimulate the production of c-AMP and so increase lipolysis. However, insulin and the prostaglandins (see page 339) depress the levels of c-AMP and so decrease the rate of lipolysis.

Oxidation of Fat

The oxidation of fat (triacylglycerol) actually involves the oxidation of the two hydrolysis products—glycerol and fatty acids.

416

Oxidation of Glycerol The glycerol part of a fat is oxidized to dihydroxyacetone phosphate, as is indicated in the following sequence. Recall that dihydroxyacetone phosphate is part of the glycolysis sequence (see page 400). This compound may be converted into glycogen in the liver or muscle tissue or into pyruvic acid, which enters the citric acid (Krebs) cycle. Thus, the glycerol part of a fat is metabolized through the carbohydrate sequence.

Oxidation of Fatty Acids There are several theories about the oxidation of fatty acids. The original one, proposed by Knoop in 1905 and still preferred today, is called the beta-oxidation theory. This theory involves the oxidation of the second carbon atom from the acid end of the fatty acid molecule—the beta carbon atom. In this process beta oxidation removes two carbon atoms at a time from the fatty acid chain. That is, an 18-carbon fatty acid is oxidized to a 16-carbon fatty acid, then to a 14-carbon fatty acid, and so on, until the oxidation process is complete. A simplified version of such an oxidation is shown in Figure 27-1.

The acetyl CoA thus produced enters the citric acid cycle and the new molecule of active fatty acid goes through the same sequence again, each time losing two carbon atoms until the entire fatty acid molecule has been oxidized. This sequence presupposes the presence of fatty acids containing an even number of carbon atoms, a condition usually encountered in nature. The $FADH_2$ and the $NADH + H^+$ enter the respiratory chain.

FIGURE 27-1. Oxidation of a fatty acid.

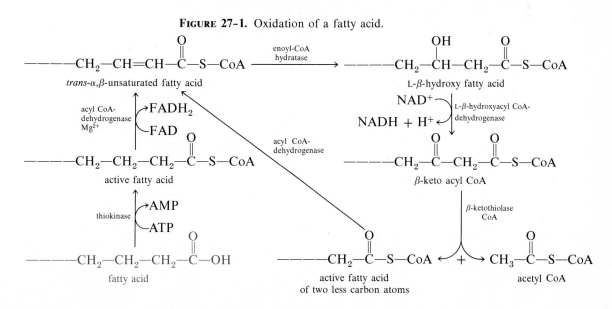

If fatty acids containing an odd number of carbon atoms are oxidized, they follow the same steps except that the final products are acetyl CoA and propionyl CoA. The propionyl CoA is changed in a series of steps to succinyl CoA, which then enters the citric acid cycle, as does the acetyl CoA. These reactions require the presence of vitamin B_{12} and also biotin.

The unsaturated fatty acids are metabolized slowly. They must first be reduced by some of the dehydrogenases found in the cells. Then they can follow the fatty acid cycle for oxidation.

Energy Produced by Oxidation of Fatty Acids

The oxidation of 1 g fat produces more than twice as much energy as the oxidation of 1 g carbohydrate. Let us see why.

The oxidation of acetyl CoA through the citric acid cycle yields 12 high-energy phosphate bonds (ATP) per molecule of acetyl CoA. If we consider the oxidation of palmitic acid, a 16-carbon fatty acid, 8 two-carbon units will be formed during the beta-oxidation cycle. These eight-carbon units will yield 8×12 or 96ATPs. However, 2 ATPs are used up in the initial activation of the fatty acid. In addition, it has been calculated that palmitic acid will produce 35ATPs as it goes through the fatty acid cycle ($7FADH_2$, each equivalent to 2ATP and 7NADH, each equivalent to 3ATPs). That is, the net number of ATP molecules produced will be $96 - 2 + 35$, or 129.

Considering each mole of ATP as requiring 7600 cal for formation, 129×7600 cal or 980 kcal are needed. The theoretic yield from 1 mole of palmitic acid is 2340 kcal, so that the efficiency of conversion is 980/2340, or 42 percent, with the remainder of the energy being produced as heat. (Other fatty acids and glycerol are also oxidized, so that the net result is that fats produce much more energy than do carbohydrates.)

Ketone (Acetone) Bodies

In a diabetic patient, or any other situation in which carbohydrate metabolism is restricted, the body uses oxaloacetate to produce glucose for the brain and muscles. This reduces the amount of oxaloacetate available for the Krebs cycle and acetyl CoA cannot be properly metabolized. When this occurs, the acetyl CoA is changed to acetoacetyl CoA, which is converted into acetoacetic acid in the liver by the enzyme deacylase. Acetoacetic acid may be changed into acetone and β-hydroxybutyric acid, as shown in reactions (27-1).

These three substances—acetoacetic acid, β-hydroxybutyric acid, and acetone—are commonly called acetone bodies, or ketone bodies. They are carried by the blood to the muscles and tissues where they are converted back to acetoacetyl CoA and then oxidized normally. However, during diabetes, the production of these ketone bodies by the liver exceeds the ability of the muscles and tissues to oxidize them, so they accumulate in the blood.

Ketosis

The excess accumulation of ketone bodies in the blood is called ketonemia. The excess accumulation of ketone bodies in the urine is called ketonuria. The overall accumulation of ketone bodies in the blood and the urine is called ketosis. During ketosis, acetone may be detected on the patient's breath because it is a volatile compound and is easily excreted through the

$$(27\text{-}1)$$

lungs. Ketosis may occur with diabetis mellitus, in starvation or severe liver damage, or on a diet high in fats and low in carbohydrates.

During diabetes mellitus the body is unable to oxidize carbohydrates and instead oxidizes fats, leading to an accumulation of ketone bodies in the blood and the urine. These ketone bodies are acidic and tend to decrease the pH of the blood. The lowering of the pH of the blood is termed acidosis and may lead to a fatal coma. During acidosis an increased amount of water intake is needed to eliminate the products of metabolism. Unless the water intake of a diabetic is increased, dehydration will occur. Dehydration of diabetics may also be caused by polyuria due to an increased amount of glucose in the urine.

Likewise, during prolonged starvation or on a high-fat, low-carbohydrate diet, the body tends to burn fat instead of carbohydrate, leading to ketosis and acidosis.

In severe liver damage, the liver cannot store glycogen in the required amounts, therefore, carbohydrates are not available for the normal oxidation of fats, which leads to ketosis.

Storage of Fat Fat in excess of that required for the normal oxidative processes of the body is stored as adipose tissue under the skin and around the internal organs. This stored fat serves several important purposes.

1. Reserve supply of food.
2. Support for the internal organs.
3. Shock absorber for the internal organs.
4. Insulation of interior of the body against sudden external changes in temperature.

Metabolism of Fats   **419**

The fat stored in the body is in equilibrium with that in the bloodstream. That is, the fats stored in the adipose tissue do not merely remain there as inert compounds until they are needed. They are continuously being used and replaced so that there is always a dynamic transfer of fats between the bloodstream and the storage tissues.

Obesity is a condition in which excess fat is deposited as adipose tissue. An obese person eats more food than his or her body can burn up so that the excess is converted to fat and stored as adipose tissue. For every 9 kcal of food eaten in excess of the body's requirements, 1 g of fat is deposited.

Most people have a tendency to become obese as they grow older. This is because they require less food for the maintenance of their bodies, especially because they exercise less than younger people.

In general obesity leads to a shortened life expectancy, as indicated in Figure 27-2. An obese person runs a higher than normal risk of developing cardiovascular disease, diabetes, or liver disease. A weight greater than 10 percent above that considered normal for a person's age and height can cause medical problems. The answer to obesity lies in proper dieting under the supervision of a doctor, because the metabolism of the body is a highly intricate mechanism that can very easily be disturbed.

Excess Mortality*

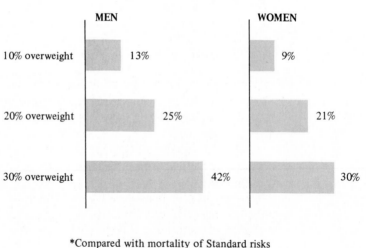

	MEN	WOMEN
10% overweight	13%	9%
20% overweight	25%	21%
30% overweight	42%	30%

FIGURE 27-2. Mortality table based on obesity. (Courtesy of Metropolitan Life Insurance Co., New York, N.Y.)

*Compared with mortality of Standard risks
(Mortality ratio of Standard risks = 100%)

Lipogenesis

Lipogenesis—the conversion of glucose to fats—takes place in the liver and in the adipose tissue, with the latter place predominating. Insulin is necessary for lipogenesis both in the liver and in the adipose tissue. Lipogenesis is reduced during fasting or during a high-fat diet, whereas it is increased during a high-carbohydrate diet.

The synthesis of fatty acids occurs in the mitochondria and in the cell cytoplasm with the latter location being predominant. The process in the mitochondria involves the lengthening of fatty acid chains of moderate length, whereas the cytoplasmic processes involve the synthesis of fatty acids from acetyl CoA.

Synthesis of Phospholipids

The phospholipids are very important because they form (along with protein) the framework of most of the cell membrane system (see page 334). The steps involved are shown in equations (27–2).

The 1,2-diglyceride may also combine with cytidine diphosphate-choline (CDP-choline) to form lecithin (phosphatidyl choline), or it may combine with CDP-ethanolamine to form cephalin (phosphatidyl ethanolamine).

Cholesterol

Cholesterol is found in all cells of the body but particularly in brain and nerve tissue. Cholesterol occurs in animal fat but not in plant fat. About 0.3 g cholesterol is ingested daily from such foods as egg yolk, meat fats, liver, and liver oils. In addition it has been estimated that the body manufactures about 1 g of cholesterol daily.

Cholesterol normally is eliminated in the bile. However, sometimes it settles out in the gallbladder as gallstones. If cholesterol deposits in the walls of the larger arteries, the condition is known as atherosclerosis, a type of hardening of the arteries. When this occurs, there is a decrease in the usable diameter of the blood vessels. The elasticity of the arterial walls decreases. There is an interference with the rate of blood flow because there is greater friction due to the irregular lining of the blood vessels. This irregular lining may also cause clots as the blood flows over that type of surface.

Cholesterol is important as a precursor of several important steroids such as vitamin D, the sex hormones, and the adrenocortical hormones (the hormones of the cortex of the adrenal glands).

Metabolism of Fats   **421**

(a)
Normal artery

(b)
Fatty deposits in
vessel wall

(c)
Plugged artery with fatty
deposits and clot

FIGURE 27-3. Comparison of normal artery wall with those containing fatty deposits. (Reprinted by permission, American Heart Association.)

Synthesis   Cholesterol is synthesized primarily in the liver, but the adrenal cortex, skin, testes, aorta, and intestines are also able to synthesize it. This synthesis takes place in the microsomal and cytosomal fraction of the cell. Acetyl CoA is the starting material and is also the source of all the carbon atoms in cholesterol.

Summary   Emulsified fats pass through the lacteals of the villi into the lymphatics through the thoracic duct to the liver. In the liver some of the fats are changed to phospholipids, which are necessary for the formation of nerve and brain tissue. Some fat is stored in the adipose tissue; some is oxidized to furnish energy.

Glycerol from a fat is oxidized to dihydroxyacetone phosphate, which is part of the glycolysis sequence. That is, the glycerol part of a fat is metabolized through the carbohydrate sequence.

Fatty acids pass through a beta-oxidation cycle in which two carbon atoms are removed at a time and converted to acetyl CoA, which then enters the citric acid cycle.

The oxidation of one molecule of a 16-carbon fatty acid yields a total of 129 ATP molecules, with an efficiency of about 42 percent.

Ketone (acetone) bodies are normally produced in the beta-oxidation process. However, the are produced only in small amounts and do not normally accumulate. If excess ketone bodies accumulate in the blood, a condition known as ketonemia exists. Accumulation of ketone bodies in the urine is termed ketonuria. The overall accumulation of ketone bodies is called ketosis; it occurs in the abnormal metabolism of carbohydrates.

Fat in excess of the body's needs is stored as adipose tissue. Stored fat serves as a reserve supply of food, as a support for the internal organs, as a shock absorber for the internal organs, and as an insulator for the body.

If excess fat is deposited in the adipose tissue, the resulting condition is termed obesity. Obesity may be due to a glandular disorder or simply to overeating.

The conversion of glucose to fats, lipogenesis, takes place in the liver and in the adipose tissue.

The synthesis of fatty acids occurs both inside and outside the mitochondria, with the latter being the predominant site.

Phospholipids may be synthesized from glycerol. If the 1,2-diglyceride formed from glycerol reacts with cytidine diphosphate choline, then the phospholipid lecithin is formed. If instead the 1,2-diglyceride combines with cytidine diphosphate ethanolamine, then the phospholipid cephalin is formed.

Cholesterol is found in all cells of the body but particularly in nerve tissue. Cholesterol is normally eliminated in the bile but if it settles out in the gallbladder, gallstones are formed. If cholesterol deposits on the walls of the arteries, atherosclerosis occurs.

Cholesterol is an important precursor for vitamin D, for the sex hormones, and for the adrenocortical hormones.

Cholesterol is synthesized in the liver beginning with acetyl CoA and proceeding through a series of steps.

Questions and Problems

1. Where are fats absorbed? How do they get to the liver?
2. What happens to fats in the liver?
3. Describe the oxidation of the glycerol part of a fat.
4. What is the beta-oxidation theory of fats? What are the end products of this cycle? What becomes of these products?
5. What types of products are formed during the oxidation of even and odd number carbon fatty acids?
6. What happens to unsaturated fatty acids before they can be oxidized?
7. Compare the energy produced by the oxidation of 1 g carbohydrate and 1 g fat.
8. In the oxidation of a fat, in which part of the sequence is most of the energy produced?
9. The oxidation of one molecule of a 16-carbon fatty acid produces how many ATP molecules?
10. What are the acetone bodies? How are they interrelated structurally?
11. Where are acetone bodies formed?
12. What is ketonemia? ketonuria? ketosis? Under what conditions might ketosis occur?
13. Where is excess fat stored? What functions does this fat have?
14. What conditions lead to obesity?
15. What is lipogenesis? Where does it occur?
16. How does lipogenesis in the mitochondria compare with the oxidation of a fat?
17. Why are phospholipids important?
18. Describe the synthesis of lecithin.
19. How does the synthesis of lecithin compare with that of cephalin?
20. Where is cholesterol found in the body? Where is it produced?
21. Why is cholesterol important in the body?
22. If cholesterol is deposited in the walls of the large arteries, what is the condition termed?
23. If cholesterol is deposited in the gallbladder, what is formed?

References

BAUM, STUART J. *Introduction to Organic and Biological Chemistry,* 3rd ed. Macmillan Publishing Company, New York, 1982, Chapter 18.

Metabolism of Fats

BENDITT, E. P. The origin of atherosclerosis. *Scientific American,* **236:**74–84 (Feb. 1977).

GREEN, D. E. Synthesis of fat. *Scientific American,* **202:**46–51 (Feb. 1960).

MARTIN, D. W., P. A. MAYES, and V. W. RODWELL. *Harper's Review of Biochemistry,* 19th ed. Lange Medical Publications, Los Altos, Calif., 1983, Chapters 14, 15.

RAWN, J. DAVID. *Biochemistry.* Harper & Row, New York, 1983, Chapter 19.

SCHAUF, G. E. The caloric theory does not apply to obesity. *Journal of the International Academy of Preventive Medicine,* **3**(2):33–41 (Dec. 1976).

28 Metabolism of Proteins

CHAPTER
OUTLINE

Functions of Protein in the Body
Nitrogen Balance
Synthesis of Protein
Body's Requirement of Protein
Catabolism of Amino Acids
  Deamination
  Transamination
  Formation of Urea

  Decarboxylation
Metabolism of the Carbon Portion of
  Amino Acids
Metabolism of Hemoglobin
Metabolism of Nucleoproteins
Metabolism of Proteins,
  Carbohydrates, and Lipids

Functions of Protein in the Body

During digestion, proteins are hydrolyzed into amino acids, which are then absorbed into the bloodstream through the villi of the small intestine. These amino acids are then transported to the tissues of the body. After a meal, the amino acid concentration of the blood rises but soon falls to its normal fasting value.

The amino acids from the digested food serve many different purposes. Among these are the following:

1. Conversion to tissue protein to build new tissue.
2. Conversion to tissue protein to replace old tissue.
3. Use in the formation of hemoglobin.
4. Use in the formation of some hormones.
5. Use in the formation of enzymes.
6. Source of the different amino acids that the body needs but does not have.
7. Source of energy when catabolized into a nitrogen part and a nonnitrogen part with subsequent oxidation.

Nitrogen Balance

The body can store carbohydrates (as glycogen in the liver and the muscles), and can store fats (as adipose tissue and in tissues around the internal organs). However, the body cannot store protein. The amino acids that result from the digestion of protein are used either for the synthesis of new tissues, for the replacement of old tissues, and for the formation of the various

425

required body substances such as hormones and enzymes, or they are converted to fat or oxidized to furnish energy.

Because the body cannot store protein and because protein contains nitrogen, the amount of nitrogen intake in the food per day should usually equal the amount of nitrogen excreted per day (for a normal adult whose weight remains constant). This takes into consideration the normal replacement of worn-out tissue where the reaction is merely one of exchange between one amino acid and another.

A person whose body excretes as much nitrogen per day as is taken in with food is said to be in nitrogen balance. Children exhibit a positive nitrogen balance because they take in more nitrogen in their food than they excrete. This is because the child has a greater need for amino acids to build growing body tissues. Any body condition marked by the growth of new tissues will exhibit a positive nitrogen balance. An example of this is seen in persons recovering from a wasting illness where the body needs to rebuild tissues and so does not excrete as much nitrogen (amino acids) as it takes in.

Conversely, if the body excretes more nitrogen than it takes in in the food, a negative nitrogen balance exists. Conditions that can produce a negative nitrogen balance are starvation, malnutrition, prolonged fever, and various wasting illnesses. However, a person can survive for a reasonable period of time in negative nitrogen balance, as when dieting, since body protein will be used for essential purposes.

However, inadequate protein intake leads to a negative nitrogen balance and the individual eventually will develop a protein deficiency disease called kwashiorkor. This disease is characterized by a wasting away of fat and muscle and a degeneration of many of the internal organs (see page 457).

Protein malnutrition also exists in seriously ill patients who cannot eat by mouth. Such patients include those who have had major surgery or trauma. If protein is not provided, along with other foods and minerals, the person will have a negative nitrogen balance and will have a much slower rate of recovery.

In such cases, a procedure called *hyperalimentation* is used whereby glucose and hydrolyzed protein are administered intravenously.

A person consuming about 300 g carbohydrate, 100 g fat, and 100 g protein (2500 kilocalories) per day will excrete about 16.5 g nitrogen per day. About 95 percent of this nitrogen is eliminated through the kidneys and the remaining 5 percent in the stool. Most of the nitrogen is excreted in the form of urea (see page 428).

Synthesis of Protein

As was discussed in Chapter 23, proteins are synthesized from amino acids through the various intermediaries such as peptides and polypeptides. The body takes the amino acids produced by the digestion of protein and recombines them into the protein that it needs in the various parts of the body. (See Chapter 33 for the mechanism of protein synthesis.)

Some amino acids that the body needs may be synthesized from other amino acids. However, there are certain amino acids that the body needs but cannot synthesize. These amino acids must be supplied in the food if the body is to function normally. These nutritionally essential amino acids are listed on page 353.

Some proteins contain all of the nutritionally essential amino acids; one that does not contain all the essential amino acids is called an **incomplete protein.** Two common incomplete proteins are gelatin, which is lacking in tryptophan, and zein (from corn), which is lacking in both tryptophan and lysine.

Body's Requirement of Protein

A certain minimum daily amount of protein is required for the normal replacement of body tissues. This amount, however, may be greatly increased by increased metabolism such as occurs in high fevers. However, for the normal adult keeping a constant weight, the recommended daily intake of protein is approximately 0.8 g per kilogram of body weight. This amounts to approximately 46 g protein per day for the adult female and 56 g per day for the adult male.

Catabolism of Amino Acids

The amino acids that the body does not need for tissue building or that are not of the correct type for this purpose are broken down to ammonia, carbon dioxide, and water, at the same time producing heat and energy.

Deamination

Deamination (also called oxidative deamination) is a catabolism reaction whereby the α-amino group of an amino acid is removed, forming an α-keto acid and ammonia. Deamination occurs primarily in the liver and the kidneys under the catalysis of the enzyme amino acid oxidase.

$$CH_3-\underset{\underset{NH_2}{|}}{CH}-COOH \xrightarrow{\text{amino acid oxidase}} CH_3-\underset{\underset{O}{\|}}{C}-COOH + NH_3$$

| alanine | pyruvic acid | ammonia |
| (an α-amino acid) | (an α-keto acid) | |

The α-keto acid produced by this process can undergo several different types of reactions.

1. It can be catabolized to carbon dioxide, water, and energy in the citric acid cycle.
2. It can be converted to carbohydrates (glycogen) or to fat.
3. It may be reconverted to a different amino acid by a process called transamination.

Transamination

Transamination is a reaction that interconverts a pair of α-amino acids and α-keto acids. This reaction is catalyzed by enzymes called transaminases or aminotransferases. All other amino acids are converted into glutamic acid by transamination. Transaminases are used for the diagnosis of a variety of disorders. By this process the body can manufacture the amino acids that it needs and does not have. An essential part of the active site of transaminases is pyridoxal phosphate, the coenzyme form of vitamin B_6.

An example of transamination is the reaction of glutamic acid (an α-amino acid) and pyruvic acid (an α-keto acid) to form α-ketoglutaric acid (another α-keto acid) and alanine (another α-amino acid).

$$\underset{\substack{\text{glutamic acid}\\(\alpha\text{-amino acid})}}{\underset{|}{CH_2}-\underset{}{CH_2}-\underset{\underset{NH_2}{|}}{CH}-COOH} + \underset{\substack{\text{pyruvic acid}\\(\alpha\text{-keto acid})}}{CH_3-\underset{\underset{O}{\|}}{C}-COOH} \xrightarrow{\text{transaminase}}$$

$$\underset{\substack{\text{α-ketoglutaric acid}\\(\alpha\text{-keto acid})}}{\underset{\underset{COOH}{|}}{CH_2}-CH_2-\underset{\underset{O}{\|}}{C}-COOH} + \underset{\substack{\text{alanine}\\(\alpha\text{-amino acid})}}{CH_3-\underset{\underset{NH_2}{|}}{CH}-COOH}$$

Formation of Urea The ammonia formed from the deamination of amino acids combines with carbon dioxide to form urea and water. This process takes place in the liver. The overall reaction may be written as shown in equation (28–1):

$$\underset{\text{ammonia}}{2NH_3} + \underset{\text{carbon dioxide}}{CO_2} \xrightarrow{\text{enzymes}} \underset{\text{urea}}{NH_2CONH_2} + \underset{\text{water}}{H_2O} \qquad (28\text{–}1)$$

However, this process is certainly not as simple as that shown in equation (28–1). It consists of a series of steps, each catalyzed by an appropriate enzyme.

Ammonia is a toxic by-product of the deamination of amino acids and as such must be removed from the body, predominantly in the form of the compound urea. In the conversion of ammonia to urea, three different amino acids are involved. These are arginine, citrulline, and ornithine. The pathways for the conversion of ammonia to urea is called the urea cycle (see Figure 28–1).

The first step in this cycle is the reaction of ammonia and carbon dioxide to form carbamoyl phosphate. In this reaction, ATP is converted to ADP. This reaction is catalyzed by magnesium ions and the presence of N-acetylglutamic acid and the enzyme carbamoyl phosphate synthetase. Lack of this enzyme produces the very serious disorder hyperammonemia. The body has only one principal way to dispose of excess nitrogen and this is by the excretion of urea.

$$NH_3 + CO_2 + H_2O + 2ATP \xrightarrow[\substack{N\text{-acetylglutamic}\\\text{acid}\\\text{carbamoyl phosphate}\\\text{synthetase}}]{Mg^{2+}} \underset{\substack{\text{carbamoyl}\\\text{phosphate}}}{H_2N-\underset{\underset{O}{\|}}{C}-O-P} + 2ADP + P$$

In the second step, carbamoyl phosphate combines with ornithine to form citrulline. This reaction is catalyzed by the liver enzyme ornithine *trans*-carbamoyl transferase. Lack of this enzyme will produce a different hyperammonemia.

Biochemistry   **428**

ornithine carbamoyl phosphate citrulline

Next, citrulline reacts with aspartic acid (derived from transamination of oxaloacetate) to form arginine succinic acid. This reaction takes place in the presence of ATP, magnesium ions, and an enzyme arginosuccinate synthetase:

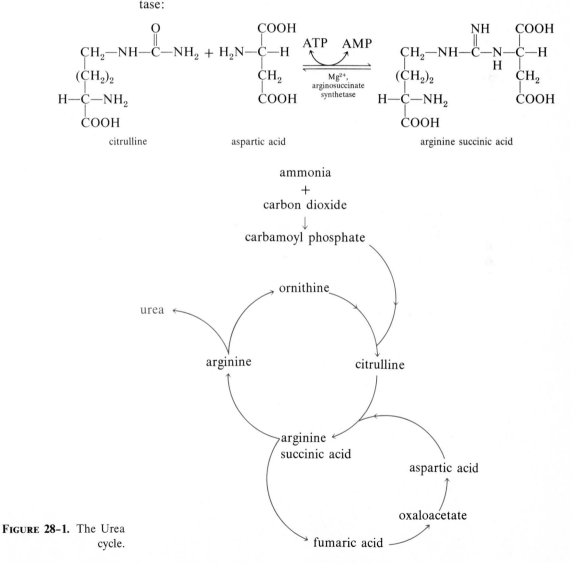

citrulline aspartic acid arginine succinic acid

FIGURE 28-1. The Urea cycle.

Metabolism of Proteins

429

Arginine succinic acid is cleaved (split) hydrolytically into arginine and fumaric acid. The fumaric acid enters the citric acid cycle.

arginine succinic acid   arginine   fumaric acid

Finally, arginine is split hydrolytically by the liver enzyme arginase into ornithine and urea. The ornithine then can go through the cycle again and the urea is excreted.

arginine   ornithine   urea

To summarize, the urea cycle is shown diagrammatically in Figure 28–1. (Note that some fumaric acid may be converted back to aspartic acid and some enters the citric acid cycle.)

The blood picks up the urea from the liver and carries it to the kidneys where it is excreted in the urine. Urea is the principal nitrogen end product of protein metabolism and contains a large percentage of the total nitrogen excreted by the body. This is the only means the body has of removing ammonia.

Decarboxylation The decarboxylation (removal of a —COOH group) of an amino acid yields a primary amine. The carboxyl group that is removed is converted to carbon dioxide. The enzyme involved in a decarboxylation reaction requires pyridoxal phosphate as a coenzyme. The decarboxylation reaction may be summarized as follows

α-amino acid   primary amine

Several naturally occurring amines are formed by the decarboxylation of amino acids. The following list includes some of these.

Biochemistry   **430**

$$\text{amino acid} \xrightarrow{\text{decarboxylation}} \textit{primary amine}$$

histidine	$\longrightarrow$ histamine
lysine	$\longrightarrow$ cadaverine
ornithine	$\longrightarrow$ putrescine
tyrosine	$\longrightarrow$ tyramine

Some decarboxylation reactions are brought about by intestinal bacterial attack on amino acids, to produce toxic amines called ptomaines (see page 393). This process is common in the spoilage of food protein.

Metabolism of the Carbon Portion of Amino Acids

Once the nitrogen has been removed from an amino acid, the carbon portion can be used as an energy source. The carbon skeletons can be converted into a variety of compounds (see Figure 28–2). The ones converted to acetyl CoA and acetoacetyl CoA are ketogenic whereas those converted to pyruvate or Krebs cycle intermediates are glucogenic, since the body can synthesize glucose from them. Amino acid catabolism thus provides energy and a wide variety of precursors and intermediates.

Metabolism of Hemoglobin

A red blood cell has a life span of about 120 days. After that period of time, the hemoglobin is catabolized. The globin (protein) part is metabolized as is any other protein. The heme is metabolized and excreted as waste products, but the iron is reused. The normal diet supplies about 12 to 15 mg of iron per day, but of this amount only about 1 mg per day may be absorbed. When hemoglobin is metabolized, 20 to 25 mg of iron are released per day. This amount must be reused or else the body will suffer a serious loss of iron. Stomach acidity is needed to aid in the absorption of iron.

When an erythrocyte (a red blood cell) ruptures, the hemoglobin ring is broken and the products formed are globin, ferrous ions, and biliverdin, a blue-green pigment. This process takes place in the reticuloendothelial cells of the liver, spleen, and bone marrow. Biliverdin is rapidly reduced to bilirubin, an orange-yellow pigment, by the enzyme bilirubin reductase, also in the reticuloendothelial cells. From there the bilirubin is transported to the liver as a bilirubin-albumin complex with the aid of serum albumin. In the liver, bilirubin is converted to bilirubin diglucuronide, which is then excreted into the bile. The bile flows into the small intestine. In the small intestine the bilirubin diglucuronide is changed to stercobilinogen and then to stercobilin for excretion into the stool and also into urobilinogen and then to urobilin for excretion into the urine.

Jaundice* is the condition in which abnormal amounts of bilirubin accumulate in the blood. Patients with jaundice exhibit a characteristic yellow-colored skin due to the presence of bilirubin.

If hemolysis takes place at an abnormally high rate, so that bilirubin accumulates in the blood, the condition is termed **hemolytic jaundice.** If the bile duct is obstructed so that bile cannot enter the intestinal tract, bilirubin again accumulates in the blood. This condition is termed **obstructive jaundice** and is characterized by white or clay-colored stools because decomposition products of bilirubin are not present. If the liver is damaged in such

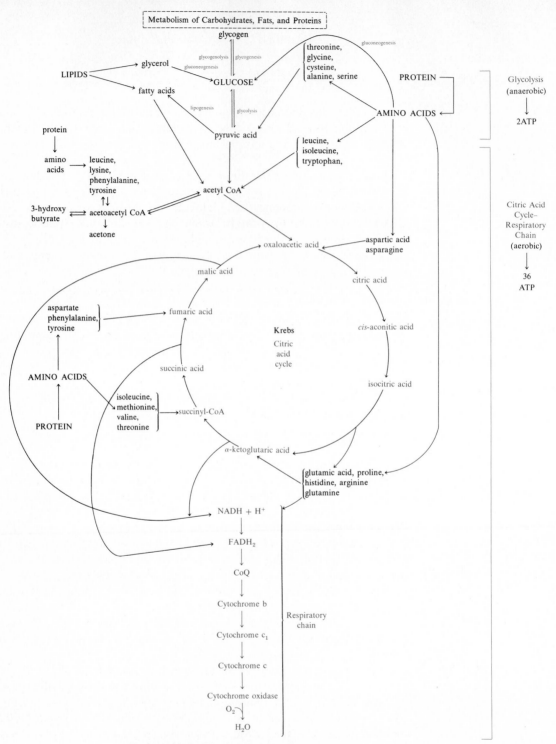

FIGURE 28-2. The interrelationships in the metabolism of carbohydrates, lipids, and proteins.

diseases as infectious hepatitis or cirrhosis, bilirubin cannot be removed and a jaundiced condition results.

Metabolism of Nucleoproteins

Nucleoproteins are composed of proteins conjugated with nucleic acids. DNA and RNA, two nucleic acids, are essential constituents of chromosomes, viruses, and cell nuclei. The following diagram illustrates the hydrolysis products of nucleoprotein.

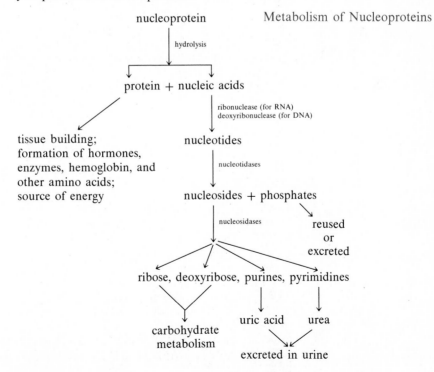

Metabolism of Proteins, Carbohydrates, and Lipids

The metabolism of protein produces compounds, such as pyruvic acid, that can enter the citric acid cycle, other products that can enter the glycogen-forming cycle, and still others that can enter the lipogenesis cycle. The inter-relationships of the metabolism of carbohydrates, lipids, and proteins are indicated in Figure 28–2.

Summary

During digestion, proteins are hydrolyzed into amino acids. These amino acids may be used for the synthesis of new tissue, for the replacement of old tissue, and for the formation of enzymes and hormones, or they may be oxidized to furnish energy. The body cannot store protein (amino acids).

A person who excretes as much nitrogen daily as he or she takes in is said to be in nitrogen balance. Children have a positive nitrogen balance because they need extra proteins for growth and so excrete less. Malnutrition and prolonged fever may lead to a negative nitrogen balance.

Amino acids that the body cannot synthesize and that must be supplied in the food are called essential amino acids. A protein that does not contain all the essential amino acids is called an incomplete protein.

For the normal adult, 46 to 56 g of protein are required per day.

Amino acids that the body does not need are catabolized into carbon dioxide and water. This catabolism may be oxidative deamination (deamination) whereby the α-amino group is removed, forming an α-keto acid and ammonia. The α-keto acid may be catabolized to carbon dioxide and water and energy through the citric acid cycle; it may be converted to glycogen or to fat; or it may undergo transamination, whereby a different amino acid is formed.

The ammonia formed from the deamination of an amino acid unites with carbon dioxide and water to form urea. This process, which takes place in the liver, proceeds through a cycle called the urea cycle.

Amino acids may also be decarboxylated to form primary amines.

When hemoglobin is metabolized, the protein part is metabolized as is any other protein. The iron is used over again and the remaining heme part goes through a series of steps eventually ending up as urobilinogen and urobilin in the urine and stercobilinogen and stercobilin in the feces.

When excessive amounts of bilirubin, one of the intermediate products of the metabolism of hemoglobin, accumulate in the blood, the condition is known as jaundice.

The end product of the metabolism of purines is uric acid, which is excreted in the urine.

The metabolism of amino acids is interrelated to that of carbohydrates and fats.

Questions and Problems

1. What are the functions of protein in the body?
2. Can the body store protein? carbohydrate? fat?
3. What is meant by the term *nitrogen balance?*
4. What might cause a positive nitrogen balance?
5. What might cause a negative nitrogen balance?
6. What is an essential amino acid? List the essential amino acids.
7. What is an incomplete protein?
8. What is the normal daily requirement of protein?
9. What is deamination? Where does it occur in the body?
10. What products are produced by a deamination reaction?
11. What is transamination? What is its function in the body?

12. What various processes may an α-keto acid undergo?
13. Where is urea formed?
14. Diagram and explain the urea cycle.
15. What is decarboxylation? What type of product is produced by the decarboxylation of an amino acid?
16. What are ptomaines? How are they produced?
17. What is biliverdin? Where is it formed?
18. What are the end products of the metabolism of hemoglobin? Which are found in the urine? in the feces?
19. What is jaundice? What can cause it?
20. Indicate the relationship between the metabolism of carbohydrates, lipids, and proteins.
21. Describe the hydrolysis of nucleoprotein. What happens to the hydrolysis products?
22. What is hyperalimentation and where is it used?
23. What causes kwashiorkor? What are its characteristic symptoms in children?

References

BAUM, STUART J. *Introduction to Organic and Biological Chemistry,* 3rd ed. Macmillan Publishing Company, New York, 1982, Chapter 19.

JANICK, J., C. H. NOLLER, and C. L. RHYKERD. The cycles of plant and animal metabolism. *Scientific American,* **235:**75–86 (Sept. 1976).

KAPPAS, A. and A. P. ALBARES. How the liver metabolizes foreign substances. *Scientific American,* **232:**22–31 (June 1975).

RAWN, J. DAVID. *Biochemistry.* Harper & Row, New York, 1983, Chapters 9, 21.

STETTEN, D. Gout and metabolism. *Scientific American,* **198:**73–81 (June 1958).

STRYER, L. *Biochemistry.* W. H. Freeman and Company, Publishers, San Francisco, Calif., 1975, Chapter 18 and pages 547–551.

29 Body Fluids: Urine

CHAPTER OUTLINE

Excretion of Waste Material
Formation of Urine
General Properties of Urine
   Volume
   Specific Gravity
   pH
   Color
   Odor
Normal Constituents
   Organic Constituents
   Inorganic Constituents

Abnormal Constituents
   Protein
   Glucose
   Other Sugars
   Acetone Bodies
   Blood
   Bile
   Phenylpyruvic Acid
Diuretics
Phenolsulfonphthalein Test
Reagent Tablets, Papers, and Dip Sticks

Excretion of Waste Material

The waste products of the body are excreted through the lungs, the skin, the intestines, and the kidneys. The liver also excretes waste products—the bile pigments and cholesterol.

The lungs eliminate water and carbon dioxide through the expired air. The skin eliminates water in the form of perspiration. Included in the perspiration are small amounts of inorganic and organic salts. The feces, excreted from the large intestine, contain undigested and undigestible material plus the excretory products from the liver—the bile pigments and cholesterol—some water, and some organic and inorganic salts. The primary excretory organs of the body, however, are the kidneys, which excrete water and water-soluble compounds including nitrogen compounds from the catabolism of amino acids.

The kidneys are important not only for their excretory function but also because they play an important role in the control and regulation of water, electrolyte, and acid-base balance in the body.

Formation of Urine

Blood flows to the kidneys through the renal arteries. From the renal arteries the blood passes into the arterioles and then into the capillaries of the kidneys. These capillaries coil up to form a **glomerulus,** a rounded ball of capillaries. Around the glomerulus is a structure called **Bowman's capsule** (see

436

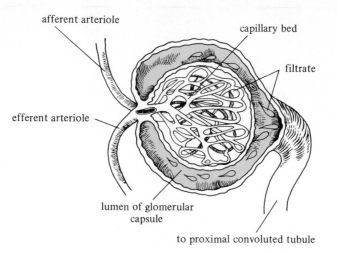

afferent arteriole

capillary bed

filtrate

efferent arteriole

lumen of glomerular capsule

to proximal convoluted tubule

FIGURE 29–1. Glomerulus and Bowman's capsule in the kidney.

Figure 29–1). Each Bowman's capsule is connected by a tubule to a larger tube, which in turn carries the urine to the bladder where it is stored until it is excreted.

As blood flows into the kidney, the various soluble components diffuse into the glomeruli (there are over a million glomeruli in each kidney). The protein material in the blood cannot pass through the membranes (recall that proteins are colloids and colloids do not pass through membranes). The driving force for this diffusion of fluid through the walls of the glomerulus is the blood pressure. The liquid in the glomerulus thus has approximately the same composition as does the blood plasma except for the protein material.

As the fluid in the glomerulus passes down the tubule, a large proportion of the water is reabsorbed into the bloodstream. Also reabsorbed are the glucose, amino acids, and most inorganic ions. The remaining liquid, containing urea and other waste products, flows to the collecting tubules and then to the bladder.

Thus, the kidneys act as a very efficient filter removing the waste materials but not the needed nutrients from the blood. Approximately 1 L of blood is filtered through the kidneys every minute. Of this amount, most of the water is reabsorbed so that the amount of urine excreted per day is less than 1 percent of the total amount of liquid filtered. If the kidneys are not functioning normally, an artificial kidney machine may be used (see page 181).

Table 29–1 compares the compositions of blood plasma and urine.

General Properties of Urine

Volume

A normal adult excretes 600 to 2500 ml of urine per day. The amount depends on the liquid intake and also on the weather conditions. In hot weather, more water is lost through perspiration, therefore, the amount of urine formed is less. Conversely, a greater amount of urine is formed during cold weather or when the humidity is high so that little evaporation of perspiration takes place. Drugs, such as caffeine (in coffee or tea) and also alcoholic beverages have a diuretic* effect—that is, they increase the flow of urine.

Body Fluids: Urine

TABLE 29-1. Comparison of Composition of
Blood Plasma and Urine

Constituent	Percentage in Blood Plasma	Percentage in Urine
Water	90–93	95
Glucose	97	0
Protein	7	0
Sodium	0.3	0.35
Ammonia	0.004	0.05
Phosphate	0.009	0.5
Urea	0.03	2.0
Sulfate	0.002	0.18

A decreased flow of urine is called **oliguria.** Such a condition may occur during a high fever when most of the water lost by the body is in the form of perspiration. Certain kidney diseases may also cause oliguria.

Anuria means a total lack of urine excretion. Anuria indicates extensive kidney damage such as may be caused by a blood transfusion of the wrong type. In this condition the blood cells disintegrate releasing hemoglobin, which clogs the glomeruli and does not allow any excretion of urine. Bichloride of mercury also affects the kidneys and may cause oliguria or anuria.

Polyuria is a condition in which the amount of urine excreted is much greater than normal. It may be due to excessive intake of water or to certain pathologic conditions. Polyuria may be caused by such diuretics as alcohol or caffeine. Urea, a normal constituent of urine, is also a diuretic. A person on a high-protein diet will excrete more urea, which in turn causes the formation of more urine.

During diabetes insipidus the hormone vasopressin, which controls the reabsorption of water in the kidneys, is lacking or deficient. In this case the amount of urine is greatly increased, sometimes as high as 30 L per day.

Patients with diabetes mellitus show a definite polyuria because glucose is a diuretic. Excessive water loss during diabetes mellitus may lead to dehydration.

Specific Gravity The specific gravity of the urine depends upon the concentration of the solutes. The greater the concentration of the solutes, the greater the specific gravity. A normal range of the specific gravity of the urine is 1.003 to 1.030. In cases of diabetes mellitus, the specific gravity will be higher because of a high concentration of sugar in the urine. In cases of diabetes insipidus, the specific gravity of the urine will be very low (close to 1.000), because of the large amounts of water being excreted.

pH Urine is normally slightly acidic, with a pH range of 4.6 to 8.0 and an average value of about 6.3. However, the pH of urine varies with the diet.

Protein foods, such as meats, increase the acidity of the urine (lower the pH) because of the formation of phosphates and sulfates. The acidity of the urine is also increased during acidosis and with fever.

Conversely, the urine may tend to become alkaline on a diet high in vegetables and fruits or because of alkalosis, a condition that may be produced by excess vomiting.

Color   Normal urine is pale yellow or amber. The color, however, varies with the amount of urine produced and also with the concentration of the solutes in the urine. The larger the volume of urine excreted, the lighter the color. The greater the concentration of solutes, the darker the color. The color of the urine is due to urobilin and urobilinogen (see page 431). Various other components of the urine may cause it to have different colors. The presence of blood in the urine gives it a reddish color. A reddish color may also be due to eating beets or rhubarb, or taking cascara, a cathartic. Homogentisic acid (an intermediary in the metabolism of phenylalanine and tyrosine) colors the urine brown. The drug methylene blue colors the urine green.

Freshly voided urine is clear and usually contains no sediment. However, on standing it may become cloudy and develop sediment because of the precipitation of calcium phosphate.

Odor   Fresh urine has a distinctive odor, but this odor may be modified by the presence of other substances. In patients having ketosis the odor of acetone may be detected. Diet may also modify the odor of urine. For example, when asparagus is eaten, the urine may have a sulfurlike odor.

Normal Constituents   Approximately 50 to 60 g of solid material are excreted daily in the urine of the average person. This solid material may be subdivided into inorganic and organic constituents (see Table 29–2). The inorganic constituents of the

TABLE 29–2. Constituents of Urine (Amount Excreted Per Day)

Constituent	Amount (g)	Approximate Percentages
Organic		
Urea	25–30	40–50
Uric acid	0.7	1
Creatinine	1.4	2.5
Creatine	0.06–0.15	0.1–0.25
Others	0.1–1	0.1–1
Inorganic		
Chloride ion	9–16	15–25
Sodium ion	4	6
Phosphates	2	3
Sulfates	2.5	4
Ammonium ions	0.7	1
Other ions and inorganic constituents	2.5	4

Body Fluids: Urine

urine make up approximately 45 percent of the total solids; the organic constituents comprise the other 55 percent.

Organic Constituents

The principal end product of the metabolism of protein, urea, comprises about one half of the total solids in the urine.

UREA

urea

URIC ACID

Uric acid, a product of the metabolism of purines (see page 528) from nucleoprotein, is only slightly soluble in water and is excreted primarily as urate salts. The structure of uric acid is

uric acid

When urine is allowed to stand, uric acid may crystallize and settle out, since it is only slightly soluble in water or acid solution.

The average daily excretion of uric acid is about 0.7 g, but an increase in nucleoproteins in the diet will cause an increased excretion of uric acid. The

FIGURE 29-2. The ravaging effects of gout are manifest in the deformed hands of a patient afflicted with this crippling disease. (Courtesy of the National Institute of Arthritus and Metabolic Diseases, National Institutes of Health, Bethesda, MD.)

Biochemistry

FIGURE 29-3. Stone in right kidney. (Courtesy Dr. Leonard Berlin, Director of Radiology, Skokie Valley Community Hospital, Skokie, IL.)

output of uric acid is also increased in leukemia, in severe liver disease, and in various stages of gout. Deposits of urates and uric acid in the joints and tissues are also characteristic of gout, so that this disease appears to be a form of arthritis (see Figure 29–2).

Under certain conditions uric acid or urates crystallize in the kidneys and are called kidney stones, or calculi* (Figure 29–3).

CREATININE

Creatinine is a product of the breakdown of creatine. The amount of creatinine excreted per day is fairly constant regardless of the protein intake. The number of milligrams of creatinine excreted in the urine within a 24-hr period per kilogram of body weight is the **creatinine coefficient** of that individual. The creatinine coefficient of the normal male is 20 to 26; that of females is 14 to 22.

The average adult excretes 1.4 g of creatinine daily and about 0.06 to 0.15 g of creatine in the same period of time. Formation of creatinine appears necessary for the excretion of most of the creatine.

Body Fluids: Urine   **441**

$$\begin{array}{ccc} \overset{\displaystyle NH}{\underset{\displaystyle \|}{C}}-NH_2 & & \overset{\displaystyle NH}{\underset{\displaystyle \|}{C}} \text{---------NH} \\ \underset{\displaystyle |}{N}-CH_2-COOH & \longrightarrow & \underset{\displaystyle |}{N}-CH_2-\overset{|}{C}{=}O + H_2O \\ CH_3 & & CH_3 \\ \text{creatine} & & \text{creatinine} \end{array}$$

CREATINE   Creatine is produced in the body from three amino acids: arginine, methionine, and glycine. Creatine is normally present in muscle, brain, and blood, both as free creatine and as creatine phosphate. Recall the reaction

$$\text{creatine-P} + \text{ADP} \longrightarrow \text{creatine} + \text{ATP}$$

Creatinuria is a condition in which abnormal amounts of creatine occur in the urine. It may occur during starvation, diabetes mellitus, prolonged fevers, wasting diseases, and hyperthyroidism. Creatinuria may also occur in pregnancy.

OTHER ORGANIC CONSTITUENTS   Also present in small amounts are amino acids, allantoin (from partial oxidation of uric acid), hippuric acid, urobilin, urobilinogen, and biliverdin. The presence of c-AMP helps diagnose parathyroid function. Patients with hyperparathyroidism excrete significantly more c-AMP and those with hypoparathyroidism excrete significantly less c-AMP than persons with normal parathyroid glands (see page 510).

Urobilinogen excretion is increased in hemolytic anemias and in liver disease. Biliverdin excretion is increased in certain liver and biliary diseases.

Tests for pregnancy are based on the fact that the implantation of a fertilized ovum in the placental tissue produces the hormone chorionic gonadotropin, which is excreted in the urine. The presence of this hormone is the basis of the "rabbit test" for pregnancy. Other tests for the presence of chorionic gonadotropin (for pregnancy) are based on the fact that this hormone will react with specific antibodies and can give a result in a doctor's office or at home in a very short time.

In addition to these constituents, the urine also normally contains very small amounts of vitamins, other hormones, and enzymes. Urinalysis for these substances is of diagnostic value.

Inorganic Constituents   The inorganic constituents of urine are the various positive and negative ions that make up the inorganic compounds being excreted. Among these are the following.

CHLORIDE IONS   Between 9 and 16 g of chloride ion are excreted daily, mostly as sodium chloride. The amount of chloride ion varies with the intake, which is primarily sodium chloride. The excretion of sodium chloride is decreased in fevers and in some stages of nephritis.*

SODIUM IONS   The amount of sodium ion excreted varies with the intake and the body's requirement. However, it is usually about 4 g per day.

PHOSPHATES   The amount of phosphates present in the urine also depends upon the diet; the amount is higher when the diet contains foods high in phosphorus (nucleoproteins and phospholipids). An increase in excreted phosphates is

Biochemistry   **442**

found in certain bone diseases and in hyperparathyroidism. A decrease in phosphates is found in hypoparathyroidism, in renal diseases, and during pregnancy.

SULFATES   The sulfates in the urine are derived from the metabolism of sulfur-containing proteins, so that the amount of sulfur is influenced by the diet. Sulfates are found both as organic and inorganic salts.

AMMONIUM IONS   The hydrolysis of urea produces ammonium ions in the urine. Ammonium compounds are present as chlorides, sulfates, and phosphates.

OTHER IONS   In addition to the sodium and ammonium ions, other positive ions present in the urine are calcium, potassium, and magnesium.

The amount of calcium ions in the urine is increased in hyperthyroidism, hyperparathyroidism, and osteoporosis and decreased in hypoparathyroidism and vitamin D deficiency.

Nitrite ions in the urine indicate the presence of reducing bacteria in urinary tract.

The normal ratio of sodium to potassium in the urine is 2 parts sodium to 1 part potassium. The ratio of sodium to potassium is increased in Addison's disease.

Magnesium concentration in urine is decreased in chronic alcoholism.

Abnormal Constituents

Protein

Because proteins are colloids and because colloids cannot pass through membranes, urine should not normally contain protein. **Proteinuria** denotes the presence of protein in the urine. Sometimes it is termed **albuminuria** because albumin is the smallest plasma protein and is the protein most frequently found in the urine. In cases of kidney disease, such as nephritis and nephrosis, and in severe heart disease, protein appears in the urine. The presence of protein due to such disorders is frequently called renal proteinuria or renal albuminuria to distinguish it from false albuminuria, which is a temporary harmless condition. False albuminuria, often called orthostatic albuminuria, is found in certain patients who stand for a long period of time. It is due to the constriction of the kidneys' blood vessels and disappears when the patient lies down. Small amounts of protein may also be found in the urine after severe muscular exercise, but they soon disappear.

The tests for the presence of protein in the urine are based on the fact that protein coagulates when heated. When a sample of urine is heated, any protein (albumin) present will precipitate out as a white cloud. However, phosphates may also precipitate when the urine is heated. To prove that the cloudy substance is albumin, the urine, after heating, is acidified with dilute acetic acid. The acid will dissolve the phosphates but not the protein so that a cloudy precipitate in the urine after heating and acidification is a verification of the presence of protein.

Glucose

The presence of glucose in the urine is called **glycosuria**. Normally there is always a very small amount of glucose present in the urine, but this amount is too small to give a positive test with Benedict's solution.

Glucose may be found in the urine after severe muscular exercise, but this condition clears up when the body returns to normal. Glucose may also be found in the urine after a meal high in carbohydrates.

Glycosuria may be due to such diseases as diabetes mellitus or renal diabetes or to liver damage.

Other Sugars Lactose and galactose may occur in the urine during pregnancy and lactation. Both of these sugars give a positive Benedict test.

Pentoses may occur in the urine after eating foods such as plums, grapes, and cherries, which contain large amounts of these carbohydrates.

Acetone Bodies Acetone (ketone) bodies are present in the urine during diabetes mellitus, in starvation, or in other circumstances with inadequate carbohydrate intake. The excretion of the acetone bodies, which are acidic compounds, requires alkaline compounds. This results in a depletion of the alkaline reserve of the blood and leads to acidosis. The kidneys produce more ammonia to neutralize these acetone bodies.

The test for the presence of acetone bodies in the urine is performed by adding sodium nitroprusside to a sample of urine and then making the mixture alkaline with ammonium hydroxide. The presence of acetone bodies is indicated by a pink-red color. Normal urine gives no color with this test.

Blood The presence of blood in the urine is called **hematuria.** It may result from lesions or stones in the kidneys or urinary tract. The presence of free hemoglobin in the urine, **hemoglobinuria,** results from hemolysis of the red blood cells caused by an injection of hypotonic solution, severe burns, or blackwater fever.

Large amounts of blood in the urine may be detected by the reddish color. Small amounts do not color the urine enough to show any color change but formerly was detected by adding benzidine and hydrogen peroxide to the urine. The presence of blood was indicated by the appearance of a blue color. Other tests for the presence of blood in urine were developed because benzidine was found to be carcinogenic.

Bile Normally, bile is excreted by the liver into the small intestine and eventually ends up in the feces. The presence of bile in the urine indicates obstruction to the flow of bile to the intestines. Bile in the urine is indicated by a greenish brown color. Bile in the urine is also indicated by the presence of a yellow foam when the urine is shaken.

Phenylpyruvic Acid Phenylpyruvic acid, an intermediate product in the metabolism of the essential amino acid phenylalanine, is not normally present in urine. However, its presence can be detected in the urine of a person with phenylketonuria (PKU) (see page 540). If this disease is not detected and treated early, mental retardation results. For this reason, some states require screening of newborns for this disease.

Biochemistry   **444**

| Diuretics | Diuretics are drugs that promote loss of water and salts through the urine. Examples of diuretics are ethyl alcohol, caffeine, mannitol, and thiazides. |

Phenol-sulfonphthalein Test

Phenolsulfonphthalein (PSP) is a red dye used to test how well the kidneys are functioning. The dye is administered by intravenous or intramuscular injection, usually the former. Urine specimens are collected at frequent intervals—after 15, 30, 60, and 120 min. If the 15-min specimen contains 25 percent or more of PSP, then the kidneys are functioning normally; 40 to 60 percent of the dye should be excreted within 1 hr; 20 to 25 percent more in the second hour.

Other kidney-function tests are based upon the amount of urea eliminated in the urine compared to the amount present in the blood (urea clearance test) or the change in the specific gravity of the urine after the patient's fluid intake is restricted (concentration test).

Reagent Tablets, Papers, and Dip Sticks

As an aid to nonlaboratory personnel to perform a variety of urine (or blood) tests easily, quickly, and economically, many tablets, papers, and dip sticks have been developed.

In all cases, it is essential that the manufacturer's directions be followed.

Reagent tablets, and some papers and dip sticks are used to test for one substance only. That is, a tablet or paper or dip stick can be used to test for glucose. To test for acetone bodies, or any other substance, another kind of tablets, paper, or dip stick must be used.

Some papers and dip sticks contain several reagent strips. These can be used to test for several substances at the same time.

In all cases, whether using tablets, papers, or dip sticks, the color produced is compared to a color chart prepared by the manufacturer in order to read the results.

Summary

The principal excretory organs of the body are the kidneys, which also control and regulate the water balance, electrolyte balance, and pH of body fluids.

The waste materials in the blood are picked up by the kidneys and are excreted in the urine.

Approximately 600 to 2500 ml of urine are excreted daily, the amount depending on fluid intake, weather conditions, humidity, and certain diuretic substances.

A decreased flow of urine is called oliguria; anuria is a total lack of urine; polyuria is excess urine formation.

The specific gravity of the urine varies between 1.003 and 1.030 and the pH ranges from 4.6 to 8.0, with an average value of 6.3. Urine is normally pale yellow or amber, but certain components may cause another color.

Approximately 50 to 60 g of solid material, both organic and inorganic, are excreted daily. The principal organic constituent of urine is urea, the end product of protein metabolism. Another important constituent is uric acid, a product of the metabolism of nucleoproteins. Gout is characterized by an increase of uric acid in the urine and blood and the deposition of uric acid or urate salts in the joints and tissues. Uric acid and urates may also crystallize in the kidneys as kidney stones.

The average adult excretes 0.06 to 0.15 g of creatine and 1.4 g of creatinine daily. Creatine is produced from three amino acids: arginine, methionine, and glycine.

Creatine is produced from creatine by a dehydration reaction. Creatinuria is the condition in which abnormal amounts of creatine occur in the urine.

Inorganic constituents of urine are the following ions: chloride, sodium, phosphate, sulfate, ammonium, and some small amounts of calcium, potassium, and magnesium.

Abnormal constituents in the urine are protein (proteinuria, or albuminuria) due to kidney disease; glucose (glycosuria) due to diabetes mellitus or liver damage; acetone bodies due to diabetes mellitus or starvation; blood (hematuria) due to lesions in the kidneys or urinary tract; and bile due to an obstruction of the flow of bile to the intestines.

Diuretics increase the output of water and salts in the urine.

Various tests may be performed to see if the kidneys are functioning normally. Among these is the phenolsulfonphthalein test (PSP) in which a red dye is administered intravenously and the amount of color measured in the urine at specified intervals of time.

Questions and Problems

1. How does the body excrete waste products?
2. What are the principal excretory organs of the body? What additional functions do they have?
3. What is a glomerulus? Bowman's capsule?
4. Describe the formation of urine. Where is the urine stored?
5. What forces the fluids through the membrane in the kidneys?
6. What happens to the nutrients and the water that also filter through the membranes in the kidneys?
7. What volume of urine does an adult excrete daily? What might affect this amount?
8. What is a diuretic?
9. What is oliguria? What might cause this condition?
10. What is anuria? What might cause this condition?
11. What might cause polyuria?
12. What does the hormone vasopressin do? If this hormone is lacking, what will be the effect on the body?
13. What is the pH range of urine? What might affect the pH of the urine?
14. What might affect the color of the urine?
15. What might cause urine to become cloudy upon standing?
16. How much solid material is excreted daily in the urine?
17. What is the principal organic constituent of the urine? Where does it come from? What is its structural formula?
18. Where does the uric acid in the urine come from?
19. Draw the structure of uric acid.
20. How much uric acid is excreted daily? What might affect this amount?
21. What is gout? What other conditions may cause an increased amount of uric acid in the urine?
22. What might cause kidney stones?
23. What is the creatinine coefficient?
24. How does the structure of creatine compare with that of creatinine?
25. Where does the body obtain its creatine?
26. Where is creatine normally present in the body?
27. What is creatinuria and what causes it?
28. Name several inorganic ions normally found in the urine.
29. How is the amount of phosphates in the urine affected by various diseases?

Biochemistry   **446**

30. What is proteinuria?
31. What might cause albuminuria?
32. What is false albuminuria?
33. Describe the test for the presence of protein in the urine. Is it necessary to acidify the urine during this test? Why?
34. What is glycosuria? What causes this condition?
35. Could other sugars besides glucose be present in the urine? under what conditions?
36. What might cause the presence of acetone (ketone) bodies in the urine?
37. Describe the test for the presence of acetone bodies in the urine.
38. What is hematuria? What might cause this condition?
39. The presence of bile in the urine might indicate what condition?
40. Describe the PSP test for kidney function.

References   MARTIN, D. W., P. A. MAYES, and V. W. RODWELL. *Harper's Review of Biochemistry,* 19th ed. Lange Medical Publications, Los Altos, Calif., 1983, Chapter 40.

NEWTON, M. and C. P. LEBLOND. The Golgi apparatus. *Scientific American,* **220:**100–107 (Feb. 1969).

ROSE, B. D. *Clinical Physiology of Acid-Base and Electrolyte Disorders.* McGraw-Hill Book Co., New York, 1977, Part One.

30 Body Fluids: The Blood

CHAPTER
OUTLINE

Functions
Composition
   Red Blood Cells (Erythrocytes)
   White Blood Cells (Leukocytes)
   Platelets (Thrombocytes)
   Blood Plasma
Plasma Substitutes
General Properties of Blood
Blood Analysis
Blood Volume
Hemoglobin
  Anemia
Plasma Lipids
Plasma Proteins
  Albumin
  Globulins
  Fibrinogen
Blood Clotting
Respiration

Transportation of Oxygen and
   Carbon Dioxide
Acid-Base Balance
  Bicarbonate Buffers
  Phosphate Buffers
  Hemoglobin Buffers
  Function of the Kidneys in
    Controlling Acid-Base Balance
  Metabolic Acidosis
  Metabolic Alkalosis
  Respiratory Acidosis
  Respiratory Alkalosis
Fluid-Electrolyte Balance
  Water Balance
  Distribution of Water in the Body
  Electrolyte Balance
  Clinical Importance of Cations and
    Anions

Functions

Blood has been called a circulating tissue. It carries oxygen, minerals, and food to the cells and carries carbon dioxide and other waste products away from the cells. It also carries hormones, enzymes, and blood cells. Blood regulates body temperature by carrying heat from the interior to the surface capillaries. The blood buffers maintain the pH of the body at its optimum value. Blood contains a clotting system that protects the body against hemorrhage and defense mechanisms against infection.

Composition

Blood consists of two parts—the suspended particles and the suspending liquid, the plasma. The suspended particles in the blood are the red blood cells, white blood cells, and platelets.

Red Blood Cells (Erythrocytes)

Normally there are 4.5 to 5.0 million red blood cells per cubic millimeter of blood. Since there are about 6 qt of blood in the human body, the total number of red blood cells is approximately 30 trillion (30,000,000,000,000).

An excess of red blood cells is called **polycythemia;** a shortage is called **anemia.** Each day 200 billion new red blood cells are formed in the bone marrow.

Erythropoietin, a hormone that stimulates red blood cell formation, is a glycoprotein with a molecular weight of approximately 35,000. Erythropoietin is formed by the action of a substance produced by the kidneys (renal erythropoietic factor) on a globulin in the blood plasma. The production of this hormone is increased by hypoxia in the kidneys, by cobalt salts, and by androgens. If the kidneys do not function properly, the patient may become anemic (see page 453).

White Blood Cells   The number of white blood cells normally present in the blood ranges from
(Leukocytes)   5000 to 10,000 per cubic millimeter. White blood cells are larger than red blood cells. White blood cells have a nucleus; red blood cells do not. There are several types of white blood cells; among these are the basophils, eosinophils, lymphocytes, monocytes, and neutrophils.

The white blood cells attack and destroy harmful microorganisms and thus serve as one of the body's defenses against infection. A white blood cell count above normal usually indicates an infection. For diagnostic purposes, a **differential count** is sometimes ordered. This count gives the percentages of each of the various type of leukocytes present.

Platelets   The number of thrombocytes or platelets ranges from 250,000 to 400,000 per
(Thrombocytes)   cubic millimeter of blood. Platelets are smaller than red blood cells and do not have a nucleus. Platelets contain cephalin (phosphatidyl ethanolamine), a phospholipid that is involved in the clotting of the blood.

Blood Plasma   Approximately 92 percent of the plasma is water. The solids dissolved or colloidally dispersed in the blood make up the other 8 percent. The most important of all plasma solids are the blood proteins. These include serum albumin, the globulins, and fibrinogen.

The plasma proteins (primarily albumin) maintain the osmotic pressure of the blood, thus regulating the water and acid-base balance in the body. The globulins (there are several) include the antibodies, which function against infection and diseases. Globulins also function in the transportation of lipids, steroids, and hormones in the plasma. Two particular globulins, transferrin and ceruloplasmin, transport iron and copper, respectively, in the plasma. Fibrinogen and prothrombin, two other globulins, function in the clotting of the blood.

Blood plasma also contains small amounts of lipids and carbohydrates (glucose), inorganic salts, waste products (such as urea, uric acid, carbon dioxide, creatinine, and ammonia), enzymes, vitamins, hormones, and antibodies. The inorganic ions present in the blood plasma serve to regulate the acid-base balance of the body.

On standing, freshly drawn blood soon forms a clot. When the clot settles, a yellowish liquid remains. This liquid is called **blood serum.** Blood serum is blood without the blood cells and without the fibrinogen necessary for the

Body Fluids: The Blood   **449**

clotting of the blood. Blood plasma may be separated from the solid parts of the blood by centrifuging, during which the cells settle at the bottom of the test tube and the plasma remains above them. To keep the blood from clotting, an anticoagulant must be added before centrifuging.

Plasma Substitutes

Plasma volume can be greatly reduced in cases of severe burns, when water intake is too low, or following severe diarrhea, excessive vomiting, or polyuria. In such cases, plasma volume can be increased by intravenous infusion of an isotonic saline solution (0.9 percent NaCl).

However, if there has been a loss of blood volume due to hemorrhaging, intravenous saline solutions are not adequate because they lack plasma protein, salts, and blood cells. In such cases, transfusions of whole blood, plasma, or plasma substitutes may be used. If whole blood is to be used for a transfusion, careful matching of blood types is a necessity.

Blood volume extenders, such as dextrans, have been used. Although such substances are able to maintain the osmotic pressure of the blood, they have an adverse effect upon the blood clotting process.

One group of plasma substitutes are the perfluorocarbons, which are clear, colorless emulsions fortified with inorganic salts and other ingredients. Such compounds have the ability to carry oxygen to the tissues and carbon dioxide from the tissues. However, they cannot assume the functions of white blood cells, platelets, clotting factors, and other blood components.

Most transfusions are given to replace lost blood volume and red blood cells, and plasma substitutes will work well in such cases. Also, such plasma substitutes can be given to all patients regardless of blood type. Plasma substitutes are particularly useful in transplantation surgery, in which large volumes of blood are required for perfusion of organs outside the body. Use of plasma substitutes in such cases saves a large volume of whole blood for other needs.

Plasma substitutes are also useful in certain types of anemias in which the ability of the blood to carry oxygen is greatly reduced.

Patients whose religious beliefs prevent them from receiving blood transfusions can be given blood substitutes.

Perfluorocarbons have a shelf life measured in years as compared to just a few weeks for whole blood. But the emulsion must be kept frozen until use or it begins to break down.

These substances are still in the experimental stage and much work must be done before they come into general usage.

General Properties of Blood

Oxygenated blood has a characteristic bright red color; deoxygenated blood has a dark purplish color.

The specific gravity of whole blood ranges from 1.054 to 1.060, whereas that of blood plasma ranges from 1.024 to 1.028.

Blood is normally slightly alkaline with a pH range of 7.35 to 7.45. If the pH of the blood falls slightly below 7.35, the condition is termed **acidosis.** If the pH of the blood rises slightly above 7.45, the condition is termed **alka-**

losis. If the pH of the blood changes more than a few tenths from the normal values, the results are usually fatal.

The viscosity of the blood is approximately 4.5 times that of water and varies according to the number of cells, the quantity of protein, the temperature, and the amount of water present in the body (see page 168).

Blood Analysis

For most laboratory tests 5 ml of blood are collected from a vein in the arm before the patient is given breakfast. If blood plasma is to be used for the test, an anticlotting agent such as potassium oxalate is added to the blood sample. If blood serum is to be tested, the blood is allowed to clot and the serum is poured off.

The usual blood chemistry tests, the normal ranges of the results, and the clinical significance of these tests are indicated in Table 30-1. Other tests include blood gas analysis (see Figure 30-1) and lactate/pyruvate determination.

Blood Volume

Approximately 8 to 9 percent of the total body weight is blood. The volume of the blood in the body amounts to 5 to 7 L in the adult. The volume

FIGURE 30-1. Blood gas analysis. (Courtesy of Ayerst Laboratories, New York, NY.)

TABLE 30-1. Normal Composition of Blood

Determination[a]	Normal Range[b] (per 100 ml)	Clinical Significance	
		Increased in	Decreased in
Calcium (s)	9–10.6 mg (4.5–5.3 mEq/L)[c]	Hyperparathyroidism, Addison's disease, malignant bone tumor, hypervitaminosis D	Hypoparathyroidism, rickets, malnutrition, diarrhea, chronic kidney disease, celiac disease
Cholesterol, total (s)	150–280 mg	Diabetes mellitus, obstructive jaundice, hypothyroidism, pregnancy	Pernicious anemia, hemolytic jaundice, hyperthyroidism, tuberculosis
Uric acid (s)	3–7.5 mg	Gout, leukemia, pneumonia, liver and kidney disease	
Urea nitrogen (b, s)	8–20 mg	Mercury poisoning, acute glomerulonephritis, kidney disease	Pregnancy, low-protein diet, severe hepatic failure
Nonprotein nitrogen (b, s)	15–35 mg	Kidney disease, pregnancy, intestinal obstruction, congestive heart failure	Low-protein diet
Creatine (s)	3–7 mg	Nephritis, renal destruction, biliary obstruction, pregnancy	
Creatinine (b, s)	0.7–1.5 mg	Nephritis, chronic renal disease	
Glucose (b)	60–100 mg	Diabetes mellitus, hyperthyroidism, infections, pregnancy, emotional stress, after meals	Starvation, hyperinsulinism, Addison's disease, hypothyroidism, extensive hepatic damage
Chlorides (s)	100–106 mEq/L	Nephritis, anemia, urinary obstruction	Diabetes, diarrhea, pneumonia, vomiting, burns
Phosphate, inorganic (p)	3–4.5 mg	Hypoparathyroidism, Addison's disease, chronic nephritis	Hyperparathyroidism, diabetes mellitus
Sodium (s)	136–145 mEq/L	Kidney disease, heart disease, pyloric obstruction	Vomiting, diarrhea, Addison's disease, myxedema, pneumonia, diabetes mellitus
Potassium (s)	3.5–5 mEq/L	Addison's disease, oliguria, anuria, tissue breakdown	Vomiting, diabetes acidosis, diarrhea
Carbon dioxide (s, p)	Adults, 24–29 mEq/L Infants, 20–26 mEq/L	Tetany, vomiting, intestinal obstruction, respiratory disease	Acidosis, diarrhea, anesthesia, nephritis
Hemoglobin (b)	Male, 14–18 g Female, 12–16 g	Polycythemia	Anemia

[a] Key to abbreviations(:)
  b = blood
  s = serum
  p = plasma
[b] Milligrams per 100 ml is also called milligrams percent.
[c] mEq/L = milliequivalents per liter.

increases in fever and pregnancy and decreases during diarrhea and hemor-rhaging. Since blood volume can be rapidly replaced, a small loss of blood because of bleeding or because of donating blood has no serious effect upon the body.

Blood volume may be determined by injecting a suitable dye into the bloodstream, waiting about 10 min, and then withdrawing a sample to de-termine the concentration of the dye. A radioactive tracer may also be in-jected into the bloodstream and the blood volume determined by the amount of dilution of the radioactivity in a sample taken a short time later.

Hemoglobin

Hemoglobin is a conjugated protein made up of a protein part, globin, and an iron-containing part, heme. Heme contains four pyrrole groups joined together with an iron ion in the center. The structure of pyrrole is

pyrrole

The structure of heme is indicated in Figure 30–2. Various hydrocarbon side chains are attached to the pyrrole rings in this compound. Four heme molecules combine with one globin molecule to form one molecule of hemo-globin.

The structures of cytochrome c, part of the oxidative phosphorylation sequence of the citric acid cycle (see page 405), and that of chlorophyll, a plant pigment, are shown in Figure 30–2 for comparison with that of heme. Note that whereas both heme and cytochrome c have an iron ion (Fe^{2+}) in the center of four pyrrole rings, chlorophyll has a magnesium ion (Mg^{2+}).

Anemia

If the hemoglobin content of the blood falls below normal, the condition is called anemia. Anemia may result from a decreased rate of production of red blood cells, from an increased destruction of red blood cells, or from an increased loss of red blood cells.

A decreased rate of production of red blood cells may be due to various diseases that destroy or suppress the activity of the blood-forming tissues. Among these diseases are leukemia, multiple myeloma,* and Hodgkin's disease. Radiation and certain drugs such as benzene and gold salts also decrease the activity of the blood-forming tissues. Another frequent cause of decreased red blood cell production is a diet lacking in iron and protein, particularly in infancy and childhood and during pregnancy. Anemia may also be related to a genetic defect that affects the production of hemoglobin (see Chapter 33). Pernicious anemia, a failure of red blood cell production, is due to a lack of vitamin B_{12} or of the intrinsic factor (see page 387).

Destruction of red blood cells may be caused by several poisons or infec-tions that can cause hemolysis. Carbon monoxide (CO) is a poisonous gas because hemoglobin combines with it approximately 210 times as fast as it

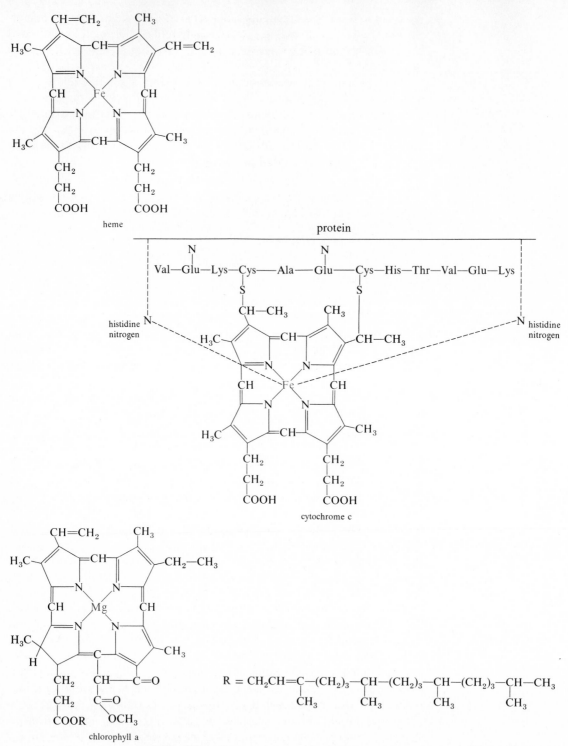

FIGURE 30-2. Structural formulas of heme, cytochrome c, and chlorophyll a.

does with oxygen. The compound formed between hemoglobin and carbon monoxide, carboxyhemoglobin, is very stable, so that only a small amount of hemoglobin is left to carry oxygen. If the CO content of the air is 0.02 percent, nausea and headache occur; if the CO content of the air rises to 0.1 percent, unconsciousness will occur within 1 hr and death within 4 hr. Other poisonous gases such as hydrogen sulfide (H_2S) and hydrocyanic acid (HCN) have similar effects on hemoglobin.

An increased loss of hemoglobin may be due to hemorrhaging.

Plasma Lipids   Plasma lipids may be divided into several classes, as shown in Table 30–2.

TABLE 30–2. Lipids in Human Blood Plasma

Lipid	Range (in mg/100 ml)
Triacylglycerols	80–120
Phospholipids	123–390
Lecithin	50–200
Cephalin	50–130
Sphingomyelins	15–35
Cholesterol (total)	107–320
Free fatty acids	6–16
Total lipids	360–820

Metabolism of lipids produces much of the body's energy. In order to metabolize lipids, they must first be transported by the bloodstream. But lipids are hydrophobic and are not soluble in blood (mostly water). The transportation of lipids in the bloodstream is accomplished by associating insoluble lipids with phospholipids (which are polar) and then combining them with cholesterol and protein to form a *hydrophillic lipoprotein complex*. In this manner triacylglycerols, which are derived from intestinal absorption of fat or from the liver, are transported as chylomicrons and very low density lipoproteins (VLDL) (see page 360). Free fatty acids, which are released from the adipose tissue, are carried in the bloodstream in an unesterified form as an albumin fatty acid complex. That is, many types of lipids are transported in the bloodstream as plasma lipoproteins.

Plasma Proteins   The plasma proteins constitute about 7 percent of the plasma and are usually divided into three groups: albumin, globulins, and fibrinogen. Approximately 55 percent of the plasma proteins is albumin, 38.5 percent globulins, and 6.5 percent fibrinogen.

Albumin   Albumin in the blood functions in the regulation of osmotic pressure. The control of osmotic pressure in turn affects the water balance in the body.

Albumin, as well as other plasma proteins, cannot pass through the walls of the blood vessels (because they are colloids and colloids cannot pass through membranes). Since albumin is the principal plasma protein and the smallest plasma protein both in size and weight (it consists of a single chain

Body Fluids: The Blood   **455**

of 610 amino acids), it accounts for most of the colloid osmotic pressure of the blood.

The effect of albumin (and other plasma proteins) on water balance (both filtration and reabsorption) has been hypothesized by Starling, as indicated in the following paragraphs and also in Figure 30–3.

When blood enters the arterial end of a capillary, it exerts a hydrostatic* (blood) pressure of 35 mm, forcing fluid outward from the blood vessel. At the same time, the colloid osmotic pressure of the plasma, 25 mm, pulls fluid back into the blood vessel. The interstitial fluid* exerts a hydrostatic pressure of 2 mm, which forces fluid out of the tissues back into the blood. Since there is almost no protein in the tissue fluids at the end of the capillary, the colloid osmotic pressure of the interstitial fluid is 0 mm. The net result of the pressure acting outward from the blood (35 and 0 mm) and the pressure acting inward toward the blood (25 and 2 mm) causes a net pressure of 8 mm, forcing fluid out of the blood at the arterial end of the capillary. Thus, there is a net outward filtration from the capillary.

At the venous end of the capillary, the following conditions exist: The hydrostatic pressure of the blood is 15 mm, forcing fluid outward. (Note that the hydrostatic pressure of the blood at the venous end is less than at the arterial end of the capillary.) The colloid osmotic pressure of the plasma remains at 25 mm, pulling fluid inward. The interstitial fluid hydrostatic pressure of 1 mm forces fluid out of the tissues back into the blood, whereas

FIGURE 30–3. Effect of albumin (and other plasma proteins) on water balance.

FIGURE 30-4. The pot-belly of this undernourished child is a sign of malnutrition. This child is receiving milk in a hospital in Tanzania. (Photograph courtesy of World Health Organization.)

the interstitial fluid colloid osmotic pressure of 3 mm causes fluid to flow back to the tissues.† The net result of two pressures acting outward at the venous end of the capillary (15 and 3 mm) and two pressures acting inward (25 and 1 mm) gives a net pressure of 8 mm inward, causing reabsorption of materials. This reabsorption is aided by the lymphatics.*

If the plasma proteins (primarily albumin) are present in decreased amounts (as in nehpritis or during a low-protein diet), the osmotic pressure of the plasma decreases. This decreased osmotic pressure of the blood causes a greater net pressure outward at the arterial end of the capillary and a lower net inward venous pressure at the venous end of the capillary. When this occurs, water (fluid) accumulates in the tissues. Such a condition is known as **edema.***

Kwashiorkor (see Figure 30–4), a protein deficiency disease, is characterized by edema in the abdomen and extremities. In children, a swollen pot-belly is characteristic. Kwashiorkor is caused by a drop in plasma protein,

† This colloid osmotic pressure is caused by small amounts of plasma protein that pass through the capillary membranes and tend to accumulate at the venous end of the capillaries.

Body Fluids: The Blood

particularly albumin. Under these circumstances, water moves from the bloodstream into the tissues, causing swelling.

Edema may also occur because of heart disease, whereby there is an increase in venous hydrostatic pressure. In many terminal illnesses, edema results. This becomes a serious problem so that tapping and draining may be necessary. Concentrated albumin infusions (25 g in 100 ml diluent) are helpful in the treatment of shock, to increase blood volume, and to remove fluid from the tissues.

The amount of albumin present in the blood is lowered in liver disease because albumin is formed in that organ.

Another function of albumin in the blood is to act as a carrier for fatty acids, trace elements, and many drugs.

Globulins   The globulins present in the plasma may be separated into different groups by a process known as electrophoresis* (see page 178), whereby the charged protein particles migrate at varying rates to electrodes of opposite charge, with albumin migrating the fastest. The distribution of the plasma proteins is shown in Figure 30–5. As can be seen in the illustration, the globulins are subdivided into alpha (α), beta (β), and gamma (γ). Alpha, beta, and gamma globulins form complexes (loose combinations) with such substances as carbohydrates (mucoprotein and glycoprotein), lipids (lipoprotein), and metal ions (transferrin for iron and ceruloplasmin for copper). The amount of transferrin is decreased in such diseases as pernicious anemia and liver disease. The amount of ceruloplasmin is decreased in Wilson's disease (see page 474). These complexes can be transported to all parts of the body.

The gamma globulins (immunoglobulins) include the antibodies with which the body fights infectious diseases. Gamma globulin has been found to contain as many as 20 different antibodies for immunity against such diseases as measles, infectious hepatitis, poliomyelitis, mumps, and influenza. The most important use of serum electrophoresis is as an aid in the diagnosis of diseases in which abnormal proteins appear in the blood (multiple myeloma* and macroglobulinemia),* or when a protein component is either present in decreased amounts or lacking altogether (agammaglobulinemia; see next paragraph).

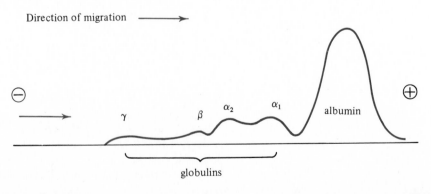

FIGURE 30–5. Distribution of plasma proteins during electrophoresis.

Some people lack the ability to make gamma globulin. These people are quite susceptible to infections because they have no antibodies to counteract such diseases. The lack of gamma globulin is called **agammaglobulinemia** and can be counteracted by the administration of gamma globulin.

Fibrinogen

Fibrinogen is the plasma protein involved in the clotting of the blood. Fibrinogen is manufactured in the liver, so that any disease that destroys liver tissue causes a decrease in the amount of fibrinogen.

Blood Clotting

When the skin is ruptured, blood flows out and soon forms a clot. When blood is taken from a vein and placed in a test tube, it soon forms a clot. Why does blood clot when it is removed from its normal place in the circulatory system? Why doesn't it clot in the blood vessels themselves?

When blood clots, a series of reactions occur in which the soluble plasma protein fibrinogen is converted into insoluble fibrin. Fibrin precipitates in the form of long threads that cling together to form a spongy mass, which entraps and holds the blood cells, forming a clot.

When a blood vessel is cut, the blood comes in contact with the tissues. The contact of the blood with the tissues liberates thromboplastin from the platelets, from the plasma, and from the tissues themselves. It should be noted that thromboplastin is not a single substance but instead refers to substances that catalyze the conversion of prothrombin to thrombin. There are many "factors" with thromboplastic activity. In the presence of thromboplastin and calcium ions, prothrombin (a globulin present in the plasma) is changed into thrombin.

The thrombin in turn acts on the fibrinogen to convert it into fibrin, which forms the clot (reactions 30–1).

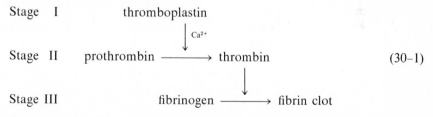

Reactions (30–1) are merely a simplified version of a very complex sequence of reactions. There are many factors involved, particularly among those having thromboplastic activity. The International Committee for the Standardization of the Nomenclature of Blood Clotting Factors has designated a system of numbering for such factors. For more detailed information, consult an advanced biochemistry textbook.

Calcium ions are necessary for the clotting of blood. The coagulation of freshly drawn blood samples may be prevented by adding a substance (such as potassium oxalate) that removes calcium ions from solution. However, since oxalates are poisonous, this method can be used only if the blood is to be analyzed in a laboratory.

To prevent clotting in blood used for transfusions, sodium citrate is added.

Body Fluids: The Blood

459

This substance removes the calcium ions from the blood by forming calcium citrate, a compound that is almost completely nondissociated.

A deficiency of vitamin K reduces the production of prothrombin, without which the blood cannot clot.

Anticoagulant drugs such as bishydroxycoumarin (Dicumarol) reduce the conversion of prothrombin to thrombin and so keep blood from clotting rapidly. Heparin speeds up the removal of thrombin from several minutes to a few seconds. Anticoagulant drugs may be used after surgery to prevent clots from forming in the cut blood vessels. A clot formed in a blood vessel is called a **thrombus.** A thrombus in a blood vessel does no harm if it remains where it was formed because it is slowly reabsorbed. However, if the clot breaks loose and travels through the blood vessels, it may lodge in and obstruct a blood vessel leading to the heart or brain, causing paralysis or death.

In addition to the previously mentioned coagulation reactions, other processes may also occur. When the skin is ruptured, a prompt vasoconstriction occurs at the site of the injury, thus reducing blood flow. Also, the platelets form a temporary plug in the injured capillaries. Prostaglandins and thromboxanes are required for this latter action. Since aspirin interferes with the action of prostaglandins, aspirin interferes with the clotting process.

Breakdown of fibrin in blood clots (fibrinolysis) occurs within a few days after formation and is the result of the action of the enzyme plasmin. Plasmin is activated by a variety of circumstances including stress, exercise, snake venom, and streptokinase from streptococci.

Respiration

The tissues require oxygen for their normal metabolic processes; they must also eliminate carbon dioxide. Oxygen is carried from the lungs to the tissues by the hemoglobin of the blood. In the tissues the oxygen is given up by the hemoglobin and the waste carbon dioxide from the tissues is picked up and carried to the lungs.

The inspired air has a higher concentration of oxygen than does the blood in the alveoli of the lungs. Gases always flow from an area of high concentration to one of lower concentration so that the oxygen flows from the lungs (high concentration) into the blood (lower concentration). In the blood the oxygen combines with the hemoglobin. Very little oxygen is actually dissolved (uncombined) in the blood. When the oxygen-rich blood reaches the tissues, it gives up its oxygen to the cells because those cells are using up oxygen and have a lower concentration of that gas than the blood. At the same time, the cells have a higher concentration of carbon dioxide than the blood; therefore, that gas flows from the cells into the bloodstream. The blood carries the carbon dioxide to the lungs. There it is in contact with air, which has a lower carbon dioxide concentration, and it passes from the blood into the lungs where it is exhaled (see page 461).

The transportation of gases in respiration includes the nine steps described in the next section.

Transportation of Oxygen and Carbon Dioxide

The transportation of oxygen and carbon dioxide is summarized in Figure 30-6 where the interrelationships of the following steps are shown.

1. As oxygen passes from the alveoli of the lungs into the bloodstream, some of it dissolves in the blood plasma. However, most of it reacts with hemoglobin (here represented by the formula HHb) to form oxyhemoglobin, HbO_2^-.

$$HHb + O_2 \longrightarrow HbO_2^- + H^+$$

   Oxygen is carried to the cells in this form.

2. At the same time, carbon dioxide, which is produced during metabolic processes in the cells, flows from the tissues into the blood. A small amount dissolves directly in the plasma, but most of the carbon dioxide diffuses into the red blood cells where it reacts with water in the cells to form carbonic acid. This reaction takes place rapidly under the influence of the enzyme carbonic anhydrase.

$$CO_2 + H_2O \xrightarrow{\text{carbonic anhydrase}} H_2CO_3$$

3. The carbonic acid thus formed ionizes to yield hydrogen and bicarbonate ions

$$H_2CO_3 \longrightarrow H^+ + HCO_3^-$$

   The hydrogen ions then react with oxyhemoglobin, as indicated in step 4.

4. In the tissues, oxyhemoglobin reacts with hydrogen ions to yield oxygen and hemoglobin (HHb).

$$HbO_2^- + H^+ \longrightarrow HHb + O_2$$

FIGURE 30-6. Transportation of oxygen and carbon dioxide.

Oxygen and Carbon Dioxide Transport

The release of oxygen to the tissues is enhanced by a decrease in the pH and by the presence of 2,3-diphosphoglyceric acid. Most of the hemoglobin travels back to the lungs to pick up more oxygen. But some of the hemoblogin reacts with carbon dioxide to form carbaminohemoglobin (here represented as $HHbCO_2$).

$$HHb + CO_2 \longrightarrow HHbCO_2$$

5. The bicarbonate ions from step 3 do not remain in the red blood cells because those cells can hold only a small amount of that ion. So, the *excess* bicarbonate ions diffuse outward into the blood plasma. Red blood cells cannot stand a loss of negative ions, so that, to counteract this, chloride ions from the blood plasma flow into the red blood cells. This process is called the **chloride shift.**

The bicarbonate ions can then act as buffers in the plasma.

6. In the lungs, the bicarbonate ions react with the hydrogen ions produced according to step 1 to form carbonic acid.

$$HCO_3^- + H^+ \longrightarrow H_2CO_3$$

7. The carbonic acid thus formed rapidly decomposes into carbon dioxide and water under the influence of the enzyme carbonic anhydrase.

$$H_2CO_3 \xrightarrow{\text{carbonic anhydrase}} H_2O + CO_2$$

8. As the bicarbonate ions are used up, in steps 6 and 7, more bicarbonate ions from the plasma flow into the red blood cells. At the same time, chloride ions migrate outward from the red blood cells. This is a **reverse chloride shift.**

9. At the same time, the carbaminohemoglobin, formed as indicated in step 4, decomposes in the lungs to yield hemoglobin and carbon dioxide.

$$HHbCO_2 \longrightarrow HHb + CO_2$$

Acid-Base Balance

The normal pH range of the blood is 7.35 to 7.45. When the pH falls below this range, the condition is termed **acidosis.** * **Alkalosis** * occurs when the pH rises above its normal value. Acidosis is more common than alkalosis because many of the metabolic products produced during digestion are acidic in nature. The ability of the blood buffers to neutralize acid is called the **alkaline reserve** of the blood. In acidosis, the alkaline reserve decreases; during alkalosis, it increases.

How does the blood maintain the pH when acid or basic substances are continuously being added to it?

The blood retains its fairly constant pH because of the presence of buffers. These buffers are present both in the blood plasma and in the red blood cells. Those in the plasma are primarily sodium buffers; those in the blood cells are mainly potassium buffers. Recall that buffers are substances (usually a weak acid and a salt of a weak acid) that resist change in pH (see page 208). The blood buffers consist of the following:

1. Bicarbonate buffers.
2. Phosphate buffers.
3. Protein buffers (including hemoglobin and oxyhemoglobin).

Bicarbonate Buffers　The bicarbonate buffer system in the red blood cells consists of carbonic acid, H_2CO_3, and potassium bicarbonate, $KHCO_3$. The bicarbonate buffer system in the blood plasma consists of carbonic acid and sodium bicarbonate, $NaHCO_3$. If we assume that a strong acid (such as HCl) is added to a sample of blood, it will react with the salt part of the buffer and undergo the following reactions:

$$HCl + KHCO_3 \longrightarrow H_2CO_3 + KCl \quad \text{(in blood cells)}$$

$$HCl + NaHCO_3 \longrightarrow H_2CO_3 + NaCl \quad \text{(in blood plasma)}$$

The carbonic acid produced (H_2CO_3) is part of the original buffer. Note that the strong acid, HCl, has been replaced by a very weak one, H_2CO_3. The other products, KCl and NaCl, are neutral salts and will not affect the pH of the system.

If we assume that a strong base such as KOH or NaOH is added to a sample of blood, the following reactions will occur with the bicarbonate buffer systems:

$$KOH + H_2CO_3 \longrightarrow KHCO_3 + H_2O \quad \text{(in blood cells)}$$

$$NaOH + H_2CO_3 \longrightarrow NaHCO_3 + H_2O \quad \text{(in blood plasma)}$$

The salts, $KHCO_3$ and $NaHCO_3$, are part of the original buffer systems and the water produced is neutral, so that the pH again is unaffected.

In both cases (reaction with a strong acid or a strong base) more of the buffer is produced plus a neutral compound.

The bicarbonate buffers and the blood protein buffers play a major part in the control of the pH; the phosphate buffers have an important role inside the cell and in the urine.

Phosphate Buffers　The phosphate buffers consist of mixtures of K_2HPO_4 and KH_2PO_4 (also Na_2HPO_4 and NaH_2PO_4), which function similarly to the bicarbonate buffers in neutralizing excess acid and base.

Body Fluids: The Blood　**463**

$$HCl + K_2HPO_4 \longrightarrow KH_2PO_4 + \quad KCl$$

$$KOH + KH_2PO_4 \longrightarrow K_2HPO_4 + \quad H_2O$$

more buffer   neutral compound

Hemoglobin Buffers

The hemoglobin buffers account for more than one half of the total buffering action in the blood. There are hemoglobin buffers and oxyhemoglobin buffers.

Hemoglobin Buffer	Oxyhemoglobin Buffer
HHb	$HHbO_2$
KHb	$KHbO_2$

These buffers, as well as other proteins that act as buffers in the bloodstream, pick up excess acid or base to help keep the pH of the blood within its normal range.

Function of the Kidneys in Controlling Acid-Base Balance

The kidneys help maintain the acid-base balance of the blood by excreting or absorbing phosphates and also by forming ammonia. The acid substances in the blood combine with ammonia and are excreted as ammonium salts through the kidneys, saving sodium and potassium ions for the buffer systems.

Metabolic Acidosis

Metabolic acidosis is characterized by a drop in plasma pH due to a decrease in HCO_3^- concentration and a compensatory drop in the partial pressure of carbon dioxide, P_{CO_2}. Metabolic acidosis may be caused by either the addition of H^+ or the loss of HCO_3^-.

The most common causes of metabolic acidosis are uncontrolled diabetes mellitus with ketosis (see page 418), renal failure, poisoning with acid substances, severe diarrhea with loss of HCO_3^-, lactic acidosis, and severe dehydration.

As the pH decreases, more H_2CO_3 is produced from the HCO_3^-. The H_2CO_3 in turn decomposes to CO_2 and H_2O.

$$HCO_3^- + H^+ \rightleftharpoons H_2CO_3 \rightleftharpoons H_2O + CO_2$$

If the blood buffers cannot control the pH, then the excess carbon dioxide produced stimulates the respiratory center of the brain, making the person breathe faster, thus removing more carbon dioxide from the blood. The increased rate of respiration (hyperventilation) continues until the amount of carbon dioxide is too small to further stimulate the respiratory center of the brain, and breathing returns to its normal rate. In addition to hyperventilation, the kidneys respond by excreting H^+ primarily as NH_4^+.

Treatment, if the kidneys are functioning normally, consists of intravenous administration of HCO_3^-. This lowers the H^+ concentration and so increases pH to normal. Fluids are administered to replace lost water. A diabetic is given insulin therapy. Hemodialysis may be required if the kidneys are not functioning normally.

Biochemistry **464**

Metabolic Alkalosis Metabolic alkalosis is characterized by an increase in plasma pH, an increase in HCO_3^- concentration and a compensatory increase in P_{CO_2}. Metabolic alkalosis is caused by a loss of H^+ or a retention of HCO_3^-.

Common causes of metabolic alkalosis are prolonged vomiting, gastric suction (both of which remove acid contents from the stomach), overdose of HCO_3^- (in the treatment of a gastric ulcer), loss of K^+ along with Cl^- in severe exercise, renal disease, massive blood transfusions, and diuretic therapy.

Normally, the kidneys are able to correct this situation by excreting large amounts of HCO_3^-. Therefore, persistence of metabolic alkalosis indicates impaired renal excretion.

Symptoms include slow respirations (hypoventilation) as the lungs try to conserve CO_2 (which comes from the H_2CO_3 needed to neutralize the excess alkalinity), numbness, convulsions, weakness, and muscle cramps.

The usual treatment involves the administration of NaCl, with KCl if the K^+ concentration is low. The increased Na^+ will enhance the excretion of HCO_3^-, thereby correcting the situation. Patients with metabolic alkalosis due to diuretic therapy can be given acetazolamide (Diamox) to increase HCO_3^- excretion.

Respiratory Acidosis Respiratory acidosis is characterized by a decrease in plasma pH, an increase in P_{CO_2}, and a variable compensatory increase in HCO_3^- concentration. Respiratory acidosis is due to impaired ventilation, either from inhibition of the respiratory center in the brain (sedatives, anesthetics, opiates, cardiac arrest) or impaired gas exchange across the lungs to the blood capillaries (poliomyelitis, emphysema, severe asthma, acute pulmonary edema, pneumonia).

Respiratory acidosis is common in "natural childbirth" and in the lamaze method.

The response to respiratory acidosis takes time. Buffers are ineffective since HCO_3^- cannot buffer H_2CO_3. The kidneys respond by increasing H^+ excretion, but this occurs over hours to days. Once renal response has developed, it is usually capable of handling excessive acidity. However, the kidneys will not be able to correct the problem. Chronic respiratory acidosis is a relatively common problem most often seen in smokers with pulmonary disease.

Symptoms of respiratory acidosis include headache, blurred vision, fatigue, and weakness. Treatment of acute respiratory acidosis includes returning the breathing to normal. This may include mechanical assistance, use of bronchodilators, and small infusions of $NaHCO_3$. Chronic respiratory acidosis is usually not treated. Care must be taken with chronic patients since opiates and anesthetics will act as further respiratory depressants and induce further hypoventilation.

Respiratory Alkalosis Respiratory alkalosis is characterized by an increase in plasma pH, a drop in P_{CO_2}, and a variable decrease in HCO_3^- concentration. Such a condition may be caused by hyperventilation (hysteria), residence at high altitudes, conges-

Body Fluids: The Blood   **465**

TABLE 30-3. Typical Changes in Plasma pH, P_{CO_2}, and HCO_3^- for Various Acid-Base Disorders.

	pH	HCO_3^-	P_{CO_2}
Metabolic acidosis	↓	↓	↓
Metabolic alkalosis	↑	↑	↑
Respiratory acidosis	↓	↑	↑
Respiratory alkalosis	↑	↓	↓

tive heart failure, pulmonary diseases, aspirin overdose, excessive exercise, and cirrhosis. The problem originates with excessive excretion of CO_2. For instance, overstimulation of the respiratory control center in the brain by chemicals (aspirin) or the need for more O_2 (congestive heart failure, residence at high altitudes) lead to excessive loss of CO_2. The kidneys will attempt to compensate by increasing HCO_3^- excretion.

Symptoms of respiratory alkalosis are hyperventilation that cannot be controlled, possible convulsions, and lightheadness. Treatment involves removal of the cause of the problem. Breathing into and out of a paper bag (to inhale CO_2 which has been exhaled) is also helpful.

Table 30-3 compares the changes in pH, P_{CO_2}, and HCO_3^- concentration for respiratory and metabolic acidosis and alkalosis. The normal pH of the blood is 7.35 to 7.45; normal P_{CO_2} is 35 to 40 mm Hg; normal HCO_3^- is 25 to 30 mEq/L.

Fluid-Electrolyte Balance

Normally, in humans, water intake is balanced by water output. If the intake of water exceeds the output, **edema** results. If the output of water exceeds the input, **dehydration** may occur (see Figure 30-7).

Water Balance

The body replenishes its water supply in three ways:

1. By the ingestion of liquids (which are primarily, if not wholly, water).
2. By the ingestion of foods such as meats, vegetables, and fruits, all of which contain a very high percentage of water.
3. By metabolic processes taking place normally in the body. When carbohydrates, fats, and proteins are metabolized, water is produced. Approximately 14 ml of water are formed for every 100 kcal of energy released by the oxidation of foods. The oxidation of 100 g of carbohy-

FIGURE 30-7. Water balance in the body.

water input   water output   greater water input   water output   water input   greater water output

Normal water balance   Edema   Dehydration

Biochemistry

drate produces 55 g of H_2O; the oxidation of 100 g fat produces 107 g of H_2O; the oxidation of 100 g protein produces 41 g of H_2O.

The total normal input of water in the body is approximately 2500 ml per day.

The body loses water in several ways:

1. Through the kidneys, as urine.
2. Through the skin, as perspiration.
3. Through the lungs, as exhaled moisture.
4. Through the feces.

The total of these methods of water loss should approximate that of the water intake, 2500 ml per day. However, the amount of water lost by these individual methods may vary considerably. For example, the amount of moisture lost through the skin (by the evaporation of perspiration) and through the lungs increases in the following circumstances:

1. During vigorous muscular exercise.
2. With an increased respiratory rate.
3. In a hot, dry environment.
4. During a fever.
5. When the skin receives severe burns.

Conversely, the amount of water lost through the kidneys increases following the ingestion of large amounts of water within a short period of time. It also increases because of the presence of large amount of waste products in the bloodstream. However, when the body loses excess water through vomiting and/or diarrhea, the ouput of water through the kidneys is immediately lessened.

Distribution of Water in the Body

The water of the body is considered to be distributed in two major areas—intracellular (within the cells), 55 percent, and extracellular (outside the cells), 45 percent. The extracellular water, in turn, may be further divided into four areas:

1. Intravascular (plasma): fluid within the heart and blood vessels (7.5 percent).
2. Interstitial and lymph: fluids outside the cells (20 percent).
3. Dense connective tissue, cartilage and bone (15 percent).
4. Transcellular fluids: extracellular fluid collections, including the salivary glands, thyroid gland, gonads, mucous membranes of the respiratory and gastrointestinal tracts, kidneys, liver, pancreas, cerebrospinal fluid, and fluid in the spaces within the eyes (2.5 percent).

Approximately 55 percent of the weight of an adult male and 50 percent of the weight of an adult female is water.

The principal difference between the blood plasma (the intravascular fluid) and the interstitial fluid is in the protein content. Proteins cannot pass through membranes and so they remain in the blood vessels. Thus, the

Body Fluids: The Blood   **467**

protein content of the interstitial fluid is very low compared to that of the intravascular fluid, although the soluble electrolytes in each are approximately the same.

There are distinct differences in salt concentration in the intracellular and extracellular fluids.

The extracellular water in the dense connective tissue, cartilage, and bone and the extracellular water in the transcellular fluids do not readily interchange fluids and electrolytes with the rest of the body water. The rest of the body water—intracellular, intravascular, interstitial, and lymph—freely moves from one area to another within the body.

Electrolyte Balance   Table 30–4 indicates the electrolyte concentrations in the intravascular, interstitial, and intracellular fluids. The ions are divided into two groups—cations (positively charged ions) and anions (negatively charged ions). Concentrations of anions and cations are expressed in units of milliequivalents per liter (mEq/L). The unit milliequivalent measures the chemical and physiologic activity of an ionized substance, the electrolyte. Since milliequivalents are based upon ions, the term milliequivalents represents the number of charged particles or the number of both positive and negative charges present in a solution of an electrolyte. Recall that the number of positive charges must always equal the number of negative charges.

Table 30–4 shows that the electrolyte concentrations of the interstitial fluid are similar to those of the intravascular fluid, except that there is more chloride ion and less protein concentration. Note also that in both the intravascular and the interstitial fluid, sodium is the principal cation and chloride the principal anion.

The intracellular fluid differs in concentrations from the intravascular and

TABLE 30-4 Electrolyte Concentrations of Body Fluids (mEq/L)

	Intravascular	Interstitial	Intracellular
Cations			
Na^+	142	145	10
K^+	4	4	158
Mg^{2+}	3	2	35
Ca^{2+}	5	3	2
	154	154	205
Anions			
Cl^-	103	115	2
HCO_3^-	27	30	8
HPO_4^{2-}	2	2	140
SO_4^{2-}	1	1	—
Protein$^-$	16	1	55
Organic acids$^-$	5	5	—
	154	154	205

Biochemistry

interstitial fluids in that potassium is the principal cation and phosphate the principal anion. Electrolyte concentrations in intracellular fluids are only approximate because they vary slightly from tissue to tissue.

Concentrations of electrolytes are frequently measured and expressed in the units milligrams per 100 ml. This may be changed to milliequivalents per liter by means of the following formula:

$$\frac{\text{mg/100 ml} \times 10 \times \text{ionic charge}}{\text{atomic weight}} = \text{mEq/L}$$

For example, suppose a laboratory reports the serum potassium concentration as 15.6 mg/100 ml. The concentration of potassium in milliequivalents per liter may be calculated by using the preceding formula and the atomic weight (39) and the ionic charge (1), or

$$\frac{15.6 \times 10 \times 1}{39} = 4 \text{ mEq/L}$$

Osmotic activity depends upon the number of particles present in a solution regardless of whether they carry a charge or not. Thus, sodium ions, potassium ions, and chloride ions cause osmotic pressure, but so does glucose, which is a nonelectrolyte (that is, it carries no charge).

Osmotic activity is expressed by the unit **milliosmol,** which is a measure of the amount of work that dissolved particles can do in drawing a fluid through a semipermeable membrane. Osmotic activity is measure by means of an instrument called an osmometer (Figure 30-8).

Body Fluids: The Blood

Sodium ions are the primary cations of the extracellular fluids. The principal functions of sodium ions are

1. To maintain the osmotic pressure of the extracellular fluid.
2. To control water retention in tissue spaces.
3. To help maintain blood pressure.
4. To maintain the body's acid-base balance by means of the bicarbonate buffer system.
5. To regulate the irritability of the nerve and muscle tissue and of the heart.

The average daily adult intake of sodium, as NaCl, is 5 to 15 g. About 95 percent of the sodium lost by the body passes through the kidneys. The body's sodium ion concentration is influenced by aldosterone, a hormone of the adrenal cortex. This hormone promotes the reabsorption of sodium ions in the kidney tubules. The antidiuretic hormone, ADH, promotes water absorption in the kidneys and so has a definite effect on extracellular sodium ion concentration.

Hyponatremia, a lower-than-normal serum sodium ion concentration, may be due to such causes as vomiting, diarrhea, hormone disorders, starvation, extensive skin burns, loss of sodium ions because of kidney damage, or use of diuretics. The clinical symptoms of hyponatremia are cold, clammy extremities, lowered blood pressure, weak and rapid pulse, oliguria, muscular weakness, and cyanosis (a dark purplish discoloration of the skin and mucous membranes due to decreased oxygenation of the blood). In addition, due to an increased plasticity of the tissues, hyponatremia frequently shows as fingerprinting over the sternum. In hyponatremia the specific gravity of the urine is less than 1.010.

Hypernatremia, a higher-than-normal serum sodium ion concentration, may be due to such causes as deficient water intake, excessive sweating, excessive water output (such as caused by diabetes insipidus), poor kidney excretion, rapid administration of sodium salts, hyperactivity of the adrenal cortex (as in Cushing's disease), and some cases of cerebral disease. The clinical symptoms of hypernatremia are dry, itchy mucous membranes, intense thirst, oliguria or anuria, rough dry tongue, and elevation of temperature. The specific gravity of the urine rises above 1.030. In an extreme case of hypernatremia the symptoms include tachycardia (rapidly beating heart), edema, and cerebral disturbances.

POTASSIUM IONS

Potassium ions are the principal cations of the intracellular fluid. Since the kidneys do not conserve potassium ions as well as they preserve sodium ions and since the body cannot store potassium ions, a depletion of this substance occurs readily in patients whose diets are low in potassium or who are excreting more potassium than they take in.

The principal functions of potassium ions in the body are

1. To maintain the osmotic pressure of the cells.
2. To maintain the electrical potential of the cells.
3. To maintain the size of the cells.

4. To maintain proper contraction of the heart.
5. To maintain proper transmission of nerve impulses.

Potassium ions move into the cells during anabolic activity and move out of the cells during catabolic activity. The concentration of potassium ion is usually measured in terms of serum potassium because this is a much easier quantity to measure than cellular potassium concentration.

Hypokalemia, a lower-than-normal serum potassium ion concentration, can occur under the following conditions:

1. Too low an intake of potassium ions
   (a) During starvation or malnutrition.
   (b) In a diet deficient in potassium.
   (c) During intravenous infusions of fluids low or lacking in potassium ions.
2. Too great an output of potassium ions
   (a) Because of the use of diuretics.
   (b) Use of corticosteroids (these hormones promote retention of sodium ions at the expense of potassium ions).
   (c) Because of prolonged vomiting.
   (d) Because of gastric suction and intestinal drainage.
   (e) Because of diarrhea.
   (f) With polyuria.

In addition, hypokalemia may be caused by a sudden shift of potassium ions from the extracellular fluid to the intracellular fluid. This could occur in such a case as the treatment of diabetic acidosis with insulin and glucose.

In general, hypokalemia occurs most frequently in conjunction with some other pathologic condition. The general symptoms of hypokalemia are general feeling of being ill, lack of energy, muscular weakness, numbness of fingers and toes, apathy, dizziness on rising, cramps, particularly in the calf muscles.

As hypokalemia develops to a greater extent, symptoms relating to the heart become evident. Among these are weak pulse, falling blood pressure, faint heart sounds, and changes in the ECG—first a flattening of the T wave, later inverted T waves with a sagging ST segment and AV block, and finally cardiac arrest.

Hypokalemia may be treated or prevented by giving the patient potassium intravenously (in the form of a potassium salt) or orally by the use of high-potassium foods such as veal, chicken, beef, pork, bananas, orange and pineapple juices, broccoli, and potatoes. Note that although there are many other foods high in potassium, they are usually also high in sodium. A patient on a high-potassium diet usually also has a low-sodium requirement, therefore, these other types of foods are not recommended.

Hyperkalemia, an increased serum potassium ion level, occurs

1. If the intake of potassium ions is too great because of too rapid an infusion of potassium ions or the administration of excess potassium ions intravenously.

2. If the output of potassium ions is too low because of renal failure or acute dehydration.
3. If there is a sudden shift of potassium ions from the intracellular fluid to the extracellular fluid because of severe burns, crush injuries (both of these could release potassium ions from the cells into the bloodstream), or during acidosis.

The symptoms of hyperkalemia are a general feeling of ill-being, muscular weakness, listlessness, mental confusion, slower heart beat, poor heart sounds, bradycardia,* and eventually cardiac arrest. Characteristic changes in the ECG are elevated T waves, widening of the QRS complex, gradual lengthening of the P-R interval, and final disappearance of the P wave.

Removal of excess potassium ions may be accomplished either by dialysis or by the administration of glucose and insulin.

CALCIUM IONS
Most of the body's calcium is found in the bones and the teeth in the form of calcium carbonate and calcium phosphate. If the blood calcium ion concentration falls, it can readily be replenished from the bone. Conversely, if the blood calcium ion concentration rises, the amount replenished from the bones decreases (see pages 508 and 510).

The daily intake (adult) for calcium varies from 200 to 1500 mg and comes primarily from milk and milk products. Ionized calcium is present in body fluids and is important in blood coagulation (see page 459), in the regulation of membrane permeability, and in the normal functioning of nerve, heart, and muscle tissue.

Because of the great amount of calcium present in the bones, calcium is not required during intravenous therapy. In addition, calcium-containing solutions are not suitable for infusions because, if mixed with citrated blood, they may cause a clot in the drip tube.

Calmodulin is a calcium-modulating protein found in all cells. It has a molecular weight of 16,700 and consists of a chain of 148 amino acids. Calmodulin affects the synthesis and action of the prostaglandins and enhances blood platelet aggregation.

Phenothiazines, which are major tranquilizers used to treat psychoses, and phenytoin, which is used in the treatment of leprosy, may inactivate calmodulin, indicating a link between these conditions and calcium metabolism.

Hypocalcemia, a low serum calcium concentration, may be due to a hypoactive parathyroid gland (see page 511), the surgical removal of the parathyroid glands, or a large infusion of citrated blood. The symptoms of hypocalcemia include tingling of the fingertips, abdominal and muscle cramps, and tetany.

Hypercalcemia, an increased serum calcium concentration, may be caused by an overactive parathyroid or by a tumor of that gland. It may also be caused by the administration of excess vitamin D. The symptoms of hypercalcemia include hypotonicity of muscles, kidney stones, deep bone pain, and bone cavitation.

Biochemistry

The serum calcium ion concentration decreases during hypoparathyroidism and rises during hyperparathyroidism (see page 511).

MAGNESIUM IONS Magnesium ion, like potassium ion, is found primarily in the intracellular fluid. Magnesium ions are essential for the proper functioning of the neuromuscular system.

Magnesium acts as an activator for more enzymes than any other metal ion in the body; it is necessary for over 100 metabolic reactions. The normal intake of magnesium is 15 to 30 mEq per day. Another unusual property of magnesium is that it is the only positively charged ion that has a higher concentration in the cerebrospinal fluid than in the blood serum.

A deficiency of serum magnesium ions, **hypomagnesemia,** because of dietary intake is unusual because magnesium is a necessary element for chlorophyll, which is found in all green plant foods. A lower-than-normal magnesium ion concentration may be caused by such factors as 1. chronic alcoholism; 2. diabetic acidosis; 3. prolonged intravenous infusion without magnesium ions; 4. hypoparathyroidism; 5. prolonged nasogastric suction; 6. acute pancreatitis; 7. severe malabsorption.

The clinical symptoms of a deficiency of magnesium ions are 1. muscular tremors; 2. convulsions; 3. delirium; 4. delusions; 5. disorientation; 6. hyperirritability; 7. elevated blood pressure.

An excess of serum magnesium ions may be caused by severe dehydration or renal insufficiency. Excess magnesium ions act as a sedative. Extreme excesses may cause coma, respiratory paralysis, or cardiac arrest.

CHLORIDE IONS The chloride ion is the primary anion of the extracellular fluid. The body's intake of chloride ion is closely related to that of the sodium ion (see page 470).

One of the principal functions of the chloride ion is as a component of gastric hydrochloric acid. The chloride ion also serves an important function in the transportation of oxygen and carbon dioxide in the blood (see page 462).

Hypochloremia, a lower-than-normal serum chloride ion concentration, occurs after prolonged vomiting, profuse sweating, and diarrhea. This condition causes an alkalosis because of an increased concentration of bicarbonate ions. Hypochloremia may also occur when there is a marked loss of potassium ions.

PHOSPHATE IONS The phosphate ion is the primary anion of the intracellular fluid. Diets that are adequate in calcium usually contain more than enough phosphorus for the body's needs.

Most of the body's phosphate is present in the bones as calcium phosphate, a substance that gives the bones their rigidity, but phosphate is found in every cell of the body. Phosphate ions are important in the acid-base balance of the body. They constitute one of the body's buffer systems. Phosphates are also of great importance in the production of ATP, the body's principal energy compound. Serum phosphate levels are low in hyperparathyroidism and high in hypoparathyroidism and celiac disease.

IRON IONS Iron ions are involved almost exclusively in cellular respiration. Iron is part of hemoglobin, myoglobin, and cytochromes as well as several oxidative enzymes. The formation of hemoglobin requires the presence of traces of copper. The best dietary sources of iron are the "organ meats," such as liver, heart, and kidneys. Other sources are egg yolk, fish, beans, and spinach.

Most of the iron present in the food we eat is in the form of ferric ions (Fe^{3+}). In the digestive system, ferric ions are reduced to ferrous ions (Fe^{2+}), which are then absorbed into the bloodstream from the stomach and duodenum. In the blood plasma, ferrous ions are oxidized to ferric ions, which then become part of a specific protein—transferrin, a β-globulin. The conversion of ferrous ions to ferric ions in the blood plasma is catalyzed by the enzyme ceruloplasmin, a copper-containing compound (see following paragraphs).

The liver, spleen, and bone marrow are able to extract the iron from transferrin and to store that iron in the form of two proteins—ferritin and hemosiderin. The bone marrow is also able to extract the iron from transferrin and to use that iron for the production of hemoglobin.

A deficiency of iron (**iron-deficiency anemia**) may result from a low intake of iron because of a diet high in cereal and low in meat, because of poor absorption of iron due to gastrointestinal disturbances or diarrhea, or because of excessive loss of blood. This type of anemia may be treated with a daily dose of ferrous sulfate in the diet, if absorption is normal.

COPPER IONS In addition to being necessary for the synthesis of hemoglobin, copper ions are necessary for certain enzymes, such as cytochrome oxidase (part of the oxidative phosphorylation sequence; see page 405) and uricase (which catalyzes the oxidation of uric acid to allantoin).

Copper is found in the brain in the form of cerebrocuprein, in the blood cells as erythrocuprein, and in the blood plasma as ceruloplasmin, an α-globulin. In **Wilson's disease,** there is a decreased concentration of ceruloplasmin in the blood. This disease is characterized by the presence of large amounts of copper in the brain along with an excessive urinary output of copper.

Copper aspirinate, a complex of copper and aspirin, has been found to be 20 times as effective as aspirin itself in the treatment of arthritis in animals. It is hoped that tests on humans will show similar results.

The average daily diet contains about 2.5 to 5 mg of copper, an amount that is considered to be adequate for the normal adult. The richest sources of copper are liver, nuts, kidney, raisins, and dried legumes.

ZINC IONS Zinc is essential for normal growth and reproduction. It has a beneficial effect on wound healing and tissue repair. Zinc complexes with insulin are present in the beta cells of the pancreas. Zinc is an essential component of several enzymes, such as alcohol dehydrogenase, alkaline phosphatase, carbonic anhydrase, and retinene reductase (found in the retina). Acetazolamide (Diamox) inhibits carbonic anhydrase activity by binding to the zinc atom present in the enzyme molecule. The absorption of zinc by the intestines involves pyridoxine, a B vitamin.

Food sources of zinc include seafood (particularly oysters and clams), meat, liver, eggs, milk, whole grain cereals. The recommended daily allowance for zinc is 15 mg/day for adults with an additional 15 mg/day during pregnancy and 10 mg/day during lactation. For children, the recommended allowance is 6 to 10 mg/day.

OTHER IONS   Zirconium chlorhydrate has been used in antiperspirant sprays, but its use has been discontinued. It was found that this compound could reach the user's lungs through inhalation. In the lungs, zirconium chlorhydrate could induce granulomas, which in turn cause growth of tumors. Aluminum chlorhydrate is still in use in antiperspirant sprays and appears to have no adverse effect upon the body.

Lithium salts are being used to treat manic-depressive psychoses and as antidepressants for some psychiatric patients. Previously, lithium chloride had been employed as a sodium substitute, with dangerous and frequently fatal results. Patients on a therapeutic dosage of lithium salts may complain of fatigue, muscular weakness, nausea, and diarrhea. Slurred speech and hand tremors are noticeable. In larger doses, the central nervous system is affected and the patient may become unconscious or even go into a coma. Abnormalities in the electroencephalogram* are also common.

Cobalt is a constituent of vitamin B_{12}, which is necessary for the formation of red blood cells. Cobalt is present in almost all foods so that a deficiency is quite rare.

Manganese is essential for normal bone structure, reproduction, and normal functioning of the central nervous system. Manganese is a constituent of several different mitochondrial enzyme systems. A deficiency of manganese is not known in humans, indicating that the average daily diet supplies a sufficient amount of this substance. Good sources of manganese are nuts, whole grain cereals, vegetables, and fruits. Poor sources are meats, poultry, and fish.

Summary   Blood carries oxygen, minerals, and food to the cells. Blood carries carbon dioxide and other waste products from the cells. Blood also carries hormones, enzymes, antibodies, and blood cells. Blood regulates body temperature and maintains the pH of the body fluids.

Blood consists of two parts: the suspended particles, red blood cells, white blood cells, and platelets; and the suspending liquid, the plasma. When freshly drawn blood is allowed to clot and settle, the yellow liquid remaining is called blood serum.

Oxygenated blood has a bright red color, whereas deoxygenated blood has a dark purplish color. Blood has a pH range of 7.35 to 7.45. If the pH falls below 7.35, the condition is called acidosis. If the pH rises above 7.45, the condition is called alkalosis. The volume of blood in the body is 5 to 7 L.

The chemical analysis of blood samples is of great clinical significance. Increased or decreased amounts of some substances may indicate a certain disease.

Blood contains hemoglobin, a conjugated protein containing iron. Hemoglobin is composed of heme and globin. Cytochrome c, part of the oxidative phosphorylation sequence in the citric acid cycle, has a structure similar to that of hemoglobin. Chlorophyll a has a structure similar to heme but with a magnesium ion at the center instead of the iron.

Body Fluids: The Blood   **475**

If the hemoglobin content of the blood falls below normal, the condition is called anemia. Anemia may result from a decreased rate of production of red blood cells, an increased destruction of red blood cells, or an increased loss of red blood cells.

Plasma proteins are divided into three groups: albumin, globulins, and fibrinogen. Albumin regulates the osmotic pressure of the blood and controls the water balance of the body. Alpha and beta globulins form loose combinations with carbohydrates, metal ions, and lipids so that these substances can be transported to all parts of the body. Gamma globulins contain the antibodies with which the body fights infectious diseases. Fibrinogen is the plasma protein involved in the clotting of the blood.

When a blood vessel is cut, thromboplastin is liberated. Thromboplastin, in the presence of calcium ions, changes prothrombin in the plasma to thrombin. Thrombin in turn acts on fibrinogen to convert it to fibrin, which forms the clot.

In respiration, the hemoglobin picks up oxygen to form oxyhemoglobin in the lungs. The oxyhemoglobin is carried to the tissues where it gives up its oxygen. At the same time the blood picks up carbon dioxide and other waste products from the cells. Bicarbonate ions are involved in the hemoglobin-oxyhemoglobin cycle and also in the carbon dioxide removal cycle. Excess bicarbonate ion in the blood cells is shifted to the plasma in a process called the chloride shift whereby chloride ions take the place of the bicarbonate ions. In the lungs, as carbon dioxide is removed from the blood, a reverse chloride shift takes place.

The blood maintains a constant pH by the use of buffers, which react with acid (or basic) substances entering the blood and form new substances that are either neutral or more buffer salts.

Buffer systems in the blood are the bicarbonate buffers, the phosphate buffers, the hemoglobin buffers, and protein.

Changes in CO_2 level in the blood and corresponding changes in HCO_3^- and pH may be caused by metabolic acidosis, metabolic alkalosis, respiratory acidosis, or respiratory alkalosis. Each condition involves different changes in these three factors.

Water intake must be balanced by water output. If water intake is greater than water output, edema occurs. If water output is greater than water intake, dehydration may occur.

Water in the body is considered to be distributed in two major areas—intracellular and extracellular. Extracellular water is further subdivided into interstitial water; intravascular and lymph water; water in dense connective tissues, cartilage, and bone; and water in transcellular fluids.

Each of the body's water compartments has its own concentration of electrolytes, all concentrations being expressed as milliequivalents per liter. An increase or decrease in the concentration of any one of the ions will have some effect on the body.

Serum osmotic pressure is affected primarily by the concentration of sodium ions, bicarbonate ions, and chloride ions. Osmotic activity is measured in the unit milliosmols.

Questions and Problems

1. What are the funtions of the blood?
2. What is the normal concentration of red blood cells in the body?
3. What is the normal concentration of white blood cells in the body?
4. What is polycythemia? anemia?
5. What is the function of the leukocytes?
6. Name several types of white blood cells.
7. What is a differential count? What is the function of the thrombocytes?

Biochemistry

8. What are the functions of the inorganic ions present in the plasma?
9. What is the difference between blood plasma and blood serum?
10. What is the normal pH range of the blood? the specific gravity range? the viscosity?
11. Under what conditions might the blood volume increase? decrease?
12. How can blood volume be measured?
13. What type of compound is hemoglobin?
14. What is heme? Diagram its structure.
15. How does the structure of heme compare with that of chlorophyll a? with cytochrome c?
16. What conditions might cause a decreased production of red blood cells?
17. What causes pernicious anemia?
18. What conditions might cause the destruction of red blood cells?
19. What might cause an increased loss of hemoglobin?
20. Name the three groups of plasma proteins. What is the function of each?
21. Describe the effect of albumin on osmotic pressure in terms of Starling's hypothesis.
22. What is edema? What might cause such a condition?
23. What are the functions of the different types of globulins?
24. What is agammaglobulinemia?
25. Describe the clotting mechanism of the blood.
26. How can blood clotting be prevented in samples taken for laboratory analysis?
27. Why should oxalates never be used to prevent blood from coagulating when that blood is to be used in a transfusion?
28. What is the effect of a deficiency of vitamin K on blood clotting?
29. What is a thrombus? What might result from the presence of a thrombus in the brain?
30. Describe the process whereby the blood carries oxygen to the tissues.
31. How does the blood carry carbon dioxide from the tissues?
32. What is the function of carbonic anhydrase?
33. What is the chloride shift? the reverse chloride shift?
34. What is the alkaline reserve of the blood?
35. What types of buffers are present in the blood?
36. Where are potassium buffers located? sodium buffers?
37. Describe the reaction (in equation form) of an acid and a base with a bicarbonate buffer.
38. How does the body replenish its water supply?
39. How does the body normally lose water?
40. Into what areas may the body's water be considered as being subdivided?
41. What are the principal functions of sodium ions in the extracellular fluid?
42. What may cause hyponatremia? What are its symptoms?
43. What may cause hypernatremia?
44. What are the principal functions of potassium ions in the body?
45. What may cause hypokalemia? What are its symptoms?
46. What may cause hyperkalemia? What are its symptoms?
47. Under what conditions may the serum calcium level change?
48. What are the symptoms of a deficiency of magnesium ions? What might cause this deficiency?
49. What are the principal functions of the chloride ion in the body?
50. What are the principal functions of the phosphate ion in the body? iron ions? copper ions?

51. A lab reports the magnesium ion concentration as 3.6 mg/100 ml. Express this as milliequivalents per liter.

52. If the colloid osmotic pressure of the plasma drops to 20 mm, all other pressures remaining the same, what will be the effect on fluid flow? What will this condition be called?

53. What clinical tests would distinguish between metabolic acidosis and respiratory acidosis? between metabolic alkalosis and respiratory alkalosis?

54. Name two causes for metabolic acidosis. How does the body try to compensate for this condition?

55. Why is NaCl used to treat metabolic alkalosis?

56. What acid-base disturbance would each of the following represent? Use normal values of: pH, 7.4; P_{CO_2}, 40 mm; HCO_3^-, 24 mEq/L.

    (a) A 30-year old woman has been vomiting persistently for 4 days. The following readings were obtained:

blood pH	7.55	HCO_3^-	40 mEq/L
P_{CO_2}	56 mm Hg		

    What is the problem? How would you treat it?

    (b) A confused, disoriented man was brought to the emergency room. No history was obtained. The following lab results were obtained:

blood pH	7.10	HCO_3^-	9 mEq/L
P_{CO_2}	23 mm Hg		

    What is the problem? What treatment might be used?

    (c) A 10-year-old boy with an acute asthma attack has the following lab results:

blood pH	7.25	HCO_3^-	30 mEq/L
P_{CO_2}	58 mm Hg		

57. What causes kwashiorkor? What are its symptoms?

58. What are the advantages and disadvantages of the use of plasma substitutes?

References

BAUM, STUART J. *Introduction to Organic and Biological Chemistry,* 3rd ed. Macmillan Publishing Company, New York 1983, Chapter 20.

DOOLITTLE, RUSSELL F. Fibrinogen and fibrin. *Scientific American,* **245:**126–135 (Dec. 1981).

GOODMAN, L. S. and A. GILMAN (eds.). *The Pharmacological Basis of Therapeutics,* 6th ed. Macmillan Publishing Company, 1980, Sec. VII.

HUGHES, D. T. D. Gaseous exchange in the lungs. *Nursing Mirror,* **139:**68–69 (Oct. 3, 1974).

INGRAM, M. and K. J. PRESTON. Automatic analysis of blood cells. *Scientific American,* **223:**72–82 (Nov. 1970).

LAMB, C. Potassium imbalance: Walking the mEq tightrope: Part 2. *Patient Care,* **9:**128 (Feb. 1,1975).

MARTIN, D. W., P. A., MAYES, and V. W. RODWELL. *Harper's Review of Biochemistry,* 19th ed. Lange Medical Publications, Los Altos, Calif., 1983, Chapters 39, 40.

PERUTZ, M. F. Hemoglobin structure and respiratory transport. *Scientific American,* **239:**92–125 (Dec. 1978).

ROSE, B. D. *Clinical Physiology of Acid-Base and Electrolyte Disorders,* 2nd ed. McGraw-Hill Book Co., New York, 1984, Part II.

ZUCKER, M. B. The functioning of blood platelets. *Scientific American,* **242:**86–103 (June 1980).

31 Vitamins

CHAPTER
OUTLINE

Fat-Soluble Vitamins
   Vitamin A
   Vitamin D
   Vitamin E
   Vitamin K
Water-Soluble Vitamins
   Vitamin B_1—Thiamine
   Vitamin B_2—Riboflavin

Niacin
Pyridoxine
Pantothenic Acid
Biotin
Folic Acid
Vitamin B_{12}—Cobalamin
Others
Vitamin C—Ascorbic Acid

Animals fed on a diet consisting only of purified carbohydrates, fats, proteins, minerals, and water will lose weight and develop certain deficiency diseases. Something else must be administered to sustain normal life. The additional substances required are called vitamins.

The name *vitamin* was originally *vitamine* because the first one found was an amine, hence the name *vital amine,* or *vitamine*. Subsequent studies of other such substances showed that they were not all amines so the "e" was dropped.

Vitamins are similar to hormones in many ways. Vitamins and hormones are carried by the bloodstream to the various parts of the body where they are needed. Vitamins and hormones are required by the body only in extremely small amounts. Neither vitamins nor hormones furnish energy by themselves, although vitamins function with certain enzymes to control energy changes in the body. One important difference between vitamins and hormones is that most vitamins must be supplied in the diet whereas hormones are synthesized by the body.

Vitamins are divided into two major groups—those that are soluble in fat solvents (the fat-soluble vitamins), and those soluble in water (the water-soluble vitamins). The fat-soluble vitamins include vitamins A, D, E, and K and are usually found associated with lipids in natural foods.

The fat-soluble vitamins are transported in the bloodstream by the lipoproteins. Fat-soluble vitamins are not excreted in the urine but do appear in the feces.

The water-soluble vitamins include vitamin C and the B-complex vitamins. Although the vitamins have a letter designation and sometimes a subscript in addition, such as vitamin B_1, the chemical names are being more and more widely used. For example, the chemical name for vitamin B_1 is thiamine.

More and more people eat a balanced diet, take vitamins, or are under medical care. This has helped to produce a healthier population. One piece of evidence that points in this direction is the constant overthrowing of previous athletic records.

Fat-Soluble Vitamins

Vitamin A

SOURCE

Vitamin A is found in fish liver oils, butter, milk, and to a small extent kidneys, fat, and muscle meats. The precursor of vitamin A (the substance from which vitamin A can be made) is called provitamin A and is found in yellow fruits and vegetables such as peaches, apricots, sweet potatoes, carrots, tomatoes, and leafy green vegetables.

STRUCTURE

Vitamin A is a high-molecular-weight alcohol known as retinol. Vitamin A has an all-*trans* structure (see page 301).

retinol, vitamin A

Provitamin A is a compound that can be converted into vitamin A. One such provitamin A is β-carotene. The conversion of β-carotene into retinal (vitamin A, aldehyde) and then to retinol (vitamin A) is indicated in the reaction shown in equation (31–1).

It should be noted that one molecule of β-carotene produces two molecules of vitamin A. Because β-carotene must be metabolized to produce vitamin A, β-carotene is only one sixth as effective as oral vitamin A itself.

Provitamin A is transformed into vitamin A in the intestinal walls of animals, such as rats and pigs, but in the liver in humans.

PROPERTIES

Vitamin A is soluble in fats but not in water. It is stable to heat, acid, and alkalis but is destroyed by oxidation. (Recall that double bonds are usually quite susceptible to oxidation). Ordinary cooking does not destroy vitamin A. The vitamin A present in butter is destroyed when the butter turns rancid (becomes oxidized).

DAILY REQUIREMENT

The recommended daily dosages of vitamin A for the normal adult male and female are 1000 and 800 retinol equivalents (5000 and 4000 IU), respectively. One retinol equivalent is 1 μg of retinol or 6 μg of β-carotene. One International Unit (IU) of vitamin A is equivalent to 0.3 μg of retinol or 0.6 μg of β-carotene. The daily requirements of vitamin A are increased to 1000 retinol equivalents (5000 IU) during pregnancy and to 1200 retinol equivalents (6000 IU) during lactation. A child requires 400 to 700 retinol equivalents (2000 to 3300 IU) daily.

Vitamin A is necessary for normal growth and development, reproduction, mucus secretion and lactation. It is necessary for the synthesis of the membranes around the lysosomes and the mitochondria and acts to regulate membrane permeability. Vitamin A plays an important role in the function-β-carotene

retinal (vitamin A aldehyde)

retinene reductase

$$NADH + H^+$$

$$NAD^+$$

retinol (vitamin A), all-*trans*

(31-1)

ing of the retina and in the maintenance of the integrity of epithelial tissues. Recent evidence suggests vitamin A can protect against a variety of cancers.

EFFECT OF DEFICIENCY Vitamin A was discovered by the observation that certain animals did not grow on a diet low in some animal fats. However, this effect on growth is characterized by a lack of other vitamins as well. A lack of vitamin A causes a shrinking and hardening of the epithelial tissues of the membranes in the eyes, digestive tract, respiratory tract, and genitourinary tract. Such a hardening is called **keratinization.**

When keratinization occurs in the lining of the respiratory tract, the patient is more likely to suffer from colds, pneumonia, and other respiratory infections because of the drying of the membranes.

When keratinization occurs in the eyes, the tear ducts become keratinized and are no longer able to secrete tears to wash the eyes. When this occurs, bacteria are able to attack the corneal tissue of the eyes, producing an infection called **xerophthalmia.** In this disease, the cornea becomes cloudy and does not allow light to pass through, so sight is lost permanently.

An early symptom of the lack of vitamin A is **nyctalopia,** or night blindness. A person with night blindness cannot see very well in dim light because of a lack of visual purple (**rhodopsin**) in the retina of the eyes. This pigment is acted on and changed by light and then regenerated in the presence of retinal, an oxidized form of vitamin A. If there is a lack or deficiency of vitamin A, the rhodopsin is regenerated very slowly; thus, there is an impairment in vision at night.

The role of vitamin A in the visual process and the part it plays in the regeneration of rhodopsin are illustrated in the following simplified cycle:

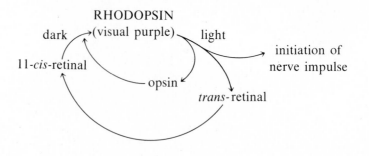

A lack of vitamin A may also produce keratinization of the epithelial cells of the genital system and might cause sterility. A lack of vitamin A causes deformities in the teeth of young animals.

All of these symptoms may be cured by the administration of vitamin A.

Retinoic acid, produced by the oxidation of retinal, serves as a carrier for polysaccharides in the synthesis of glycoproteins. A derivative of retinoic acid, 13-*cis*-retinoic acid, has been used in the treatment of severe acne.

STORAGE AND ABSORPTION Vitamin A is stored in the liver until is needed. Mother's milk contains 10 to 100 times as much vitamin A as does ordinary milk. Zinc is necessary for vitamin A to be mobilized from the liver indicating that vitamin A metabolism may be adversely affected by a zinc deficiency.

Mineral oil should never be taken immediately before or after a meal as it coats the mucosa and interferes with the absorption of carotenes.

Hypervitaminosis A, an intake of vitamin A far in excess of normal daily requirements, has such early symptoms as irritability, loss of appetite, fatigue, and itching. These symptoms usually disappear within a week after the withdrawal of the vitamin.

Acute cases of hypervitaminosis A have been observed following ingestion of polar bear liver, which contains up to 35,000 IU of vitamin A per gram. Symptoms are drowsiness, sluggishness, vomiting, severe headache, and generalized peeling of the skin after 24 hr. Membranes have increased permeability and decreased stability, leading to mitochondrial swelling, lysosomal rupture, and eventually death.

Eating too many carrots on a daily basis may result in *carotenosis,* a benign condition characterized by a yellowing of the skin.

Since vitamin A is fat soluble, it cannot be absorbed from the intestinal tract without the presence of bile. Any interference with the flow of bile to the intestines will also cause a deficiency of this fat-soluble vitamin.

Vitamin D

Vitamin D is sometimes called "the sunshine vitamin." The richest sources of vitamin D are oils from such fish as cod or halibut and the flesh of such

SOURCE

oily fish as sardines, salmon, and mackerel. Milk is not a very good source of vitamin D, although its vitamin D content may be increased by irradiation with ultraviolet light. The vitamin D content of the body may be increased by exposure of the skin to ultraviolet rays from the sun. Care must be taken to avoid overexposure and consequent sunburn.

STRUCTURE

The D vitamins are a group of sterols with considerable differences in their potency. The two most important vitamins in the D group are vitamin D_2 (ergocalciferol, or activated ergosterol) and vitamin D_3 (activated 7-dehydrocholesterol or cholecalciferol). Vitamin D_1, originally called vitamin D, was found to be a mixture of vitamins D_2 and D_3.

The structure of vitamin D_2, ergocalciferol, is

ergocalciferol (vitamin D_2)

Vitamin D_3 is similar to vitamin D_2, the difference being in the structure of the side chain. Vitamin D_3 is made by the irradiation of 7-dehydrocholesterol so it is frequently called "activated 7-dehydrocholesterol."

7-dehydrocholesterol

vitamin D_3

Ergosterol, the precursor of vitamin D_2 occurs in plants, whereas 7-dehyrocholesterol, the precursor of vitamin D_3, occurs in the skin of humans and animals. 7-Dehydrocholesterol in the skin is isomerized to vitamin D_3 under the influence of ultraviolet light.

Vitamin D must acquire two hydroxyl groups in order to be biologically active. The first hydroxyl group is added in the liver and the second in the kidneys, as indicated in reactions (31–2) for vitamin D_3. The same reactions occur with vitamin D_2. Patients who cannot convert vitamin D to its active form, because of liver or kidney disease, often develop osteomalacia,* osteoporosis,* or other bone diseases. Such patients can now be treated with synthetic active-form vitamin D.

vitamin D_3

25-hydroxy vitamin D_3

(31–2)

1,25-dihydroxy vitamin D_3

PROPERTIES   The D vitamins are soluble in fats and insoluble in water. They are stable to heat, resistant to oxidation, and unaffected by cooking. Vitamin D_2 has a greater potency in humans than vitamin D_3, whereas the reverse is true in chickens.

DAILY REQUIREMENT   The daily requirement for children is 400 IU. Daily requirements for adults are not stated because, in most instances, exposure to sunlight is sufficient to supply the body's need. However, 400 IU are recommended daily for women during pregnancy and lactation. One international unit of vitamin D is defined as the biologic activity of 0.025 μg of ergocalciferol.

Biochemistry

The principal action of vitamin D is to increase the absorption of calcium and phosphorus from the small intestines. It also increases the release of calcium and phosphate in the bones, and is necessary for normal growth and development. A lack of vitamin D may cause hypocalcemia and hypophosphatemia. Vitamin D is required for the proper activity of the parathyroid hormone (see page 510) and so is used therapeutically in the treatment of hypoparathyroidism.

Rickets, a disease primarily of infancy and childhood, was previously thought to be due to a deficiency of vitamin D. This disease is now believed to be due to a lack of sunshine on the skin. Why? Because sunshine is necessary for the synthesis of calciferol in the skin.

Rickets is characterized by an inability to deposit calcium phosphate in the bones. The bones become soft and pliable; they bend and become deformed. The joints become enlarged and the ribs become beaded. The knobby or beaded appearance of the ribs is called **rachitic rosary.** A child who has rickets does not grow. He or she develops such symptoms as nervousness, irritability, a bulging abdomen, loss of weight, loss of appetite, anemia, and a delayed development of the teeth. Injection of small amounts of calciferol, or one of its derivatives, or adequate exposure to sunlight can prevent or cure rickets (see Figure 31–1).

FIGURE 31–1. The classical signs of rickets are seen in this child from West Benghal: big abdomen caused by weak abdominal muscles, big forehead, soft leg bones and vertebrae, the rachitic rosary on the ribs, and the swelling of the wrists. (Photograph courtesy of Pan American Health Organization, World Health Organization.)

Vitamins　　　　　　　　　　　　　　　　　　　　　**485**

A diet low in phosphorus and vitamin D may produce **osteomalacia,*** or adult rickets. Since adult rickets is a rare condition, this suggests that adults need less vitamin D than children do. When an adult develops rickets, there is no bulging of the joints since the growth of the bones in an adult is already complete. There is, however, some softening of the bones with accompanying deformities. This disease occurs must often in women after repeated pregnancies during which there are been a deficiency of vitamin D.

A lack of calcium and vitamin D in the diet may cause **osteoporosis*** in the adult. This disease, like osteomalacia, is characterized by decalcification and softening of the bones but to a much greater extent.

Hypervitaminosis D may show such early symptoms as weakness, lassitude, fatigue, nausea, vomiting, and diarrhea, all of which are associated with hypercalcemia. Later symptoms include calcification of soft tissues, including the kidneys and the lungs. Treatment of hypervitaminosis D consists of the immediate withdrawal of the vitamin, increased fluid intake, a diet low in calcium, and the administration of glucocorticoids.

Vitamin E

SOURCE Vitamin E is found in milk, eggs, fish, muscle meats, cereals, leafy vegetables such as lettuce, spinach, and parsley, and plant oils such as cottonseed oil, corn oil, and peanut oil. Wheat germ oil is particularly rich in vitamin E.

STRUCTURE There are several vitamins E. The most important is called α-tocopherol; β- and δ-tocopherols are less active and γ-tocopherol is inactive.

As indicated by the ending of the name, *-ol,* vitamin E is an alcohol. The structure of alpha-tocopherol is

α-tocopherol

PROPERTIES α-Tocopherol, the most important and most active of the E vitamins, is a colorless to pale yellow oil. It is soluble in fats and fat solvents but insoluble in water. Vitamin E is stable to heat but is destroyed by ultraviolet light and by oxidizing agents.

The activity of the tocopherols appears to be due to their antioxidant properties. They are very effective in preventing the oxidation of vitamin A and unsaturated fatty acids. There is also evidence that vitamin E functions as a cofactor in oxidative phosphorylation reactions. Vitamin E is believed to protect the lung tissues from damage by oxidants present in polluted air.

Vitamin E also plays an important role in a selenium metabolism. Selenium is required for pancreatic function. This includes absorption of lipids along with vitamin E. Selenium is present in the enzyme glutathione peroxidase, which helps destroy peroxides and reduces the requirement of vitamin E for maintenance of membranes. Selenium also aids in the retention of vitamin E in plasma lipoprotein.

Biochemistry

Conversely, vitamin E reduces selenium requirements in the body by preventing the loss of that element.

Premature infants suffering from hemolytic anemia show very low levels of α-tocopherol in their blood. When given vitamin E supplements, people suffering from hemolytic anemia improve greatly. It is now believed that vitamin E is essential in infant metabolism. The U.S. Food and Drug Administration requires that commercial milk substitutes sold as infant foods contain adequate amounts of vitamin E. Recent evidence has shown that vitamin E is helpful in the diets of pregnant and lactating women. Vitamin E also is useful in treating older persons suffering from circulatory problems.

Vitamin E is required in higher animals such as cattle and poultry for fertility. The name *tocopherol* is derived from the Greek *tokos* meaning "childbirth" and *pherein* meaning "to bear."

DAILY REQUIREMENT

The international unit of vitamin E is defined as the activity of 1 mg of *dl*-α-tocopherol acetate. The recommended daily requirement of vitamin E is 15 IU for the adult male and 12 IU for the adult female.

EFFECT OF DEFICIENCY

Vitamin E is known to prevent sterility in animals. A deficiency of vitamin E in male rats produces sterility because the animal is unable to produce spermatozoa. (Mated female rats lacking in vitamin E will produce embryos that develop normally for a few weeks then die and are reabsorbed.) Vitamin E has not proven useful in treating sterility in humans.

Some animals on a vitamin E-deficient diet develop muscular dystrophy, resulting in paralysis. Administration of vitamin E helps these animals overcome such effects. Vitamin E has not been found effective in treating muscular dystrophy in humans, and there is no evidence that vitamin E has any therapeutic use at all.

Severely impaired absorption of fat in the intestines can cause vitamin E deficiency in humans. The symptoms of such a disease are muscular weakness, creatinuria, and fragile red blood cells.

There appears to be a relationship between vitamins A and E. Vitamin E may help in the absorption, storage, and utilization of vitamin A. Vitamin E also appears to offer protection against large overdoses of vitamin A. No definite side effects of large doses of vitamin E are known.

Vitamin K

SOURCE

Vitamin K is found in the green leafy tissues of such plants as spinach, cabbage, and alfalfa. Vitamin K is also found in putrefied fish meal, liver, eggs, and cheese. Fruits contain very little vitamin K.

STRUCTURE

There are two naturally occurring K vitamins, K_1 and K_2. Vitamin K_1 is a yellow oil whose structure is

vitamin K_1

Vitamin K_2 differs from K_1 only in the nature of the side chain. Vitamin K_1 is produced in plants and K_2 by intestinal bacteria. A synthetic compound, menadione, exhibits vitamin K activity. It is converted in the body to vitamin K.

menadione

Compare the structure of the K vitamins with that of coenzyme Q (page 377), which functions in oxidative phosphorylation.

PROPERTIES

The K vitamins are soluble in fats and insoluble in water. They are stable to heat but are destroyed in acid and alkaline solutions. They are also unstable to light and oxidizing agents.

DAILY REQUIREMENT

There is no generally accepted figure for the daily human requirement of vitamin K, but the amount needed appears to be extremely small. The average diet supplies sufficient vitamin K; in addition, intestinal bacteria are able to synthesize this vitamin for their host.

A deficiency of vitamin K will occur only as a result of prolonged use of a broad-spectrum antibiotic couples with poor dietary intake of foods, particularly those lacking or low in vitamin K. Vitamin K deficiency does occur in breastfed infants because they do not have intestinal bacteria and because breast milk is a poor source of vitamin K. Vitamin K is usually given as a supplement during the first five months after birth. Some infants are born with a deficiency of prothrombin and are subject to bleeding. Other infants have no ability to manufacture vitamin K in the intestine. Without proper care such infants may die because of brain hemorrhage. This condition may be alleviated by administering vitamin K to the mother before delivery or to the infant shortly after birth.

EFFECT OF DEFICIENCY

A deficiency of vitamin K may also occur when fat absorption is impaired as in biliary or pancreatic disease or in the atrophy of intestinal mucosa.

Vitamin K is known as the antihemorrhaging vitamin. It is necessary for the production of prothrombin in the liver. When there is a deficiency of vitamin K, there is a lack of prothrombin and thus a prolonged clotting time for the blood. Vitamin K is also necessary as a cofactor for oxidative phosphorylation reactions.

Vitamin K is absorbed from the small intestine with the help of bile. In conditions in which bile does not enter the small intestine, such as in obstructive jaundice, vitamin K is not absorbed. This condition leads to a tendency to bleed for a long period of time after an injury or when undergoing surgery. This effect may be overcome by administering both bile and vitamin K to the patient.

Vitamin K is also used therapeutically as an antidote for anticoagulant drugs such as Dicumarol.

Large doses of vitamin K can cause hemolysis in infants and aggravate hyperbilirubinemia.

Water-Soluble Vitamins

The water-soluble vitamins include the B-complex vitamins and vitamin C. The B complex represents a whole series of vitamins, many of which act as cofactors or coenzymes in various oxidative reactions. Each member of the B-complex vitamins has a different physiologic activity. The B complex, also called the vitamin B family, contains the following vitamins:

1. Vitamin B_1—thiamine
2. Vitamin B_2—riboflavin
3. Niacin
4. Pyridoxine
5. Pantothenic acid
6. Biotin
7. Folic acid
8. Vitamin B_{12}—cobalamin

Since these vitamins are water soluble, they can be excreted in the urine, and thus rarely accumulate in toxic amounts.

Because they are water soluble, the B vitamins must be provided continually in the diet. The only exception is vitamin B_{12}, cobalamin, because the human liver can store several years' supply of this vitamin.

Vitamin B_1—Thiamine

SOURCE

Thiamine occurs in yeast, milk, eggs, meat, nuts, and whole grains. Vegetables and fruits contain very little vitamin B_1. Synthetic vitamin B_1 is now being added to enrich the vitamin content of flour and bread.

STRUCTURE

Thiamine has been crystallized as a hydrochloride with the following structure:

thiamine hydrochloride

PROPERTIES

Thiamine is soluble in water and also in alcohol up to 70 percent. It is insoluble in fats and fat solvents. Thiamine is stable in acid solution but is destroyed in alkaline and neutral solutions. Thiamine is quite stable to heat; it can be sterilized for 30 min at 120°C without appreciable loss in activity. Thiamine hydrochloride, a salt produced by treating thiamine with hydrochloric acid, is more soluble than thiamine itself and so is generally used whenever this vitamin is required.

DAILY REQUIREMENT

It is difficult to determine the amount of thiamine required daily. It depends upon several factors. The body's requirement of thiamine increases during a fever, increased muscular activity, hyperthyroidism, pregnancy, and lactation. The thiamine requirement of the body also increases during a diet high in carbohydrates, whereas it decreases with a diet in fat and protein. Thiamine cannot be stored in the body to any significant degree.

The recommended thiamine daily intake 0.3 to 0.5 mg for infants, 0.7 to 1.2 mg for children, 1.0 to 1.1 mg for adult females, and 1.2 to 1.4 mg for adult males.

EFFECT OF DEFICIENCY A deficiency of vitamin B_1 (thiamine) causes a lack of appetite, failure of growth, and loss in weight.

Alcoholism is the most common cause of thiamine deficiency in the United States. This is due to low vitamin intake plus the high calorie content of alcohol.

As the lack of thiamine continues, a disease called beriberi develops in humans (in animals this disease is called polyneuritis). Beriberi occurs mainly in the Orient where fish and polished rice (both lacking in vitamin B_1) are the chief diet. In beriberi there is a degeneration of certain nerves leading to the muscles. When pressure is applied along the nerves, severe pain is felt. The muscles served by these nerves become stiff and atrophy from disuse. Cardiovascular symptoms also occur. These are palpitation, tachycardia, an enlarged heart, and an abnormal electrocardiogram. Finally, death may occur because of heart failure. Beriberi can be prevented or treated by a diet containing thiamine.

Thiamine is necessary for the normal metabolism of carbohydrates. The vitamin is changed in the liver to thiamine pyrophosphate (TPP), which acts as a coenzyme (cocarboxylase) for the decarboxylation of pyruvic and α-keto acids and also acts in transketolase reactions. In the Krebs cycle, cocarboxylase is necessary for the conversion of pyruvic acid to acetyl CoA and also for the conversion of α-ketoglutaric acid to succinyl CoA (see page 406). In thiamine pyrophosphate, the —OH group is replaced by two phosphate groups. During a deficiency of thiamine, pyruvic acid accumulates in the blood and carbohydrates are not properly metabolized.

Thiamine also functions in the utilization of pentoses in the hexose-monophosphate shunt and in some amino acid syntheses.

Vitamin B_2—Riboflavin

SOURCE Riboflavin occurs in many of the same sources as thiamine. It is found in yeast, milk, liver, kidneys, heart meats, and leafy vegetables. Cereals contain very little riboflavin unless it is added artificially.

DAILY REQUIREMENT The daily requirement of riboflavin is 0.8 to 1.4 mg for children, 1.4 to 1.7 mg for adult males and 1.2 to 1.3 mg for adult females, with increased amount needed during pregnancy and lactation.

STRUCTURE Riboflavin or vitamin B_2 has been found to consist of a five-carbon sugar alcohol (ribitol) and a pigment (flavin). Its structure is on page 491.

PROPERTIES Riboflavin is an orange-red crystalline solid, slightly soluble in water and alcohol but insoluble in fats and fat solvents. In water solution riboflavin forms a greenish yellow fluorescent liquid. Riboflavin is destroyed by light and alkaline solutions but is fairly stable to heat and so is not destroyed by cooking.

riboflavin

Riboflavin acts as a coenzyme in two different forms—flavin adenine dinucleotide (FAD) and flavin mononucleotide (FMN). These riboflavin coenzymes act as acceptors for the transfer of protons between NAD^+ and $NADP^+$ and the cytochromes, which transport electrons in the mitochondria (see page 407).

(see page 407).

EFFECT OF DEFICIENCY
A deficiency of riboflavin in humans produces lesions in the corners of the mouth (cheilitis), inflammation of the tongue (glossitis), and lesions on the lips and around the eyes and nose. There is also an inflammation of the skin (dermatitis) and a clouding of the cornea of the eye.

Because riboflavin is so sensitive to light, newborn infants with hyperbilirubinemia when treated with phototherapy show signs of ribloflavin deficiency. This condition persists even when riboflavin supplements are given.

In rats a deficiency of riboflavin produces dermatitis, clouding of the corneas, and loss of hair.

Niacin

SOURCE
Niacin (formerly known as nicotinic acid or vitamin B_5) is widely distributed in plants and animals. It is found in liver, kidney, and heart meats as well as in yeast, peanuts, and wheat germ. Milk, eggs, and fruit contain some niacin but are generally classified as poor sources of that vitamin.

STRUCTURE AND PROPERTIES
Niacin and niacinamide (nicotinamide), which it readily forms in the body, have the following structures.

niacin
(nicotinic acid)

niacinamide
(nicotinamide)

Niacin is slightly soluble in water but quite soluble in alkali. It is insoluble in fats. Niacin is stable to alkalis in acid and to heat and light, and it is not destroyed by cooking.

Niacinamide, along with thiamine and riboflavin, serves as a coenzyme in tissue oxidation. It functions in the mitochondria in the form of NAD^+

(nicotinamide adenine dinucleotide) and $NADP^+$ (nicotinamide adenine dinucleotide phosphate) (see page 376).

DAILY REQUIREMENT

The recommended daily intake of niacin is 16 to 19 mg for males and 13 to 15 mg for females with a slight increase in requirements for adolescents and during pregnancy and lactation. However, these requirements can be greatly affected by the protein of the diet because the amino acid tryptophan can supply much of the body's needed niacin (60 mg of tryptophan equals 1 mg of niacin). Some niacin may also be synthesized by intestinal bacterial action and thus become available for use in the body.

EFFECT OF DEFICIENCY

Niacin was originally called nicotinic acid or the antipellagra factor. The word **pellagra** comes from the Italian words *pelle agra* meaning rough skin. A deficiency of niacin in humans produces serious consequences, although a deficiency in this vitamin is usually accompanied by a deficiency in other substances also. In pellagra there is a dermatitis (skin rash or lesions) and an inflammation of the mouth and tongue (glossitis). These symptoms are accompanied by diarrhea and then dementia (see Figure 31–2).

FIGURE 31–2. This extremely malnourished child has the rough skin, dark in patches, characteristic of the niacin-deficiency disease pellagra. Irritation and inflammation of the mouth and gastrointestinal tract are also characteristic of pellagra. (Photograph courtesy of World Health Organization.)

A lack of niacin in dogs produces tongue lesions called black tongue. A diet containing niacin is effective in curing pellagra in humans and also niacin deficiency diseases in animals.

Pellagra was quite common in the South where the diet consisted chiefly of corn and fat pork. Corn has a low tryptophan content and can give very little niacin. Fat pork also has very little niacin. Thus there was a deficiency of this vitamin, leading to pellagra. With an improvement in the diet, especially with the addition of foods containing niacin (or tryptophan), pellagra is not as common in the United States as it was previously.

High doses of niacin (nicotinic acid) but not niacinamide can produce such symptoms as skin flushing, gastrointestinal distress, and pruritus as well as lower serum cholesterol levels.

Pyridoxine

STRUCTURE

Pyridoxine was originally called vitamin B_6, or the rat antidermatitis factor. Subsequent work showed that vitamin B_6 was a mixture of pyridoxine, pyridoxal, and pyridoxamine. The generally accepted term for these compounds is pyridoxine because these compounds are readily interconvertible. The stuctures are

pyridoxal   pyridoxine   pyridoxamine

Pyridoxine is found in yeast, liver, egg yolk, and the germ of various grains and seeds. It is also found to a limited extent in milk and leafy vegetables.

DAILY REQUIREMENT

The recommended requirement of pyridoxine for the adult is 2 mg per day.

EFFECT OF DEFICIENCY

A deficiency of pyridoxine in rats produces dermatitis in the paws, nose, and ears. A deficiency in dogs and pigs produces anemia. If the deficiency of pyridoxine is continued for a long period of time, these animals suffer from epileptiform fits. A deficiency of pyridoxine in infants produces convulsions. A deficiency of this vitamin in adults produces such symptoms as dermatitis, sore tongue, irritability, and apathy. A diet containing pyridoxine (or vitamin B_6) will alleviate these symptoms.

The generation of niacin from the amino acid tryptophan requires the presence of the coenzyme pyridoxal phosphate. Therefore, pellagra frequently accompanies pyridoxine deficiency.

A widely used antituberculosis drug, isonicotinic acid hydrazide (isoniazid) can induce isolated pyridoxine deficiency by forming a compound with pyridoxal. This compound is excreted in the urine, thus producing a deficiency of pyridoxal.

The antihypertensive drug hydralazine and the chelating agent penicillinamine will also cause pyridoxine deficiencies. Pyridoxine should not be taken by patients receiving levodopa treatment for Parkinson's disease because pyridoxine enhances the drug's deactivation.

Pyridoxal phosphate and pyridoxamine phosphate serve as coenzymes for the decarboxylation of amino acids, taking part in the reactions occurring primarily in the gray matter of the central nervous system. It is believed that a deficiency of these coenzymes interferes with decarboxylation reactions in the central nervous system and so leads to epileptiform seizures. Pyridoxal phosphate and pyridoxamine phosphate also serve as coenzymes in amino acid metabolism. Further, pyridoxine is involved in the absorption of zinc by the intestines.

Pantothenic Acid

SOURCES

Pantothenic acid has a widespread distribution in nature. Its name comes from the Greek word meaning "from everywhere." Good sources of pantothenic acid are egg yolk, yeast, kidney, and lean meats. Other fairly good sources are lean beef, skimmed milk, broccoli, sweet potatoes, and molasses.

STRUCTURE AND PROPERTIES

Pantothenic acid is a viscous yellow oil, soluble in water but insoluble in fat solvents such as chloroform. It is stable in acid and alkaline solution. Pantothenic acid is one of the constituents of CoA, which is involved in the metabolism of carbohydrates, fats, and proteins and in the synthesis of cholesterol (see pages 375 and 422).

The structures of pantothenic acid and of CoA are

pantothenic acid

pyrophosphate

coenzyme A

The daily human requirement of pantothenic acid is not known, but estimates of 4 to 7 mg are usually considered adequate and are easily met from an ordinary diet.

EFFECT OF DEFICIENCY Pantothenic acid was originally known as chick antidermatitis factor because it was a substance that prevented dermatitis in chicks.

Rats and dogs who were given a diet deficient in pantothenic acid showed a loss of pigmentation from their hair. The black hair of such animals turned gray but returned to its original black color upon the addition of pantothenic acid to the diet. There is no evidence that this vitamin is of significant value in restoring hair color in humans. There is little evidence of pantothenic acid deficiency in humans.

A deficiency of pantothenic acid in animals cause degeneration in the adrenal cortex and a failure in reproduction.

Biotin Biotin, another member of the vitamin B complex, is widely distributed in nature. Rich sources of this vitamin are liver, egg yolk, kidneys, yeast, and milk. Biotin was formerly known as the anti-egg-white injury factor. This name was given to it because rats fed raw egg white failed to grow and also developed dermatitis. Raw egg white contains a protein, avidin, that combines with biotin and renders it unavailable to the animal.

The structure of biotin is

biotin

An artifically produced deficiency of biotin in humans causes scaly dermatitis, nausea, muscle pains, and depression. These symptoms are rapidly relieved by the administration of a diet containing biotin.

Biotin is supplied by the action of intestinal bacteria, in humans as well as in animals, so that a deficiency of this vitamin is unlikely in most cases, except on a severely restricted diet. Biotin functions as a coenzyme for carboxylation reactions in the formation of fatty acids (see page 418).

Folic Acid Folic acid (folacin) occurs in green leaves, yeast, liver, kidneys, and cauliflower. The structure of folic acid (which contains a pteridine nucleus, *p*-aminobenzoic acid, and glutamic acid) is shown on page 496.

Actually, this compound, which is also called pteroylglutamic acid (PGA), is only one of several related compounds in the folic acid group. Others are pteroic acid, pteroyltriglutamic acid, and pteroylheptaglutamic acid.

A deficiency of folic acid causes megaloblastic* anemia and gastrointestinal disturbances.

folic acid (folacin)

Folic acid in its reduced form, tetrahydrofolic acid, acts as a coenzyme for the transfer of methyl groups in the formation of such compounds as choline and methionine.

Folic acid is primarily involved in reactions involving transfer of methyl groups. This type of reaction plays an essential role in the synthesis of hemoglobin, nucleic acids, and methionine.

Treatment with antileukemic drugs such as methotrexate involve inhibiting the conversion of folic acid into its active form tetrahydrofolate. Without this folate cancer cells (as well as other cells) cannot grow.

Vitamin B$_{12}$—Cobalamin

SOURCE

Plants do not contain vitamin B$_{12}$ (cobalamin). Microorganisms are able to synthesize it. The best sources of cobalamin are liver, kidneys, fish, eggs, milk, oysters, and clams.

STRUCTURE AND PROPERTIES

Cobalamin is an odorless, tasteless, reddish crystalline compound, soluble in water and alcohol and insoluble in fat solvents such as ether and acetone. One unusual property of this vitamin is that it contains the element cobalt (4.35 percent).

A cyano group (CN$^-$) is usually attached to the central cobalt atom during isolation of the vitamin. This compound is known as cyanocobalamin. The cyano group must be traded for a methyl group in the body before cobalamin can be activated. The structure of cyanocobalamin is shown on p. 497.

DAILY REQUIREMENT

The recommended daily amount of vitamin B$_{12}$ (cobalamin) is 3 μg.

EFFECT OF DEFICIENCY

Vitamin B$_{12}$ is important in the transfer of methyl groups. Thus, many symptoms of vitamin B$_{12}$ and folate deficiency are similar. Vitamin B$_{12}$ is involved in the maintenance of the myelin sheath, in the synthesis of nucleic acids and hemoglobin, and in the metabolism of lipids and carbohydrates. Pernicious anemia is an anemia that resembles megaloblastic anemia. Pernicious anemia has several neurologic complications. It results from a dietary lack of vitamin B$_{12}$ (strict vegetarianism) or of the intrinsic factor.

Vitamin B$_{12}$ (cobalamin) is also called the anti-pernicious anemia factor. It is absorbed from the small intestine in the presence of hydrochloric acid and the intrinsic factor (see page 307). In the absence of the intrinsic factor, vitamin B$_{12}$ cannot be absorbed, and this leads to pernicious anemia. Injection of a small amount of cobalamin will produce remarkable improvement in that disease.

cyanocobalamin

DERIVATIVES   Coenzyme B_{12} is one of several coenzymes derived from vitamin B_{12}. These coenzymes are required for hydrogen transfer and isomerization in the conversion of methyl malonate to succinate, thus involving both carbohydrate and fat metabolism.

Coenzyme B_{12} differs from vitamin B_{12} in that a 5-deoxyadenosine group replaces the CN group attached to the central cobalt.

Others   There are several substances frequently classified along with the B vitamins although they are not truly vitamins. Among these are choline, inositol, *p*-aminobenzoic acid, and lipoic acid.

CHOLINE   Choline is an essential substance as far as the body is concerned, although it is generally not classified as a vitamin because it can be synthesized in the required amounts in the body and it is required in much larger amounts than vitamins.

Choline is a viscous, colorless liquid, soluble in water and alcohol but insoluble in ether. Its structure is

choline

A deficiency in choline leads to such symptoms as fatty liver. Young rats on a diet deficient in choline also had hemorrhagic degeneration of the kidneys. Older rats who survived these symptoms developed cirrhosis. Chicks and young turkeys develop perosis or slipped tendon disease.

Vitamins   **497**

Choline is a constituent of lecithin (phosphatidyl choline) and sphingo-myelin and is important in brain and nervous tissue. A deficiency of choline will not develop in a person on a high-protein diet because proteins supply the amino acids from which the body can synthesize this compound.

Choline is a constituent of acetylcholine, which is present in nerve cells and aids in the transmission of nerve impulses by the following means: When a nerve cell is stimulated, it releases acetylcholine. This acetylcholine in turn stimulates the adjacent nerve cell also to release acetylcholine. This process continues as a chain reaction until the impulse reaches the brain. Once a nerve cell has passed its impulse on the next cell, the enzyme acetylcholinesterase hydrolyzes acetylcholine into acetic acid and choline. The nerve cells then use these two compounds to regenerate the acetylcholine for the next impulse.

INOSITOL   Inositol is found in liver, milk, vegetables, yeast, whole grains, and fruits. The molecular formula for inositol is $C_6H_{12}O_6$, so it is an isomer of glucose. Its structure is

inositol (hexahydroxycyclohexane)

It was found that mice, on a synthetic diet containing all of the known vitamins, still failed to grow. Also there was an effect on their hair and impaired lactation. Pantothenic acid, which affect hair in mice, did not help these animals. However, these symtpoms were overcome by the addition of a compound obtained from cereal grain. This compound was inositol. Inositol is required for the growth of yeasts, mice, rats, guinea pigs, chickens, and turkeys.

Inositol, along with folic acid and p-aminobenzoic acid, is not a true vitamin. However, it is included with the B group even though no specific role in human nutrition has been established.

p-AMINOBENZOIC ACID   p-Aminobenzoic acid (PABA) is a growth factor for certain microorganisms. It forms part of the folic acid molecule and is believed to be necessary for the formation of that vitamin. However, humans are incapable of using p-aminobenzoic acid to produce folic acid. p-Aminobenzoic acid is formed upon the hydrolysis of folic acid. The structure of p-aminobenzoic acid is

p-aminobenzoic acid

sulfanilamide

Compare the structure of sulfanilamide with that of *p*-aminobenzoic acid beside it. Sulfonamides exert their antibacterial action by acting as antimetabolites to *p*-aminobenzoic acid. One theory is that the sulfa drugs are similar in structure to *p*-aminobenzoic acid and attach themselves to an enzyme required in the metabolism of *p*-aminobenzoic acid, thus blocking the use of that substance (see page 374). Persons taking sulfa drugs should be cautioned against taking vitamins containing PABA.

p-Aminobenzoic acid is not regarded as a vitamin for humans, but it is included here because it is necessary for the synthesis of folic acid by some microorganisms.

LIPOIC ACID   Lipoic acid was first detected in the studies of the growth of lactic acid bacteria. It is fat soluble and so was called lipoic acid. Its structure is

lipoic acid

As far as is known, lipoic acid is not required in the diet of higher animals and no deficiency effects have been noted.

Actually, lipoic acid is not a true vitamin; however, because its coenzyme function in carbohydrate metabolism is closely related to that of thiamine, it is classified along with the B-vitamin group. Lipoic acid functions, along with thiamine, in the initial decarboxylation of α-keto acids to form acetyl CoA for the citric acid cycle.

Vitamin C—   Fresh fruits and vegetables such as oranges, lemons, grapefruit, berries, mel-
Ascorbic Acid   ons, tomatoes, and raw cabbage are excellent sources of vitamin C. Dry cereals, legumes, milk, meats, and eggs contain very little of this vitamin.

SOURCE

STRUCTURE AND   Vitamin C, ascorbic acid, is a white crystalline substance soluble in water
PROPERTIES   and alcohol but insoluble in most fat solvents. Ascorbic acid is a strong reducing agent and is easily oxidized in air, especially in the presence of such metallic ions as Fe^{3+} or Cu^{2+}. Ascorbic acid is rapidly destroyed by heating. For this reason, cooking of foods in copper pots should be avoided because this will destroy the vitamin C content of the foods being cooked.

It can easily be oxidized to dehydroascorbic acid. Both ascorbic acid and dehydroascorbic acid are biologically active, and both have been synthesized in the laboratory. Their structures are

ascorbic acid   dehydroascorbic acid

The recommended daily intake of ascorbic acid for an adult is 60 mg; the amount is increased to 80 mg during pregnancy and 100 mg during lactation.

Plants and all animals except guinea pigs, humans, and other primates are able to synthesize ascorbic acid and are resistant to diseases caused by a lack of this vitamin. A deficiency of vitamin C produces a disease known as scurvy. The symptoms in humans are swollen, bleeding gums, pain in the joints, decalcification of the bones, loss of weight, and anemia.

A deficiency of vitamin C prevents the body from forming and maintaining the intercellular substance that cements the tissues together. A lack of this intercellular substance in the capillaries leads to rupturing and subsequent hemorrhaging in these vessels, to the formation of weak bones and atrophy of the bone marrow, accompanied by anemia, and also accounts for loosening of the teeth and spongy gums. All of these symptoms are relieved by the addition of ascorbic acid to the diet.

Vitamin C is also believed to function in oxidation-reduction reactions and in cellular respiration.

Linus Pauling, Nobel prize winner in chemistry, has suggested that the common cold can be prevented or treated by the administration of large doses of ascorbic acid. To date there have been many efforts to prove or disprove this hypothesis, but since the cause of a cold itself is not known, the controversy still continues.

Summary

The body requires vitamins in addition to carbohydrates, fats, and proteins but in much smaller amounts. Vitamins must be supplied in the diet, whereas hormones are synthesized by the body.

Vitamins are divided into two type: the fat soluble and the water soluble.

Vitamin A is found in fish liver oils, in butter, and in milk. Vitamin A is an alcohol. The recommended daily adult dose of vitamin A is 1000 retinol equivalents (5000 IU) for the adult male and 800 retinol equivalents (4000 IU) for the adult female. Vitamin A has an all-*trans* structure.

A lack of vitamin A produces keratinization in the membranes of the eyes, digestive tract, respiratory tract, and genitourinary tract. Nyctalopia is also due to a deficiency of vitamin A. Vitamin A is stored in the liver.

Vitamin D is found in fish liver oils such as cod or halibut. The vitamin D content of milk is increased by irradiation. The D vitamins are sterols with a structure similar to that of cholesterol. Vitamin D functions to increase the absorption of calcium and phosphorus from the small intestine. Vitamin D also functions in the deposition of calcium phosphate in the teeth and bones. A lack of vitamin D produces rickets.

Vitamin E is found in many foods; wheat germ is particularly rich in this substance. The E vitamins have antioxidant properties and act as a cofactor in oxidative phosphorylation reactions. Vitamin E prevents sterility in animals but its necessity in humans has not yet been determined.

Vitamin K is known as the antihemorrhaging vitamin. It is necessary for the production of the prothrombin in the liver.

Vitamin B_1 (thiamine) occurs naturally in yeast, milk, and whole grains and also may be made synthetically. A deficiency of this vitamin causes a lack of appetite, failure of growth, and loss in weight. A prolonged deficiency of vitamin B_1 leads to the disease known as beriberi (or polyneuritis in animals). Thiamine is also necessary for the normal metabolism of carbohydrates. This vitamin acts as a coenzyme for the decarboxylation of pyruvic acid. The coenzyme, known as cocarboxylase, is necessary in the Krebs cycle for the conversion of α-ketoglutaric acid to succinyl CoA.

Vitamin B_2 (riboflavin) is found in the same sources as thiamine. Riboflavin acts as a coenzyme in two different forms: flavin adenine dinucleotide (FAD) and flavin mononucleotide (FMN). These coenzymes act as acceptors for the transfer of protons between NAD^+ and $NADP^+$ and the cytochromes.

Niacin (or nicotinic acid) is widely distributed in nature. A deficiency of this vitamin produces a condition known as pellagra. Niacin is an important constituent of two coenzymes: nicotinamide adenine dinucleotide (NAD^+) and nicotinamide adenine dinucleotide phosphate ($NADP^+$). These coenzymes are involved in most oxidation-reduction reactions in the mitochondria.

Pyridoxine is involved in the decarboxylation of amino acids and is also required for certain transaminase reactions.

Pantothenic acid is one of the constituents of CoA, which is involved in the metabolism of carbohydrates, fats, and proteins as well as in the synthesis of cholesterol.

Biotin functions in the activation of carbon dioxide for carboxylation reactions in the formation of fatty acids.

Folic acid is concerned with the transfer of methyl groups in the formation of such compounds as choline and methionine.

Vitamin B_{12}, cobalamin, is called the anti-pernicious anemia factor. It is also involved in the synthesis of certain amino acids and of choline, and is necessary for the formation of coenzyme B_{12}.

Choline is a constituent of lecithin and so is important in brain and nerve tissue. Choline is also a constituent of acetylcholine, which aids in the transmission of nerve impulses.

p-Aminobenzoic acid is formed upon the hydrolysis of folic acid. This substance is a growth factor for certain microorganisms.

Inositol is required for the growth of yeasts, mice, and rats.

Lipoic acid is closely related to thiamine in the initial oxidation of α-keto acids.

Vitamin C, ascorbic acid, may be synthesized by plants and most animals but not by humans. A lack of this vitamin produces a disease known as scurvy. A lack of ascorbic acid also causes a lack of the intercellular substance that cements the tissues together.

Questions and Problems

1. Compare vitamins with hormones
2. Which vitamins are water soluble? fat soluble?
3. What are the sources of vitamin A?
4. Why should mineral oil never be taken immediately before or after a meal?
5. What is beta-carotene? How is it used in the body?
6. What are the effects of a deficiency of vitamin A?
7. Where is vitamin A stored in the body? How is it absorbed?
8. Why does the body need vitamin A? What causes hypervitaminosis A? What are the symptoms?
9. Describe the role of vitamin A in the visual process.
10. What are the sources of vitamin D?
11. Why is vitamin D called the sunshine vitamin?
12. What type of compound is vitamin D? Are all the D vitamins equally potent?

13. What are the daily adult requirements of vitamin A? D?
14. What are the functions of vitamin D in the body?
15. What are the effects of a lack of vitamin D? of an excess?
16. What are the sources of vitamin E? What are its properties? functions?
17. What are the sources of vitamin K? What are its properties? functions?
18. What are the sources of vitamin B_1? What are its properties? functions?
19. What are the effects of a lack of thiamine?
20. What are the sources of riboflavin?
21. What are the sources of niacin? pyridoxine?
22. What are the effects of a deficiency of niacin? pyridoxine? How does the body use these substances?
23. What are the sources of pantothenic acid? its properties? the effects of a deficiency?
24. What are the functions of lipoic acid, biotin, folic acid, *p*-aminobenzoic acid, inositol, and cobalamin?
25. What are the sources of vitamin C? its properties? its functions?
26. What are the effects of a deficiency of ascorbic acid?
27. How do sulfonamides exert their antibacterial effect?
28. What is carotenosis?
29. How are nerve impulses transmitted?
30. How does vitamin E affect selenium metabolism?

References

BAUM, STUART J. *Introduction to Organic and Biological Chemistry,* 3rd ed. Macmillan Publishing Company, New York, 1982, Chapter 21.

DOWLING, J. E. Night blindness. *Scientific American,* **215:**78–84 (Oct. 1966).

GOODMAN, L. S. and A. GILMAN (eds.). *The Pharmacological Basis of Therapeutics,* 7th ed. Macmillan Publishing Company, New York, 1985, Sec. XVIII.

LESLIE, C. R. The action of vitamin C on blood vessels. *Health,* **11:**13–15 (Winter 1974/1975).

LOOMIS, W. F. Rickets. *Scientific American,* **223:**76–91 (Dec. 1970).

———. Zinc: A trace element essential in vitamin A metabolism. *Science,* **181:**954–955 (Sept. 7, 1973).

MARTIN, D. W., P. A. MAYES, and V. W. RODWELL. *Harper's Review of Biochemistry,* 19th ed. Lange Medical Publications, Los Altos, Calif., 1983, Chapters 10, 11, 41.

WALTERS, J. D. and R. P. HUEMER. Prevalence of vitamin deficiencies. *Journal of the International Academy of Preventive Medicine,* **3**(2):59–61 (Dec. 1976).

WHALEY, A. M. A comparison of infant sudden unexpected death syndrome with some signs of thiamine deficiency. *Journal of the International Academy of Preventive Medicine,* **3**(2):64–69 (Dec. 1976).

32 Hormones

CHAPTER
OUTLINE

Cyclic Adenosine Monophosphate
Hormones of the Gastrointestinal System
Hormones of the Pancreas
  Insulin
  Glucagon
Hormones of the Thyroid Gland
  Hypothyroidism
  Hyperthyroidism
Hormones of the Parathyroid Glands
Hormones of the Adrenal Glands
  Hormones of the Adrenal Cortex

Hormones of the Adrenal Medulla
Hormones of the Pituitary Gland
  Hormones of the Anterior Lobe
  Hormone of the Intermediate Lobe
  Hormones of the Posterior Lobe
Hormones of the Hypothalamus
The Female Sex Hormones
  Estrogenic or Follicular Hormones
  Progestational Hormones
The Male Sex Hormones
Hormones of the Kidney

Hormones exert a very important influence on the regulation of body processes. Hormones are produced in the endocrine glands and are secreted directly into the bloodstream. Hormones may be proteins, polypeptides, amino acids, or steroids.

There is an internal balance and interaction among the various endocrine glands.

Hormones act in several different ways. Some stimulate RNA production in target cell nuclei and thus increase the production of enzymes. Some hormones stimulate enzyme synthesis in the ribosomes through the translation of information carried by messenger RNA. Others are involved in the transportation of various substances across membranes. Hormones also affect the levels of c-AMP, which in turn activates many kinase enzymes (see following section). The action of most protein hormones is inhibited by an absence or a large decrease in the concentration of calcium ions.

Both vitamins and hormones are necessary in only very small amounts; however, unlike vitamins, hormones are produced in the body. Hormones are produced in a particular organ and are carried by the bloodstream to some other body part, where they cause a specific physiologic effect. The level of hormones in the bloodstream ranges from $10^{-6}\,M$ to $10^{-12}\,M$.

Cyclic Adenosine Monophosphate

Cyclic adenosine monophosphate (c-AMP) is present in almost every type of body cell. It is produced through the activity of the enzyme adenylate cyclase (found in the membranes of the cell walls) on ATP.

When a hormone, a chemical messenger, reaches its target cell, it interacts with the cell membrane and triggers the production or release of the E prostaglandins, which in turn activate the enzyme adenylate cyclase, causing the production of more c-AMP. This c-AMP, diffusing into the cell, acts as a messenger and instructs the cell to respond to the hormone in a certain characteristic manner.

The concentration of c-AMP in the cells is controlled primarily by two different methods: (1) the regulation of its rate of synthesis and (2) changing it into an inactive form, AMP, through the action of certain enzymes.

Abnormalities in the metabolism of c-AMP may explain the effects caused by certain diseases. For example, the bacteria that cause cholera produce a toxin that stimulates the intestinal cells to accumulate c-AMP. The excess c-AMP instructs the cells to secrete a salty fluid. The accumulation and subsequent loss of large amounts of this salty fluid and the resulting dehydration, if unchecked, can cause cholera to be fatal.

c-AMP activates a protein kinase that catalyzes phosphorylation and thus activates RNA polymerase. RNA polymerase, in turn, stimulates RNA production, which then functions as a messenger for protein synthesis (see page 532). In this way, c-AMP influences the synthesis of protein.

The role of c-AMP in the breakdown of liver and muscle glycogen to glucose is indicated on page 400.

The structure of c-AMP is as follows.

cyclic adenosine monophosphate, c-AMP

c-AMP is not found in plants.

A similar compound, cyclic guanosine monophosphate (c-GMP), is involved in the actions of the F prostaglandins, whose effects run counter to those of the E prostaglandins. It has been suggested that c-AMP and c-GMP function reciprocally in regulating cellular activity, but much more research needs to be done in this area.

Hormones of the Gastrointestinal System

The pyloric mucosa produces a hormone called **gastrin.** Gastrin is absorbed into the bloodstream and carried back to the stomach where it stimulates the secretion of hydrochloric acid in the gastric juice and also produces a greater motility of the stomach. Gastrin also stimulates the secretion of pepsin and the intrinsic factor (see page 387). Gastrin is a polypeptide containing 17 amino acids.

Secretin is formed in the mucosa of the small intestine when the acidic chyme enters the duodenum. Secretin stimulates the pancreas to release the pancreatic juices into the small intestine. Secretin is a polypeptide containing 27 amino acids, 14 of which are identical to those found in glucagon (page 506).

Cholecystokinin-pancreozymin (CCK-PZ) is secreted when fat enters the duodenum. CCK-PZ stimulates the contraction and emptying of the gallbladder into the small intestine. It also stimulates pancreatic enzyme secretion. CCK-PZ is a polypeptide containing 33 amino acids.

In addition to these established gastrointestinal hormones, several others have been postulated as being hormones involved in the gastrointestinal system. Among these are the following:

Enterogastrone, involved with inhibition of gastric acid secretion.
Motilin, stimulates gastric motility.
Enteroglucagon, involved in glycogenolysis.
Gastric inhibitory polypeptide (GIP), inhibits gastric acid secretion and gastric motility; stimulates release of insulin by pancreas.
Chymodenin, stimulates secretion of chymotrypsin.

Hormones of the Pancreas

The pancreas secretes digestive enzymes (see Chapter 25). It also secretes two hormones that affect carbohydrate metabolism. These hormones are insulin and glucagon.

Insulin

Insulin is a protein secreted by the beta cells of the islets of Langerhans in the pancreas. Insulin has been isolated and crystallized. Crystalline insulin contains a small amount of zinc, which it obtains from the zinc-rich tissues in the pancreas. Small amounts of chromium are also needed for the synthesis of insulin. The amount of chromium in the body decreases with age. The amino acid sequence in insulin is indicated on page 355.

Insulin increases the rate of oxidation of glucose, facilitates the conversion of glucose to glycogen in the liver and the muscles, and increases the synthesis of fatty acids, protein, and RNA. Insulin functions to decrease blood sugar to its normal fasting level after it has been increased by digestion of carbohydrates by facilitating the transportation of glucose through the membranes into the cells.

Normally, the blood sugar level rises to 120 to 160 mg per 100 ml of blood after a meal containing carbohydrates. This level is returned to its normal fasting value by the action of insulin. If the islets of Langerhans are underactive or degenerated, little or no insulin is produced, so that the blood sugar level remains high. This condition is termed hyperglycemia and is associated with diabetes mellitus. In diabetes mellitus, there is an increased blood sugar level; glucose appears in the urine, and there is formation of acetone bodies accompanied by acidosis. Injection of insulin will produce a rapid recovery from these symptoms. It will not, however, cure diabetes because these same symptoms will reappear after a short time. Thus insulin must be taken by diabetics for the rest of their lives.

Since insulin is a protein, it cannot be taken orally because it would be digested. Therefore, insulin is given by subcutaneous injection. Injections of insulin must be given two or three times a day to a patient with diabetes mellitus. However, when insulin is combined with protamine (a protein), the product, called protamine zinc insulin, is utilized much more slowly and is effective for more than 24 hr. Thus only one injection is needed daily.

Another hormone, somatostatin (see page 519), is being tried either by itself or in combination with insulin for the control of diabetes. Somatostatin inhibits the release of glucagon, one of the hormones that is responsible for maintaining high blood sugar levels.

If too large a dose of insulin is administered, the blood sugar level falls far below its normal fasting value. This condition is called hypoglycemia and is characterized by such symptoms as dizziness, nervousness, blurring of vision, and then unconsciousness. Such a state is called insulin shock and may be relieved by the administration of sugar, either orally or by injection. Hypoglycemia also occurs when there is a tumor on the islets of Langerhans in the pancreas. Insulin is degraded primarily in the liver and kidneys by the enzyme glutathione insulin transhydroxylase.

Insulin is available in sterile solutions where 1 ml contains 100 units (U-100); 1 unit of insulin is the amount required to reduce the blood sugar level of a normal 2-kg rabbit after a 24-hr fast from 120 to 45 mg per 100 ml.

Although insulin cannot be taken orally, there are certain hypoglycemic* substances that will lower blood sugar level. These substances are effective in treating adult diabetes but not juvenile diabetes. They function by stimulating the beta cells of the islets of Langerhans to produce insulin. Examples of such hypoglycemic agents are tolbutamide (Orinase) and chlorpropamide (Diabinese). The structural formula of tolbutamide is

tolbutamide

Recent evidence indicates that these so-called hypoglycemic agents have many toxic side effects. Adult patients with a mild type of diabetes frequently can control it just as well by means of a proper diet.

Glucagon When crude insulin was first used to lower blood sugar levels, it was noted that a temporary hyperglycemia occurred first and then, soon afterward, came the hypoglycemic effects expected of insulin. The unknown substance present in the crude insulin that gave the hyperglycemic effects was called the hyperglycemic-glycogenolytic factor, or HGF. This factor is now known as glucagon. Glucagon has been isolated and crystallized. It is a polypeptide containing 29 amino acids in a single chain.

Glucagon has a different arrangement of amino acids than insulin. It contains no disulfide bridges as does insulin. Glucagon contains methionine and tryptophan, which insulin does not. However, insulin contains cysteine, proline, and isoleucine, whereas glucagon does not.

Glucagon is formed in the alpha cells of the islets of Langerhans in the pancreas. Significant amounts of glucagon also come from A cells in the stomach and other parts of the GI tract.

Glucagon causes an increase in the sugar content of the blood by stimulating phosphorylase activity in the liver. The reactions involved are as follows:

$$\text{glycogen} + \text{phosphate} \xrightarrow{\text{phosphorylase}} \text{glucose-1-phosphate}$$

$$\text{glucose-1-phosphate} \xrightarrow{\text{phosphoglucomutase}} \text{glucose-6-phosphate}$$

$$\text{glucose-6-phosphate} \xrightarrow{\text{phosphatase}} \text{glucose} + \text{phosphate}$$

Glucagon increases the formation of c-AMP, which activates phosphorylase, and so increases the glucose content of the blood, causing hyperglycemia.

Glucagon stimulates the formation of glucose from amino acids (gluconeogenesis). It also increases the release of potassium ions from the liver. In the adipose tissue glucagon increases the breakdown of lipids to fatty acids and glycerol.

Glucagon has been used to treat hypoglycemic effects due to an overdose of insulin or after the inducement of insulin shock in the treatment of psychiatric patients.

Glucagon is also used in a diagnostic test for glycogen storage disease.

Hormones of the Thyroid Gland

The thyroid gland is an H-shaped gland consisting of one lobe on each side of the trachea with a piece of tissue connecting the two lobes. In the adult the thyroid gland weighs approximately 25 to 30 g.

The hormones of the thyroid gland regulate the metabolism of the body. They also affect the growth and development of the body.

The thyroid is filled with many small follicles that contain colloid. This colloid contains the thyroid gland's stored hormones. Actually, the thyroid is the only endocrine gland in the body that is capable of storing appreciable amounts of hormone.

The thyroid gland contains the element iodine—one of the elements necessary for the proper functioning of the body. Iodine is found in the body in two different forms: as iodide ions and in the thyroid hormones.

Older, indirect methods for evaluating thyroid activity such as basal metabolic rate (BMR), protein-bound iodine (PBI), and butanol extractable iodine (BEI) have been replaced by radioimmunoassay methods that are direct and more reliable.

The colloid of the thyroid contains the protein **thyroglobin,** a glycoprotein. This protein liberates **triiodothyronine** and **thyroxine,** the principal thyroid hormones. T_3 is the major active form of the thyroid hormone and is three to five times as biologically active as T_4. Some mono- and diiodotyrosine are also formed, but these compounds are quickly deiodinated in the bloodstream and the freed iodine is used to form more thyroglobin. The structures of these hormones are

thyroxine (T_4)

triiodothyronine (T_3)

The C cells in the thyroid gland produce the hormone calcitonin (thyrocalcitonin), which, along with the parathyroid hormone, regulates the calcium ions in the blood. It has been shown that the parathyroid hormone sustains the blood supply of calcium ions whereas calcitonin prevents the blood calcium ion concentration from rising above the required level.

Pure calcitonin was first isolated in 1968 and its structure determined shortly thereafter. This hormone is a polypepetide containing a single chain of 32 amino acids. Calcitonin has now been synthesized in the laboratory, and its mode of action in the body has been investigated. It produces its effect by inhibiting the release of calcium ions from the bone to the blood. The release of calcitonin is stimulated by high levels of Ca^{2+} in the blood.

Medullary thyroid carcinoma, a disorder of the C cells of the thyroid, causes an abnormally high production of calcitonin.

Hypothyroidism   Hypothyroidism refers to a condition in which the thyroid gland does not manufacture sufficient thyroxine for the body's needs. It is usually due to a lack of iodine in the diet, particularly in parts of the country where the water and foods contain litle iodine. Hypothyroidism may also be due to a disease of the thyroid gland or to its congenital absence.

The symptoms of hypothyroidism are sluggishness, gain of weight, slower heartbeat, reduced metabolic rate, and loss of appetite. Hypothyroidism is easily remedied by the use of iodized salts as part of the normal diet.

CRETINISM   If the thyroid gland is absent or fails to develop in an infant, the effects produced are called cretinism and the individual is called a cretin. Cretins have a greatly retarded growth, both physically and mentally. They are

Biochemistry

usually abnormal dwarfs with coarse hair, thick dry skin, obese with pro-truding abdomens. They are also underdeveloped mentally and sexually.

A cretin may develop normally if given thyroid hormones before he or she reaches adulthood (see Figure 32-1).

If the thyroid gland should atrophy after an individual reaches adulthood, the same symptoms as in cretinism appear, except that the individual remains adult in size. One very noticeable symptom is in the development of thick, coarse, dry skin. Such a condition is known as **myxedema.*** Persons with myxedema are also sluggish, have a lower pulse and metabolic rate, lower body temperature and are frequently anemic. They are also very sensitive to cold.

Myxedema may usually be cured by the administration of thyroxine.

SIMPLE GOITER   Simple goiter,* also called colloid goiter or endemic goiter, is a condition in which the thyroid gland enlarges, usually because of a lack of iodine in

FIGURE 32-1. Cretin B is much shorter than her twin A. After therapy with thyroid hormones the difference, although present, is greatly reduced. (Courtesy of Warner-Chilcott Laboratories, Morris Planes, N.J.)

the diet. The decreased production of thyroid hormones causes an increased production of TSH, the thyroid-stimulating hormone, which in turn over-stimulates the thyroid gland. Simple goiter is accompanied by a definite increase in the amount of colloid material in the thyroid gland and also an increase in the size of the neck itself.

Simple goiter occurs in areas where there is a deficiency of iodine in the food and drinking water. The condition may be successfully prevented or cured by the addition of iodine compounds (usually iodized salt) to the diet.

HASHIMOTO'S DISEASE   Hashimoto's disease is a type of hypothyroidism in which all aspects of thyroid function may be impaired. This disease is caused by an attack on the thyroid gland by the body's own immune system.

Hyperthyroidism   Hyperthyroidism occurs when the thyroid gland produces excess thyroxine. The symptoms are an increased metabolic rate, bulging of the eyes (exophthalmos), nervousness, loss of weight, a rapid, irregular heartbeat and an elevated body temperature. Such a condition is also called Graves' disease, Basedow's disease, or exophthalmic goiter. Hyperthyroidism may also be due to a tumor in the thyroid gland (toxic adenoma or Plummer's disease).

Hyperthyroidism may be controlled or cured by surgical removal of part of the thyroid gland, by the oral administration of radioactive iodine, or by the use of antithyroid drugs. Hypertrophy of endocrine glands may lead to toxic adenomas with a malignant potential if not treated promptly.

Radioactive iodine, used in the treatment of hyperthyroidism, is usually administered in the form of sodium iodide, NaI. The body coverts the inorganic radioactive iodide into thyroglobin in the thyroid gland, thus subjecting that gland to radiation that will cut down its activity.

Hormones of the Parathyroid Glands   There are four small parathyroid glands attached to the thyroid gland. In humans these glands are reddish brown and together weigh 0.05 to 0.3 g. In early experimental thyroidectomies (removal of the thyroid glands) in animals, the parathyroid glands were also inadvertently removed. This caused the death of the animals.

The parathyroid glands produce **parathyroid hormone,** a hormone that influences the metabolism of calcium and phosphorus in the body. This hormone is a protein with a molecular weight of approximately 9500 and consists of a single polypeptide chain of 84 amino acids. The parathyroid gland cannot store this hormone, so it is synthesized and secreted continuously. Recall that calcitonin (page 508) is also involved in the regulation of calcium. Administration of vitamin A decreases parathyroid hormone, possibly by increasing calcium uptake into the parathyroid gland.

Surgical removal of the parathyroid glands causes **hypoparathyroidism,** characterized by such symptoms as muscular weakness, irritability, and tetany owing to a decrease in the calcium content of the blood plasma. Death occurs because of convulsions caused by the lack of calcium. At the same time as the calcium content of the plasma is decreasing, the calcium content of the urine is also decreasing and the phosphate content of the plasma is increasing.

The symptoms of hypoparathyroidism may be relieved by treatment with vitamin D or calcium salts, or both.

Hyperparathyroidism is an increase in the production of hormones by the parathyroid glands. It is usually due to a tumor of that gland (parathyroid adenoma) and produces such symptoms as decalcification of the bones followed by deformation and fractures of these bones, nausea, and polyuria. Deposits of calcium occur in soft tissues and renal stones frequently occur.

In hyperparathyroidism, the calcium content of the blood plasma is high and the phosphate content low. The extra calcium in the blood is obtained by withdrawal of that element from the bones, thus causing those bones to become decalcified. Urine calcium, phosphate, and c-AMP are increased.

Hyperparathyroidism is usually treated by the surgical removal of the tumor of the parathyroid glands.

Hormones of the Adrenal Glands

The adrenal (suprarenal) glands are located close to the upper pole of the kidneys and weigh about 3 to 6 g each. The adrenal glands are divided into two distinct portions: the cortex, which is the outer portion, and the medulla, which is the inner portion (see Figure 32-2). Each of these portions is distinct both structurally and physiologically and each produces its own hormones.

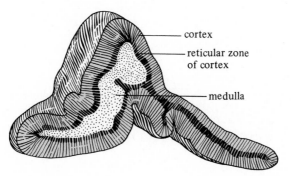

FIGURE 32-2. Adrenal glands showing cortex and medulla.

Hormones of the Adrenal Cortex

The hormones of the adrenal cortex are steroid in nature and fall into three categories:

1. **Glucocorticoids,** which primarily affect the metabolism of carbohydrates, lipids, and protein. Examples are corticosterone, cortisone (11-dehydroxycorticosterone), and cortisol (hydrocortisone).
2. **Mineralocorticoids,** which primarily affect the transportation of electrolytes and the distribution of water in the tissues. The most potent of this group is aldosterone.
3. **Androgens** or **estrogens,** which primarily affect secondary sex characteristics. The principal androgen is dehydroepiandrosterone.

The steroids of the adrenal cortex function in the cell nucleus for the synthesis of RNA and protein. The steroid nucleus contains four fused carbon rings, numbered as indicated in formula (32-1).

steroid nucleus

(32–1)

corticosterone

cortisone

cortisol

aldosterone

dehydroepiandrosterone

EFFECT OF A DEFICIENCY OF THE HORMONES OF THE ADRENAL CORTEX

If the adrenal glands are removed from an animal, it will soon die because of a lack of the hormones produced by the adrenal cortex. In humans, a hypofunctioning of the adrenal glands, because of a tuberculosis of those glands or in association with pernicious anemia, diabetes, or hypothyroidism, results in Addison's disease. It is characterized by an excessive loss of sodium chloride in the urine, low blood pressure, low body temperature, hypoglycemia, elevation of serum potassium, muscular weakness, a progressive brownish pigmentation of the skin, nausea, and loss of appetite.

The preceding symptoms, except for the pigmentation, are owing to a lack of the salt- and water-regulating hormones—the mineralocorticoids, primarily aldosterone. These hormones stimulate the kidney tubules to reabsorb sodium ions. If there is a lack of these hormones, sodium ions are not reabsorbed and are eliminated in the urine. Along with the sodium ions, chloride ions are also eliminated so that the urine is abnormally high in sodium chloride. Accompanying the sodium chloride loss by the body is a loss of water through osmosis. This loss in water in turn decreases both blood volume and blood pressure. The blood becomes more concentrated and excretion of urea, uric acid, and creatinine is decreased, thereby increasing the concentration of these substances in the blood. Dehydration occurs rapidly and death occurs from circulatory collapse.

Another function of the hormones of the adrenal cortex is to stimulate the process of gluconeogenesis, the formation of glucose from amino acids. This process takes place in the liver. In the absence of the adrenocortical hormones, the *glucocorticoids,* the blood sugar falls and the glycogen stored in the liver and the muscles decreases considerably.

All of these symptoms may be relieved, except the skin discoloration, by the use of cortisonelike compounds—either naturally occurring extracts or synthetically prepared ones.

EFFECTS OF HYPERACTIVITY OF THE ADRENAL CORTEX

Hyperactivity of the adrenal cortex (hyperadrenocorticism) is caused by a tumor on the adrenal cortex, by an overdosage of cortisone or ACTH, or by an increased production of ACTH (see page 516).

In children, hyperactivity of the adrenal cortex is manifested by early sexual development. Hyperactivity of the adrenal cortex in the adult female, which occurs more often than in the adult male, causes a decrease in feminine characteristics. The voice deepens, the breasts decrease in size, the uterus atrophies, and hair appears on the face. In the adult male, hyperactivity of the adrenal cortex is manifested by an increase in male characteristics—an increase in amount of body hair, increased size of sex organs, deeper voice.

Other effects of hyperadrenocorticism are hyperglycemia and glycosuria, retention of sodium ions and water, increased blood volume, edema, depletion of potassium ions (hypokalemia), and excessive gluconeogenesis.

Hormones of the Adrenal Medulla

Even though the medulla of the adrenal glands secretes two hormones—**epinephrine** (adrenaline) and **norepinephrine** (noradrenaline)—it is not essential to human life. That is, it may be removed without causing death. Norepinephrine is a precursor of epinephrine. The structure of these two hormones is

norepinephrine   epinephrine

The D form of these hormones is much more physiologically active than the L form. Epinephrine produces several marked effects on the body.

1. It relaxes the smooth muscles of the stomach, intestines, bronchioles, and bladder. This relaxing effect on the muscles of the bronchioles makes epinephrine especially useful in the treatment of asthma and hay fever.

2. It elevates blood pressure by stimulating the action of the heart and also by constricting the arterioles of the skin and dilating the arterioles of the skeletal muscles. Epinephrine is sometimes used during minor surgery when it is administered along with a local anesthetic. The constriction of the arterioles by epinephrine prevents the anesthetic from spreading too rapidly from the site of the injection. Epinephrine can be injected directly into the heart muscle when that organ stops beating or when it does not start to beat in a newborn baby.

3. It causes glycogenolysis in the liver and skeletal muscle, producing a rise in blood sugar level. This effect is due to the activation of adenylate cyclase, which increases the production of c-AMP. c-AMP, in turn, activates a protein kinase, which results in increased phosphorylation, thus catalyzing glycogenolysis in the liver. Epinephrine production is increased during anxiety, fear, or other stress. This extra epinephrine in turn causes a rise in blood sugar, frequently exceeding the renal threshold. In this case, glucose appears in the urine. Such a condition is called emotional glycosuria and disappears as soon as the stress is relieved.

Norepinephrine raises blood pressure by constricting the arterioles. It does not affect the heart itself and does not relax the muscles of the bronchioles as does epinephrine. Norepinephrine is found in the sympathetic nerves where it acts as a neurotransmitter.

The medulla of the adrenal glands rarely becomes diseased. To date, no deficiency effects of its hormones are known. However, certain tumors of the medulla of the adrenal glands stimulate these glands to produce excess hormones. The symptoms caused are intermittent hypertension leading to permanent hypertension and eventually to death from such complications as coronary insufficiency, ventricular fibrillation, and pulmonary edema.

Hormones of the Pituitary Gland

The pituitary gland (**hypophysis**) is located at the base of the brain. It consists of two parts: the anterior and intermediate lobes (the **adenohypophysis**) and the posterior lobe (the **neurohypophysis**). Each of these parts secretes or parts secretes or releases its own hormones. The pituitary gland has often been called the "master gland" of the body because it seemed to exert a direct influence upon most of the other endocrine glands. It is now known that almost all of the secretory activity of the pituitary gland is controlled by a small area of the brain known as the **hypothalamus** (see Figure 32–3).

Hormones of the Anterior Lobe

Six hormones have been isolated from the anterior lobe of the pituitary gland:

1. Growth hormone (GH)
2. Thyrotropic hormone (TSH)
3. Adrenocorticotropic hormone (ACTH)
4. Lactogenic hormone (LTH)

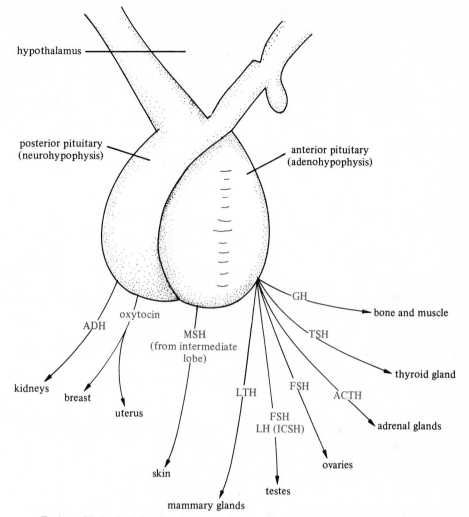

FIGURE 32–3. Relationship between hypothalamus and the pituitary gland.

5. Luteinizing hormone (LH), also known as the interstitial cell-stimulating hormone (ICSH)
6. Follicle-stimulating hormone (FSH)

GROWTH HORMONE   Growth hormone (GH), also called somatotropin, is a protein with a molecular weight of about 21,500 and containing 191 amino acids. It is present in much higher quantities than other pituitary hormones. Growth hormone stimulates the growth of the long bones at the epiphyses, stimulates the growth of soft tissue, and increases the retention of calcium ions. The growth hormone also increases protein synthesis, leading to a positive nitrogen balance. In the muscle, growth hormone increases amino acid transportation across membranes, also leading to increased protein, DNA, and RNA syn-

Hormones   **515**

thesis. Growth hormone causes mobilization of fatty acids from fat deposits, providing cellular fuel. In the muscles, growth hormone antagonizes the effects of insulin; it inhibits glucose metabolism by muscle tissue.

Growth hormone also stimulates the mammary glands and increases the production of somatomedins from the liver. Somatomedins, in turn, foster sulfate incorporation into the cartilage.

Underactivity of the anterior lobe of the pituitary gland in children leads to a deficiency of the growth hormone, causing dwarfism. These children develop normally but do not grow in size. Unlike cretins, they are not mentally retarded, but they may be sexually underdeveloped.

An overactivity of the anterior lobe of the pituitary gland, possibly due to a tumor, results in an overproduction of growth hormone. When this occurs in a child, growth is stimulated and gigantism results. If the overactivity of this gland occurs during adulthood, the individual does not grow in size but the bones in the hands, feet, and face grow, producing a condition known as acromegaly.*

Secretion of growth hormone is regulated by the growth hormone-releasing factor (GHRF) from the hypothalamus.

THYROTROPIC HORMONE

The thyrotropic hormone is also called the thyroid-stimulating hormone, hence, the abbreviation TSH. This hormone is a glycoprotein with a molecular weight of approximately 30,000. The release of TSH from the pituitary gland is regulated by TRF, the thyrotropic-releasing factor, from the hypothalamus.

A deficiency of TSH causes the thyroid gland to atrophy. As a result, thyroxine production ceases with a consequent drop in metabolic rate.

If this hormone is injected into an animal, the symptoms of hyperthyroidism appear—increased metabolic rate, increased heart rate, and exophthalmos.*

ADRENOCORTICO-TROPIC HORMONE

The adrenocorticotropic hormone (ACTH) is a polypeptide with a molecular weight of 4500. ACTH contains 39 amino acids, but it has been shown that only the first 23 are required for activity. The remaining 16 vary according to the animal source. The release of ACTH by the pituitary gland appears to be regulated by the corticotropin-releasing factor (CRF) of the hypothalamus in response to various biologic stresses. ACTH has been prepared synthetically and is used medically.

ACTH stimulates the synthesis and release of the hormones by the adrenal cortex. ACTH, as do many other hormones, controls its target tissue through c-AMP. Administration of ACTH to a normal person causes retention of sodium ions, chloride ions, and water, elevation of blood sugar, and increased excretion of potassium ions, nitrogen, phosphorus, and uric acid.

LACTOGENIC HORMONE (PROLACTIN) OR LUTEOTROPIN (LTH)

This hormone was first identified by its property of stimulating the formation of "crop milk" in the crop glands of pigeons. The arrangement of the amino acids in prolactin has been determined. It is a protein with a molecular weight of about 23,000.

Prolactin initiates lactation. In mammals, a hormone produced by the placenta stimulates the growth of the mammary glands and, at the same time, inhibits the secretion of prolactin. At parturition the inhibiting effect of the placenta is not present so that prolactin is secreted and thus initiates lactation.

GONADOTROPIC HORMONES

The gonadotropic hormones LH and FSH (and also prolactin) are secreted by the anterior lobe of the pituitary gland. Removal of the anterior lobe in a male causes atrophy of the testes, prostate gland, and seminal vesicles. Removal in a female causes atrophy of the ovaries, uterus, and fallopian tubes.

LH and FSH as well as TSH consist of an α and a β chain of amino acids. The α chain is the same in all three, so that biologic specificity must reside in the β chain. Both LH and FSH stimulate c-AMP synthesis in appropriate target organs.

LUTEINIZING HORMONE (LH)

LH is also known as the interstitial cell-stimulating hormone (ICSH). This hormone is a glycoprotein with a molecular weight of about 40,000. It is the first pituitary gonadotropin whose sequence of amino acids has been precisely determined.

LH stimulates the development of the testes in males and also causes an increased production of testosterone. In male animals who have had the pituitary gland surgically removed (hypophysectomy), administration of LH increases the weight of the seiminal vesicles and also of the ventral lobe of the prostate gland.

In females, LH plays an important role in causing ovulation. It not only causes the production of the corpus luteum but sustains it and stimulates the production of progesterone. In hypophysectomized females, an injection of LH stimulates repair of interstitial ovarian tissues and also increases ovarian weight.

FOLLICLE-STIMULATING HORMONE (FSH)

FSH is a glycoprotein with a molecular weight of 25,000. It stimulates and initiates the development of the follicles of the ovary and prepares those follicles for the action of LH. It also stimulates the secretion of estrogen. In males it causes the growth of the testes and stimulates the production of spermatozoa.

Hormone of the Intermediate Lobe

The pars intermedia or intermediate lobe of the pituitary gland secretes a hormone called **intermedin** or the **melanocyte-stimulating hormone** (MSH). It is a polypeptide with alpha and beta parts.

MSH increases the deposition of melanin in the human skin, thus producing darker pigmentation. When the adrenal cortex is underactive, as in Addison's disease, more MSH is produced. This leads to an increased synthesis of melanin with the accompanying brown pigmentation of the skin. Epinephrine and, even more strongly, norepinephrine inhibit the action of the melanocyte-stimulating hormone.

Hormones of the Posterior Lobe

The posterior lobe of the pituitary gland contains two hormones—**vasopressin** and **oxytocin**—which are produced in the hypothalamus and stored in this lobe of the pituitary gland.

VASOPRESSIN

Vasopressin, also called the antidiuretic hormone (ADH), stimulates the kidneys to reabsorb water. When the water content of the body is high, very little of this hormone is secreted so that more water is eliminated. Conversely, when the water content of the body is low, more of this hormone is secreted, causing the kidney tubules to reabsorb more water. Thus, this hormone serves to regulate the water balance in the body.

Diabetes insipidus (see page 438) is caused by the absence of the antidiuretic hormone, which causes excess daily elimination of water (up to 30 L). Diabetes insipidus may be controlled by the administration of ADH.

Vasopressin, ADH, stimulates the peripheral blood vessels to constrict and causes an increase in blood pressure. Because of this effect, it has been used to overcome low blood pressure caused by shock following surgery.

Vasopressin is a polypeptide whose arrangement of amino acids is indicated below.

$$
\begin{array}{c}
\text{Cys—Tyr— Phe} \\
\quad| \qquad\qquad\; | \\
\text{Cys—Asn—Gln} \\
\quad| \\
\text{Pro—Arg—Gly}
\end{array}
$$

vasopressin

OXYTOCIN   Oxytocin is also a polypeptide whose structure is similar to that of vasopressin except that isoleucine occurs in place of phenylalanine, and leucine in place of arginine.

Oxytocin contracts the muscles of the uterus and also stimulates the ejection of milk from the mammary glands. Oxytocin is used in obstetrics when uterine contraction is desired.

Hormones of the Hypothalamus

The hypothalamus secretes certain neurohormones, some of which act as stimulators and others as inhibitors for the secretion of hormones by the anterior pituitary. These hormones are also called **releasing hormones** or **factors**. They have a relatively short life span in the bloodstream. Their half-life is about 2 to 3 min compared to 10 to 15 min for the growth hormone. Therefore, levels of releasing factors are 100 to 1000 times lower in the bloodstream than for the growth hormone.

The first of the hypothalamic hormones to be isolated (and later synthesized) was the thyrotropic-releasing hormone (TRH), also known as the thyrotropic-releasing factor (TRF), which controls the release of the thyroid-stimulating hormone (TSH). TRH is a tripeptide containing three amino acids: glutamic acid, histidine, and proline. The structure of TRH is

TRH, pyroglutamylhistidylproline amide

TRH is highly specific and causes an increase of TSH within 1 min. It may be administered orally. TRH is used to distinguish between lesions in the pituitary and the hypothalamus. TRH also affects the central nervous system. Synthetic analogs of TRH have been prepared that enhance the effect on the central nervous system while not affecting the thyrotropin-releasing influence.

The second hypothalamic releasing factor that was isolated was the luteinizing hormone releasing hormone (factor), LH-RH, which controls the release of the leuteinizing hormone from the anterior pituitary. It is a decapeptide (10 amino acid chain), whose amino acid sequence is

$$\text{Glu-His-Trp-Ser-Tyr-Gly-Leu-Arg-Pro-Gly}$$

An injection of LH-RH causes an increase in circulating LH in 1 to 2 min. LH-RH also increases the amount of FSH and so may be identical with the follicle-stimulating hormone releasing hormone (factor), FSH-RH.

Another releasing factor is corticotropin (ACTH) releasing hormone, CRH, which has recently been synthesized. It contains 41 amino acids. Other releasing factors are growth hormone releasing hormone (factor), GH-RH; prolactin releasing hormone, PRH; melanocyte-stimulating hormone releasing hormone (factor), MRH, and follicle-stimulating hormone releasing hormone (factor), FSH-RH. The structures of these hormones have not been determined although they appear to be simple peptides.

In addition to the releasing factors, the hypothalamus also contains **release-inhibiting factors**—hormones that inhibit the release of the "releasing factors."

Among the release-inhibiting factors are the growth hormone release-inhibiting factor, GH-RIH (GIF). GIF, also called somatostatin, is a tetradecapeptide (14 amino acid chain). This factor inhibits the release of the growth hormone. GIF also inhibits the release of insulin (see page 506), glucagon, gastrin, TSH, and FSH.

Release-inhibiting factors whose structures have not been determined are prolactin release-inhibiting factor, PRIH or PIF, melanocyte-stimulating hormone release-inhibiting factor, MRIH or MIF, and follicle-stimulating hormone release-inhibiting factor (FSH-RIH or FSH-RIF). Other release-inhibiting factors have been postulated but have not been isolated or identified.

The hypothalamus also produces two hormones that are stored in and secreted by the posterior lobe of the pituitary gland. They are the antidiuretic hormone (ADH) and oxytocin (see page 518).

In addition the hypothalamus contains polypeptides called **endorphins.** One of these compounds, β-endorphin, exhibits morphinelike activity in the brain and has been used in the treatment of psychiatric patients. The α- and γ-endorphins have not yet been tried on humans, but in rats α-endorphin produced analgesia whereas γ-endorphin induced violent behavior.

A subclass of the endorphins is the **enkephalins,** which are pentapeptides. However, the enkephalins act separately in the body instead of in conjunction with the endorphins.

Two predominant enkephalins in the brain differ only in the end amino acid:

Tyr-Gly-Gly-Phe-Leu leucine enkephalin
Tyr-Gly-Gly-Phe-Met methionine enkephalin

Morphine and other opiates (see page 288) bind to opiate receptors in the brain. Endorphins and enkephalins also bind to these same receptors.

The enkephalins are involved with the sensation of pain. It is believed that enkephalins bind to the opiate receptors and prevent the transmission of pain impulses. Morphine also binds to opiate receptors and increases the pain-killing effect of enkephalins.

Opiates such as morphine are addictive. Why? In the cells, the synthesis of c-AMP (see page 503) is catalyzed by the enzyme adenylate cyclase. Opiates and enkephalins inhibit the production of this enzyme so that the amount of c-AMP in the cells decreases. Therefore, the cells try to compensate by synthesizing more of the enzyme. When this occurs, more opiate must be used in order to have the same pain-killing effect. Eventually, the body will adjust to the new amount of opiate and again c-AMP will begin to increase. So, the addict requires more and more of the drug.

Conversely, if the opiate is withdrawn, the synthesis of adenylate cyclase is no longer inhibited and large amounts of c-AMP are produced. It is the high concentration of c-AMP that produces the symptoms of withdrawal.

The increased production of endorphins at about 20 to 30 min into a run may be responsible for a "runner's high" and for the addiction to running experienced by many runners.

It is believed that acupuncture works by triggering nerve impulses that stimulate the release of endorphins and enkephalins.

The Female Sex Hormones

The ovary secretes two different types of hormones. The follicles of the ovary secrete the follicular or estrogenic hormones. The corpus luteum that forms in the ovary from the ruptured follicle secretes the progestational hormones.

Estrogenic or Follicular Hormones

The maturing follicles of the ovaries produce the estrogenic hormones, which are also called **estrogens.** These hormones are **estradiol, estrone,** and **estriol.** Of these three hormones, estradiol is the parent compound and also the most active. The other two hormones are derived from estradiol. Estriol is the main estrogen found in the urine of pregnant women and also in the placenta. Estrone is in metabolic equilibrium with estradiol. Note the similarities of structures of these three hormones. One international unit (1 IU) of estrogen activity is equal to 0.1 mg of estrone.

Estradiol, estrone, and estriol are concerned with the maturation of the eggs (ova) and the maintenance of the secondary sex characteristics. In lower animals, the estrogens produce estrus, the urge for mating. The estrogens also suppress production of FSH, the follicle-stimulating hormone, by the pituitary gland. FSH initially starts the development of the follicle. Once

estrone

estradiol

estriol

the follicle begins to develop, further production of FSH is not needed and is inhibited by the estrogenic hormones. However, the estrogenic hormones stimulate the production of LH, the luteinizing hormone.

Synthetic estrogens such as diethylstilbestrol and ethinyl estradiol have been developed. These synthetics may be given orally, but naturally occurring estrogens are destroyed in the digestive tract. Estrogens may be used in treatment of underdeveloped female characteristics.

diethylstilbestrol

ethinyl estradiol

Progestational Hormones The corpus luteum is produced in the follicle after the matured ovum is discharged into the uterus. The corpus luteum produces a hormone called **progesterone.** This hormone causes development of the endometrium of the uterus, preparing the uterus to receive and maintain the ovum, and it stimulates the mammary gland. Progesterone inhibits estrus, ovulation, and the production of LH, the hormone that initially stimulated ovulation, which led to the formation and maintenance of the corpus luteum. If the ovum is not fertilized, the corpus luteum breaks down and menstruation follows. If the ovum is fertilized, progesterone from the corpus luteum aids in the development of the placenta.

Progesterone is excreted as **pregnanediol** and found in the urine.

Hormones

521

progesterone   pregnanediol

In addition to progesterone, the corpus luteum also produces another hormone, **relaxin,** which is a polypeptide with a molecular weight of 5521. Relaxin also occurs in the placenta. It causes ligaments of the symphysis pubis to distend, increases dilation of the cervix in pregnant women at parturition, and also helps, along with estrogen and progesterone, to maintain gestation.

The Male Sex Hormones

Male hormones are produced primarily in the testes, although small amounts are also produced in the adrenal glands. The male hormones are called **androgens.** The principal male hormone is **testosterone.** This hormone is changed to another hormone, **androsterone.** Both are found in the urine. Androsterone is used as the international unit of androgen activity; 1 IU is equal to 0.1 mg of androsterone.

testosterone   androsterone

The male hormones are responsible for the development of the male sex organs and the secondary male characteristics. Note that the structures of the male sex hormones are similar to those of the female sex hormones. Both are derived from a common substance, cholesterol.

Hormones of the Kidney

In addition to their excretory function, the kidneys act as endocrine glands. Among the hormones produced by the kidneys are **renin** (see page 380), which increases the force of the heartbeat and constricts the arterioles, and **erythropoietin** and **erythrogenin,** which causes the bone marrow to stimulate the production of red blood cells. The kidneys play an important role in the activation of vitamin D (see page 484). The kidneys also produce prostaglandins PGE_1, PGE_2, PGE_{20}, and possibly others. PGE_1 antagonizes the effects of vasopressin; PGE_2 increases excretion of sodium; and PGE_{20} decreases venous tone.

Summary   Hormones are produced in the body's endocrine glands and secreted directly into the bloodstream, which carries them to the body parts on which they produce their effects.

Cyclic adenosine monophosphate (c-AMP) acts as a messenger that instructs the cells to respond to a particular hormone.

The pyloric mucosa produces gastrin, which stimulates the secretion of hydrochloric acid and also produces a greater motility of the stomach.

The mucosa of the small intestine produces secretin, which stimulates the pancreas to release the pancreatic juices, and cholecystokinin-pancreozymin, which stimulates the contraction and emptying of the gallbladder.

The pancreas secretes insulin, which increases the rate of oxidation of glucose and also facilitates the conversion of glucose to glycogen in the liver and the muscles.

The pancreas also secretes glucagon, which causes an increase in blood sugar content by stimulating phosphorylase activity in the liver.

The hormones of the thyroid gland regulate the metabolism of the body and also affect the growth and development of the body. The thyroid hormones contain the element iodine. The hormonal iodine carried by the blood is termed protein-bound iodine, or PBI. Hypothyroidism occurs when the thyroid gland does not manufacture sufficient thyroxine. The symptoms of hypothyroidism are sluggishness, gain in weight, slower heartbeat, reduced metabolic rate, and loss of appetite.

If the thyroid gland is absent or fails to develop in an infant, the effect produced is called cretinism. If the thyroid gland in an adult should atrophy, the effect produced is called myxedema. If the thyroid gland enlarges, the condition is called simple goiter.

If the thyroid gland produces excess thyroxine, hyperthyroidism results; the symptoms are increased metabolic rate, bulging of the eye, nervousness, loss of weight, and a rapid, irregular heartbeat. Certain drugs may be given to counteract the effects of an overactive thyroid gland.

Another hormone of the thyroid gland, calcitonin, keeps the calcium concentration of the blood from becoming too high by inhibiting the release of calcium ions from the bone.

The parathyroid glands produce a hormone, parathormone, which influences the metabolism of calcium and phosphorus in the body.

The adrenal glands are divided into two portions: the cortex and the medulla.

The hormones of the adrenal cortex are divided into three categories: the glucocorticoids, which primarily affect the metabolism of carbohydrate, fat, and protein; the mineralocorticoids, which primarily affect the transportation of electrolytes and the distribution of water in the body; and the androgens or estrogens, which primarily affect secondary sex characteristics. A hypofunctioning of the adrenal glands produces Addison's disease, which is characterized by an excessive loss of NaCl in the urine, low blood pressure, elevation of serum potassium, muscular weakness, brownish pigmentation of the skin, nausea, and loss of appetite.

The medulla of the adrenal glands secretes epinephrine and norepinephrine. Norepinephrine is a precursor of epinephrine. Epinephrine relaxes the smooth muscles, elevates blood pressure, and causes glycogenolysis in the liver.

The pituitary gland consists of two parts: the anterior and posterior lobes. The flow of hormones from the pituitary gland is under the control of the hypothalamus.

The hormones of the anterior lobe of the pituitary gland are the growth hormone (GH), the thyrotropic hormone (TSH), the adrenocorticotropic hormone (ACTH), lactogenic hormone (LTH), luteinizing hormone (LH), and follicle-stimulating hormone (FSH).

The posterior lobe of the pituitary secretes the hormones vasopressin and oxytocin. Vasopressin stimulates the kidneys to reabsorb water. Oxytocin contracts the muscles of the uterus and stimulates the ejection of milk from the mammary glands.

The pars intermedia of the pituitary gland secretes the hormone intermedin, which increases the deposition of melanin in the skin.

The hypothalamus secretes neurohormones, some of which stimulate and others of which inhibit the secretion of hormones by the anterior pituitary.

The ovaries secrete two different types of hormones. The follicles secrete the follicular or estrogenic hormones. The corpus luteum that forms in the ovary from the ruptured follicle secretes the protestational hormones.

The male sex hormones are produced in the testes. The principal male hormone is testosterone. Both male and female sex hormones are derived from cholesterol.

The hypothalamus also contains endorphins and enkephalins, which have morphinelike activity.

The kidneys, in addition to their excretory function, also act as endocrine glands.

Questions and Problems

1. Compare hormones with vitamins.
2. In what different ways can hormones act?
3. Where is gastrin produced? What is its function?
4. Where is secretin formed? What is the function of secretin? of CCK-PZ?
5. What hormones are produced by the pancreas?
6. Insulin contains what metallic element?
7. Why can insulin not be taken orally?
8. What is protamine zinc insulin?
9. What are the functions of insulin in carbohydrate metabolism?
10. What is hyperglycemia?
11. Will insulin cure diabetes mellitus? Why?
12. What might cause hypoglycemia? What will relieve such a symptom?
13. What is the function of glucagon?
14. What unusual element is found in the thyroid gland?
15. List the symptoms of diabetes mellitus.
16. List the symptoms of hyperthyroidism.
17. What is a cretin? How may this defect be overcome?
18. What causes myxedema?
19. What are the symptoms of a goiter?
20. What are the symptoms of hypothyroidism?
21. What function do the parathyroid hormones perform?
22. What are the symptoms of hypoparathyroidism? of hyperparathyroidism?
23. What three types of hormones are produced by the adrenal cortex? What is their function? Give an example of each.
24. What causes Addison's disease?
25. Indicate the symptoms of a lack of the adrenocortical hormones.
26. What are the effects of hyperadrenocorticism?
27. What are the hormones of the medulla of the adrenal glands? What is the function of each?
28. List the hormones of the anterior lobe of the pituitary gland. What is the function of each?
29. Compare dwarfism with cretinism.
30. What are the symptoms of an overactive anterior lobe of the pituitary gland?
31. What are the hormones of the posterior lobe of the pituitary gland? What is the function of each?

32. What is MSH? Where is it formed? What is its function?
33. What types of hormones are produced by the hypothalamus? What do they do?
34. What type of structure do the hypothalamic hormones have?
35. Where are the estrogenic hormones produced? the progestational hormones?
36. Where are the male sex hormones produced?
37. Why is the pituitary gland no longer considered to be "the master gland" of the body?
38. Where are vasopressin and oxytocin produced? stored?
39. How do enkephalins prevent transmission of pain?
40. Why are opiates addictive?
41. Why does acupuncture work?
42. What hormones are produced by the kidneys? What are their functions?
43. What role does *c*-AMP play in the cells? *c*-GMP?

References

CHEUNG, WAI YIU. Calmodulin. *Scientific American,* **246:**62–81 (Jan. 1982).

GUILLEMIN, R., and R. BURGUS. The hormones of the hypothalamus. *Scientific American,* **227:**24–33 (Nov. 1972).

GUILLEMIN, R., R. BURGUS, and W. VALE. The hypothalamic hypophysiotropic thyrotropin releasing factor (TRF). *Vitamins and Hormones,* **29:**1 (1971).

IVERSON, L. The chemistry of the brain. *Scientific American,* **241:**134–149 (Sept. 1979).

LLINAS, RUDOLFO R. Calcium in synaptic transmission. *Scientific American,* **247:**56–65 (Oct. 1982).

MARTIN, D. W., P. A. MAYES, and V. W. RODWELL. *Harper's Review of Biochemistry,* 19th ed. Lange Medical Publications, Los Altos, Calif., 1983, Chapters 34–36.

MCEWEN, B. S. Interactions between hormones and nerve tissue. *Scientific American,* **235:**48–58 (July 1976).

NATHANSON, J. A., and P. GREENGADR. Second messengers in the brain. *Scientific American,* **237:**108–119 (Aug. 1977).

O'MALLEY, B. W., and W. T. SCHRADER. The receptors of steroid hormones. *Scientific American,* **234:**32–43 (Feb. 1976).

PETERSON, R. E., and R. GUILLEMIN. The hormones of the hypothalamus. *American Journal of Medicine,* **57:**591–600 (Oct. 1974).

RUBENSTEIN, E. Diseases caused by impaired communication among cells. *Scientific American,* **242:**102–121 (March 1980).

SNYDER, S. H. Opiate receptors and internal opiates. *Scientific American,* **236:**44–56 (March 1977).

33 Heredity

C H A P T E R
O U T L I N E

Nucleic Acids
  Heterocyclic Bases
  The Adenosine Phosphates
The Watson–Crick Model of DNA
The DNA Code
Replication of DNA
Transfer of Information
The Triplet Code
Decoding the Code
  Regulation of Protein Synthesis
Mutations
Genetic Diseases

Consequences of Inherited Enzyme
  Deficiency
Common Genetic Diseases
Sickle Cell Anemia
Phenylketonuria
Galactosemia
Wilson's Disease
Albinism
Hemophilia
Other Genetic Diseases
Recombinant DNA (Gene Splicing)

A human being grows from one fertilized egg cell. As this organism divides and grows, it develops gradually into recognizable form. How do the cells "know" where the head should be, where the arms should be, that there should be two arms and not one or three? Why not claws instead of fingers, scales instead of skin?

Originally it was believed that the chromosomes somehow transmitted information from one generation to the next. The next step forward in the study of heredity was the theory that the chromosomes contained genes—each gene giving a particular characteristic to that individual; that is, there were genes for tallness or shortness, for blue eyes or brown eyes, for light hair or dark hair.

Recent studies have shown that genes are composed of deoxyribonucleic acid (DNA). In 1953 J. D. Watson (see Figure 33–1) and F. H. C. Crick of Cambridge University proposed a double helix structure for the DNA molecule. Before we discuss this structure and explain what a double helix is, let us review a little about nucleic acids.

Nucleic Acids

Nucleic acids were first isolated from the cellular nucleus, hence the name. Nucleic acids are macromolecules, huge polymers with molecular weights over 100 million.

There are two main types of nucleic acids, **deoxyribonucleic acid (DNA)** and **ribonucleic acid (RNA)**. DNA is primarily responsible for the transfer of genetic information whereas RNA is primarily concerned with the synthesis of protein.

526

FIGURE 33-1. Dr. J. D. Watson, Harvard University, who was awarded the Nobel Prize for Medicine and Physiology in 1962, along with Dr. F. H. C. Crick and Dr. M. H. F. Wilkins, for their discovery of the molecular structure of deoxyribonucleic acid (DNA).

Hydrolysis of nucleic acids gives nucleotides, which may be considered the units that make up the polymer. Nucleotides can be further hydrolyzed to nucleosides and phosphoric acid. Hydrolysis of nucleosides yields a sugar and a heterocyclic base, as indicated in the following diagram:

nucleic acid

$\Updownarrow$

nucleotide

$\Updownarrow$

nucleoside + phosphoric acid

$\Updownarrow$

heterocyclic base + sugar

The sugar in both types of nucleic acids is a pentose. In RNA the sugar is ribose whereas in DNA it is deoxyribose. The prefix *deoxy-* means "without oxygen." Note in the following structural diagrams that deoxyribose contains one less oxygen atom than does ribose.

ribose   deoxyribose

Heterocyclic Bases   The heterocyclic bases present in nucleic acids are divided into two types—purines and pyrimidines. The two purines present in both DNA and RNA are **adenine** and **guanine.** The pyrimidine **cytosine** is present in both DNA and RNA whereas **thymine** is found in DNA only and **uracil** is present in RNA only. The structures of these heterocyclic bases are indicated in the following sections.

THE PYRIMIDINES   Pyrimidine is a six-membered heterocyclic ring containing two nitrogen atoms. Three important pyrimidines found in nucleic acids are thymine (2,6-dioxy-5-methylpyrimidine), cytosine (2-oxy-6-aminopyrimidine), and uracil (2,6-dioxypyrimidine). Their structures are as follows:

pyrimidine   thymine   cytosine   uracil

Other important compounds containing pyrimidines are thiamin (vitamin B_1) and the barbiturates.

THE PURINES   The purines, which are found in nucleic acids, are derivatives of a substance, purine, that does not occur naturally.

purine

As indicated by their structures, adenine is 6-aminopurine and guanine is 2-amino-6-oxypurine.

adenine   guanine

The end product of the metabolism of purines is uric acid. The uric acid concentration in the blood is increased during the disease called gout. In this disease, uric acid crystals are deposited in and around the joints and in the cartilage, chiefly in the large toe and in the ear cartilage.

Other purines include caffeine and theophylline. Caffeine is a stimulant for the central nervous system and also a diuretic. Caffeine is found in coffee and tea. Its chemical name is 1,3,7-trimethyl-2,6-dioxypurine. Theophylline, 1,3-dimethyl-2,6-dioxypurine, is found in tea and is used medicinally as a diuretic and for bronchial asthma.

uric acid   caffeine   theophylline

The Adenosine Phosphates

One important nucleotide is adenosine monophosphate (AMP). It is formed by the reaction of adenosine (a nucleoside) with one molecule of phosphoric acid. If two phosphate groups react with adenosine, adenosine diphosphate (ADP) is formed, and ATP, adenosine triphosphate, is formed when three phosphate groups react.

AMP (adenosine monophosphate)
ADP (adenosine diphosphate)
ATP (adenosine triphosphate)

ATP, ADP, and AMP are involved in various metabolic processes involving the storage and release of energy from their phosphate bonds.

The Watson–Crick Model of DNA

The Watson–Crick model of DNA proposed a double-coiled chain consisting of two strands intertwined around one another. The sugar and phosphate groups form the backbone of the strands and the heterocyclic groups the connecting links. Watson and Crick also proposed that an adenine of one chain was bonded to a thymine of the opposite chain and a guanine of one chain was bound to a cytosine of the other chain.

The Watson–Crick model of DNA may also be shown as indicated in Figure 33–2, representing it as a spiral ladder with the two sides being held

Heredity

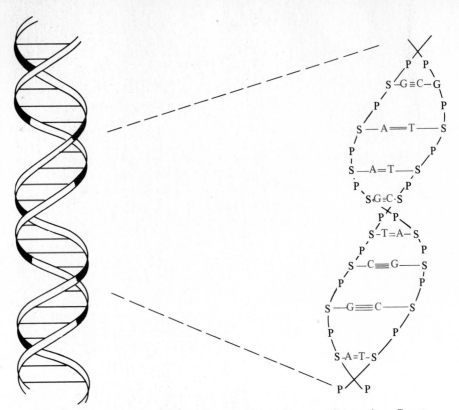

FIGURE 33-2. Structure of DNA. P, phosphate; S, sugar; G, guanine; C, cytosine; A, adenine; T, thymine.

together by rungs consisting of heterocyclic nitrogen compounds (adenine thymine, guanine, and cytosine).

If the chain is untwisted and straightened out, it may be represented as follows

The solid lines indicate ordinary chemical bonding and the dotted lines indicate hydrogen bonding. Recall that hydrogen bonds are much weaker than ordinary chemical bonds. Note that there are two hydrogen bonds between adenine and thymine and three hydrogen bonds between guanine and cytosine.

The DNA Code   All DNA molecules have the same sequence of deoxyribose and phosphates in the ladder part of the chain. The difference lies in the order of the adenine, thymine, cytosine, and guanine parts of the chain. This difference in sequence of the heterocyclic compounds constitutes the genetic code.

This code consists of only four letters—A, T, G, and C—representing adenine, thymine, guanine, and cytosine, respectively. In the DNA molecule these letters of the code are grouped in threes (which we shall discuss later). Thus the code might by ATC, TAC, AAA, CCT, and so on.

Simple bacterial viruses contain about 5500 nucleotides in their DNA molecules; 5500 nucleotides, grouped in threes can produce 5500/3 or approximately 1800 coded pieces of information. These 1800 coded pieces of information are sufficient to describe that particular virus. If each piece of information corresponded to one letter of our alphabet, it would take 1800 letters to describe, genetically, that virus; 1800 letters corresponds roughly to the number of letters on one page of this book.

One DNA molecule in a human contains approximately 5,000,000,000 nucleotides, or enough to form 1,700,000,000 coded pieces of information (of three nucleotides to a group). If each of these coded pieces corresponded to a letter of our alphabet, it would take approximately 2500 volumes, each the size of this book, to describe a human being genetically.

Replication of DNA

When a cell divides, it produces two new cells with identical characteristics. This means that the DNA originally present must duplicate (or replicate) itself. How does the DNA molecule direct the synthesis of another identical DNA molecule?

Watson and Crick theorized that the DNA molecule unwinds, and each half acts as a template for nucleotide units to collect on and form a new chain. Recall that if adenine (A) is present on one chain, it can attract and hold only thymine (T), and cytosine (C) can attract and hold only guanine (G). Thus each half of the chain is highly specific in what it attracts. It forms complementary chains that coil up again and form two new DNA molecules.

FIGURE 33-3. Unwinding of DNA.

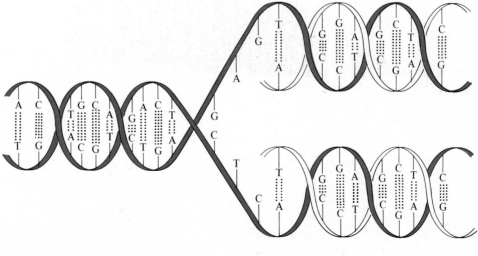

This may be represented diagrammatically, as shown in Figure 33–3. This representation is necessarily quite general and approximate. The actual mechanism of DNA unwinding and untwisting for replication is quite complex, involving several enzymes such as DNA polymerase and DNA ligase, and is beyond the scope of this book.

Transfer of Information

The preceding paragraph indicates how the DNA molecule duplicates itself, but how does the DNA molecule transfer its coded information to the cell's ribosomes where the actual production of the protein called for by the code takes place?

The information contained in the DNA molecule is carried by another molecule called messenger RNA. During replication, DNA "unzips" and synthesizes two new chains to produce two identical molecules. When the DNA molecule synthesizes messenger RNA, the DNA again "unzips"; however, only one part of one strand of DNA acts as a template for the information of messenger RNA (see Figure 33–4). The enzyme required is called RNA polymerase.

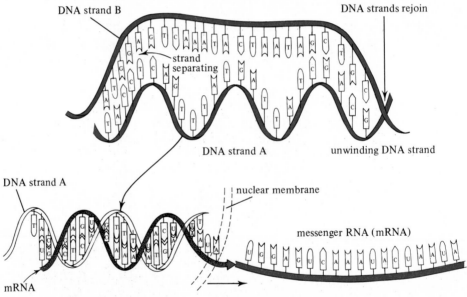

FIGURE 33–4. Formation of messenger RNA from DNA.

When messenger RNA is produced, there is one major difference in the attraction of nucleotides between it and DNA. In RNA, the partner of adenine (A) is uracil (U) and not thymine (T). Another difference is that RNA contains the pentose ribose, whereas DNA contains the pentose deoxyribose.

There are at least three types of RNA: (1) messenger RNA, (2) ribosomal RNA, and (3) transfer RNA. **Messenger RNA (mRNA)** is concerned with the transmission of genetic information from DNA to the site of protein synthesis, the ribosomes; it is found in the nucleus and the cytoplasm of the cell. **Ribosomal RNA (rRNA),** which is the major fraction of the total RNA, combines with protein to form the ribosomes; therefore, ribosomes are an example of nucleoprotein. It is in the ribosomes that the translation of the DNA message takes place. **Transfer RNA (tRNA)** holds a specific amino acid for incorporation into a protein molecule, as indicated in the following paragraphs. A fourth type of RNA, **heterogeneous RNA (hRNA),** may be a precursor for mRNA. This hRNA is found in the nucleus of the cell.

Let us see how mRNA and tRNA function in the ribosomes in the synthesis of a protein. The mRNA moves from the nucleus to the cytoplasm and then to the ribosomes, where it acts as a template for the information of protein. In the cytoplasm is tRNA, which is a spiral form of RNA containing relatively few nucleotides. At one end of the tRNA are three nucleotides that are specific for a certain code on the mRNA. Amino acids in the cytoplasm are activated by ATP and are coupled to the other end of tRNA. This may be designated as shown in Figure 33–5.

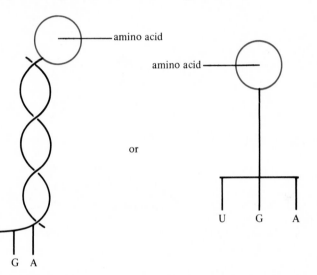

FIGURE 33–5. Diagrammatic forms of transfer RNA (tRNA).

If mRNA contains the coded units ACU, the tRNA that would attach itself must have the code UGA. [Recall that in RNA the adenine (A) is bonded to uracil (U) and cytosine (C) to guanine (G).] If the coded message in mRNA is UGC, the corresponding code in tRNA must be ACG:

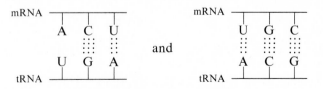

As the mRNA travels across the ribosome, the first coded group (of three letters) picks up and holds a corresponding tRNA. As the second coded group of the mRNA passes, it too picks up a corresponding tRNA. Attached to the opposite end of each tRNA is an amino acid. The amino acid attached to the end of the second tRNA becomes bonded to the amino acid at the end of the first tRNA. The amino acid at the end of the third tRNA in turn becomes bonded to the second amino acid.

Thus, as each tRNA attaches itself to the mRNA, the tRNA gives up its amino acid to form a chain of amino acids, or a protein. After giving up its amino acid, the tRNA leaves the mRNA and goes in search of another amino acid that it can pick up and use to repeat the sequence.

Thus, as the mRNA passes through the ribosome, it directs the gathering, in specified sequence, of the tRNAs, which in turn bond together their amino acids to form a protein.

This effect may be illustrated diagrammatically as shown in Figure 33–6.

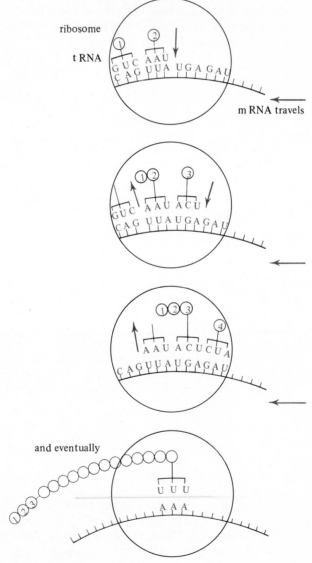

FIGURE 33-6. mRNA directs the proper sequence of tRNA's to form a protein.

In these diagrams, the first coded group in the mRNA—group CAG—attracts tRNA coded GUC. Attached to tRNA coded GUC is an amino acid that we have simply labeled 1. As the mRNA passes further along into the ribosome, the next coded group, code UUA, attracts tRNA coded AAU. The amino acid attached to the end of this tRNA is labeled 2. Amino acid 2 bonds itself to amino acid 1 as illustrated. At the same time, the tRNA coded GUC that held amino acid 1 goes off in search of another amino acid labeled 1 so it can be used again whenever the code calls for it. The third coded group in the mRNA, code UGA, attracts tRNA, coded ACU, with its attached amino acid 3. Then amino acid 3 bonds to amino acid 2, which is already bonded to amino acid 1. So the chain of amino acids begins and continues as illustrated in the fourth figure. This process continues until the end of the coded groups of the mRNA. At this time, the protein is complete and moves out of the ribosome into the cytoplasm.

The Triplet Code

The DNA code consists of four letters. A, T, C, and G, grouped in threes. It is believed that the code in the DNA molecule specifies individual amino acids. Since there are 20 primary amino acids that occur in nature, there must be at least 20 different coded groups in the DNA molecule.

The 20 primary amino acids and their abbreviations are as follows:

alanine—Ala	glycine—Gly	proline—Pro
arginine—Arg	histidine—His	serine—Ser
asparagine—Asn	isoleucine—Ile	threonine—Thr
aspartic acid—Asp	leucine—Leu	tryptophan—Trp
cysteine—Cys	lysine—Lys	tyrosine—Tyr
glutamic acid—Glu	methionine—Met	valine—Val
glutamine—Gln	phenylalanine—Phe	

Decoding the Code

How can the DNA code be decoded? That is, how can we tell which amino acid is specified by a certain coded group?

In 1961 it was found that if a synthetic RNA composed only of uracil nucleotides was substituted for mRNA in a protein-synthesis system, a polypeptide was formed that contained only the amino acid phenylalanine. Since the synthetic mRNA contained only uracil, it must have the code group UUU. The corresponding group in the DNA molecule must be AAA. Thus we can say that the coded group AAA in the DNA molecule corresponds to the code UUU in mRNA, which in turn specifies the amino acid phenylalanine. Another synthetic mRNA, consisting solely of adenine nucleotides, produced a polypeptide containing only lysine. Thus the mRNA code for lysine is AAA and the corresponding DNA code must be TTT.

Table 33–1 indicates the amino acids and their coded groups.

Some experiments indicated that there may be more than one code group for a specific amino acid. That is, alanine is indicated by the mRNA codes GCU, GCC, GCA, and also GCG. Note that all of these code groups begin with the letters "GC." In general, the first two "letters" of the code are more important than the third.

Heredity

TABLE 33-1. Genetic Code in mRNA

First Letter	Second Letter				Third Letter
	A	C	G	U	
A	Lys	Thr	Arg	Ile	A
	Asn	Thr	Ser	Ile	C
	Lys	Thr	Arg	Met[b]	G
	Asn	Thr	Ser	Ile	U
C	Gln	Pro	Arg	Leu	A
	His	Pro	Arg	Leu	C
	Gln	Pro	Arg	Leu	G
	His	Pro	Arg	Leu	U
G	Glu	Ala	Gly	Val	A
	Asp	Ala	Gly	Val	C
	Glu	Ala	Gly	Val	G
	Asp	Ala	Gly	Val	U
U	[a]	Ser	[a]	Leu	A
	Tyr	Ser	Cys	Phe	C
	[a]	Ser	Trp	Leu	G
	Tyr	Ser	Cys	Phe	U

[a] Chain terminator.
[b] Chain initiator.

The genetic code is universal. That is, all known organisms use this same code for the synthesis of their proteins.

Figure 33–7 indicates the synthesis of a polypeptide chain from mRNA, indicating the various amino acids specified by that mRNA.

Regulation of Protein Synthesis

When mRNA acts as a template for the synthesis of protein, only a small amount of the total information in DNA is used at one time to produce a certain type of protein. What determines whether mRNA is formed from a certain segment of the DNA? What "turns on" the DNA and what "turns it off"?

Since protein is not synthesized continuously but only as needed, DNA must normally be in a "repressed state." A **repressor**, which is a polypeptide, binds to a small segment of the DNA. This segment is called the **operator site**. As long as the repressor is bonded to the DNA, no mRNA is produced and so production of protein is inhibited. When a particular protein is needed, an **inducer** is formed. The inducer combines with the repressor, changing its shape so that it can no longer bind to the DNA. Once the repressor is removed from the DNA, synthesis of mRNA and hence protein can begin. When sufficient protein has been produced, the inducer is removed and the repressor once again binds to the DNA, stopping protein synthesis.

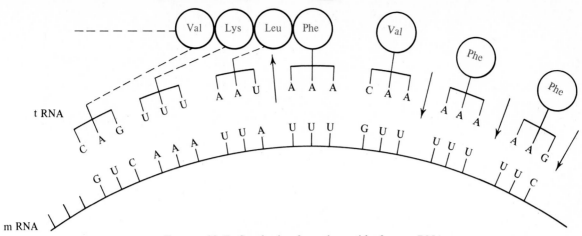

FIGURE 33-7. Synthesis of a polypeptide from mRNA.

Certain drugs, such as tetracyclines and streptomycin, bind to the ribosomes of bacteria and prevent synthesis of protein. Hence these drugs are effective antibiotics.

Mutations Suppose that one of the letters (nucleotides) in a DNA code group was substituted by another letter. Then the message would be miscopied and a mutation would occur. Such a change in the sequence of nucleotides may (1) give no detectable effect, particularly if the change is in the third letter of the code (see page 536); (2) cause a different amino acid to be incorporated into the chain (the results may be acceptable, partially acceptable, or totally unacceptable to the function of that protein); or (3) cause the termination of the chain prematurely so that the protein cannot functionally normally.

A mutation will also occur if one of the code letters is omitted or if one is added or if the order of the code letters is rearranged. Mutations occur because of exposure to radiation (in industry, medically, because of naturally occurring radiations and cosmic rays, or because of fallout) and possibly because of certain chemicals.

Genetic Diseases Most genetic diseases are caused by a defective gene, which results in a loss of activity of some enzyme. Even though the body has thousands of enzymes, the loss of only one may be disastrous.

Consequences of Inherited Enzyme Deficiency Consider a simple enzymatic reaction in which compound X is changed to compound Y under the influence of enzyme x_1, and then compound Y is changed to compound Z under the influence of enzyme y_1.

$$X \xrightarrow[x_1]{} Y \xrightarrow[y_1]{} Z$$

If the enzyme y_1 is deficient, one of the following consequences might occur:

$$X \xrightarrow{x_1} Y \underset{y_1}{\not\longrightarrow} Z$$

A. The body would be lacking in compound Z, with the resulting effect of that lack.

$$X \xrightarrow{x_1} Y \underset{y_1}{\not\longrightarrow} Z$$
$$\searrow R$$

B. Compound Y might be changed to a harmful by-product R.

$$\begin{array}{c} Y \\ X \xrightarrow{x_1} Y \underset{y_1}{\not\longrightarrow} Z \\ Y \end{array}$$

C. Compound Y might accumulate and may be harmful if present in large amounts.

In the preceding cases, the genetic disease is caused by a lack of enzyme y_1, which in turn is due to a defective gene—one that might have been copied incorrectly, or changed, or even be lacking altogether. We shall see in the following paragraphs how a single simple change in the sequence of a code group in mRNA can lead to a genetic defect.

Common Genetic Diseases

The most common genetic disease in the United States is cystic fibrosis, which affects 1 individual in 2000. Another genetic disease, phenylketonuria, affects 1 in 10,000. Most states now require routine screening of newborn infants for this latter disease. Tay–Sachs disease affects 1 in 1000 among persons of Eastern European Jewish origin. One out of every 10 black persons in the United States carries a sickle cell gene.

Paget's disease, a disease of the bones, occurs frequently among people of English descent. Polynesians are prone to have clubfoot and Finns to kidney disease. There is a higher-than-average frequency of deafness in Eskimos and of glaucoma in Icelanders. American Indians and Mexicans are very susceptible to diabetes and gallbladder disease. Impacted wisdom teeth occur frequently among Europeans and Asians but rarely among Africans. Today there are at least 1200 distinct inherited genetic diseases that have been identified.

Sickle-Cell Anemia

Notice the arrangement for the 146 amino acids in the beta chain of normal hemoglobin, shown in structure 33–1. Each of these 146 amino acids was designated by a certain arrangement of three nucleotides in mRNA. Altogether these must have been 438 (3×146) nucleotides, arranged in the proper sequence in order to form this molecule of the beta chain of hemoglobin.

Look at amino acid 6, the one in color. This amino acid, Glu, is glutamic acid. The mRNA code group for glutamic acid is either GAA or GAG. If the middle codon of this group is changed from A to U, the sequence becomes either GUA or GUG, both of which designate the amino acid valine (Val). That is, if there is a change in only one of the nucleotides, from A to U, on the sixth codon of the 146 amino acid chain of the beta chain of hemoglobin, a different type of molecule is produced. This type of hemoglobin is called hemoglobin-S and causes the genetic disease sickle cell anemia.

The red blood cells normally have a concave shape when deoxygenated (see Figure 33–8a). Red blood cells containing hemoglobin-S look like a

Val-His-Leu-Thr-Pro-Glu-Glu-Lys-Ser-Ala-Val-Thr-Ala-Leu-Try-Gly-Lys ⌐

Val ⌐

Val-Val-Leu-Leu-Arg-Gly-Leu-Ala-Glu-Gly-Gly-Val-Glu-Asp-Val-Asn ⌐

Tyr

Pro-Try-Thr-Gln-Arg-Phe-Phe-Glu-Ser-Phe-Gly-Asp-Leu-Ser-Thr-Pro ⌐

Asp

Leu-Val-Lys-Lys-Gly-His-Ala-Lys-Val-Lys-Pro-Asn-Gly-Met-Val-Ala ⌐

Gly

Ala-Phe-Ser-Asp-Gly-Leu-Ala-His-Leu-Asp-Asn-Leu-Lys-Gly-Thr-Phe ⌐

Ala

Asn-Glu-Pro-Asp-Val-His-Leu-Lys-Asp-Cys-His-Leu-Glu-Ser-Leu-Thr ⌐

Phe

Arg-Leu-Leu-Gly-Asn-Val-Leu-Val-Cys-Val-Leu-Ala-His-His-Phe-Gly ⌐

Lys

Val-Gly-Ala-Val-Val-Lys-Gln-Tyr-Ala-Ala-Gln-Val-Pro-Pro-Thr-Phe-Glu ⌐

Ala

Asn-Ala-Leu-Ala-His-Lys-Tyr-His

$$(33\text{--}1)$$

FIGURE 33–8. (a) Normal red blood cells. **(b)** Red blood cells of an individual with the sickle cell trait. (Courtesy of Dr. M. Eisenberger, Chicago, IL.)

sickle (see Figure 33–8b). These sickle cells are more fragile than normal red blood cells, leading to anemia. They can also occlude capillaries, leading to thrombosis. The points and abnormal shapes of the sickle cells cause slowing and sludging of the red blood cells in the capillaries, with resulting hypoxia of the tissues. This produces such symptoms as fever, swelling, and pain in various parts of the body. Eventually the spleen is affected. Many victims of severe sickle cell anemia die in childhood.

Sickle cell anemia is a hereditary condition found primarily among Hispanics and blacks. Many of these people have the sickle cell trait but are relatively unaffected by it until there is a sharp drop in blood oxygen level, such as might be caused by strenuous exercise at high altitudes, underwater swimming, and drunkenness.

Phenylketonuria   Phenylketonuria (PKU) results when the enzyme phenylalanine hydroxylase is absent. A person having PKU cannot convert phenylalanine to tyrosine, and so the phenylalanine accumulates in the body, resulting in injury to the nervous system. In infants and in children up to age 6, an accumulation of phenylalanine leads to retarded mental development.

This disease may be readily diagnosed from a sample of blood or urine. Treatment consists of giving the patient a diet low in phenylalanine.

Galactosemia   Galactosemia results from the lack of an enzyme uridyl transferase that catalyzes the formation of glucose from galactose. This disease may result in an increased concentration of galactose in the blood. Galactose in the blood is reduced in the eye to galacticol, which accumulates and causes a cataract. Ultimately, if galactose continues to accumulate, liver failure and mental retardation will occur. This disease may be controlled by the administration of a diet free of galactose.

Wilson's Disease   Wilson's disease is caused by the body's failure to eliminate excess Cu^{2+} ions because of lack of ceruloplasmin (see page 474) or a failure in the bonding of copper ions to the copper-bonding globulin, or both factors. In this disease copper accumulates in the liver, kidneys, and brain. There is also an excess of copper in the urine. If deposition of copper in the liver becomes excessive, cirrhosis may develop. In addition, accumulation of copper in the kidneys may lead to damage of the renal tubules, leading to increased urinary output of amino acids and peptides.

Albinism   Albinism is caused by a missing enzyme, tyrosinase, which is necessary for the formation of melanin, the pigment of the hair, skin, and eyes. Consequently, albinos have very white skin and hair. Although this disease is not serious, persons affected by it are very sensitive to sunburn.

Hemophilia   Hemophilia is caused by a missing protein, an antihemophilic globulin, which is important in the normal clotting process of the blood. Consequently, any cut may be life threatening to hemophiliacs, but the primary

Biochemistry   **540**

damage is the crippling effect of repeated episodes of internal bleeding into body joints.

Other Genetic Diseases

Niemann–Pick disease is caused by a lack of the enzyme sphingomyelinase, which causes an accumulation of sphingomyelin in the liver, spleen, bone marrow, and lymph nodes. This disease affects the brain and causes mental retardation and early death.

Gaucher's disease is caused by a lack of the enzyme glucocerebrosidase, which is necessary for the cleavage of glucocerebrosides into glucose and ceramide. This disease is characterized by the accumulation of glycolipids in the spleen and liver. In children, Gaucher's disease causes severe mental retardation and early death (see page 338). In adults, the spleen and liver enlarge progressively but the disease is compatible with long life.

Tay–Sachs disease is due to a lack of the enzyme hexosaminidase-A, leading to the accumulation of glycolipids in the brain and the eyes. Red spots show up in the retina and there is also muscular weakness. This disease is fatal to infants before the age of 4.

Recombinant DNA (Gene Splicing)

The term recombinant DNA refers to DNA molecules that have been artificially created by splicing segments of DNA from one organism into the DNA of a completely different organism. Almost any organism (animal, plant, bacteria, virus) can serve as a DNA donor. Theoretically, any organism also can serve as a DNA acceptor, but to date the bacterium *Escherichia coli* (*E. coli*) has been used almost exclusively as a DNA acceptor. *E. coli* was selected because its genetic makeup has been thoroughly studied. Most of *E. coli's* 3–4 thousand genes are contained within a large, single, ringed chromosome. In addition to this large chromosome, there are *plasmids,* smaller closed loops of DNA consisting of only a few genes. It is these plasmids that act as DNA acceptors for *E. coli,* since the plasmids are known to multiply independently within the host cell as the cell itself replicates.

How does gene splicing work? First, the *E. coli* is placed in a detergent solution to break open the cells. The plasmids are extracted with *restriction enzymes* which cut the plasmid DNA at specific points. DNA from another organism (also cleaved by a similar method) is inserted into the *E. coli* plasmid. The plasmid ring is then closed and the plasmid put back into *E. coli.* The new cells are isolated and allowed to replicate (*E. coli* duplicates itself every 20–30 minutes). As the cells replicate, they synthesize the proteins coded for by their DNA, including those coded for by the inserted DNA (see Figure 33–9).

Recombinant DNA research has produced human insulin, interferon, growth hormone, somatostatin, and some vaccines. Theoretically, gene splicing could be used to find cures for genetic diseases, for cancer, and to manufacture various enzymes, hormones, antibodies, etc., that are difficult to isolate and produce pharmaceutically.

Opponents of recombinant DNA research point out the considerable risks involved. They fear that a man-made strain of *E. coli* might be accidentally released and cause a world-wide epidemic and death of large populations.

Heredity

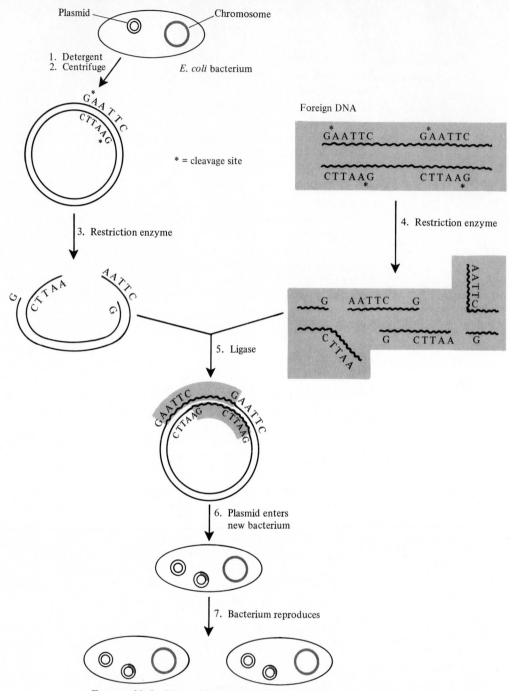

Figure 33-9. Recombinant DNA in *Escherichia coli*. (From S. J. Baum, *Intro-duction to Organic and Biological Chemistry,* 3rd. ed., Macmillan Publishing Company, New York, 1982.)

They also believe that this type of research might be used politically to control human behavior.

Summary   Originally it was believed that the cell's chromosomes transmitted information from one generation to the next. Then it was believed that the chromosomes contained genes, with each gene giving a particular characteristic to that individual. However, recent studies have shown that genes are composed of deoxyribonucleic acid (DNA), which stores and transfers hereditary characteristics.

The two types of nucleic acids are deoxyribonucleic acid (DNA), which is primarily responsible for the transfer of genetic information, and ribonucleic acid (RNA), which is primarily responsible for protein synthesis.

The Watson–Crick model of DNA proposes a double-coiled chain consisting of two strands intertwined around one another. The chains are composed of alternating sugar (deoxyribose) and phosphates with the sugar being bonded to one of four different heterocyclic compounds—adenine, guanine, cytosine, and thymine (A, G, C, T). The model suggests that the adenine of one chain is always bonded to a thymine of the opposite chain and that cytosine is always bonded to guanine.

All DNA molecules have the same sequence of deoxyribose and phosphates in the ladder part of the chain. The difference lies in the order of adenine, thymine, guanine, and cytosine.

When a cell divides, the DNA molecule uncoils and each half acts as a template for the formation of a new chain.

During replication, the DNA molecule uncoils and both halves produce molecules identical to the original. However, when the DNA molecule synthesizes RNA, although the coil again unwinds, only one half acts as the template to produce RNA. There are three kinds of RNA: ribosomal RNA (rRNA), messenger RNA (mRNA), transfer RNA (tRNA), and possibly heterogeneous RNA (hRNA).

When mRNA is formed from DNA, guanine is still bonded to cytosine but adenine is bonded to uracil (U) rather than to thymine.

Messenger RNA moves through the cytoplasm to the ribosomes, where it acts as a template for the formation of protein. The ribosomes contain tRNA; tRNA carries a specific amino acid to the mRNA. The identity of this amino acid is determined by the code on the end of the tRNA, and this code is specific for another code on the mRNA.

As the mRNA moves through the ribosome, the first of its coded groups picks up and holds a corresponding coded group on tRNA. The second, third, and succeeding groups on mRNA do likewise. The specific amino acids carried by the tRNA becomes bonded to one another to form the designated protein, and the tRNAs are released to find more of the specific amino acids and begin the procedure again.

The DNA code consists of four letters (A, T, C, and G) arranged in groups of three.

The three-letter coded groups specify the 20 primary amino acids occurring in nature.

If one of the code letters is changed or is missing, the information copied would be incorrect and a mutation would occur. Mutations occur because of exposure to radiation, both naturally occurring and that in industry and medicine, and possibly because of certain chemicals.

DNA directs the synthesis of enzymes (which are also proteins). If the message is transferred incorrectly, the proper enzyme will not be synthesized and so will be lacking in the body. This lack of a specific enzyme may lead to a genetic disease such as phenylketonuria, galactosemia, albinism, pentosuria, hemophilia, and others.

Questions and Problems

1. What is the relationship between chromosomes, genes, and DNA?
2. What are nucleic acids?
3. Diagram briefly the Watson–Crick model of DNA.
4. What types of bonds are present in the DNA molecules? Are they all equal in strength?
5. How does DNA replicate?
6. What are the three types of RNA? What is the function of each?
7. What is the difference in nucleotides in mRNA and DNA?
8. How do mRNA and tRNA function in the formation of protein?
9. What is the most common genetic disease in the United States?
10. How many primary amino acids occur in nature?
11. Name the primary amino acids and indicate their abbreviations.
12. How many units are present in one unit of the DNA code?
13. Describe briefly how the DNA code was decoded.
14. What amino acid does each of the following coded groups of mRNA represent?

ACG, GCA, UUU, GUU, CCC, CGA

15. What is a mutation in terms of the DNA molecule?
16. What is sickle cell disease? What causes it?
17. How do normal blood cells differ from sickle cells in (a) shape and (b) arrangement of amino acids?
18. What causes the following genetic diseases?

Phenylketonuria
Hemophilia
Galactosemia
Albinism
Wilson's disease
Tay–Sachs disease

What are the symptoms of each disease?
19. Explain how a genetic disease might occur if an enzyme is deficient.

References

BISHOP, J. MICHAEL. Oncogenes. *Scientific American,* **246**:80–93 (March 1982).

BRADY, R. O. Hereditary fat-metabolism diseases. *Scientific American,* **229**:88–97 (Aug. 1973).

CRICK, F. H. The genetic code. *Scientific American,* **207**:66–74 (Oct. 1962).

———. The genetic code: III. *Scientific American,* **215**:55–60 (Oct. 1966).

CROCE, C. M. and H. KOPROWSKI. The genetics of human cancer. *Scientific American,* **238**:117–125 (Feb. 1978).

DARNELL, JAMES E. JR. The processing of RNA. *Scientific American,* **249**:90–101 (Oct. 1983).

FRIEDMANN, T. Prenatal diagnosis of genetic disease. *Scientific American,* **225**:34–42 (Nov. 1971).

FUCHS, F. Genetic amniocentesis. *Scientific American,* **242**:47–53 (June 1980).

GRIVELL, LESLIE A. Mitochondrial DNA. *Scientific American* **248**:78–89 (March 1983).

Biochemistry

HINKLE, P. C. and R. E. McCARTY. How cells make ATP. *Scientific American,* **238:**104–123 (March 1978).

LAKE, JAMES A. The ribosome. *Scientific American,* **245:**84–97 (Aug. 1981).

MARTIN, D. W., P. A. MAYES, and V. W. RIDWELL. *Harper's Review of Biochemistry,* 19th ed. Lange Medical Publications, Los Altos, Calif. 1983, Chapters 25–30.

NICOLSON, G. L. Cancer metastasis. *Scientific American,* **240:**66–76 (March 1979).

NOMURA, MASAGASU. The control of ribosome synthesis. *Scientific American* **250:**102–114 (Jan. 1984).

PESTKA, SIDNEY. The purification and manufacture of human interferon. *Scientific American,* **249:**36–43 (Aug. 1983).

RAWN, J. DAVID. *Biochemistry.* Harper & Row, New York, 1983, Chapters 24–27.

RICH, A. and S. H. KIM. The three-dimensional structure of transfer RNA. *Scientific American,* **238:**52–62 (Jan. 1978).

ZIMMERMAN, HENRY and ISAAC ZIMMERMAN. *Organic Chemistry,* 2nd ed. Macmillan Publishing Company, New York, 1983, Chapter 16.

A APPENDIX Exponential Numbers

Changing Exponential Numbers to Common Numbers

Mathematicians have developed a shorthand method for expressing very large or very small numbers. This system involves the use of a base number, 10, raised to some power. A power, or exponent, indicates how many times the base number, 10, is repeated as a factor. Thus,

1×10^2 (10 repeated as a factor 2 times) $= 1 \times 10 \times 10 = 100$
1×10^3 (10 repeated as a factor 3 times) $= 1 \times 10 \times 10 \times 10 = 1000$
1×10^5 (10 repeated as a factor 5 times) $= 1 \times 10 \times 10 \times 10 \times 10 \times 10 = 100,000$

Negative exponents are used to indicate numbers less than 1. A negative exponent indicates the reciprocal of the same number with a positive exponent:

$$1 \times 10^{-1} = 1 \times \frac{1}{10^1} = 0.1$$

$$1 \times 10^{-2} = 1 \times \frac{1}{10^2} = 0.01$$

$$1 \times 10^{-4} = 1 \times \frac{1}{10^4} = 0.0001$$

Note: The positive exponent indicates how many places the decimal point must be moved to the right (from the number 1). Also, note that the negative exponent indicates how many places the decimal point must be moved to the left (from the number 1).

Any number that is not an exact power of 10 may be expressed as a product of two numbers, one of which is a power of 10. The other number is always written with just one figure to the left of the decimal point.

EXAMPLE A-1. Express 6.2×10^3 as a common number.
A positive three ($+3$) exponent indicates that the decimal point should be moved three places to the right. Thus

$$6.2 \times 10^3 = (6.200) = 6200$$

■

EXAMPLE A-2. Change 8.45×10^5 to common numbers.

A $+5$ exponent indicates that the decimal point should be moved five places to the right.

$$8.45 \times 10^5 = (8.45000) = 845,000 \qquad \blacksquare$$

EXAMPLE A-3. Change 1.27×10^{-2} to common numbers.

A -2 exponent indicates that the decimal point should be moved two places to the left.

$$1.27 \times 10^{-2} = (001.27) = 0.0127 \qquad \blacksquare$$

EXAMPLE A-4. Change 3.5×10^{-9} to common numbers.

$$3.5 \times 10^{-9} = (0000000003.5) = 0.0000000035 \qquad \blacksquare$$

Changing Common Numbers to Exponential Numbers

When changing a common number to an exponential number, the decimal point is moved so that there is just one digit in front of it. The exponent corresponds to the number of places the decimal point must be moved. If the decimal point is moved to the left, the exponent is positive; if to the right, it is negative.

EXAMPLE A-5. Change 4000 to an exponential number.

The decimal point must be moved to the left three places in order for just one digit to remain before that decimal point. Three places to the left indicates an exponent of 3 $(+3)$.

$$4000 = (4000) = 4 \times 10^3 \qquad \blacksquare$$

EXAMPLE A-6. Change 604 to exponential numbers.

$$604 = (604) = 6.04 \times 10^2 \qquad \blacksquare$$

EXAMPLE A-7. Change 0.00037 to exponential numbers.

$$0.00037 = (0.00037) = 3.7 \times 10^{-4}$$

where the negative exponent indicates that the decimal point has been moved to the right. $\qquad \blacksquare$

B Functional Groups

Class of Compound	Functional Group	Typical Aliphatic Example	
		Formula	Name
Alkane	$-\overset{\mid}{\underset{\mid}{C}}-\overset{\mid}{\underset{\mid}{C}}-$	$CH_3CH_2CH_3$	Propane
Alkene	$-\overset{\mid}{C}=\overset{\mid}{C}-$	$CH_3CH{=}CH_2$	Propene
Alkyne	$-C{\equiv}C-$	$CH_3C{\equiv}CH$	Propyne
Alcohol	$-OH$	CH_3OH	Methanol (methyl alcohol)
Ether	$-O-$	$CH_3CH_2OCH_2CH_3$	Ethyl ether
Aldehyde	$-\overset{\overset{\textstyle O}{\|}}{C}-H$	CH_3CHO	Ethanal (acetaldehyde)
Ketone	$\overset{}{C}{=}O$	$CH_3\overset{\overset{\textstyle O}{\|}}{C}CH_3$	Propanone (acetone)
Acid	$-\overset{\overset{\textstyle O}{\|}}{C}-OH$	$CH_3\overset{\overset{\textstyle O}{\|}}{C}OH$	Ethanoic acid (acetic acid)
Amine	$-NH_2$	CH_3NH_2	Methylamine
Amide	$-\overset{\overset{\textstyle O}{\|}}{C}-NH_2$	$CH_3\overset{\overset{\textstyle O}{\|}}{C}-NH_2$	Acetamide
Ester	$-\overset{\overset{\textstyle O}{\|}}{C}-O-$	$CH_3\overset{\overset{\textstyle O}{\|}}{C}OCH_2CH_3$	Ethyl acetate

Acetal Compound formed by the reaction of one molecule of an aldehyde with two molecules of alcohol. The general formula is

$$\text{R}-\underset{\underset{\text{OR}''}{|}}{\overset{\overset{\text{OR}'}{|}}{\text{C}}}-\text{H}$$

Acidosis Condition in which the pH of the blood drops from 7.35.

Acromegaly Pathologic enlargement of the bones of the face, hands, and feet resulting from an overactive anterior lobe of the pituitary gland.

Activation energy Minimum amount of energy molecules must possess in order for a reaction to occur.

Adhesion The attraction or joining of two dissimilar substances.

Aerobic Requiring oxygen.

Aerosol Gaseous suspension of fine solid or liquid particles.

Alkalosis Condition in which the pH of the blood rises from 7.45.

Alloy Solid solution of two or more metals.

Alveoli Air sacs in the lungs.

Amoebicide Substance that destroys amoeba.

Amphipathic Molecules having a hydrophobic and a hydrophillic end.

Amphoteric Capable of reacting either as an acid or a base.

Anaerobic Not requiring the presence of oxygen.

Analgesic A pain killer.

Anion A negatively charged ion.

Antimetabolite Substance that inhibits utilization of metabolites.

Antineoplastic agents Agents that inhibit the growth of malignant cells.

Antiseptic Capable of destroying disease-causing microorganisms.

Antispasmodic Capable of preventing spasms or convulsions.

Antitoxin An antibody capable of neutralizing a poison of biologic origin.

Apoenzyme Protein part of an enzyme.

Asphyxiation Unconsciousness or death caused by lack of oxygen.

Astringent Substance that draws together or contracts tissue.

Atherosclerosis Thickening of arterial wall, characterized by deposition of fatty substances.

Autoradiograph Self-picture taken by a radioactive substance.

Bactericidal Property of killing bacteria.

Bacteriostatic Inhibition of growth of bacteria without destruction.

Bradycardia Slower-than-normal heart rate.

Bronchioles Thin-walled extensions of the bronchial tubes in the lungs.

Calculi Stones, such as those found in the gallbladder or kidney.

Capillary action Rise of fluid through a small opening.

Carcinogenic Cancer-causing.

Cathartic Laxative.

Catheter Slender, flexible tube inserted into a body channel.

Cation Positively charged ion.

Chain reaction Self-sustaining nuclear reaction yielding products that cause further reactions of the same kind.

549

Chemotherapeutic agents Chemicals used in treatment of disease, particularly cancer.

Chorea A nervous disorder marked by uncontrollable and irregular body movements.

Coenzyme Small molecule that combines with the apoenzyme to form an active enzyme.

Cohesion Property of a substance sticking to itself.

Crenation Shrinking of red blood cells in a hypertonic solution.

Curie Standard of radiation; 1 curie (Ci) equals 37 billion nuclear disintegrations per second.

Diabetes mellitus Disorder of carbohydrate metabolism characterized by inadequate secretion or utilization of insulin.

Diuretic Substance that increases output of urine.

Eczema Noncontagious inflammation of the skin, marked by the outbreak of lesions that become encrusted and scaly.

Edema Accumulation of fluid in the tissues.

Electroencephalogram Graphic record of the electrical activity of the brain.

Electrophoresis Separation of charged particles under the influence of an electric field.

Emphysema Pathologic enlargement of the alveoli in the lungs.

Endothermic Absorbing energy.

Equilibrium Dynamic state in which the rates of opposing reactions are equal.

Euphoria Feeling of well-being.

Excoriated Chafed.

Exogenous Developed from external causes.

Exophthalmos Abnormal protrusion of the eyeball.

Fission Splitting of the nucleus of an atom.

Fusion Combining of small nuclei to make a larger one.

Glycosidic linkage Bond formed between two monosaccharides.

Goiter Enlargement of the thyroid gland visible as a swelling in the front of the neck.

Halogen Any one of group VIIA nonmetals.

Hemiacetal Compound formed by the reaction of one molecule of an aldehyde with one molecule of an alcohol; general formula is

$$\begin{array}{c} OR' \\ | \\ R-C-H \\ | \\ OH \end{array}$$

Hemiketal Compound formed by the reaction of one molecule of a ketone with one molecule of alcohol; general formula is

$$\begin{array}{c} OR'' \\ | \\ R-C-R' \\ | \\ OH \end{array}$$

Hemolysis Destruction of red blood cells caused by a hypotonic solution.

Hertz Unit of frequency equal to 1 cycle per second.

Hybaroxic High pressure oxygen.

Hydrophillic Having an affinity for water.

Hydrophobic Antagonistic to water.

Hydrostatic Referring to the pressures liquids exert.

Hypercalcemia Increased serum calcium concentration.

Hypertension High blood pressure.

Hypertonic Higher salt concentration than the blood.

Hypnotics Sleep inducers.

Hypoacidity Lower-than-normal acidity.

Hypoglycemia Abnormally low blood sugar level.

Hypotonic Salt concentration less than that of the blood.

Hypoxia Deficiency in the amount of oxygen reaching body tissues.

Interstitial fluid Fluid between tissues.

Isoelectric point pH at which amino acids are neutral.

Isotonic Having the same salt concentration as the blood.

IUPAC International Union of Pure and Applied Chemistry.

Jaundice Yellowish pigmentation of the skin caused by deposition of bile pigments.

Ketal Compound formed by the reaction of one molecule of a ketone with two molecules of alcohol; general formula is

$$R-\underset{\underset{OR'''}{|}}{\overset{\overset{OR''}{|}}{C}}-R'$$

Lacrimator Causing production of tears.

Lacteals Lymphatic vessels arising from the villi of the small intestine.

Laked Bursting of red blood cells so that hemoglobin is released into the plasma.

Lymphatics Vessels that carry lymph.

Macrocytic Referring to abnormally large red blood cells.

Macroglobulinemia Disease characterized by an increase in blood serum viscosity and presence of highly polymerized globulins.

Mammography X-ray examination of the breasts.

Medulla Inner part of a biologic structure, such as the adrenal medulla.

Megaloblastic Referring to very large immature cells.

Metastases Spreading of disease from original sites.

Mitochondria Microscopic bodies, found in all cells, that play an important part in metabolic reactions and energy production.

Multiple myeloma Disease of the bone marrow.

Mutagenic Causing biologic mutation.

Myocardial infarction Formation of dead tissue resulting from an obstruction of blood vessels supplying the myocardium.

Myxedema Disease caused by decreased activity of the thyroid gland in adults.

Neoplasms Abnormal new growth of tissues; tumors.

Nephritis Inflammation of the kidneys.

Occlusions Substances containing trapped liquid and gaseous material.

Osmolarity Measure of the concentration of particles in solution.

Osmosis Flow of solvent through a semipermeable membrane until concentrations on both sides are equal.

Osteolysis Bone destruction.

Osteomalacia Softening of the bones because of a deficiency of vitamin D, calcium, or phosphorus.

Osteomyelitis Inflammation of the bone marrow.

Osteoporosis Reduction in the quantity of bone.

Paranoia Chronic psychosis characterized by delusion of persecution or of grandeur.

Plasmolysis Shrinking of red blood cells because of addition of a hypertonic solution.

Pneumonitis Inflammation of the lungs.

Positron Positive electron.

Pruritus Itching.

Psychedelics Substances causing hallucinations.

Psychoneuroses Neuroses based on emotional conflict.

Rad Unit of radiation equal to 100 ergs per gram of irradiated tissue.

Rem Unit of radiation equivalent to the absorption of 1 roentgen by a human.

Resonance When two or more structures of a compound can be written that differ only in the position of the valence electrons, then those structures exhibit resonance.

Roentgen Unit of radiation involving X rays that produce 1 electrostatic unit of positive or negative charge in 1 cm^3 of air.

Semipermeable membrane A selective membrane.

Specific heat Amount of heat required to raise the temperature of 1 g of a substance 1°C.

Substrate Molecules on which an enzyme acts.

Surfactant Surface-active agent.

Syndrome A group of signs and symptoms that collectively indicate a disease.

Tachycardia Excessively rapid heart beat.

Tetrahedral Having four sides with equal triangular faces.

Therapeutic Having healing powers.

Thromboses Blood clots.

Tincture Alcoholic solution.

Vasoconstrictor Substance that constricts blood vessels.

Villi Projections arising from a mucous membrane.

Virucide Substance that destroys viruses.

Viscosity A measure of resistance to flow.

Volatile Easily vaporized.

Answers to Odd-Numbered Questions

CHAPTER 1
(page 11)

1. 37°C.   3. 185°F, 358 K.   5. They are identical.
7. Kilogram, cubic meter; kilogram, liter.
9. g, gram; cm, centimeter; mm, millimeter; kl, kiloliter; m, meter.
11. (a) 50.8 cm   (b) 10.0 kg   (c) 42.7 lb   (d) 25.0 in.
    (e) 3.9 in.   (f) 110 lb   (g) 162.6 cm   (h) 80.0 kg
13. 60 in.; 149.6 lb; 99°F.   15. 255 g.   17. 14.7 ml.
19. Kilowatts, thousands of watts; milliseconds, thousandths of a second; megacuries, millions of curies; microamperes, millionths of an ampere.
21. 3,750 cm^3; 3.75 L; 0.00375 kl.
23. Weight depends on gravity and varies; mass depends on the amount of matter and is constant.   25. 36 mg.

CHAPTER 2
(page 25)

1. (a) Solids have a definite shape; liquids and gases do not.
   (b) Solids and liquids have a definite volume; gases do not.
   (c) Solids have a high or low density; liquids usually have a low density; gases have a very low density.
   (d) Solids have particles that are closely adhering and tightly packed; liquids have particles that are mobile and relatively close to one another; gases have particles that are independent and relatively far apart.
   (e) Solids and liquids are incompressible; gases are highly compressible.
   (f) Solids and liquids expand slightly when heated; gases expand greatly when heated.
3. Heat of vaporization is the number of calories required to change 1 g of liquid to gas at the boiling point; heat of fusion is the number of calories required to change 1 g of solid to liquid at the melting point.
5. Potential energy is stored energy, energy of position; kinetic energy is active energy, energy of motion.
7. 6000 cal; 1.5 g protein.
9. Elements and compounds must be homogeneous. Mixtures may be.
11. (a) Mg   (b) Ca   (c) I   (d) C   (e) P
    (f) Zn   (g) Cu   (h) Br   (i) Hg   (j) B
13. No. Some substances will burn or decompose when heated (paper, wood, etc).

15. (a) Zn, Cr   (b) Ca, P   (c) Fe, Cu.
17. The particles no longer retain their orderly arrangement.
19. Because the particles are free to move in liquids and gases while they are fixed in a solid.   21. Calorie.
23. Metals conduct heat and electricity; nonmetals do not. Metals have a luster, are ductile, and malleable; nonmetals are not. Metals are usually solid at room temperature; nonmetals may be solid, liquid, or gas at room temperature.

CHAPTER 3
(page 40)

1.

N $1s^22s^22p^3$ Be $1s^22s^2$ F $1s^12s^22p^5$

S $1s^22s^22p^63s^23p^4$ Ne $1s^22s^22p^6$ Si $1s^22s^22p^63s^23p^2$

3.

	Electrons in Outer Energy Level	Electron Energy Levels
(a) Be	2	2
(b) P	5	3
(c) Br	7	4
(d) Ca	2	4
(e) Rb	1	5
(f) As	5	4
(g) Ra	2	7
(h) Zr	2	5
(i) Mn	2	4
(j) Ac	2	7
(k) Rn	8	6

5. An atom is the smallest portion of an element that retains all of the properties of that element.
7. In the nucleus.   9. Periods.
11. No; yes.   13. Left and center; right side; extreme right column.
15. Electrons in the outer energy level; elements with eight electrons in their outer energy level (except for helium).
19. It has six electrons in its outer energy level; it has four energy levels of electrons; it is a nonmetal.

CHAPTER 4
(page 69)

1. Helium nuclei; high speed electrons, electromagnetic radiation.
3. (a) $^{12}_{6}C$ (b) $^{24}_{11}Na$ (c) $^{30}_{16}S$.
5. Isotopes produced artificially by bombardment with various types of particles; ^{14}C, tracing the path of carbon as it passes through the body in various types of compounds. ^{131}I, for thyroid diagnosis and treatment; ^{59}Fe, for measurement of absorption of iron from the digestive tract.
7. 64 mg.

9. Used to take photos of various body parts and also for the treatment of superficial skin conditions.

11. Radiation causes ionization within the cell and also may produce substances that impair cellular metabolism; radiation may also cause sterility, leukemia, and cataracts.

13. From the natural background, from medical diagnosis and treatment, and from fallout.

15. ^{99m}Tc is injected into the bloodstream. A short while later a sample of blood is withdrawn and its radioactivity measured. From the amount of radiation originally present and that in the sample withdrawn, the blood volume may be calculated.

17. Ultrasonography uses high-frequency sound waves in place of X rays.

19. The CAT scanner rotates in a circle around a patient, taking sharp, detailed X rays of narrow cross sections of a body part. This information is fed into a computer, which produces a visible image of the section scanned.

21. When an alpha particle is emitted, atomic number decreases by 2 and mass number decreases by 4; when a beta particle is emitted, atomic number increases by 1 while mass number does not change; when a gamma ray is emitted, there is no change in either the atomic number or the mass number.

23. Nuclear fission involves breaking apart the nucleus while fusion involves building up a nucleus. Both produce large amounts of energy.

25. The energy comes from the "loss" in mass; the amount of energy may be calculated by using Einstein's equation, $E = mc^2$.

27. Positron emission transverse tomography, a method of using positron-emitting substances to trace biologically active chemicals through the brain.

29. A method of measuring minute concentrations of substances present in the blood; It is based upon the body's antigen-antibody system.

31. By causing the ionization of water or by knocking an electron out of the water molecule; it alters the chemical balance within the cells causing damage to the cell and its systems.

33. 2 mrem.

CHAPTER 5
(page 88)

1. A molecule is a combination of two or more atoms.

3. A representation whereby the symbol indicates all of the atom except the electrons in the outer energy level. Each electron in the outer energy level is indicated by a dot.

5. Eight electrons in the outer energy level.   7. ionic.

9. (a) Potassium iodide   (b) calcium sulfate   (c) zinc sulfide
   (d) sodium nitrate   (e) aluminum chloride

11. H:H   H:Cl: H:S:H   H:P:H   H:C:H   :H N:
                                       H   H

13. Single covalent bond—one in which electrons are shared equally as in Cl_2; double covalent bond—two pair of electrons shared, as in CO_2; triple covalent bond—three pairs of shared electrons, as in N_2.

15. (a) phosphorus trichloride   (b) sulfur dioxide
    (c) dinitrogen pentoxide   (d) carbon disulfide
    (e) iodine chloride.

Answers to Odd-Numbered Questions   555

17. (a) Ag_2SO_4 (b) $KHCO_3$ (c) $(NH_4)_2S$ (d) HNO_3.

19. H_2, one molecule of hydrogen; 2H, two atoms of hydrogen; CO_2, one molecule of carbon dioxide; CO, one molecule of carbon monoxide.

21. An empirical formula represents the relative number of each type of atom present in each molecule of a given compound; a molecular formula represents the actual number of atoms present in each molecule of a given compound.

23. A metallic atom, because the ion has the same nuclear charge but fewer electrons, and thus these electrons are pulled in closer; a nonmetal ion, because the ion has a greater charge in its electron energy levels than in its nucleus, so that the energy levels are not held as closely as in the neutral atom.

25. A nonpolar molecule may contain symmetrically placed polar bonds.

27. Na^+; K^+.

29. If the two elements have equal electronegativities, the bond will be nonpolar; if the electronegativities are unequal, the bond will be polar.

31. It has one electron that it can lose from its outer energy level.

33. No; the sum of the oxidation numbers must be zero.   35. P_4O_{10}.

CHAPTER 6
(page 100)

1. (a) $2Mg + O_2 \longrightarrow 2MgO$
   (b) $Zn + 2HCl \longrightarrow ZnCl_2 + H_2$
   (c) $C + O_2 \longrightarrow CO_2$
   (d) $NaCl + AgNO_3 \longrightarrow AgCl + NaNO_3$
   (e) $ZnSO_4 + 2NaOH \longrightarrow Zn(OH)_2 + Na_2SO_4$
   (f) $3Fe + 2O_2 \longrightarrow Fe_3O_4$
   (g) $Mg + 2AgNO_3 \longrightarrow Mg(NO_3)_2 + 2Ag$
   (h) $2Al(OH)_3 + 3H_2SO_4 \longrightarrow Al_2(SO_4)_3 + 6H_2O$

3. Nature of the reacting substances, temperature, concentration of reacting substances, presence of catalyst, surface area.

5. One mole is the number of atoms in 12.000 g of ^{12}C; 342 g.   7. 2.5.

9. A dynamic state in which the rates of forward and reverse reaction are equal; Le Chatelier's principle states that when a stress is applied to a reaction at equilibrium, the equilibrium will be displaced in such a direction as to relieve that stress.

11. 20 g.   13. 3.01×10^{24}; 9.03×10^{24}.   15. 80 g.

17. By adding N_2 or H_2, by removing NH_3, by decreasing temperature; reverse of previous steps.

19. It increases the chances of collision between reactants.

21. Dynamic; both forward and reverse reaction continue, but at the same rate so that there is no net change.

CHAPTER 7
(page 115)

1. (a) Molecules are far apart so that there is a small mass and a large volume.
   (b) Molecules are far apart and can be forced closer together.
   (c) Collisions between molecules are perfectly elastic so that no energy is lost.
   (d) There is enough space between molecules of one gas for another gas to enter.

(e) Molecules are in rapid motion in all directions and continue moving unless confined by the walls of a container.

(f) At constant pressure, as the temperature is increased the molecules move faster, and in order to maintain a constant pressure they must occupy a larger volume.

(g) At constant temperature, when the volume of a gas is decreased, the same number of molecules is confined in a smaller volume; thus, they strike the walls of the container more often, thus increasing the pressure.

3. 579 mm Hg.   5. 2.23 ft^3.

7. When the pressure in a chest respirator is increased, the volume of the lungs is decreased, thus forcing air out; when the pressure in the respirator is decreased, the air in the lungs expands.

9. Because the partial pressure of CO_2 is higher in the blood than in the lungs and gases always flow from a high pressure area to one of lower pressure.

11. CH_4.   13. Automobiles, tobacco smoke, the burning of fossil fuel.

15. (a) First, eye irritation and irritation of respiratory passages, followed later by increased airway resistance and acute bronchitis and pneumonitis.

(b) Eye irritation and danger to persons with respiratory and cardiac problems.

(c) Impairment of vision and judgment, and possibly strokes and hypertension.

(d) Airway spasms, particularly dangerous to persons having lung problems.

(e) Causes spasms in lung tissue and also destruction of cells in the lungs.

17. Since molecules are moving in all directions, they should exert a pressure equally in all directions.

19. When the bulb is squeezed, the pressure of air inside the bulb is increased. This increased pressure is transmitted to the mercury in the cuff. As the blood exerts a pressure against the cuff, this change in pressure is indicated on the dial attached to the sphygmomanometer.

21. Each molecule in a gas acts independently of the others. If the concentration of one type of molecule is higher, then more of that type will strike the walls of the container in a given period of time, causing a greater (partial) pressure.

23. Divers work under high pressure, causing more air to dissolve in the blood. If the pressure is reduced too quickly, the dissolved gases bubble out too rapidly, causing bubbles in the blood and blockage of some blood vessels.

25. A barometer consists of a glass tube filled with mercury, the open end of which was inverted into a dish of mercury. The mercury in the tube falls until the pressure of the air just balances the pressure of the column of mercury in the tube. As air pressure increases or decreases, the mercury level in the barometer rises or falls correspondingly.

27. 0.125 mol.

29. Acid rain is formed by the action of rain with oxides of nitrogen and sulfur in the air. Acid rain affects marble and also mortar between bricks; it affects trees, fruits, and vegetables.

31. It prevents the sun's high-energy ultraviolet radiation from reaching the earth's surface; chlorofluorocarbons and oxides of nitrogen.

CHAPTER 8
(page 129)

1. Oxygen is heavier than air, so a bottle is kept mouth upward to prevent the oxygen from escaping.

3. An oxide.

5. Care should be taken in handling and storing flammable fluids such as ether and alcohol. Smoking should not be allowed in a room where oxygen is in use, nor should body rubs with alcohol or powder be given in the presence of oxygen equipment in use.

7. Laboratory: heating $KClO_3$, electrolysis of water. Commercial: liquefaction of air.

9. Oxygen is used for patients with pulmonary diseases, for patients having hypoxia, for cases of asphyxia, or for those who have been nearly drowned. Care must be taken not to allow smoking or active electrical equipment in rooms where oxygen is in use.

11. To stimulate breathing.

13. Caused by bubbles of nitrogen forming in the blood vessels when a diver has the air pressure reduced too suddenly. It may be overcome by building up the pressure around the diver and then slowly releasing it.

15. Colorless gas with almost no odor or taste, heavier than air, and a low solubility in blood; it is nonflammable but does support combustion; care must be taken with its use to avoid a fire, as with oxygen.

17. Because it forms a strong bond with hemoglobin so that the blood is unable to carry sufficient oxygen to the tissues.

19. In acidic or neutral solutions.

21. When a metal reacts with oxygen, an oxide is formed; when an active metal reacts with oxygen, a peroxide is formed; when a very active metal reacts with oxygen, a superoxide is formed.

23. 0; -2; -1; $-\frac{1}{2}$.

25. It is removed through the action of the enzyme catalase.

27. No; oxidation can involve other elements such as in the reaction of sodium with chlorine.

29. The presence of oxyhemoglobin.

CHAPTER 9
(page 139)

	Oxidizing Agent	Reducing Agent
1. (a)	Cl_2	KI
(b)	H_2SO_4	Al
(c)	$AgNO_3$	Cu
(d)	O_2	H_2

3. Electrons can never be lost by one substance unless another substance gains those electrons.

5. (a) Reaction of sodium with chlorine (Na is oxidized).
   (b) Reaction of carbon with oxygen ($C + O_2 \longrightarrow CO_2$).
   (c) CH_3CH_2OH being oxidized to CH_3CHO.

7. See page 138.

9.	Oxidized	Reduced	Oxidizing Agent	Reducing Agent
(a)	Zn	HCl	HCl	Zn
(b)	P	HNO_3	HNO_3	P
(c)	$MnCl_2$	Br_2	Br_2	$MnCl_2$
(d)	$Mn(NO_3)_2$	$NaBiO_3$	$NaBiO_3$	$Mn(NO_3)_2$

CHAPTER 10
(page 156)

1. Because of a lack of dissolved gases and minerals.
3. Water expands upon freezing and so is less dense.
5. Increasing the pressure increases the boiling point, so food will cook properly.
7. It takes energy for a solution to evaporate. The energy comes from the liquid or from the skin, thus lowering the temperature.
9. H:$\ddot{\text{O}}$:   It is polar because it has a + and a − end.
    H
11. No.   13. Acid.
15. Because ordinary water may contain bacteria and other microorganisms that might be harmful.
17. Boiling kills bacteria; boiling does not remove impurities.
19. A salt combined with a definite amount of water of crystallization.
21. The property of a hydrate giving off water.
23. Bicarbonates of calcium and magnesium; removed by boiling.
25. Hard water is passed through a tank containing a zeolite. The calcium and magnesium compounds are changed to sodium compounds, which do not cause hardness. The calcium and magnesium compounds remain behind in the tank.
27. Any water that is not pure; oil and dead fish floating on the surface of water; bad taste to drinking water, foul odor along a waterfront, tainted fish that cannot be eaten, unchecked growth of aquatic weeds along the shore.
29. Bacteria, sewage, and wastes from paper mills, food-processing plants, and other industrial wastes.
31. Decreases the amount of oxygen dissolved in water and increases the rate of chemical reaction; may also be fatal to certain types of marine life. Caused by water used as a coolant in an industrial plant.
33. Molecules escaping from the surface of a liquid into the air above; directly.
35. The higher the vapor pressure of a liquid, the lower the boiling point.
37. Digestion involves the hydrolysis of carbohydrates, fats, and proteins.
39. No; it should not be used by persons on restricted sodium intake.

CHAPTER 11
(page 184)

1. (a) 5 g boric acid dissolved in sufficient water to make 100 ml.
   (b) 1 g $KMnO_4$ dissolved in sufficient water to make 300 ml.
   (c) 117 g NaCl dissolved in sufficient water to make 2 L.
   (d) 4.5 g NaCl dissolved in sufficient water to make 500 ml.
3. Because blood cells are affected by other types of solutions.
5. Clear, homogeneous, do not settle, have variable composition, can be separated by physical means, pass through filter paper.
7. Not clear, homogeneous, do not settle, pass through filter paper but not membranes, exhibit Brownian movement, Tyndall effect.
9. The scattering of light by colloidal particles when a beam of light is passed through a colloidal dispersion.
11. The net downward force exerted on surface molecules of a liquid.
13. Raises boiling point and lowers freezing point.
15. If concentrations in blood and dialysate are the same, no waste products will be removed.
17. By adding an emulsifying agent.

Answers to Odd-Numbered Questions   **559**

19. They are smaller than openings in filter paper but larger than openings in membranes.
21. Alcoholic solution.
23. Add another crystal of solute. If it dissolves, solution was unsaturated; if it doesn't, solution was saturated.
25. pH and mineral content of dialysate will affect the body; also temperature control is important to avoid chilling the blood.
27. By adding excess solute to a saturated solution, warming, filtering off excess solute, and then allowing the solution to cool to room temperature; no; if shaken or if one crystal of the solute is added, excess solute will crystallize immediately and a saturated solution will remain.
29. 2.92 g.   31. Take 101 g KOH, dissolve in water, and dilute to 1.5 L.
33. KNO_3
35. A solid solution of two metals; an alloy containing mercury; alloys are used in artificial joints; amalgams in dental fillings.
37. (a) Take 100 ml 10 percent stock solution and dilute to 500 ml.
    (b) Take 20 ml 1:10 stock solution and dilute to 200 ml.
39. Adhesion, attraction of unlike molecules; cohesion, attraction of like molecules; flow of a liquid through a small tube or small openings; resistance of a liquid to flow.
41. In reverse osmosis, water flows from a dilute to a concentrated solution. This process is caused by the application of hydrostatic pressure to the system.
43. (a) 500 milliosmols   (b) 400 milliosmols   (c) 550 milliosmols.

CHAPTER 12
(page 191)

1. Use a conductivity apparatus. If it conducts electricity, it is an electrolyte.
3. Decreases freezing point more than a nonionized solute does; each ion of an electrolyte has an effect upon the freezing point of the liquid.
5. (a) When electrolytes are placed in water, the molecules break up into ions.
   (b) Some ions have a positive charge, others a negative charge.
   (c) The sum of the positive charges equals the sum of the negative charges.
   (d) The conductance of electricity by solutions of electrolytes is due to the presence of ions.
   (e) Nonelectrolytes do not conduct electricity because of the absence of ions.
   (f) The greater effect of electrolytes on boiling point and on freezing point is due to the increased number of particles (ions) present.
7. Positively charged ions are attracted toward the negative electrodes. Negatively charged ions are attracted toward the positive electrodes.
9. One that is highly or completely ionized; HNO_3 or H_2SO_4.
11. See table in text.
13. Sodium chloride solution has twice the osmolarity of an equimolar glucose solution and so should have twice the effect on an increase in the boiling point.
15. Strong electrolytes are highly ionized and in general undergo irreversible reactions; weak electrolytes behave oppositely.

CHAPTER 13
(page 202)

1. (a) A substance that yields hydrogen ions in solution.
   (b) A substance that yields hydroxide ions in solution.

Answers to Odd-Numbered Questions   **560**

(c) Reaction of an acid with a base to produce a salt and water.

(d) A measurement indicating the strength of an acid or a base.

3. Yield hydroxide ions in solution, have a bitter taste and a slippery feeling, react with indicators, neutralize acids.

5. Turns it from red to blue.

7. Otherwise they would react with the metal of the container.

9. Wash thoroughly with water and neutralize with sodium bicarbonate.

11. Calcium hydroxide, an antacid and antidote used for oxalic acid poisoning; magnesium hydroxide, an antacid and laxative; ammonium hydroxide, a heart and respiratory stimulant.

13. Blood, 7.35–7.45; urine, 5.5–7.0; saliva, 6.2–7.4.

15. For an acid, both definitions are essentially the same since a proton is a hydrogen ion; for bases, the Bronsted definition is broader because substances other than hydroxide ions can also accept protons.

17. Strong acids and bases are highly or completely ionized; weak acids and bases are slightly ionized.

19. KOH yields OH^- ions in solution; C_2H_5OH does not.

21. Because of the presence of dissolved CO_2, which forms the weak acid H_2CO_3.

23. 0.325 N KNO_3.   25. 19.7 ml.

CHAPTER 14
(page 210)

1. (a) Product, other than water, formed by reaction of an acid and a base.

(b) Reaction of a salt with water.

(c) Solution that maintains a constant pH upon addition of acid or base.

3. Any carbonates and phosphates, except those of sodium, potassium, and ammonium.

5. $Zn + CuSO_4 \longrightarrow ZnSO_4 + Cu$

7. $2HCl + Na_2CO_3 \longrightarrow 2NaCl + H_2O + CO_2$

9. Any 10 from Table 14-4.

11. Acids or bases react with a buffer to produce a neutral compound plus more buffer so that the pH does not change.

13. They maintain a constant pH for the blood cells so enzymes can function best.

15. (a) 7   (b) above 7   (c) below 7.

CHAPTER 15
(page 219)

1. He showed that an organic compound could be made from inorganic reagents.

3. A bond refers to a pair of shared electrons.

5. Because one molecular formula may represent two or more structural formulas. Each different structural formula represents a different compound with different properties.

7.

9. 3.

11. The angle from the center of the tetrahedron where the carbon is to any of the four hydrogens around it. The angle is 109.5°.

CHAPTER 16
(page 238)

1. (a) Pentane; ethane.
   (b) Butyne; propyne.
   (c) Octene; ethene.

3. An alkane from which one hydrogen has been removed. Ethyl, C_2H_5— or

$$
\begin{array}{cc}
 & H \quad H \\
 & | \quad\;\; | \\
H- & C-C- \\
 & | \quad\;\; | \\
 & H \quad H
\end{array}
$$

5. Single bonds between carbon atoms.

7. By substitution; $CH_4 + Cl_2 \longrightarrow CH_3Cl + HCl$

9. Petroleum and natural gas.

11. 2,2,4-trimethylpentane; $2C_8H_{18} + 25O_2 \longrightarrow 16CO_2 + 18H_2O +$ energy

13. (a) $\underset{\underset{Cl}{|}}{CH_3-CH-CH_3}$ (b) $CH_3-CH_2-CH_2-CH_2-CH_3$

     (c) $\underset{\underset{I}{|}}{CH_3-\overset{\overset{CH_3}{|}}{C}-CH_2-CH_3}$ (d) $\underset{\underset{Cl}{|}}{CH_2}-CH_2-\underset{\underset{Cl}{|}}{CH_2}$

15. (a) 2,3-dibromobutane   (b) 3-bromo-1-butene
   (c) 4-ethylcyclopentene   (d) 5-chloro-2-pentene

17. Polymers are formed when many molecules of a substance are joined together to make a very large molecule; polymers are used for synthetic heart valves, blood vessels, syringes, and drug containers. Starch is a polymer, as is cellulose.

CHAPTER 17
(page 249)

1. ROH

3. (a)   (b)   (c)

(d) propanol

(e) 1,2,3-propanetriol

5. Seventy percent alcohol coagulates protein slowly enough that it can penetrate all the way through a cell before coagulation takes place.

7. It evaporates more slowly but it is cheaper and nonflammable.

9. Alcohol rendered unfit for human consumption; used for industrial purposes.

11. By fermentation of sugar.

13. Because it is a constituent of the body's fat.

15. Primary, methanol or methyl alcohol; secondary; 2-propanol or isopropyl alcohol; tertiary, 2-methyl-2-propanol.

17.

$$H-\overset{H}{\underset{H}{C}}-\overset{H}{\underset{H}{C}}-OH + HO-\overset{H}{\underset{H}{C}}-\overset{H}{\underset{H}{C}}-H \xrightarrow{H_2SO_4} H-\overset{H}{\underset{H}{C}}-\overset{H}{\underset{H}{C}}-O-\overset{H}{\underset{H}{C}}-\overset{H}{\underset{H}{C}}-H + H_2O$$

19. May produce nausea; irritating to membranes of respiratory tract; flammable.

21. By reaction of carbon monoxide and hydrogen; from fermentation of molasses or from the reaction of ethene and water.

23. $CH_3-CH_2-CH_2-CH_2-O-CH_2-CH_2-CH_2-CH_3 + H_2O$

   $CH_3-CH_2-CH=CH_2 + H_2O$

CHAPTER 18
(page 267)

1.

$$H-\overset{H}{\underset{H}{C}}-OH + [O] \longrightarrow H-\overset{H}{C}=O; \text{ methanal (formaldehyde).}$$

3. RCHO.   5. A ketone.

7. A polymer of acetaldehyde; used as a hypnotic.

9.

$$H-\overset{H}{\underset{H}{C}}-\overset{H}{\underset{OH}{C}}-\overset{H}{\underset{H}{C}}-H + [O] \longrightarrow H-\overset{H}{\underset{H}{C}}-\overset{}{\underset{O}{C}}-\overset{H}{\underset{H}{C}}-H$$

11. A ketone.

13.

$$H-\overset{H}{C}=O + [O] \longrightarrow H-\overset{OH}{C}=O; \text{ methanoic acid (formic acid).}$$

15. RCOOH.

17. Citric acid in citrus fruits; acetic acid in vinegar; lactic acid in sour milk.

19. $HCOOH + C_2H_5OH \longrightarrow HCOOC_2H_5 + H_2O$; ethyl formate.

21. Organic compound derived from ammonia. Primary amine, RNH_2; secondary amine, R_2NH; tertiary amine, R_3N.

23. Organic acids that have an amine attached to them; acts as both acid and base.

25. They have an acid part (COOH) and a basic part (NH$_2$).

27.

H$-$C$-$OH + H$-$N$-$H $\xrightarrow{\text{heat}}$ H$-$C$-$NH$_2$ + H$_2$O; formamide.

29. Because it may be considered as being formed from carbonic acid and two molecules of ammonia.

31. (a) 3-chlorobutanal   (b) 2,2-dichloropropanoic acid
(c) 3-methylbutanal   (d) 3-methylbutanone
(e) 2-aminopropanoic acid   (f) 4-methyl-3-hexanone
(g) N-ethylmethanamide.

33. Aldehydes are easily oxidized by Cu(OH)$_2$ whereas ketones are not.

35. A compound formed by the reaction of one molecule of a ketone with one (two) molecule(s) of an alcohol; they are important in the structure of monosaccharides.

CHAPTER 19
(page 284)

1.

3. Decrease red and white blood cell count; it is also carcinogenic.

5. Because all six positions on the benzene ring are identical.

7. (a)   Br   (b)   I   (c)   Cl

9. m-Chloroiodobenzene; o-dibromobenzene; p-bromoiodobenzene.

11.   CH$_3$

; urinary preservative.

13.   OH

15.

phenanthrene has the basic structure from which are derived the sex hormones, vitamin D, and cholesterol.

Answers to Odd-Numbered Questions   **564**

17. Methyl derivation of phenol; 3; as antiseptics.
19. By mild oxidation of toluene;

21. By oxidation of toluene;

23. To relieve pain in muscles; and joints; an antipyretic and to relieve pain of arthritis and headache.
25. Antipyretic; analgesic; to treat rheumatic fever and arthritis.

27.

29. The *p*-aminobenzenesulfonamide group.

31.

33. By substitution; by addition; by substitution.
35. Five; product of burned coal or wood; it is carcinogenic.
37. Food preservatives.
39. Estrone, testosterone, androsterone, progesterone.

CHAPTER 20
(page 294)

1. A ring compound that contains some element other than carbon in the ring.
3. Morphine narcotics obtained from the poppy plant.
5. Depress the central nervous system, producing analgesia, sedation, drowsiness, lethargy, and euphoria.
7. Used in cough medicines to depress the cough center of the brain; it is methylmorphine.
9. With methadone, which eliminates the desire for heroin and also reduces withdrawal symptoms.
11. As an anticonvulsant in the treatment of epilepsy.
13. An overwhelming compulsion to sleep; treated with amphetamines.
15. They produce visions or hallucinations.
17. It is believed to interfere with the action of serotonin, a hormone that plays an important part in the thought process.

Answers to Odd-Numbered Questions

19. Glucose, biotin, thiamine.
21. Hallucinogens stimulate sensory perception; psychomimetics mimic psychoses.

CHAPTER 21
(page 319)

1. A polyhydroxy aldehyde or ketone or substances that yield these compounds on hydrolysis.
3. Structural isomers have the same molecular formula, same functional groups, but different structural formulas.

example: C—C—C—C—C   and   C—C—C—C
|
C

5. Functional isomers have the same structural formulas but different functional groups.

example: CH_3OCH_3 and CH_3CH_2OH

7. (a)   (b)

9. By using the formula 2^n, where n is the number of asymmetric carbon atoms.
11. Ordinary light vibrates in all planes, polarized light in only one plane.
13. They refer to the configuration of the OH group on the carbon atom next to the end of the chain containing the primary alcohol group; D on the right, L on the left.
15. D
17. A polysaccharide that on hydrolysis yields hexoses; a polysaccharide that on hydrolysis yields pentoses.
19. They are formed as monosaccharides from CO_2 in the air and H_2O from the ground under the action of sunlight and chlorophyll.
21. Three-carbon simple sugars; 5-carbon simple sugars; 6-carbon simple sugars.
23. All have same molecular formula; glucose and galactose are both aldehydes with a different arrangement about carbon atom #4; fructose is a ketone.
25. Found in fruit juices, particularly grape.
27. In the bloodstream and the tissues.
29. Clinitest, Fehling's solution, Benedict's solution.
31. No; glucose and fructose will, galactose will not because of a lack of a particular enzyme in yeast.
33. Glucuronic acid.   35. Sorbitol.
37. No; yeast contains sucrase and maltase but not lactase.
39. Sucrose has no free carbonyl group so is not a reducing sugar; lactose and maltose have a free carbonyl group so they are reducing sugars.
41. In sprouting grain.
43. Polysaccharides have a high MW, mono- and disaccharides have a low MW; polysaccharides are tasteless, mono- and disaccharides are sweet; polysaccharides are insoluble in water, mono- and disaccharides are soluble; polysaccharides give a negative test with $Cu(OH)_2$, mono- and disaccharides give

a positive test except for sucrose; polysaccharides and disaccharides do not pass through membranes, monosaccharides pass through membranes.

45. Add I_2 and see if blue color develops; add starch and see if blue color develops.

47. As a supporting and structural substance.

49. As a reserve supply of carbohydrate.

51. Hydrolysis products of starch; used as glues.

53. A compound formed by the reaction of one molecule of an aldehyde with one molecule of an alcohol.

55. A three-dimensional representation of structure in which the horizontal lines indicate bonds extending forward from the plane and the vertical lines indicate bonds extending backward from the plane.

57.

α-D-galactose

59. A bond between two monosaccharides that is either a ketal or an acetal.

61. The —OH on carbon #1 may be either above or below the plane.

CHAPTER 22
(page 343)

1. Insoluble in water, soluble in organic solvents, yield fatty acids on hydrolysis or combine with fatty acids to form an ester, take part in metabolism, contain C, H, and O.

3. In a fat the alcohol is glycerol; in a wax the alcohol has a high molecular weight. A fat is a highly saturated compound; an oil is unsaturated.

5. A compound derived from simple and compound lipids on hydrolysis. Examples are fatty acids, glycerol, other alcohols, and sterols.

7. Saturated have single bonds between carbon atoms; unsaturated have one or more double bonds.

9. Linoleic; without it infants lose weight and develop eczema.

11. Chaulmoogric acid.   13. Vegetable fats.

15.

$$\begin{array}{l} \text{H} \\ \text{H—C—OOCC}_{15}\text{H}_{31} \\ \text{H—C—OOCC}_{17}\text{H}_{35} \\ \text{H—C—OOCC}_{17}\text{H}_{33} \\ \text{H} \end{array}$$

17. Odorless and tasteless when pure, insoluble in water but soluble in organic solvents; fats are solid and oils are liquids.
19. Salt of a fatty acid (soap) and glycerol.
21. Acrolein test; heat fat or oil with $KHSO_4$ and see if odor of acrolein is present.
23. Soaps are salts of fatty acids; detergents are salts of long-chain alcohol sulfates.
25. Presence of air bubbles.
27. To remove debris and bacteria from the skin.
29. A compound containing fatty acids, glycerol, a nitrogen compound, and phosphoric acid.
31. A compound produced when one molecule of fatty acid is removed from lecithin under the influence of the enzyme lecithinase A. It is very poisonous.
33. They form a bilayer, which helps control passage into and out of the cell.
35. Deposits of excess lipids from bloodstream; reduce intake of lipids or use hyperlipidemic drugs.
37. Cholesterol.
39. Because the body manufacturers its own cholesterol; a diet low in cholesterol, particularly one containing unsaturated fish and vegetable oils.
41. Soap has a fat-soluble and a water-soluble end. The fat-soluble end dissolves in oil or grease and the water-soluble end sticks out into the water. The water-soluble end ionizes, leaving the oil drop with a negative charge that repels all other oil drops that have a like charge. Thus, the oil is emulsified and easily washed away.
43. Detergents that are degraded by natural conditions and do not cause pollution.
45. They stimulate the movement of calcium ions from bone.
47. In the fluid-mosaic model, proteins are embedded throughout the membrane and transport polar molecules and ions through the membrane.
49. Prostacyclin stimulates protection of c-AMP; thromboxanes inhibit production of c-AMP.

CHAPTER 23
(page 368)

1. C, H, O, N.   3. From CO_2 and water by photosynthesis.
5. Nitrogen in the air is fixed by bacteria into soil nitrates, which are picked up by plants and changed to plant protein. Plant protein becomes animal protein, then waste, which is denitrified and changed back to air nitrogen.
7. Equal; less.
9. Compounds containing an acid group, COOH, and an amine group, NH_2; see text.
11. Because they contain both acid and basic groups; they contain an asymmetric carbon; L.
13. Becomes minimum.

15.
$$(CH_3)_2CH-\underset{\underset{NH_2}{|}}{CH}-\overset{\overset{O}{\|}}{C}-\boxed{OH + H}NH-CH_2COOH \longrightarrow$$

valine   glycine

$$(CH_3)_2CH\underset{\underset{NH_2}{|}}{CH}-\overset{\overset{O}{\|}}{C}-NHCH_2COOH$$

valyl glycine

$$NH_2-CH_2CO\boxed{OH} + (CH_3)_2CHCH-\overset{\displaystyle O}{\overset{\|}{C}}-OH \longrightarrow NH_2CH_2-\overset{\displaystyle O}{\overset{\|}{C}}-NHCH-COOH$$

$$\boxed{H}NH \qquad\qquad\qquad CH(CH_3)_2$$

glycine   valine   glycyl valine

17. Alanine, arginine, asparagine, cysteine, glutamic acid, glutamine, glycine, histidine, isoleucine, leucine, lysine, phenylalanine, proline, serine, threonine, tyrosine, valine.

19. Proteoses, peptones, polypeptides, tripeptides, dipeptides, amino acids.

21. According to composition, function, or shape.

23. Nucleoproteins, glycoproteins, phosphoproteins, chromoproteins, lipoproteins, metalloproteins.

25. Seventy percent alcohol goes all the way through a cell before it coagulates the protein inside.

27. Egg white; otherwise the stomach would digest the antidote.

29. Xanthoproteic test: HNO_3 for protein containing a benzene ring.
Biuret test: $NaOH + CuSO_4$ for two or more peptide linkages.
Million's test: $Hg + HNO_3$ for protein containing tyrosine.
Hopkins–Cole test: glyoxalic acid for protein containing typtophan.
Ninhydrin test: ninhydrin for free amino acid or peptides.

31. A drop of unknown is placed at the bottom of a piece of filter paper suspended in a solvent. As the solvent rises in the paper, it carries the components of the unknown upward at different rates, depending upon their relative solubilities. Then paper is turned at right angles and placed in another solvent to repeat the process in a second direction.

33. Column is packed with an inert material coated with a thin layer of a high-boiling, nonvolatile liquid. Sample is injected into the top of the column, which is then heated as an inert carrier is passed through. The mixture in the unknown separates gradually as the more volatile components vaporize first.

35. In certain microorganisms; used as antibiotics.

37. A dipolar ion formed when the carboxyl group of an amino acid donates a hydrogen ion to the amino group of the same amino acid.

39. Because the amino acids are all of the L configuration.

41. Salt bridges, hydrogen bonds, disulfide bonds, hydrophobic bonds.

43. Storage, ferritin; transportation, hemoglobin, serum albumin; enzyme, pepsin; hormone, insulin.

CHAPTER 24
(page 385)

1. Enzymes increase the speed of a reaction.

3. An increase in temperature increases its rate of reaction.

5. Each enzyme has an optimum pH at which it functions best.

7. Increase in concentration leads to increased rate.

9. Essential for metabolism of carbohydrates, fats, proteins; pantothenic acid, adenine, ribose, phosphoric acid, mercaptoethanolamine.

11. Hydrolytic enzymes, oxidation-reduction enzymes, transferases, isomerases, ligases, lyases.

13. Enzymes that catalyze hydrolysis of esters; gastric lipase in gastric juice and pancreatic lipase in pancreatic juice; both catalyze hydrolysis of fats to fatty acids and glycerol.

15. An enzyme for the hydrolysis of nucleic acids.
17. An enzyme that catalyzes the transfer of functional groups; an enzyme that catalyzes the interconversion of optical, geometric, and structural isomers.
19. A coenzyme found in the mitrochondria; it functions in electron transport and oxidative phosphorylation.
21. With three points of attachment on an active site, only one optical isomer will fit.
23. Nonspecific inhibitors affect all enzymes in the same manner; specific inhibitors affect only one enzyme or group of enzymes.
25. Use of chemicals to destroy infectious microorganisms and cancerous cells without damaging the hosts cells; antibiotics such as penicillin and tetracycline and antimetabolites such as sulfanilamide.
27. Levels of some enzymes increase or decrease during diseases and so blood levels are analyzed for abnormal concentrations of those enzymes.
29. Competitive inhibitors compete for the active site of the enzyme. Noncompetitive inhibitors prevent the enzyme from functioning by bonding to another part of that enzyme, not the active site.
31. In the lock-and-key theory the active site is rigid. In the induced-fit theory, the active site is flexible and can change upon binding to a substrate.
33. They are key metabolic enzymes whose activity can be changed by molecules other than the substrate; to ensure that biolgic processes remain coordinated at all time.

CHAPTER 25
(page 394)

1. To produce simple molecules that can be absorbed into the bloodstream through the intestinal walls.
3. In the mouth, stomach, and small intestine.
5. 1–2; presence of HCl.
7. A higher-than-normal acid condition in the stomach; may be indicative of gastric uclers, hypertension, or gastritis.
9. Pepsinogen is an inactive form of the enzyme pepsin.
11. It stimulates the pancreas to release the pancreatic juice into the small intestine.
13. A substance secreted by the parietal cells in the walls of the stomach; vitamin B_{12} must react with the intrinsic factor before it can be absorbed. A lack of the intrinsic factor is associated with pernicious anemia.
15. Trypsinogen, for hydrolysis of protein; chymotrypsinogen, for hydrolysis of protein; carboxypeptidase, for hydrolysis of polypeptides and dipeptides; steapsin, for hydrolysis of fat; amylopsin, for hydrolysis of starch to maltose.
17. In the liver; in the gallbladder.
19. 7.8 to 8.6; bile salts, bile pigments, and cholesterol.
21. From the breakdown of hemoglobin; in urine and feces.
23. Jaundice is produced with yellow pigmentation of skin.
25. Digestion of carbohydrates begins in the mouth with ptyalin, which acts on starch; digestion is completed in the small intestine through the aid of enzymes in the pancreatic and intestinal juices; absorbed through villi in small intestine.
27. Digestion of protein begins in the stomach through the action of pepsin; it is continued in small intestine through the action of trypsin, and chymotrypsin; absorbed through villi of small intestine.
29. Serves as a place for reabsorption of water and some salts and for formation of feces.

31. Action of bacteria on waste products.
33. An intestinal enzyme that changes trypsinogen to trypsin in the small intestines.

CHAPTER 26
(page 414)

1. Glucose.
3. Synthesis of glycogen from glucose; in muscles and liver.
5. Point at which blood sugar spills over into urine.
7. By oxidation; by conversion to glycogen; by conversion to fat; through the action of hormones.
9. $A—P \sim P \sim P \longrightarrow A—P \sim P$; 7600 cal per mole.
11. Glycogenesis occurs primarily in the liver and the muscles. First, glucose is changed to glucose-6-P under the influence of the enzyme glucokinase, the hormone insulin, and ATP. Glucose-6-P is changed to glucose-1-P through the action of the enzyme phosphoglucomutase. Glucose-1-P reacts with UTP to form UDPG under the influence of the enzyme UDPG pyrophosphorylase. Finally, UDPG under the influence of the enzyme glycogen synthetase and insulin and cyclic AMP form glycogen.
13. No; because the enzyme glucose-6-phosphatase is found in the liver but not in the muscle.
15. It supplies most of the body's energy for muscular contraction.
17. No; only one fifth of it.
19. By conversion of blood glucose to muscle glycogen.
21. It provides five-carbon sugars for synthesis of nucleic acids and $NADP^+$.
23. It is the main fuel of the cycle.
25. Most of the energy is produced in the Krebs cycle.
27. Formation of glucose from noncarbohydrate substances; high-protein diet, decreased carbohydrate diet, starvation, severe diabetes.
29. Because the reaction of pyruvic acid to acetyl CoA is not reversible.
31. During periods of emotional stress; it promotes glycogenolysis.
33. After a fast a patient is given glucose orally and blood sugar levels are checked periodically to see how fast blood sugar levels return to normal; test for diabetes.
35. An enzyme that binds oxygen in the electron transport system, then reduces it with electrons received from other cytochromes, and finally converts the O_2 to H_2O; it contains the elements Fe and Cu; it is essential to life because it controls a critical step in the body's metabolic process.

CHAPTER 27
(page 423)

1. Through lacteals of villi of small intestine into lymphatics to thoracic duct to liver.
3. Glycerol is oxidized to dihydroxyacetone phosphate, which is part of the glycolysis sequence and so becomes part of carbohydrate metabolism.
5. Acetyl CoA; acetyl CoA and propionyl CoA.
7. Carbohydrate 4 kcal; fat, 9 kcal.   9. 129.   11. Liver
13. In adipose tissue under skin and around internal organs; reserve supply of fuel, support for internal organs, shock absorber for internal organs, insulation.
15. Conversion of glucose to fat; in the mitochondria and the cytoplasm.
17. They form part of the framework of cell membranes.
19. In lecithin a 1,2-diglyceride reacts with CDP-choline; in cephalin, a 1,2-diglyceride reacts with CDP-ethanolamine.

21. It is a precursor for vitamin D, sex hormones, and hormones of the adrenal cortex.
23. Gallstones

CHAPTER 28
(page 434)

1. To build new tissue; to replace old tissue; to form hemoglobin, enzymes, and hormones; to produce energy.
3. When intake of nitrogen equals output.
5. Starvation, malnutrition, prolonged fever, wasting illness.
7. One that does not contain all the essential amino acids.
9. Process of removing alpha amino group of an amino acid to form an alpha-keto acid; in the liver.
11. A reaction whereby an amino group from an amino acid is transferred to a keto acid; to manufacture amino acids the body needs.
13. In the liver.
15. Removal of a carboxyl group from an amino acid; primary amine.
17. A blue-green pigment from hemoglobin produced in reticuloendothelial cells of liver, spleen, and bone marrow.
19. Hemolytic jaundice is caused by accumulation of bilirubin in blood caused by hemolysis; obstructive jaundice is caused by a blocked bile duct.
21. Nucleoproteins are hydrolyzed to protein and nucleic acid; the protein part is used as any other protein is in the body; the nucleic acids yield ribose and deoxyribose, which enter the carbohydrate cycle, and also urea and uric acid, which are excreted in the urine.

CHAPTER 29
(page 446)

1. Through the lungs, skin, intestines, and kidneys.
3. A coil of capillaries in the kidneys; a structure around the glomerulus in the kidneys.
5. Blood pressure.
7. 600–2500 ml; weather conditions, drugs, muscular activity.
9. A decreased output of urine; high fever and certain kidney diseases.
11. Excessive water intake; diuretics and high-protein diet.
13. 4.7 to 8.0; diet.
15. Precipitation of calcium phosphate.
17. Urea; from metabolism of protein; $H_2N\overset{\overset{\displaystyle O}{\|}}{C}NH_2$.
19.

21. Deposits of uric acid and urates in joints and tissues; leukemia, severe liver disease.
23. Number of milligrams of creatinine excreted within a 24-hr period per kilogram of body weight.
25. From arginine, methionine, and glycine.
27. A condition in which abnormal amounts of creatine occur in the urine.

Answers to Odd-Numbered Questions

29. High, on diet high in nucleoprotein; high in hyperparathyroidism; low in hypoparathyroidism and renal diseases.

31. Nephritis, nephrosis, severe heart disease.

33. Sample of urine is heated and acidified with dilute acetic acid. Protein forms a cloud. Without acidification, phosphates give a false test.

35. Lactose and galactose during pregnancy; pentoses after a meal containing plums, grapes, or cherries.

37. Add sodium nitroprusside and then NH_4OH until alkaline. A red-pink color is positive.

39. Obstruction to flow of bile from liver.

CHAPTER 30
(page 476)

1. To carry oxygen, minerals, food to cells and carbon dioxide and wastes from cells. Also to carry hormones, enzymes, blood cells, and antibodies. Blood acts as a buffer and helps regulate body temperature.

3. 5-10 thousand/mm³.   5. Defense against infection.

7. The percentage of each type of leukocyte present; they are involved in the clotting of the blood.

9. Blood serum is blood plasma without the fibrinogen for clotting.

11. Increases during fever and pregnancy; decreases in diarrhea and hemorrhaging.

13. A conjugated protein.

15. Chlorophyll *a* has a Mg in its center while hemoglobin has an Fe, and both have different side chains; cytochrome *c* has an Fe in its center like hemoglobin but has sulfur bonding to protein.

17. Lack of vitamin B_{12} or the intrinsic factor.   19. Hemorrhaging.

21. Albumin causes most of the colloid osmotic pressure of the blood and draws water back into the bloodstream.

23. Alpha and beta globulins aid in transportation of carbohydrates, lipids, and metal ions; gamma globulins contain the antibodies.

25. When a blood vessel is cut, the tissues liberate thromboplastin; in the presence of thromboplastin and Ca^{2+}, prothrombin is changed to thrombin, which in turn acts on fibrinogen to change it to fibrin, the clot.

27. It is poisonous.

29. A clot formed in a blood vessel; paralysis or death.

31. CO_2 is carried as H_2CO_3, as $NaHCO_3$, and as $HHbCO_2$.

33. Since blood cells can carry only a limited amount of HCO_3^- ion, much of that ion diffuses out into the plasma while Cl^- comes in; this is the chloride shift. The reverse takes place in the lungs.

35. Bicarbonate, phosphate, protein buffers.

37. $HCl + KHCO_3 \longrightarrow KCl + H_2CO_3$

$NaOH + H_2CO_3 \longrightarrow H_2O + NaHCO_3$

39. Through the skin, as urine, through lungs, through feces.

41. To maintain osmotic pressure of extracellular fluid, to control water retention in tissue spaces, to help maintain blood pressure, to help maintain acid–base balance, to regulate irritability of nerve and muscle tissue.

43. Deficient water intake, excessive water output, poor kidney excretion, rapid administration of sodium salts, hyperactivity of adrenal cortex.

45. Too low an intake, or too great an output of potassium, or sudden shift of K^+ from extracellular to intracellular fluids; general feeling of being ill, lack

Answers to Odd-Numbered Questions   573

of energy, muscular weakness, apathy, dizziness on rising, cramps, numbness of fingers and toes.

47. A hypoactive parathyroid may cause hypocalcemia; a hyperactive parathyroid may cause hypercalcemia.

49. In the formation of HCl in the stomach and in the transportation of oxygen by the blood.

51. $$\frac{3.6 \times 10 \times 2}{24} = 3 \text{ mEq/L}$$

53. P_{CO_2} and HCO_3^-; pH.

55. To enhance the excretion of HCO_3^-.

57. A drop in plasma protein caused by protein deficiency; swollen abdomen and extremities.

CHAPTER 31
(page 501)

1. Both are carried by the bloodstream; both are required in small amounts; neither furnishes energy; vitamins are supplied in food, hormones are produced by the body.

3. Fish liver oils, butter, milk.

5. Provitamin A; it is changed in the body into two molecules of vitamin A.

7. In the liver; absorbed with aid of bile.

9. Light changes rhodopsin to all *trans*-retinal and opsin. *Trans*-retinal is changed to 11-*cis*-retinal, and back to rhodopsin to begin the cycle anew.

11. Because it is produced by exposure of the skin to ultraviolet rays of the sun.

13. One thousand and 800 retinol equivalents for male and female, respectively; 400 IU vitamin D.

15. Rickets, osteomalacia, osteoporosis; calcification of soft tissues.

17. Green leafy tissues, liver, eggs, cheese, edible fats and oils; insoluble in water, stable to heat, destroyed by acid and alkaline solutions, unstable to light and oxidants; necessary for production of prothrombin for blood-clotting process.

19. Lack of appetite, failure of growth, loss of weight, beriberi.

21. Liver, kidneys, heart meats, yeast, peanuts, wheat germ; yeast, liver, egg yolk, germ of grain, and seeds.

23. Egg yolk, yeast, kidney and lean meats, skimmed milk, broccoli, sweet potatoes, molasses; soluble in water, insoluble in fat solvents, stable in acid and alkaline solution; causes degeneration in adrenal cortex and a failure in reproduction.

25. Fresh fruits and vegetables, dry cereals, milk, meats, eggs; soluble in water and alcohol, insoluble in fat solvents, strong reducing agent rapidly destroyed by heat; functions in oxidation-reduction reactions in cellular respiration, in formation of intercellular substance that cements tissues together.

27. By acting as competitive inhibitor.

29. When a nerve cell is stimulated, it releases acetylcholine, which stimulates the adjacent nerve cell to also release acetylcholine. This process continues until the impulse reaches the brain. After the impulse has passed, acetylcholine is regenerated to be used again.

CHAPTER 32
(page 524)

1. Both are necessary in small amounts and both are highly specific, but hormones are produced in the body whereas vitamins are not.

3. The pyloric mucosa; stimulates secretion of HCl and produces greater motility in stomach.
5. Insulin and glucagon.   7. It is a protein and would be digested.
9. Increases rate of oxidation of glucose, facilitates glycogenesis, and increases synthesis of fatty acids, protein, and RNA.
11. No; it temporarily reduces blood sugar level.
13. Increases blood sugar level.
15. Increased blood sugar level, sugar in urine, acetone bodies in blood, acidosis.
17. Individuals who have a retarded growth because of absence or failure of development of thryoid gland; cured by administration of thyroid hormones before adulthood.
19. Increase in size of thyroid and neck.
21. It influences the metabolism of calcium and phosphorus.
23. Glucocorticoids; affect metabolism of carbohydrates, fats, and protein; corticosterone, cortisone, cortisol.
    Mineralocorticoids; affect transportation of electrolytes and distribution of water; aldosterone.
    Androgens or estrogens; affect secondary sex characteristics; dehydroepiandrosterone.
25. Excessive loss of NaCl, low blood pressure, low body temperature, hypoglycemia, elevation of serum potassium, muscular weakness, nausea, loss of appetite, brownish pigmentations of skin.
27. Epinephrine; relaxes smooth muscles and elevates blood pressure, norepinephrine; raises blood pressure.
29. Dwarfs develop normally but do not grow in size; they are not retarded but may be sexually retarded.
31. Vasopressin; stimulates kidney to reabsorb water. Oxytocin; contracts muscles of uterus.
33. Neurohormones; stimulators and inhibitors for release of hormones.
35. Follicles of ovary; corpus luteum.
37. Because its hormones are controlled by the hypothalamus.
39. By binding to opiate receptors in the brain.
41. By triggering impulses that stimulate the release of endorphins and enkephalins.
43. Act as a chemical messenger to regulate enzyme activity; involved in action of F prostaglandins.

CHAPTER 33
(page 544)

1. Chromosomes contain genes and genes are made of DNA, which holds the hereditary information.

3.

5. The DNA unwinds and each half acts as a template for nucleotides to collect on and form a new chain, which then coils up to form two new chains of DNA.

7. In RNA, adenine bonds to uracil; in DNA, adenine bonds to thymine.
9. Cystic fibrosis.   11. See page 535.
13. A synthetic RNA composed only of uracil was substituted for mRNA in a system. The polypeptide formed contained only phenylalanine. Thus, the RNA, which had the code UUU, has the corresponding code of AAA on DNA and specifies phenylalanine.
15. A miscopying of the genetic code or omission or change in sequence of the letters of the code.
17. (a) Normal red blood cells have a concave shape; sickle cells have a sickle shape.
    (b) Hemoglobin and hemoglobin-S differ only in #6 amino acid of a 146-amino acid chain.
19. If an enzyme is deficient, the body might lack the compound produced through the action of that enzyme.

Index

Abdomen X rays, 65
Abortion, 340
Abscesses, 56
Absolute zero, 10
Acetal, 256, 312
Acetaldehyde, 132, 251, 252, 256, 257
Acetamide, 265
Acetaminophen, 280
Acetanilide, 281
Acetazolamide, 465, 474
Acetic acid, 133, 192, 256, 257, 258, 265, 266, 281, 298, 393, 443, 498
Acetoacetic acid, 411, 418, 419
Acetoacetyl CoA, 418, 419, 431, 432
Acetone, 133, 146, 254, 322, 328, 411, 419, 432, 439, 496
Acetone bodies, 418, 419, 444, 445, 505
Acetophenone, 278
Acetyl coenzyme A, 259, 262, 376, 406, 407, 408, 417, 418, 419, 421, 422, 431, 432, 490, 499
Acetyl group, 258, 376
Acetylation, 288
Acetylation reaction, 375, 376
Acetylcholine, 498
Acetylcholinesterase, 498
Acetylene, 126, 233, 236
Acetylsalicylic acid, 195, 196, 280
Achroodextrin, 316
Acid-base balance, 190, 436, 449, 462, 464, 470, 473
Acid-base titration, 198
Acid rain, 113
Acid phosphatase, 383
Acidosis, 209, 411, 419, 439, 444, 450, 452, 462, 463, 505
Acids, 147, 164, 192, 204, 206, 245, 256, 279, 428
  strong, 195, 205, 463
  uses of, 195
Aconitase, 408
Acrolein test, 329

Acromegaly, 516
ACTH, 513, 514, 515, 516
ACTH-releasing hormone, 519
Actin, 361
Activated ergosterol, 483
Activated glucose, 399
Activation energy, 97
Activators, 372, 473
Active acetate, 407
Active fatty acid, 417, 421
Active metals, 126, 147
Active site, 372, 375, 383
Active transport, 169, 391
Activity series, 193, 206
Acupuncture, 520
Acute glomerulonephritis, 452
Acute hepatitis, 383
Acute pancreatic disease, 382, 383
Addison's disease, 412, 443, 452, 512, 517
Addition reactions, 235
Adenine, 287, 399, 494, 528, 530, 531, 532, 535
Adenohypophysis, 340, 514
Adenosine, 529
Adenosine diphosphate, 262, 397, 529
Adenosine monophosphate, 262, 529
Adenosine triphosphate, 262, 379, 397, 398, 399, 529
Adenylate cyclase, 400, 503, 504, 514, 520
ADH, 470, 515, 517, 518, 519
Adhesion, 168
Adhesives, 317
Adipose tissue, 327, 340, 391, 416, 419, 420, 425, 455, 507
ADP, 262, 287, 397, 398, 400, 401, 402, 403, 404, 405, 409, 417, 421, 428, 442, 529
Adrenal cortex, 341, 411, 422, 470, 495, 511, 512, 513, 516, 517
Adrenal glands, 53, 339, 511, 514
Adrenaline, 290, 291, 513

Adrenocorticotropic hormone, 421, 514, 516
Adriamycin, 382
Adsorption, 177
Adult rickets, 486
Aeration, 151
Aerobic sequence, 405, 407, 432
Aerosol mask, 123
Agammaglobulinemia, 458, 459
Air pollution, 112, 149
Alanine, 349, 354, 366, 380, 381, 427, 428, 432, 535
Alanine racemase, 380
Albinism, 540
Albumin, 54, 55, 195, 354, 359, 361, 363, 431, 443, 449, 455, 457, 458
Albumin-fatty acid complex, 455
Albuminoids, 359
Albuminuria, 443
Alcohol, 119, 146, 159, 168, 240, 246, 250, 322, 362, 379, 384, 438, 445, 489, 499
  secondary, 244, 245, 250, 255
Alcohol dehydrogenase, 474
Alcoholism, 252, 290, 443, 473, 490
Aldehydes, 245, 250, 256, 278, 298, 304, 309, 325
Aldohexose, 307, 308
Aldolase, 402, 403
Aldopentose, 299
Aldoses, 299, 304, 305, 308
Aldosterone, 380, 470, 511, 512
Alimentary glycosuria, 308
Aliphatic compounds, 218, 331
Alkaline, 439
Alkaline phosphatase, 383, 474
Alkaline reserve, 444, 463
Alkaloidal reagents, 363, 373
Alkaloids, 275, 286, 293
Alkalosis, 209, 439, 450, 462, 473
Alkanes, 221, 234, 247
Alka-Seltzer, 194
Alkenes, 230, 232, 235, 245, 247

Alkoxy derivatives, 247
Alkyl groups, 224
Alkyl halides, 246
Alkylating agents, 382
Alkynes, 233, 235
Allantoin, 442, 474
Allergic sensitivity, 382
Allosteric enzyme, 383
Allotropic forms, 127
Alloy, 161
Alpha-amino acids, 265, 348, 364, 427, 428, 430
Alpha-globulin, 458
Alpha-glycerophosphate, 417, 421
Alpha helix, 355
Alpha-ketoacids, 427, 428, 490, 499
Alpha-ketoglutaric acid, 406, 408, 432, 490
Alpha-naphthol, 274
Alpha particles, 44, 45, 61
Aluminum chlorohydrate, 475
Alveoli, 109, 168, 460, 461
Amalgam, 161
Amebicide, 128
Amide bond, 265, 382
Amides, 265, 283
Amines, 262, 281, 377, 479
  secondary, 262, 263, 265
Amino acid oxidase, 427
Amino acids, 145, 262, 265, 347, 348, 352, 355, 357, 363, 375, 377, 378, 379, 380, 386, 391, 392, 393, 410, 412, 425, 426, 428, 431, 432, 436, 437, 442, 444, 490, 493, 494, 503, 505, 507, 508, 510, 513, 515, 516, 517, 520, 533, 534, 535, 537
  nutritionally essential, 427
Aminoacetic acid, 263
Aminoethanoic acid, 263
Aminopeptidase, 380, 387, 391, 392
Aminopropane, 263
Aminotransferases, 427
Ammonia, 110, 153, 196, 263, 265, 283, 427, 428, 429, 444, 449, 464
Ammonia, spirits of, 198
Ammonium chloride, 208
Ammonium ions, 190, 439, 443, 464
Ammonium salts, 264
AMP, 262, 287, 404, 429, 504, 529
AMP cyclic, 262, 286, 399, 412, 416, 442, 503, 507, 514, 516, 520
Amphetamines, 264, 290, 291
Amphipathic, 333
Amphoteric compounds, 265, 352
Amu, 29
Amyl acetate, 261
Amyl butyrate, 261
Amylase, 383
Amylodextrin, 316
Amylopectin, 316, 318

Amylopsin, 379
Amylose, 316, 318
Anabolic activity, 471
Anaerobic sequence, 400
Anaerobically, 258, 259, 432
Analgesic, 196, 280, 281, 288, 293, 519
Androgens, 449, 511, 522
Androsterone, 279, 522
Anemia, 55, 208, 281, 339, 449, 450, 452, 453, 474, 485, 487, 493, 500, 509, 538, 540
Anesthesia, 293, 452
Anesthetic, 123, 128, 227, 229, 236, 248, 264, 293, 465, 514
  local, 293
Angiotensin, 380
Angiotensinogen, 380
Anhydrous, 148
Aniline, 281
Anions, 75, 158, 468, 469, 470
Anorexia, 65
Antabuse, 253
Antacids, 194, 197, 208
Anterior lobe, 514
Anthracene, 275
Antibacterial action, 264, 277, 331, 499
Antibiotics, 348, 380, 382, 488, 537
Antibodies, 55, 64, 347, 442, 449, 458, 459, 541
Anticoagulant, 258, 317, 450, 460, 488
Anticlotting agent, 451
Anticonvulsant, 290
Antidepressant, 475
Antidermatitis factor, 493
Antidiuretic hormone, 470, 517, 518, 519
Antidote, 488
Anti-egg-white injury factor, 495
Antifreeze, 167, 244
Antigen, 56
Antihemophilic globulin, 540
Antihemorrhaging vitamin, 488
Antihyperlipidemic drugs, 341
Antihypertensive drug, 493
Antileukemic drugs, 496
Antimetabolites, 380, 382, 499
Antimony potassium tartrate, 259
Antineoplastic agents, 382
Antioxidants, 329, 486
Antipellagra factor, 492
Antipernicious anemia factor, 496
Antiperspirant sprays, 475
Antipyretic, 196, 280, 281, 293
Antiseptic, 126, 138, 241, 261, 264
Antispasmodic, 288
Antithyroid drugs, 510
Antitoxins, 180
Antituberculosis drug, 493
Anuria, 438, 452, 470

Apoenzyme, 375
Arabinose, 306, 359
Arachidic acid, 323
Arachidonic acid, 323, 339, 340
Arginase, 430
Arginine, 350, 353, 357, 366, 428, 429, 430, 432, 442, 518, 535
Arginine succinic acid, 429, 430
Arginosuccinate synthetase, 429
Argyrol, 177
Aromatic compounds, 218, 269
Arrhenius, Svante, 187
Arsenic, 22
Arterial blood, 109
Arteries, hardening of, 421
Arterioles, 380, 436
Arteriosclerosis, 341
Arthritis, 383, 441
Artificial kidney machine, 181, 437
Artificial radioactivity, 47
Asbestos, 112
Ascorbic acid, 195, 499
Asparagine, 350, 432, 535
Aspartame, 315
Aspartic acid, 357, 429, 432, 535
Asphyxiation, 123
Aspirin, 194, 195, 196, 280, 339, 460, 466, 474
Asthma, 293, 340
Astringent, 243
Asymmetric carbon atoms, 302, 304, 335
Atherosclerosis, 341, 360, 421
Atom, 28, 73
  stability of, 72
  structure of, 29, 31
Atomic mass units, 29
Atomic numbers, 30
Atomic orbitals, 34
Atomic weight, 30
ATP, 262, 287, 379, 397, 398, 399, 400, 401, 402, 403, 404, 405, 407, 409, 411, 417, 418, 421, 428, 429, 432, 442, 473, 500, 529
Autoclave, 107, 142, 146
Autoradiograph, 43
Avidin, 495
Avogadro's number, 84

Bacteria, 393, 504, 541
Bacterial cell wall, 381
Bacterial infections, 382
Bacteriocide, 128, 282
Bacteriostatic, 282
Baking soda, 208
Balancing chemical equations, 91
Balancing oxidation-reduction equations, 134
Barbiturates, 263, 286, 289, 528
Barium sulfate, 56, 207, 208
Barometer, 103

Basal metabolic rate, 124, 507
Basedow's disease, 510
Bases, 147, 164, 193, 196, 197, 204, 206, 257, 264
    commonly used, 197
    strong, 205, 463
Basophils, 449
Beeswax, 332
BEI, 507
Bends, 111, 125
Benedict's solution, 253, 255, 309, 310, 397, 412, 443, 444
"Bennies," 290
Benzaldehyde, 278
Benzalkonium chloride, 264
Benzamide, 283
Benzedrine, 290, 291
Benzene, 144, 146, 160, 269, 328, 348, 363, 453
Benzidine, 444
Benzocaine, 261
Benzoic acid, 274, 283
Benzpyrene, 128, 275
Beriberi, 490
Beta-amino acid, 265
Beta-carotene, 480
Beta cells, 411
Beta globulins, 458, 474
Beta-glucosidase, 339
Beta-hydroxy butyric acid, 411, 418, 419
Beta-hydroxy fatty acid, 417
Beta-keto acyl CoA, 417
Beta-naphthol, 274
Beta oxidation theory, 417
Beta particles, 44, 45, 61
Beta pleated sheets, 356
BHA, 277
BHT, 277
Bicarbonate buffers, 463, 470
Bicarbonate ions, 190, 194, 386, 461, 462, 466, 473
Bichloride of mercury, 178, 362, 438
Bichloroacteic acid, 195
Bilayer, 334
Bile, 168, 201, 286, 328, 388, 391, 392, 421, 431, 444, 482, 488
Bile acids, 275
Bile pigments, 388, 392, 436
Bile salts, 341, 388, 392, 416
Biliary disease, 488
Biliary obstruction, 452
Bilirubin, 286, 388, 431, 433
Bilirubin digluconuride, 431, 433
Bilirubin reductase, 431
Biliverdin, 388, 431, 433, 442
Binary compounds, 77
Biodegradable, 332
Biologic effects of radiation, 61
Biologic half-life, 52, 308
Biotin, 292, 418, 489, 495
Bishydroxycoumarin, 460

Biuret test, 364
Black tongue, 493
Black water fever, 444
Blackstrap molasses, 242
Bleach, 126, 363
Bleaching powder, 138
Blindness, 241
Blood, 168, 173, 201, 439, 444, 448
    analysis, 451
    anticoagulant, 258, 317
    buffers, 190, 448, 464
    cells, 450
    citrated, 472
    clotting, 22, 190, 208, 280, 317, 336, 361, 383, 416, 425, 448, 449, 451, 459, 472, 488, 540
    composition, 448, 452
    extenders, 317
    gas analysis, 451
    plasma, 438, 449, 450, 455, 461, 462, 511
    plasma volume, 463, 467, 474
    platelets, 280, 339, 340, 472
    pressure, 104, 247, 293, 318, 380, 437, 456, 470, 471, 472, 473, 512, 514, 518
    properties, 450
    proteins, 449
    serum, 366, 449
    sugar, normal fasting, 396, 505, 506
    sugar level, 396, 411, 412, 413, 506, 513, 514, 515, 516
    types, 360, 450
    viscosity, 168, 451
    volume, 54, 318, 451, 512, 513
"Blue babies," 340
BMR, 124, 507
Body fluids, 436, 448
    concentration of, 468
Body's protein requirements, 427
Boiler scale, 152
Boiling, 150, 167, 187
Boiling point, 15, 146, 167, 187
Bonding, 72, 215, 217
Bonds
    single, 79
    strength of, 80
    triple, 79, 233
Bone
    diseases, 484
    marrow, 431
    scans, 54
    and teeth, 55, 56, 467, 472, 473, 485, 486, 511, 538
Borax, 153
Boric acid, 192, 195, 196
Bowman's capsule, 436, 437
Boyle's law, 104
Bradycardia, 472
Brain scans, 54
Branching enzyme, 399, 400, 401

Breast cancer, 58
Bromoform, 228
Brompton's cocktail, 289
Bronchial asthma, 528
Bronchial secretions, 176
Bronchitis, 113
Bronchodilators, 465
Bronsted acid, 192
Bronsted base, 196
Brownian movement, 179
Buffers, 208, 372, 386, 462, 463, 464, 465, 473
Buret, 198
Burns, 452, 467, 470, 472
Butanal, 251
Butane, 223
Butanoic acid, 257
Butanol extractable iodine, 507
Butanone, 254, 255
Butene, 232
Buttocks, excoriated, 393
Butyric acid, 257, 323, 330, 393

Cadaverine, 264, 393, 431
Cadmium, 22
Caffeine, 287, 293, 437, 438, 445, 528, 529
Calciferol, 341, 485
Calcitonin, 508, 510
Calcium, 22, 58, 190, 258, 315, 330, 340, 386, 391, 443, 452, 460, 472, 485, 503, 508, 510, 511, 515
    carbonate, 208, 472
    citrate, 460
    chloride, 208
    hydroxide, 197, 205
    hypochlorite, 138
    phosphate, 439, 472, 473, 485
    sulfate, 208
Calculi, 441
Calmodulin, 472
Calorie, 18, 19, 143
Calorie value of some foods, 19
c-AMP, 262, 287, 399, 412, 416, 442, 503, 507, 514, 516, 517, 520
Cancer, 54, 60, 111, 113, 121, 233, 292, 363, 373, 380, 383, 387, 481, 496, 511, 541
Cane sugar, 242, 314
Cannabis, 292
Capillaries, 392, 540
Capillary action, 168, 364
Capric acid, 323
Caproic acid, 323
Caprylic acid, 323
Carbaminohemoglobin, 462
Carbamoyl phosphate, 428, 429
Carbamoyl phosphate synthetase, 428
Carbohydrases, 377, 379, 390
Carbohydrates, 298, 334, 338, 348,

Carbohydrates (cont.)
359, 377, 379, 427, 444, 449,
458, 466, 479, 490, 494, 496,
505, 511
absorption of, 391
classification, 298
digestion, 389, 396
metabolism, 246, 254, 375, 378,
396, 398, 407, 411, 433, 434,
490, 494, 496, 497, 499, 511
origin, 299
Carbon dioxide, 109, 119, 121, 194,
245, 310, 393, 404, 406, 407,
408, 427, 428, 430, 436, 448,
449, 450, 452, 460, 461, 462,
464, 473
Carbon-14, 32, 55
Carbon-12, 30, 32
Carbon-13, 60
Carbon monoxide, 112, 123, 127,
128, 241, 453, 455
Carbon tetrachloride, 119, 128, 144,
160, 228, 322
Carbonate buffers, 209
Carbonic acid, 192, 461, 462, 463
Carbonic anhydrase, 370, 372, 461,
462, 474
Carbonyl group, 251, 254, 265, 298
Carboxyl group, 257, 357
Carboxyhemoglobin, 455
Carboxylation, 495
Carboxypeptidase, 380, 387, 391, 392
Carcinogenic, 128, 270, 275, 302, 444
Cardiac arrest, 465, 471, 473
Cardioplegic solution, 172
Cardiovascular disease, 113, 420
Caries, 208
Carnauba wax, 332
Carotenes, 482
Carotenosis, 482
Cartilage, 467
Casein, 354, 359, 363, 377, 391
Casts, 148, 208
CAT scanner, 57
Catabolic activity, 471
Catabolism, 427, 431, 436, 471
Catalase, 127, 379
Catalyst, 95, 97, 99, 120, 330, 370
Cataract, 63, 64, 311, 540
Cathartic, 175, 208, 258, 259, 439
Cations, 75, 188, 468, 469, 470
Cavities, 56, 161
CCK-PZ, 387, 505
CDP-choline, 421
CDP-ethanolamine, 421
Celiac disease, 330, 452, 473
Cell membrane, 333, 411, 421
Cellobiose, 312, 313
Cellulose, 300, 313, 316, 392
Celsius, 8
Centigrade, 8
Centrosome, 378

Cephalin, 335, 336, 337, 416, 421,
449, 455
Ceramide, 451
Cerebrocuprein, 474
Cerebron, 338
Cerebrosides, 325, 338
Cerebrospinal fluid, 290, 467, 473
Cerebrum, 325
Ceruloplasmin, 359, 382, 383, 449,
458, 474, 540
Ceryl alcohol, 332
Cesium-129, 55
c-GMP, 504
Chain initiator, 536
Chain reactions, 66
Chain terminator, 536
Charles' law, 106
Chaulmoogric acid, 323, 324
Cheilitis, 491
Chelating agent, 493
Chemical bonding, 72, 530
Chemical change, 16
Chemical equations, 90
balancing of, 91
interpreting of, 96
Chemical properties, 16, 147
Chemical reactions, types of, 92
Chemical, inorganic, 156, 386, 437
Chemotherapeutic agents, 382
Chemotherapy, 380
Chest respirator, 104
Chest X ray, 65
"Chick antidermatitis factor," 495
Chiral, 302
Chloracetophenone, 279
Chloral hydrate, 229
Chloride ions, 190, 439, 442, 452,
465, 469, 473, 512, 516
Chloride shift, 462
Chlorine, 22, 138, 151, 235
Chloroalkanes, 228
Chlorobenzene, 270
Chloroethane, 234
Chlorofluorocarbons, 114
Chloroform, 228, 289, 494
Chlorophyll, 286, 287, 299, 453, 473
Chlorpropamide, 506
Cholocalciferol, 483
Cholecystokinin-pancreozymin, 387,
505
Cholera, 155, 504
Cholesterol, 244, 275, 334, 341, 348,
360, 388, 389, 421, 436, 452,
455, 493, 494, 522
Cholic acid, 388
Choline, 335, 338, 496, 497, 498
Chorionic gonadotropin, 442
Chromium, 22, 55, 505
Chromatography, 24, 364
Chromatogram, 366
Chromoprotein, 359
Chromosomes, 378, 433, 526, 541

Chylomicrons, 360, 455
Chymodenin, 505
Chymotrypsin, 380, 391, 392, 505
Chymotrypsinogen, 387, 391
Cigarette smoke, 113
Cinnamic aldehyde, 278
Cirrhosis, 242, 431, 466, 497, 540
cis-aconitic acid, 406, 408, 432
cis-configuration, 324
cis-retinal, 380, 482
cis-trans isomerism, 301
Citrate, 404
Citrate of magnesia, 208
Citrate synthetase, 408
Citric acid, 192, 194, 258, 406, 408,
432
Citric acid cycle, 259, 376, 378, 380,
398, 405, 406, 407, 417, 418,
427, 430, 432, 434, 453, 499
Citrulline, 428, 429
CK BB, 53
Cleansing action, 330
Clinitest tablets, 253, 255, 310
Clots, 449, 459
Clotting factors, 459
Clotting time, 488
Clubfoot, 538
CoA, 287, 376, 408, 494
Coagulation, 362, 460
Cobalamin, 377, 489, 496
Cobalt, 22, 449, 475, 496
Cobalt-52, 54
Cobalt-60, 54, 56
Cocaine, 289, 293, 490
Cocarboxylase, 490
Codeine, 288
Coefficient, 73
Coenzyme, 375, 376, 382, 405, 430,
490, 491, 493, 494, 495, 496,
497, 498
Coenzyme A, 287, 375, 406, 407, 408,
421, 432, 494
Coenzyme Q, 278, 377, 407, 409, 488
Cofactor, 486, 488
Cohesion, 168
Collagen, 359, 360, 361
Colloid, 177, 316, 317, 361, 437, 443,
449, 455, 507, 508, 510
Colloid goiter, 509
Colloid osmotic pressure, 456
Color, 439
Color tests, 363
Column chromatography, 364
Coma, 419, 473, 475
Combination reactions, 92
Combined gas laws, 107
Combustion, 118
Common cold, 500
Competitive inhibitor, 374
Compound lipids, 325
Compounds, 21, 77
Concentrated solution, 161

Concentration, 99, 372, 396
    effects of, 95
Condensed structural formulas, 223
Conductivity, 186, 188
Congestive heart failure, 452, 466
Coniine, 286
Conjugated protein, 358, 453
Connective tissue, 467
Conservation of energy and matter,
    law of, 18
Contractile protein, 361
Contraction, muscular, 347
Control rods, 66
Conversion units, 4
Convulsions, 465, 466, 493
Copper, 22, 182, 287, 309, 359, 407,
    449, 458, 474, 499, 540
Copper aspirinate, 474
Copper complex ions, 309
Copper II ions, 253
Cornea, 491
Coronary arteries, 122
Coronary heart disease, 360
Corpus luteum, 340, 517, 520, 521
Corticosteroids, 471
Corticosterone, 511, 512
Corticotropin-releasing hormone,
    516, 519
Cortisol, 511, 512
Cortisone, 511, 512
Cosmic rays, 537
Cotton, 316
Cough drops, 244, 288
Covalent bonds, 77
Covalent compounds, 143
    naming, 80
CPK, 383
Cream of tartar, 259
Creatine, 402, 439, 441, 442, 452
Creatine kinase, 383
Creatine phosphate, 402
Creatinine, 439, 441, 442, 449, 452,
    512
    coefficient, 175
    phosphokinase, 383
Creatinuria, 442, 487
Crenation, 175
Cresols, 276
Cretins, 508, 516
CRF, 516
CRH, 519
Crick, F. H. C., 526
Cristae, 378
Crop milk, 516
Cupric ions, 253
Cuprous oxide, 253
Curie, 47
Cushing's disease, 470
Cyanide poisoning, 373, 407
Cyanocobalamin, 496
Cyanosis, 470
Cyanotic congenital heart disease, 340

Cyclamate, 315
Cyclic alcohol, 244
Cyclic AMP, 262, 340, 373, 399, 412,
    416, 442, 503, 511, 515, 519
Cyclic compounds, 218, 227, 269
Cyclic fatty acids, 323
Cyclic GMP, 504
Cycloalkanes, 227
Cycloalkenes, 231
Cyclobutane, 228
Cyclobutene, 231
Cyclohexanol, 275
Cyclopropane, 227
Cysteine, 138, 246, 351, 358, 432, 507
Cystic fibrosis, 376, 538
Cystine, 246, 366
Cytidine diphosphate-choline, 421
Cytochrome oxidase, 287, 373, 407,
    409, 432, 474
Cytochromes, 190, 287, 359, 407, 409,
    432, 453, 491
Cytoplasm, 306, 378, 379, 420, 421,
    532

D-amino acids, 392
D-form, 513
D-series, 304, 348, 373, 392
d-sublevel, 34
Dacron, 237, 244
Dakin's solution, 139
Dalton's law, 108
Deacylase, 418, 419
Deafness, 538
Deaminases, 377
Deamination, 427, 428, 500
Decalcification, 486, 511
Decane, 223
Decapeptide, 380, 519
Decarboxylase, 419
Decarboxylation, 393, 418, 430, 490,
    494, 499
Decay curve, 51
Decomposition reactions, 92
Decompression sickness, 111
Decongestant, 293
Deep sea divers, 125
Defective gene, 537
Definite proportions, law of, 23
Dehydrating agent, 245, 246, 329
Dehydration, 141, 170, 173, 175, 246,
    411, 419, 438, 464, 466, 473,
    504, 513
Dehydroascorbic acid, 499
7-Dehydrocholesterol, 483, 484
11-Dehydrocorticosterone, 511
Dehydroepiandrosterone, 511, 512
Dehydrogenases, 377, 379, 418
Deionized water, 155
Dementia, 492
Demerol, 288
Denaturants, 242

Denaturation, 138, 240, 361, 362,
    372, 373
Density, 6, 142
Dental surgery, 123
Dental X rays, 56, 57, 65
5-Deoxyadenosine, 497
Deoxyribonuclease, 380, 433
Deoxyribonucleic acid, 262, 287, 304,
    526
Deoxyribose, 304, 433, 527, 530, 532
Depression, 290, 411
Derived lipids, 325
Derived protein, 355
Derived units, 3
Dermatitis, 491, 492, 493
DES, 302
Detergents, 152, 167, 264, 331, 541
Deuterium, 67
Deuteron, 46
Dextran, 317, 450
Dextrin, 316, 317, 379, 390, 392
Dextroamphetamine, 290
Dextrose, 307
Diabetes insipidus, 8, 438, 470, 518
Diabetes mellitus, 208, 254, 308, 310,
    311, 411, 412, 413, 418, 419,
    420, 438, 442, 444, 452, 464,
    505, 506
Diabetic acidosis, 452, 471, 473
Diabetic coma, 411
Diabinese, 506
Diacylglycerol, 326, 421
Diagnostic instrumentation, 57
Dialysis, 180, 363, 471
Dialyzate, 182
Diamox, 465, 474
Diaphragm, 104
Diarrhea, 63, 65, 281, 289, 390, 393,
    450, 452, 453, 467, 470, 471,
    473, 474, 475, 486, 492, 512
Diatomic molecules, 73
Dichloroacetic acid, 195
Dichlorobenzene, 270, 271, 300
Dichloromethane, 228
Dicumarol, 460, 488
Diet
    low protein, 452
    low sodium, 360
Diethyl ether, 247
Diethyl ketone, 255
Diethylstilbesterol, 302, 521
Differential count, 449
Diffusion, 103, 110, 168, 169, 437
Digestion, 161, 386, 416
Diglycerides, 326, 391, 421
1,2-Diglycerides, 421
Dihydroxyacetone, 254
Dihydroxyacetone phosphate, 402,
    403, 404, 410, 417
Dihydroxybenzene, 276, 277
Diiodotyrosine, 508
Dilute solutions, 161

Dilution, 166
Dimethyl benzene, 274
Dimethyl ether, 216, 247, 301
Dimethyl ketone, 255
Dimethylamine, 263, 265
Dipeptidase, 387, 391, 392
Dipeptides, 353, 354, 355, 364, 391
Dipalmityl lecithin, 336
Dipsticks, 445
Diphosphoglycerate, 402, 403, 404
Disaccharides, 256, 298, 299, 307,
    312, 391
Disease-causing agents, 155
Disinfectants, 196, 276, 362
Dissociation, 187, 199
Distillation, 150
Distribution of charges, 143
Disubstitution products, 271
Disulfide bonds, 138, 358, 362, 363,
    507
Disulfides, 246
Diuretics, 175, 208, 293, 437, 438,
    444, 465, 470, 471, 528
Divinyl ether, 248
DNA, 63, 144, 262, 287, 304, 347,
    433, 514, 526, 527, 528, 529,
    530, 531, 532, 535, 536, 541,
    542
DNA code, 535, 537
DNA transfer of information, 532
DNA donor, 541
DNA ligase, 532
DNA polymerase, 532
DNA replication, 531
DOMAGK, 282
Double bond, 79, 301, 380
Double displacement reaction, 92,
    206
Double helix structure, 526
2,3-DPG, 404
Dramine, 287
Drowsiness, 288
DTPA, 54
Dulcitol, 311
Duodenum, 388
Dwarfs, 509

ECG, 471, 472, 490
Eczema, 323
Edema, 113, 141, 457, 458, 465, 466,
    470, 513, 514
Effectors, 383
Effervescences, 194
Efflorescent, 148
Eicosanoids, 339
Einstein's equation, 66
Elaidic acid, 324
Elastic collisions, 102
Electrical charge, 177
Electrical potential, 470
Electrocardiogram, 490

Electrolysis, 21, 90, 120, 147
Electrolyte balance, 436, 468
Electrolyte concentrations of body
    fluids, 468
Electrolytes, 187, 188, 468, 511
    effect on B.P. and F.P., 187
    strong and weak, 188, 205, 463
Electron, 29, 44, 131
Electron cloud, 33, 59, 270
Electron-dot structures, 73
Electron transport, 377, 378, 398,
    407, 409, 491
Electronegativity, 79
Electrons, arrangement of, 33
Electrophoresis, 178, 366, 458
Electrostatic field, 44
Elements, 20
    in human body, 21
Embalming fluid, 252
Embden-Meyerhof pathway, 400
Emotional glycosuria, 308, 514
Emotional stress, 194, 412
Emphysema, 118, 465
Emulsification, 328, 388, 390, 416
Emulsifying agent, 183, 328, 331, 336
Emulsions, 416
    permanent, 182, 328
    temporary, 182, 328
End point, 198
Endocrine glands, 503, 510, 514, 522
Endoplasmic reticulum, 378
Endorphins, 519
Endothermic, 17, 300
Energy, 17, 90, 121, 402, 405, 466
    of activation, 97, 370
    levels, 33, 72, 73
    measurement of, 18
    nuclear, 65
    sources, 65
    sublevels, 34
    transformation, 17
English-metric conversions, 5
Enkephalins, 519
Enolase, 402, 403, 410
Enterogastrone, 505
Enteroglucagon, 505
Enterokinase, 391
Enzyme-inhibitor complex, 374
Enzyme-substrate complex, 373, 375
Enzymes, 22, 138, 190, 243, 299, 304,
    328, 347, 355, 360, 361, 370,
    387, 425, 426, 442, 448, 449,
    461, 474, 479, 503, 504, 506,
    532, 537, 540, 541
Eosinophils, 449
Ephedrine, 293
Epilepsy, 51, 290, 493, 494
Epimerase, 308
Epimeres, 308
Epinephrine, 291, 411, 412, 416, 513,
    517
Epiphyses, 515

Epithelial tissue, 392, 481
Epsom salts, 149, 208
Equations, 90
    balancing, 91
Equilibrium, 93, 127, 145, 161, 259,
    420
Equilibrium constant, 93, 199
Equilibrium reactions, 93, 127
Equivalent, 166
Equivalent weight, 164
Erg, 48
Ergocalciferol, 483, 484
Erythrocuprein, 474
Erythrocytes, 431, 448
Erythrodextrin, 316
Erythrogenin, 522
Erythropoietin, 449, 522
Erythrose, 304
Escherichia coli, 541, 542
Esophagus, 387
Essential amino acids, 352, 427, 444
Essential fatty acid, 323, 339
Esterases, 379
Esters, 245, 257, 259, 322, 324, 379
Estradiol, 342, 520, 521
Estriol, 520, 521
Estrogen, 511, 517, 520, 522
Estrogenic hormones, 520
Estrone, 279, 520, 521
Ethanal, 133, 252, 253
Ethanediol, 244
Ethanoic acid, 256, 257, 260, 265,
    266
Ethanol, 132, 240, 241, 244, 245, 275
Ethanolamine, 336, 421
Ethene, 230, 231, 232, 235, 236, 237,
    243, 245
Ether, 103, 119, 146, 159, 160, 168,
    227, 245, 246, 322, 328, 496
Ethinyl estradiol, 521
Ethoxyethane, 247
Ethoxy group, 247
Ethyl, 224
Ethyl alcohol, 160, 216, 240, 241,
    244, 247, 251, 258, 260, 301,
    310, 348, 445
Ethyl aminobenzoate, 261
Ethyl butyrate, 261
Ethyl chloride, 230, 234
Ethyl ether, 247
Ethyl formate, 260, 261
Ethyl methanoate, 261
Ethyl propanoate, 261
Ethyl propionate, 261
Ethylamine, 266
Ethylene, 236, 237
Ethylene glycol, 244
Ethyne, 233, 236
Euphoria, 288
Evaporation, 24, 143, 144, 242, 467
Excoriated buttocks, 393
Excretion, 436

Index

Exogenous poison, 182
Exophthalmic goiter, 510
Exophthalmos, 510, 516
Exothermic, 17, 300
Expectorant, 208
Exponential numbers, 546
Extracellular fluid, 470, 471, 472, 473
Extracellular ions, 190
Extracellular water, 467
Eye tumors, 55
Eyes, 467

f-sublevel, 34
FAD, 407, 408, 491
$FADH_2$, 407, 408, 417, 418, 432
Fahrenheit temperature, 8
Fallout, 65
False albuminuria, 443
Families, 37
Fats, 262, 323, 324, 326, 379, 386,
    387, 391, 392, 397, 411, 416,
    419, 420, 421, 426, 427, 466,
    479, 490, 494, 511, 516
  absorption, 391, 416
  digestion, 53, 390
  emulsification, 388
  metabolism, 410, 416, 417, 494,
    497, 511
  and oils, 322, 323, 325
  oxidation, 416
  properties, 327
  storage, 419
  structure, 325
  uses, 327
Fat-soluble vitamins, 479, 480
Fatty acids, 302, 322, 378, 379, 386,
    391, 392, 405, 411, 416, 417,
    418, 421, 432, 455, 458, 495,
    505, 507, 516
  essential, 323
  oxidation, 417
  saturated, 322
  unsaturated, 322
Fatty liver, 497
Feces, 316, 389, 392, 393, 436, 444,
    467
Fehling's solution, 253, 309, 310
Female sex hormones, 275, 520
Fermentation, 242, 310, 314, 393
Ferritin, 361, 474
Ferrous ion, 431
Ferrous sulfate, 208
Fertility, 487
Fever, 242, 426, 438, 439, 442, 453,
    467, 489, 540
Fibrin, 359, 361, 459, 460
Fibrinigin, 348, 354, 361, 449, 455,
    458, 459
Fibrinolysis, 460
Fibrous protein, 361
Film badges, 49

Filtration, 151
Fire prevention, 119
Fischer projection, 303
Fission, 65
Flavin, 490
Flavin adenine dinucleotide, 491
Flavin mononucleotide, 491
Flavoproteins, 359
Flavoring agents, 261
Fluid-electrolyte balance, 466
Fluid-mosaic model, 344
Fluorine, 22
FMN, 491
Folacin, 495, 496
Folate deficiency, 496
Follicle-stimulating hormone, 515,
    517, 520
Follicle-stimulating hormone-
    release-inhibiting hormone,
    519
Follicle-stimulating hormone-
    releasing hormone (factor),
    519
Follicles, 57
Follicular hormones, 520
Food preservative, 277, 279
Formaldehyde, 132, 138, 242, 251,
    252, 256
Formalin, 252
Formic acid, 132, 252, 256, 257, 260,
    266
Formula weight, 83
Formulas, 73, 82, 216
  empirical, 85
  structural, 216, 222
  writing, 82
Freezing point, 167, 187
Freon, 230
Fructose, 149, 307, 309, 311, 312,
    315, 379, 391, 392, 396
Fructose-6-P, 402, 403, 404, 410
Fructose-1,6-diphosphate, 402, 403,
    404, 410
Fructosemia, 309
Fructosuria, 412
Fruit sugar, 309
FSH, 515, 517, 519, 520, 521
FSH-RF, 519
FSH-RH, 519
FSH-RIH, 519
Fumarase, 380, 408
Fumaric acid, 380, 406, 408, 429,
    430, 432
Function groups, 240, 245, 246, 250,
    256, 548
Functional isomers, 301
Fundamental particles, 29
Fundamental units, 2
Fussion, 67

GABA, 347
Galacticol, 540

Galactokinase, 308
Galactonic acid, 311
Galactose, 307, 308, 311, 312, 315,
    338, 359, 379, 391, 392, 396,
    444, 540
Galactosemia, 308, 540
Galactosuria, 308, 412
Galacturonic acid, 311
Gallbladder, 53, 387, 388, 389, 421,
    505, 538
Gallium-67, 55
Gallstones, 341, 389, 421
Gamma-aminobutyric acid, 347
Gamma rays, 45, 54, 61
Gammaglobulin, 64, 361, 458, 459
Gangliosides, 338
Gangrene, 123
Gas exchange, 465
Gas laws, 104
Gas-liquid chromatography, 366
Gaseous state, 15, 102, 117
Gasoline, 236, 242
Gastric acid, 505
Gastric digestion, 387, 392
Gastric inhibitory polypeptides, 505
Gastric juice, 195, 201, 372, 379, 387,
    391, 392, 504
Gastric lipase, 379, 387, 390, 392
Gastric sunction, 465, 471
Gastric ulcer, 387, 465
Gastrin, 387, 504, 519
Gastritis, 387
Gaucher's disease, 338, 541
GDP, 406, 408
Geiger counter, 48
Gelatin, 427
Gels, 180, 316
Gene splicing, 541
General formula, 223, 231, 233, 240,
    247, 251, 254, 257, 262, 263,
    298
Genes, 526
Genetic code, 530, 536
Genetic diseases, 537, 538, 541
Genetic changes, 63, 64
Genetic disorders, 412
Genetic regulation, 347
Geometric isomers, 301, 380
Germicidal soaps, 330, 331
Germicide, 128, 177, 196, 208, 252,
    276, 330
GH, 514, 515
GHRF, 516
GHRH, 519
GHRIH, 519
GIF, 519
Gigantism, 516
GIP, 505
Glacial acetic acid, 258
Glauber's salt, 149, 208
Glaucoma, 538
Globin, 359, 388, 431, 433, 453

Globular protein, 361
Globulins, 354, 359, 361, 449, 455, 458, 459, 474, 540
Glomerulonephritis, 452
Glomerlus, 436, 437
Glossitis, 491, 492
Glucocerebrosidase, 541
Glucocerebrosides, 541
Glucocorticoids, 486, 511, 513
Glucogon, 411, 412, 416, 505, 506, 519
Glucokinase, 399, 400, 401, 402, 403, 411
Gluconeogenesis, 397, 398, 407, 410, 412, 507, 513
Gluconic acid, 310, 311
Glucosamine, 317
Glucosans, 315
Glucose, 51, 118, 131, 149, 217, 253, 259, 292, 298, 304, 307, 312, 315, 316, 333, 348, 379, 390, 391, 392, 396, 397, 398, 399, 400, 401, 402, 403, 404, 405, 410, 411, 412, 418, 419, 431, 432, 437, 438, 443, 444, 449, 452, 469, 471, 472, 498, 504, 505, 507, 516, 540, 541
Glucose-1-P, 399, 400, 401, 402, 404, 507
Glucose 6-P, 399, 400, 401, 402, 403, 404, 405, 410, 507
Glucose tolerance test, 412
beta-Glucosidase, 339
Glucuronic acid, 311, 317
Glutamic acid, 351, 357, 366, 427, 428, 432, 495, 496, 518, 535, 538
Glutamic oxaloacetic transaminase, 382, 383
Glutamic pyruvic transaminase, 382, 383
Glutamine, 351, 432, 535
Glutaraldehyde, 256
Glutathione insulin transhydroxylase, 506
Glutathione peroxidase, 486
Glyceraldehyde, 252, 253, 302, 303, 304, 348, 371, 402, 405
Glyceraldehyde-3-P, 402, 403, 404, 405, 410
Glyceraldehyde-3-P dehydrogenase, 402, 403
Glycerin, 243
Glycerol, 168, 243, 324, 325, 328, 333, 337, 379, 386, 391, 392, 410, 416, 417, 418, 432, 507
Glycerose, 304
Glycerophosphatidic acid, 421
Glyceryl distearate, 325
Glyceryl monostearate, 325
Glyceryl trinitrate, 261
Glyceryl tripalmitate, 328
Glyceryl tristearate, 326

Glycine, 265, 348, 351, 353, 432, 442, 535
Glycogen, 316, 317, 396, 397, 399, 400, 402, 404, 405, 411, 412, 417, 419, 421, 425, 427, 434, 504, 505, 507, 513
Glycogen synthetase, 399, 400, 401
Glycogenesis, 317, 396, 397, 398, 399, 400, 401, 405, 410, 411, 412, 432, 505, 514
Glycol, 244
Glycolipids, 308, 324, 338, 360, 541
Glycolysis, 348, 400, 403, 404, 405, 410, 417, 432
Glycophorin, 360
Glycoprotein, 308, 359, 360, 386, 449, 458, 482, 507, 516, 517
Glycosidic linkage, 312, 399
Glycosuria, 308, 397, 411, 443, 444, 513
Glycyl-alanine, 354
Glyoxalic acid, 364
Goiter, 509
Gold, 55, 453
Golgi body, 378
Gonadotropic hormones, 517
Gonads, 467
GOT, 383
Gout, 440, 441, 452, 528
GPT, 383
Graham's law, 110
Grain alcohol, 241
Gram, 3, 143
Gram equivalent weight, 164
Granulomas, 475
Grapesugar, 507
"Grass," 292
Grave's disease, 510
Growth hormone, 514, 515, 518, 541
Growth hormone release-inhibiting factor, 519
Growth hormone-releasing factor, 516, 519
GTP, 406, 407, 408
Guanine, 287, 528, 529, 530, 531, 533
Guanosine triphosphate, 407

Half-life, 51, 52, 308
Hallucinogens, 291
Haloalkanes, 228
Halogen derivatives, 270
Halothane, 128, 229, 248
Hardness, permanent temporary, 153
Hardness, water, 152, 163, 330, 331
Hashimoto's disease, 510
Hashish, 292
Haworth projection, 306
Hay fever, 513
HCN, 123, 455
HDL, 360
Headache, 455, 465
Heart disease, 51, 443, 458

Heart failure, 490
Heat, 155, 362, 373, 448
of fusion, 15
of vaporization, 16
Heavy metal salts, 362
Helium, 44, 126
alpha-Helix, 355
Heller's ring test, 363
Hematuria, 444
Heme, 358, 388, 407, 431, 453
Hemiacteal, 255, 256, 306, 312
Hemiketal, 255, 256, 309, 312
Hemocyanin, 348, 359
Hemodialysis, 180, 464
Hemoglobin, 22, 112, 121, 126, 128, 190, 286, 287, 347, 348, 354, 355, 358, 359, 361, 388, 405, 407, 411, 425, 431, 433, 438, 444, 452, 453, 455, 460, 461, 462, 474, 496, 538
buffers, 463, 464
metabolism, 431
Hemoglobin-S, 538
Hemoglobinuria, 444
Hemolysis, 173, 326, 431, 444, 453, 489
Hemolytic anemia, 442, 487
Hemolytic jaundice, 431, 487
Hemophilia, 540
Hemorrhage, 173, 280, 380, 448, 450, 453, 455, 488, 497, 500
Hemosiderin, 474
Henry's law, 110
Heparin, 311, 317, 460
Hepatic failure, 452
Hepatitis, 383
Heptane, 223, 236
Heptene, 232
Heredity, 520
Heroin, 288, 289
Hertz, 59
Heterocyclic bases, 527, 528, 529, 530
Heterocyclic compounds, 218, 286
Heterogeneous RNA, 533
Hexachlorophene, 273
Hexane, 222, 223
Hexene, 232
Hexosans, 299, 315, 316
Hexose monophosphate shunt, 304, 398, 405, 410, 490
Hexoseaminidase-A, 339, 541
Hexoses, 299, 306, 315, 316
Hexylresorcinol, 277
HGF, 506
High-density lipoproteins, 360
High-energy phosphate bonds, 405, 418
Hippuric acid, 442
Histamine, 263, 393, 431
Histidine, 351, 353, 393, 431, 432, 518, 535
Histones, 359
Hodgkin's disease, 382, 453

Home permanents, 138
Homogentistic acid, 439
Hopkin's-Cole test, 364
Hormones, 340, 347, 360, 380, 387, 400, 411, 412, 442, 471, 479, 503, 516, 541
    adrenal cortex, 341, 411, 426, 448, 449, 511
    adrenal glands, 412, 511
    adrenal medulla, 412, 513
    anterior lobe, 514, 517, 518
    gastrointestinal system, 504
    hypothalmus, 518
    intermediate lobe, 514, 517
    kidneys, 522
    pancreas, 505
    parathyroid glands, 510
    pituitary, 411, 514
    posterior lobe, 514, 517
    in regulating blood sugar, 411
    sex, 341, 421, 520
    thyroid gland, 411, 507, 508
Huntington's chorea, 347
Hyaline membrane disease, 168
Hybaroxic cancer radiation, 56, 111, 123
Hydralazine, 493
Hydrates, 147, 298
Hydrocarbons, 112, 221, 236, 332
    naming, 224
Hydrochloric acid, 192, 194, 205, 264, 363, 387, 391, 392, 463, 473, 496, 504
Hydrocortisone, 511
Hydrocyanic acid, 128, 455
Hydrogen, 55, 132, 133, 393
    replaceable, 164
Hydrogen bonding, 144, 247, 356, 357, 358, 362, 363, 530
Hydrogen cyanide, 123, 129
Hydrogen ions, 192, 256, 461
Hydrogen peroxide, 126, 137, 379
Hydrogen sulfide, 127, 129, 455
Hydrogenation, 235, 328
Hydrolases, 377, 379, 386
Hydrolysis, 149, 189, 205, 298, 299, 306, 307, 309, 313, 315, 317, 322, 324, 328, 329, 347, 360, 375, 377, 379, 380, 386, 387, 389, 391, 416, 425, 433, 490, 527
Hydrolytic enzymes, 379, 386
Hydrophillic, 180, 331, 333, 334
Hydrophillic lipoprotein complex, 455
Hydrophobic, 180, 331, 333, 334, 363, 455
Hydroquinone, 277
Hydrostatic pressure, 171, 456, 458
Hydroxides, 193, 196
Hydroxybutyric acid, 432
Hydroxyl group, 240
Hydroxypropanal, 301

Hygroscopic, 148
Hyperacidity, 194, 387
Hyperadrenocorticism, 513
Hyperalimentation, 426
Hyperammonemia, 428
Hyperbilirubinemia, 489, 491
Hypercalcemia, 340, 411, 472, 486
Hyperglycemia, 412, 505, 506, 507, 513
Hyperglycemic-glycogenolytic factor, 506
Hyperinsulinism, 412, 452
Hyperkalemia, 471
Hypernatremia, 470
Hyperparathyroidism, 442, 443, 452, 473, 511
Hypertension, 112, 293, 340, 383, 387, 514
Hyperthermia, 122
Hyperthyroidism, 53, 54, 442, 443, 452, 489, 510, 516
Hypertonic solution, 175
Hypertrophy, 510
Hyperventilation, 464, 465, 466
Hypervitaminosis, 452, 482, 486
Hypnotic, 252, 279, 288, 289
Hypoacidity, 195, 387
Hypocalcemia, 472, 485
Hypochloremia, 473
Hypochlorous acid, 195, 196
Hypoglycemia, 309, 413, 506, 512
Hypoglycemic effects, 506, 507
Hypokalemia, 380, 471, 513
Hypomagnesia, 473
Hyponatremia, 470
Hypoparathyroidism, 442, 443, 452, 472, 485, 510
Hypophosphatemia, 485
Hypophysectomy, 517
Hypophysis, 514
Hypopituitarism, 412
Hypothalamus, 514, 516, 517, 518, 519
Hypothermia, 121
Hypothyroidism, 53, 452, 505, 512
Hypotonic solution, 173, 444
Hypoventilation, 465
Hypoxia, 60, 123, 128, 449, 540
Hysteria, 465

^{131}I, 53
ICSH, 515, 517
Idiopathic pentosuria, 412
Immiscible, 182
Immune response, 126
Immune system, 510
Immunity, 55, 64
Immunoglobulins, 360, 458
Incubator, 106
Indicators, 193, 197, 198
Indole, 393

Induced-fit model, 374
Inducer, 536
Inert gases, 36
Infectious hepatitis, 382, 383, 433, 458
Influenza, 458
Inhalation therapy, 176
Inhibiting enzymes, 380
Inhibitors, 99, 372, 383, 518
Initiator, 237
Inorganic compounds, 215
Inositol, 337, 497, 498
Insecticide, 293
Insulin, 22, 333, 340, 348, 354, 355, 361, 397, 399, 400, 401, 411, 416, 420, 464, 471, 472, 474, 505, 507, 516, 519, 541
Insulin shock, 506, 507
Insulin therapy, 464
Interferon, 360, 541
Intermediate lobe, 514, 517
Intermedin, 517
Intermittent partial pressure, 110
International system, 2
International units, 480, 484, 487, 497, 520
Interpreting chemical equations, 96
Interstitial cell-stimulating hormones, 515, 517
Interstitial fluid, 456, 467, 468
Interstitial water, 467
Intestinal bacteria, 431, 488
Intestinal digestion, 387, 392
Intestinal enzymes, 391
Intestinal juice, 379, 380, 387, 390, 392
Intestinal obstruction, 452
Intracellular ions, 190
Intracellular water, 467, 468
Intravascular fluid, 467, 468, 470, 471, 472, 473
Intravenous infusion, 174, 237, 471, 472
Intrinsic factor, 387, 453, 496, 505
Inulin, 309
Invert sugar, 314
Iodide ions, 190
Iodine, 22, 53, 124, 316, 317, 327, 507, 508, 509, 510
Iodine number, 327
Iodized salts, 508, 510
Iodoform, 228
Ion exchange, 153
Ion pairs, 48, 63
Ionic bonds, 75, 188
Ionic compounds, naming, 77
Ionization, 59, 63, 186, 240
    evidence of, 189
    theory, 187
    of water, 199
Ions, 74, 75, 189
    importance of, 190
    size of, 75

Iron, 22, 55, 190, 388, 407, 431, 449, 453, 458, 473, 499
Iron-deficiency anemia, 474
Irradiation, 483
Islets of Langerhans, 411, 505, 506, 507
Isoamyl acetate, 261
Isobutyraldehyde, 252
Isocitric acid, 406, 408, 432
Isoelectric point, 349, 353
Isoenzymes, 383
Isoleucine, 349, 353, 432, 507, 518, 535
Isomerases, 380
Isomerization, 497
Isomers, 216, 217, 300, 380
  structural, 300, 380
Isoniazid, 493
Isonicotinic acid hydrazide, 493
Isooctane, 236
Isopropyl alcohol, 133, 240, 243, 245, 253, 300
Isopropyl amine, 263
Isopropyl mercaptan, 246
Isotonic solution, 173, 450
Isotopes, 32
Isozyme, 383
IUPAC, 224, 240, 243, 244, 246, 247, 251, 254, 256, 261, 265, 270, 271, 326

Jaundice, 389, 431
Javelle water, 139
Joule, 18, 66
Juvenile diabetes, 506

Kaolin, 177
Kekule, 269
Kelvin temperature scale, 8, 106
Kerasin, 338
Keratin, 138, 359, 361
Keratinization, 481, 482
Ketohexose, 299, 309
Ketol, 256, 312
Ketone bodies, 255, 262, 325, 411, 418, 419, 444
Ketonemia, 418
Ketones, 245, 253, 278, 298, 304
  reactions of, 255
Ketonuria, 418
Ketoses, 299, 309
Ketosis, 411, 418, 439, 464
Kidney disease, 438, 452, 484, 538
Kidney stones, 441, 472
Kidneys, 380, 427, 438, 441, 445, 449, 464, 465, 466, 467, 470, 484, 486, 497, 506, 518, 522, 540
Kilocalorie, 18
Kilopascals, 104
Kinetic energy, 17, 102
Kinetic molecular theory, 102

Knock-out drops, 229
Knoop, 417
Krebs cycle, 376, 404, 405, 408, 410, 417, 418, 431, 432, 490
Krypton, 2, 55
K_w, 199
Kwashiorkor, 426, 457

L-amino acid, 392
L-series, 304, 335, 348, 356, 373, 392, 513
Lacrimator, 279
Lactalbumin, 348, 359
Lactase, 314, 379, 387, 390, 392
Lactate, 400, 402, 403, 404, 405, 410
Lactate dehydrogenase, 383, 402, 403
Lactate/pyruvate determination, 451
Lactation, 444, 475, 480, 484, 487, 490, 492, 498, 500, 516, 517
Lactic acid, 258, 259, 315, 393, 400, 404, 405, 408, 410, 412
Lactic acid bacteria, 499
Lactic acid cycle, 405
Lactic acidosis, 464
Lactogenic hormone (Prolactin), 515, 516
Lactoglobulin, 359
Lactose, 258, 312, 314, 315, 379, 390, 392, 444
Laked blood, 173
Lamaze method, 465
Lanolin, 332
Lauric acid, 323
Lauryl alcohol, 332
Lauryl hydrogen sulfate, 332
Laxative, 197, 236
LD_{50}^{30}, 64
LDH, 383
Lead aerosols, 112
Le Chatelier's principle, 95
Lecithin, 335, 337, 416, 421, 455, 498
Lecithinase-A, 336
Leprosy, 472
Lesions, 329, 491
LET, 48
Lethargy, 288
Leucine, 349, 353, 432, 518, 535
Leucine enkephalin, 520
Leukemia, 63, 64, 382, 383, 441, 452, 453
Leukocytes, 64, 444
Leukotrienes, 339
Levodopa, 494
Levulose, 309
Lewis structure, 73
LH, 515, 517, 521
LH-RH, 519
Life span, 64
Ligase, 380
Lime-soda process, 153
Lime water, 197
Linear energy transfer, 48

Linoleic acid, 323, 339
Linolenic acid, 323
Linseed oil, 119, 323
Lipases, 377
Lipids, 322, 324, 334, 348, 359, 375, 377, 432, 434, 449, 455, 458, 479, 486, 496
  simple, 324
Lipogenesis, 380, 420, 442, 434
Lipoic acid, 377, 497, 499
Lipolysis, 416
Lipoprotein, 327, 359, 360, 455, 458, 479, 486
  low-density, 360
Liquid air, 120
Liquid mixtures, 158
Liquid oxygen, 126
Liquids, 14
Lister antiseptic, 276
Liter, 3
Litharge, 323
Lithium salts, 474
Litmus, 193, 197, 200
Liver, 53, 54, 335, 383, 387, 388, 391, 392, 393, 396, 398, 400, 411, 412, 416, 418, 420, 425, 427, 428, 430, 431, 441, 442, 444, 452, 458, 459, 467, 474, 480, 482, 484, 488, 490, 504, 506, 507, 513, 514, 516, 541
Lock-and-key theory, 373
Logarithm, 200
LOX, 126
LSD, 291
LTH, 514, 515, 516
Lubricant, 236, 243, 386, 390
Lugol's solution, 139
Luminal, 290
Lunar caustic, 208, 362
Lungs, 436
Luteinizing hormone, 515, 517, 519, 521
Luteinizing hormone-releasing hormone, 519
Luteotropin, 516
Lyases, 380
Lye, 197
Lymph, 392, 467, 468
Lymphocytes, 65, 499
Lysergic acid diethylamide, 291
Lysine, 351, 353, 357, 381, 393, 427, 431, 432, 535
Lysol, 276
Lysolecithin, 336
Lysosome, 378, 379, 480, 482
Lyxose, 306

Maalox, 194
Macroglobulinemia, 458
Magnesium, 22, 190, 372
Magnesium citrate, 175, 208, 258
Magnesium hydroxide, 197

Magnesium ions, 330, 401, 403, 417, 428, 429, 443, 453, 473
Magnesium sulfate, 175, 208
Magnetic resonance imaging, 60
Malaria, 293
Male sex hormones, 275, 522
Malic acid, 380, 406, 408, 432
Malignancies, 51
Malignant bone tumor, 452
Malnutrition, 309, 426, 452, 471
Malonyl CoA, 380
Malt, 243
Malt sugar, 315
Maltase, 313, 314, 377, 379, 387, 390, 392
Maltose, 312, 313, 314, 315, 316, 377, 379, 389, 390, 392
Mammography, 58
Manganese, 475
Manic-depressive psychoses, 475
Mannitol, 311, 445
Mannose, 359
Marihuana ("Mary Jane"), 292
Mass, 2
Mass action, law of, 93
Mass number, 30
Master gland, 514
Matter, 13, 28
Maximum density, 142
Mayonnaise, 336
MB isoenzyme, 56
Measles, 458
Megaloblastic anemia, 383, 496
Melanin, 517, 540
Melanocyte-stimulating hormone, 517
Melanocyte-stimulating hormone-release-inhibiting factor, 519
Melanocyte-stimulating hormone-releasing hormone, 519
Melting point, 15, 81
Membranes, 334, 360, 378, 421, 437, 443, 480, 481, 482, 486, 504, 505
Menadione, 458
Menstruation, 521
Mental illness, 51
Mental retardation, 338, 444
Menthol, 244
Meperidine, 288
Mercaptans, 246
Mercaptoethanolamine, 276, 494
Mercaptopurine, 382
Mercerized cotton, 317
Mercuric chloride, 362
Mercuric nitrate, 364
Mercurous nitrate, 364
Mercury, 103, 156, 364
Mercury, poisoning, 452
Mescaline, 291
Messenger RNA, 503, 532, 536, 537, 538
MET, 124

Meta compounds, 272
Metabolic acidosis, 465
Metabolic alkalosis, 465
Metabolic rate, 507, 516
Metabolism, 114, 207, 300, 322, 327, 335, 375, 396, 415, 416, 419, 433, 444, 455, 460, 487, 494, 496, 507, 510, 511, 516, 528
Metal oxides, 147, 193
Metalloprotein, 458
Metals, 20, 73, 206, 458
Metastases, 55
Metathesis reactions, 92
Methadone, 288, 289
Methamphetamine, 290
Methanal, 252, 256
Methane, 221, 223, 236, 393
Methanethiol, 246
Methanoic acid, 256, 257, 265
Methanol, 240, 241, 244, 256, 260
Methionine, 349, 353, 432, 442, 496, 507, 535
Methionine enkephalin, 520
Methoxy group, 247
Methoxy methane, 247
Methoxyflurane, 128, 248
Methyl, 224, 496
Methyl acetate, 260, 261
Methyl alcohol, 160, 240, 241, 244, 247, 250, 251, 252, 256, 260
Methyl amine, 263
Methyl chloride, 228
Methyl ethanoate, 260, 261
Methyl ether, 247
Methyl ethyl ether, 247
Methyl ethyl ketone, 255
Methyl groups, 496
Methyl hexane, 300
Methyl iodide, 264
Methyl isopropyl ether, 247
Methyl mercaptan, 246
Methyl morphine, 288
Methyl propanal, 252
Methyl propyl ketone, 255
Methyl salicylate, 261, 279
Methyl malonate, 497
Methylene blue, 439
Metric system, 2, 143
Mevinolin, 341
Microcurie, 47
MIF, 519
Milk of magnesia, 175, 176, 197
Milk sugar, 315
Millicurie, 47
Milliequivalents, 468
Milliequivalents per liter, 166, 452, 466, 468, 469
Milligram percent, 163
Milliosmol, 171, 469
Millon's test, 364
Mineral oil, 236, 327, 482
Mineralocorticoids, 511, 512
Minerals, inorganic, 156, 386, 437

Mirror images, 302
Miscible, 182
Mist, 126
Mitochondria, 138, 334, 376, 377, 378, 405, 407, 420, 421, 475, 480, 482, 491
Mitochondrial enzymes, 475
Mixed ethers, 247
Mixtures, 23
Moderator, 66
Molar gas volumes, 111
Molar solution, 163
Mole, 84, 163
Molecular formula, 85, 217, 223
Molecular weight, 83, 84, 348
Molecules, 72, 102
Molybdenum, 22
Monatomic, 73
Monoacylglycerols, 326
Monocytes, 449
Monoglycerides, 326, 391
Monohydric alcohol, 243
Monohydroxy alcohol, 243
Monoiodotyrosine, 508
Monosaccharides, 255, 298, 299, 304, 312, 315, 386, 390, 391, 392, 396
Monosodium glutamate, 352
Monosubstitution products, 271
Morphine, 288, 289, 386, 520
Mortality table, 420
Motilin, 505
MRH, 519
MRIH, 519
MSG, 352
MSH, 515, 517
Mucin, 359, 360, 386
Mucoprotein, 458
Mucosa, 381, 387, 390
Multiple myeloma, 453, 458
Mumps, 458
Muscular dystrophy, 487
Muscular relaxant, 247
Muscle contraction, 404
Mutagenic substances, 128
Mutations, 63
Myelin, 334, 496
Myocardial infarction, 55, 382, 383
Myoglobin, 287, 474
Myosin, 361
Myricyl alcohol, 332
Myristic acid, 323
Myxedema, 452, 509

N-acetylglutamic acid, 428
NAD$^+$, 286, 377, 402, 403, 406, 407, 408, 417, 491
NADH, 370, 402, 403, 406, 407, 408, 409, 417, 418, 432
NADH dehydrogenase, 376
NADP$^+$, 370, 405, 491, 492
NADPH, 405

Naloxone, 289
Naphtha, 270
Naphthalene, 274
Naphthol, 274
Narcolepsy, 290
Narcotic, 230
Narcotic analgesics, 288
Nasal cannula, 121
Nasal mask, 121
Nasal spray, 244
Nasogastric suction, 473
Natural gas, 236
Natural radioactivity, 47
Nausea, 65, 248, 291, 455, 486, 511
Nebulizer, 176
Nembutal, 289, 290
Neoplasms, 95
Nephritis, 361, 442, 443, 452, 457
Nephrosis, 443
Nerves, 347
Nervon, 338
N-ethylformamide, 266
N-ethylmethanamide, 266
Neuraminic acid, 359
Neurohormones, 514
Neurohypophysis, 514
Neuromuscular blocking drugs, 236
Neurotransmitter, 514
Neutralization, 149, 193, 204
Neutron, 29, 30, 45, 59, 66
Neutrophils, 449
Niacin, 266, 283, 286, 489, 491
Niacinamide, 266, 283, 491
Nickel, 22
Nicotinamide, 376, 377, 491, 493
Niotinamide adenine dinucleotide,
    377, 402, 492
Nicotinamide adenine dinucleotide
    phosphate, 377, 405, 492
Nicotine, 286, 293
Nicotinic acid, 491, 492, 493
Niemann-Pick disease, 337, 541
Night blindness, 481
Ninhydrin test, 364
Nitric acid, 192, 193, 205, 243, 363,
    364
Nitrobenzene, 285
Nitrogen, 125
Nitrogen balance, 425, 515
Nitrogen cycle, 347
Nitrogen oxides, 112, 114, 123, 128
Nitroglycerin, 243, 261
Nitrous oxide, 123, 128, 227, 229,
    248
NMR, 60
N,N-dimethylacetamide, 266
N,N-dimethylethanamide, 266
Noble gases, 20, 36, 72
Nonane, 223
Noncompetitive inhibitors, 375
Nonelectrolytes, 187, 240, 469
Nonmetal oxides, 147
Nonmetals, 20, 73, 147

Nonpolar amino acids, 349, 350, 357
Nonpolar compounds, 160
Nonpolar covalent bonds, 79
Nonpolar liquids, 160
Nonprotein nitrogen, 542
Nonspecific inhibitors, 373
Nonvolatile solute, 167
Noradrenalin, 513
Norepinephrine, 513, 517
Normal solutions, 164, 198
Normality, 164
Novocain, 264
Noxious, 128
N-radiography, 59
Nuclases, 360, 380, 512
Nuclear energy, 65
Nuclear fission, 65
Nuclear magnetic resonance, 60
Nuclear reaction, 45
Nuclear reactors, 66
Nucleic acids, 22, 264, 287, 304, 359,
    380, 405, 433, 496, 526, 527,
    528
Nucleohistone, 359
Nucleolus, 378
Nucleoprotein, 286, 359, 387, 433,
    440, 442, 533
    metabolism, 433
Nucleosides, 433, 527, 528, 531
Nucleotides, 405, 433, 527, 531, 533,
    537, 538
Nyctalopia, 481
Nylon, 237

Obesity, 290, 420, 509
Obstructive jaundice, 431, 452, 488
Octane, 223
Octane number, 236
Octapeptide, 380
Octene, 231, 232
Octet rule, 72
Octyl acetate, 261
Odor, 439
Oil of Wintergreen, 261
Oils, 123, 322, 323, 324, 325
    structure of, 325
Oleic acid, 323, 324
Oleomargarine, 328
Oliguria, 438, 452, 470
Operator site, 536
Opiate antagonists, 289
Opiates, 288, 465, 520
Optical activity, 300, 335, 373
Optical isomers, 302, 304, 380
Orbitals, 34
Organelles, 379
Organic acid, 256
Organic chemistry, introduction, 214
Organic compounds, 215
Organic peroxides, 379
Orinase, 506
Ornithine, 393, 428, 429, 430, 431

Ornithine transcarbomyl transferase,
    428
Orthostatic albuminuria, 443
Osmol, 167, 171
Osmolarity, 167, 171
Osmometer, 469
Osmosis, 169, 512
Osmotic activity, 469
Osmotic pressure, 171, 190, 207, 353,
    449, 450, 455, 457, 469, 470
Osteolysis, 340
Osteomalacia, 484, 486
Osteomyelitis, 55
Osteoporosis, 443, 484, 486
Oxalic acid, 139, 197, 258
Oxaloacetate, 418, 429, 432
Oxaloacetic acid, 406, 407, 408
Oxidases, 379
Oxidation, 118, 131, 132, 250, 253,
    254, 256, 310, 329, 418, 426,
    480, 489, 491
Oxidation number, 81, 82, 131
Oxidation-reduction, 131, 133, 134,
    338, 500
Oxidative deamination, 427
Oxidative phosphorylation, 377, 378,
    407, 409, 453, 474, 486, 488
Oxides, 112, 117
Oxidizing agents, 133, 139, 250, 254,
    363, 488
Oxidoreductases, 138, 378
Oxygen, 109, 111, 112, 117, 132, 133,
    299, 347, 379, 402, 404, 407,
    409, 411, 432, 448, 450, 455,
    473
    medical uses of, 120
    transportation, 404, 461, 462
Oxygen-carbon dioxide cycle, 300
Oxygen-demanding wastes, 155
Oxyhemoglobin, 121, 461, 463
Oxyhemoglobin buffer, 463, 464
Oxynervon, 338
Oxytocin, 515, 517, 518, 519
Ozone, 112, 113, 127
Ozone layer, 113, 127

P-sublevel, 34
Pa, 104
PABA, 282, 323, 375, 382, 498, 499
P_{CO_2}, 464, 465, 466
Paget's disease, 538
Palmitic acid, 328, 418
p-Aminobenzoic acid, 282, 375, 382,
    496, 498
Pancreas, 340, 411, 467, 505
Pancreas scans, 55
Pancreatic amylase, 379, 387, 390,
    392
Pancreatic disease, 488
Pancreatic function, 486
Pancreatic juice, 372, 379, 380, 387,
    390, 391, 392, 505

Pancreatic lipase, 379, 387, 388, 391, 392
Pancreatitis, 473
Pantothenic acid, 376, 377, 489, 494, 498
Papaverine, 288
Paper chromatography, 364
Para compounds, 272
Para-aminobenzenesulfonic acid, 281
Para-aminobenzoic acid, 282, 382, 495, 496, 497, 498
Paracasein, 391
Paraffin wax, 332
Paraldehyde, 252
Paranoia, 290
Parathyroid adenoma, 511
Parathyroid function, 442
Parathyroid glands, 472
Parathyroid hormone, 485, 508, 510
Parietal cells, 387
Parkinson's disease, 51, 494
Pars intermedia, 517
Partial pressure, 109, 464, 465
Particulate matter, 112
Parts per billion, 112, 163
Parts per million, 112, 163
Pascals, 104
Passive transport, 167
Pauling, Linus, 500
PBI, 507
Pellagra, 492, 493
Penicillin, 286, 381
Penicillin amine, 493
Penicillinase, 382
Pentane, 222, 223
Pentanol, 245
Pentanone, 255
Pentapeptide, 519
Pentene, 232, 245
Pentobarbital, 289, 290
Pentosans, 299, 315
Pentose shunt, 405
Pentoses, 299, 304, 315, 359, 444, 527
Pentosuria, 412
"Pep pills," 290
Peptic ulcers, 340
Pepsin, 361, 372, 375, 377, 379, 391, 392, 504
Pepsinogen, 387, 391, 392
Peptidases, 379, 380
Peptide bonds, 266, 353, 363, 364, 381
Peptide linkage, 353, 355, 364
Peptides, 426, 540
Peptones, 355, 391
Percentage composition, 84, 358
Percentage solution, 162
Perfluorocarbons, 450
Perfumes, 261
Pericardial studies, 54
Periodic table, inside front cover, 37, 38
Periods, 37

Pernicious anemia, 55, 387, 452, 453, 458, 496, 512
Perosis, 497
Peroxidases, 379
Peroxides, 247, 486
Peroxyacyl nitrates, 113
Peroxybenzoyl nitrate, 112
Perspiration, 143, 436, 437, 438, 467
Petroleum, 236
PETT, 51
PGA, 495
pH, 199, 363, 387, 388, 411, 419, 438, 450, 462, 463, 464, 465, 466
  optimum, 372, 386, 390, 391, 448
pH meter, 200
pH values, 200
Phenacetin, 281
Phenanthrene, 275
Phenobarbital, 289, 290
Phenol, 275
Phenol coefficient, 276
Phenol derivatives, 276
Phenolphthalein, 193, 197
Phenolsulfonaphthalein, 445
Phenothiazines, 472
Phenyl mercuric acetate, 261
Phenylalanine, 349, 353, 363, 432, 439, 444, 518, 535, 540
Phenylalanine hydroxylase, 540
Phenylketonuria, 444, 538, 540
Phenylpyruvic acid, 444
Phenytoin, 472
Phosgene, 119, 123
Phosphatases, 372, 379, 417, 507
Phosphate bonds, 405, 529
Phosphate buffers, 209, 463
Phosphate esters, 262, 333
Phosphate ions, 438, 469
Phosphates, 153, 190, 359, 376, 379, 397, 399, 401, 438, 442, 443, 452, 464, 473, 507, 510, 511, 530
Phosphatidyl choline, 335, 416, 421, 498
Phosphatidyl ethanolamine, 336, 421, 449
Phosphatidyl serine, 336
Phosphoenol pyruvate, 336
Phosphofructokinase, 383, 402, 403
Phosphoglucoisomerase, 402, 410
Phosphoglucomutase, 399, 400, 401, 402, 410, 507
Phosphoglycerate, 402, 403, 404, 410
Phosphoglycerides, 333, 334, 338, 387, 392
Phosphoglyceroisomerase, 402
Phosphoglycerokinase, 402, 403, 410
Phosphoglyceromutase, 402, 403
Phosphohexoseisomerase, 400
Phospholipids, 22, 262, 325, 333, 337, 360, 416, 421, 442, 449, 455
Phosphoprotein, 359
Phosphoric acid, 192, 325, 335, 336,

338, 376, 379, 527, 529
Phosphorus, 22, 55, 60, 485, 510, 511, 516
Phosphorylase, 262, 400, 401, 402, 412, 507
Phosphorylation, 378, 398, 399, 405, 407, 411, 504, 514
Phosphosphingosides, 333, 337
Phosphotriose isomerase, 402, 403
Phototherapy, 491
Photosynthesis, 17, 299, 300
Physical change, 16, 24
Physical constance, 143
Physical properties, 16
Physiological saline solutions, 173, 208
Picric acid, 363
PIF, 519
Pigmentation, 495
Pinocytotic vesicle, 378
Pituitary gland, 515, 517, 519
PKU, 444, 540
Placenta, 516, 520
Placque, 38
Plant nutrients, 155
Plasma, 448
  enzyme levels, 382
  lipids, 445
  proteins, 450, 455, 456, 457, 459
  substitutes, 450
  volume, 450
Plasmids, 541, 542
Plasmin, 460
Plasmogens, 337
Plasmolysis, 175
Plaster of paris, 148, 208
Platelets, 64, 448, 449, 459, 460
beta-Pleated sheet, 356
Plummer's disease, 541
Pneumonia, 113, 121, 281, 452, 465, 481
Poisons, 453, 464
Polar amino acids, 349, 350, 358
Polar liquids, 160, 331
Polar covalent bonds, 79
Polar molecules, 143, 160
Polarized light, 302, 304, 312
Poliomyelitis, 155, 458, 465
Pollutants, 155, 163
Polyatomic ions, 76
Polyatomic molecules, 73
Polycythemia, 449, 452
Polyethylene, 236, 237
Polyhydroxyaldehydes, 298
Polyhydroxyketones, 298
Polymerization, 236, 300
Polymers, 230, 236, 265, 526
Polyneuritis, 490
Polypeptides, 354, 355, 361, 379, 380, 391, 392, 426, 503, 505, 507, 508, 510, 516, 518, 519, 522, 536, 537
Polypropylene, 236, 237

Polysaccharides, 256, 298, 299, 307, 315, 316, 317, 381, 391, 396, 452
Polystyrene, 237
Polyuria, 419, 438, 450, 471, 511
Polyvinylchloride, 230, 237
Porphyn, 287
Porphyrins, 287
Positron emission transverse tomography, 51
Posterior lobe, 515, 517, 519
Postoperative shock, 173
"Pot," 292
Potassium, 22, 452
Potassium bicarbonate, 463
Potassium bisulfate, 329
Potassium buffers, 463
Potassium chlorate, 139
Potassium hydrogen tartrate, 259
Potassium hydroxide, 205, 330
Potassium iodide, 208
Potassium ions, 386, 443, 452, 464, 465, 470, 471, 472, 473, 507, 512, 513, 516
Potassium oxalate, 459
Potassium permanganate, 139, 258
Potassium sodium tartrate, 208, 259
Potential energy, 17, 72
Precipitate, 90, 152, 330
Precipitated chalk, 208
Prefixes, 226
Pregnancy, 63, 340, 412, 442, 444, 452, 453, 475, 480, 484, 487, 489, 490, 492, 500, 520
Pregnanediol, 521, 522
Premature infants, 125
Pressure, 103, 159
Pressure cooker, 142
Pressure–temperature relationship, 107
PRH, 519
PRIH, 519
Primary alcohol, 244, 245, 250, 253, 256, 304
Primary amine, 262, 263, 265, 430
Procaine hydrochloride, 264
Procaine penicillin G, 176
Products, 90
Progestational hormones, 520, 521
Progesterone, 279, 517, 521, 522
Prolactin, 516, 517
Prolactin release-inhibiting factor, 519
Prolactin-releasing hormone, 519
Prolamines, 362
Proline, 350, 432, 507, 518, 535
Prontosil, 282
Proof, 242
Propanal, 252
Propane, 221, 223
Propanethiol, 246
Propanetriol, 243
Propanoic acid, 257, 301

Propanol, 240, 243, 244, 245, 254
Propanone, 254, 255
Propene, 230, 231, 232, 236, 237
Propionaldehyde, 252
Propionic acid, 257,
Propionyl CoA, 418
Propyl, 224
Propyl alcohol, 240, 243, 244, 300
Propylbutanoate, 261
Propylbutyrate, 261
Propylene, 236, 237
Propyne, 233
Prostacyclin, 339, 340
Prostaglandins, 280, 323, 339
Prostate gland, 383, 517
Protamine, 506
Protamine zinc insulin, 506
Proteases, 377, 379
Protein, 236, 241, 265, 334, 346, 348, 371, 373, 375, 377, 379, 380, 386, 391, 392, 397, 411, 432, 434, 437, 443, 451, 467, 468, 474, 479, 490, 495, 503, 505, 506, 510, 511, 515, 516, 532, 534
  absorption, 392
  amphoteric nature, 352
  body's requirements, 427
  buffers, 463
  classification, 358, 359, 361
  colloidal nature of, 361
  color tests, 363
  composition, 348, 359
  conjugated, 375
  denaturation, 138, 240, 373
  digestion, 391
  functions, 346, 361, 425
  inadequate, 426
  incomplete, 427
  kinase, 400, 504, 514
  metabolism, 375, 407, 410, 425, 433, 440, 494, 511
  molecular weight, 347
  percentage composition, 358
  primary structure, 355
  properties, 361
  protective, 361
  secondary structure, 355, 373
  shape, 361
  simple, 358
  sources, 346
  structural, 361
  structure, 355, 373
  synthesis, 426, 505, 515, 526, 533, 536, 537
Protein-bond iodine, 507
Proteinases, 379
Proteinuria, 443
Proteosis, 355, 391
Prothrombin, 317, 449, 459, 460, 488
Proton, 9, 45, 192, 196, 264, 491
Protoplasm, 180
Provitamin A, 480

Pruritus, 493
PSP, 445
Psychedelics, 263, 288, 291
Psychoactive drugs, 288
Psychomimetics, 291
Psychoneuroses, 292
Psychoses, 291, 472, 475
Pteridine nucleus, 495, 496
Pteroic acid, 495
Pteroylglutamic acid, 495
Pteroylheptaglutamic acid, 495
Pteroyltriglutamic acid, 495
Ptomaines, 393, 431
Ptyalin, 377, 389, 392
Pulmonary disease, 466
Pulmonary edema, 465, 514
Pulmonary respiration, 109, 124
Pulse rate, 248, 440
Purine, 287, 376, 433, 528
Putrescine, 264, 393, 431
PVC, 230, 237
Pyloric obstruction, 452
Pyridine, 286
Pyridoxal, 493
Pyridoxal phosphate, 427, 430, 493, 494
Pyridoxamine, 493, 494
Pyridoxine, 377, 474, 489, 493
Pyrimidine, 286, 287, 433, 528
Pyrogallol, 298
Pyroglutamylhistidylproline amide, 518
Pyrophosphate, 401, 401, 494
Pyrophosphate bonds, 380
Pyrrole, 286, 287, 453
Pyruvate, 400, 402, 403, 404, 410, 431
Pyruvic acid, 258, 400, 405, 406, 407, 408, 417, 428, 432, 434, 490
Pyruvic carboxylate, 410
Pyruvic kinase, 402, 403

Quarks, 29
Quaternary ammonium salts, 264, 335
Quaternary structure, 358
Quinine, 293
Quinone, 277

Rabbit test, 442
Rachitic rosary, 485
Rad, 48
Radiation, 363, 453, 537
  biologic effects, 61, 64
  detection and measurement, 48
  in medical treatment, 65
  sickness, 63
  sources, 65
  standards, 64
  pipes, 44
  units, 47
Radioactive iodine, 510

Radioactive material, 155, 508
Radioactive tracer, 453
Radioactivity, 42
Radioimmunoassay, 53, 55, 507
Radioisotopes, 49, 53
Radiopaque, 56, 207
Rancidity, 329
Rat antidermatitis factor, 493
Ratio solutions, 163
Rayon, 237, 317
RDS, 168
Reactants, 90
Reacting substances, nature of, 97
Reaction rates, 93, 97
Reactors, 66
Reagent papers, 445
Reagent tablets, 445
Receptor sites, 333, 360
Recombinant DNA, 543
Red blood cells, 55, 63, 334, 370,
    388, 402, 404, 431, 444, 448,
    449, 461, 462, 463, 475, 487,
    522, 538, 540
Reducing agents, 133, 138, 253, 363,
    399
Reducing properties, 314
Reducing sugars, 314
Reduction, 132, 253, 311
Relative weight, 30
Relaxant, 293
Relaxin, 522
Release-inhibiting factors, 519
Releasing hormones (factors), 518
REM, 48
Renal albuminuria, 443
Renal arteries, 436
Renal diabetes, 444
Renal disease, 443, 452, 465
Renal erythropoeitin factor, 449
Renal failure, 464, 472
Renal proteinuria, 443
Renal scans, 54
Renal stones, 511
Renal threshold, 397, 411, 412, 514
Renin, 56, 380, 383, 522
Rennin, 377, 391
Replacement reaction, single, 92, 194
Replication, DNA, 531
Repressor, 536
Reserpine, 293
Resonance, 269, 270
Resorcinol, 276
Respiration, 104, 247, 460
Respirator, 104
Respiratory acidosis, 465
Respiratory alkalosis, 465
Respiratory center, 464, 465
Respiratory chain, 417, 432
Respiratory disease, 452, 481
Respiratory distress syndrome, 168
Respiratory paralysis, 473
Restriction enzymes, 541
Reticuloendothelial cells, 388

Retinal, 380, 482
Retinal isomerase, 380
Retinene reductase, 474
Retinoic acid, 482
Retinol, 244, 480
Retinol equivalent, 480
Retrolental fibroplasia, 125
Reverse chloride shift, 462
Reverse osmosis, 171
Reversible denaturation, 361
Reversible reactions, 93
Rhamnose, 298
Rheumatic fever, 280
Rhodopsin, 302, 482
Ribitol, 490
Riboflavin, 377, 489, 490
Ribonuclease, 380, 433
Ribonucleic acid. See RNA
Ribose, 304, 306, 376, 433, 494, 527,
    532
Ribosomal RNA, 532, 533
Ribosomes, 378, 503, 532, 533, 535,
    537
Ribulose, 306
Rickets, 452, 485
RNA, 144, 262, 287, 304, 433, 503,
    504, 505, 511, 514, 526, 527,
    528, 532, 533, 535
RNA polymerase, 504, 532
Rochelle salts, 208, 259
Roentgen, 48
Rolaids, 194
Rubber, 236, 243
Rubbing alcohol, 243
Rubidium, 55, 82
"Runners' high," 520

s-Sublevel, 34
Saccharic acid, 311
Saccharin, 315
Sal ammoniac, 208
Salicylic acid, 279
Saline cathartic, 175
Saliva, 201, 359, 386, 392
Salivary amylase, 379, 386, 389, 390,
    392
Salivary digestion, 386, 392
Salivary glands, 467
Salt bridge, 357, 362, 363
Salting out, 363
Salts, 204, 254, 257, 392, 436, 443,
    449, 463, 467
  heavy metal, 362
  insoluble, 160, 354
  neutral, 463
  reaction, 205
  solubility, 160, 204
  uses, 207, 208
Saponification, 328, 330
Saturated fatty acids, 323
Saturated hydrocarbons, 221, 234
Saturated solutions, 161

Scan, 48, 50
Schistosomiasis, 259
Scintillation counter, 48
SCN, 386
Scouring soap, 330
Scuba diving accidents, 111
Scurvy, 196, 500
Secobarbital, 289, 290
Seconal, 289, 290
Secretin, 387, 505
Sedation, 288
Sedatives, 293, 465, 473
  hypnotics, 288, 289
Sedimentation, 151
Selenium, 22, 55, 486, 487
Seminal fluids, 339
Semipermeable membrane, 169, 469
Serine, 337, 352, 432, 535
Serotonin, 292
Serum albumin, 361, 431, 449
Serum electrophoresis, 458
Serum globulin, 348, 354, 359
Serum potassium, 512
Sewage, 155
Sex hormones, 275, 279, 341, 421
Shock, 173, 458, 518
Sialic acid, 359
Sickle cell, 280, 355
Sickle cell anemia, 280, 383, 538
Siderophilin, 359
Silicon, 22
Silver complex ion, 253
Silver mirror test, 253, 310
Silver nitrates, 208, 362
SI units, 2
Skatole, 393
Smog, 112
Smoke, cigarette, 113
Soap, 152, 167, 197, 243, 259, 277,
    328, 330
Sodium, 22, 190, 442, 452, 470, 473
Sodium acetate, 257
Sodium benzoate, 279
Sodium bicarbonate, 195, 208, 209,
    463
Sodium chloride, 208, 512
Sodium citrate, 208, 258, 459
Sodium fluoride, 208
Sodium glycocholate, 388
Sodium hydroxide, 197, 205, 257, 330
Sodium hypochlorite, 139
Sodium iodide, 510
Sodium ions, 439, 442, 452, 464, 469,
    470, 471, 473, 512, 513, 516,
    522
Sodium lauryl sulfate, 372
Sodium nitroprusside, 255, 444
Sodium pertechnate, 54
Sodium phenoxide, 275
Sodium salicylate, 274
Sodium stearate, 259, 328, 330
Sodium sulfate, 208
Sodium taurocholate, 388

Sodium thiosulfate, 139
Solid solution, 161
Solid state, 14
Sols, 180
Solubility, 159, 204
Solute, 158, 163, 247
Solutions, 158
  buffer, 208
  conductivity, 186, 188
  dilution, 166
  importance of, 161
  special properties, 167
  strength, 161
Solvent, 158, 159, 242, 247
Somatomedins, 516
Somatostatin, 506, 519, 541
Somatotropin, 515
Sorbitol, 311
Specific gravity, 7, 143, 450, 470
Specific inhibitors, 373
"Speed," 290
Spermaceti, 332
Spermatozoa, 517
Sphingolipids, 337
Sphingomyelin, 337, 416, 455, 498, 541
Sphingomyelinase, 337, 541
Sphingosine, 325, 333, 337
Sphygmomanometer, 104
Spirits of ammonia, 198
Spleen, 388, 431, 474
Sponge baths, 242
Spontaneous combustion, 118
Stain remover, 139
Standard meter, 2
Standard pressure, 104
Stannous fluoride, 208
Starch, 180, 236, 243, 307, 315, 316, 379, 386, 389, 390, 392, 396
Starling's hypothesis, 456
Starvation, 209, 407, 419, 426, 442, 444, 452, 470, 471
State, change of, 15
States of matter, 13
Steapsin, 379, 388
Stearic acid, 259, 323, 330
Stem, 77
Stercobilin, 431, 433
Stercobilinogen, 431, 433
Sterile solution, 150
Sterility, 63, 482, 487
Sterilization, 362
Steroids, 325, 341, 449, 503, 512
Sterols, 325, 483
Stimulants, 288, 290, 528
Stimulators, 518
Storage protein, 361
STP, 111, 291
Streptococci, 460
Streptokinase, 460
Streptomycin, 537
Styrene, 237

Substitution reactions, 92, 234
Substrate, 370, 377, 379, 381, 405
Succinate, 497
Succinic acid, 406, 408, 432
Succinic dehydrogenase, 408
Succinyl CoA, 406, 408, 418, 432, 490
Succinyl CoA synthetase, 408
Sucrase, 314, 379, 387, 390, 392
Sucrose, 149, 243, 298, 309, 312, 314, 315, 348, 379, 390, 392
Sugar, 396, 506, 527
  sweetness of, 315
Sulfa drugs, 282, 499
Sulfacetamide, 282
Sulfadiazene, 282
Sulfamethoxazole, 282
Sulfanilamide, 281, 282, 375, 382, 499
Sulfanilic acid, 281
Sulfapyridine, 282, 286
Sulfates, 439, 443, 516
Sulfhydryls, 246
Sulfur oxides, 112, 129, 138
Sulfuric acid, 192, 195, 205, 245, 246, 247, 364
Sunshine vitamin, 483
Superoxide, 126
Superoxide dismutase, 127
Supersaturated solution, 162
Suppositories, 243
Surface-active agent, 336
Surface area, 99, 159, 378
Surface tension, 168, 331, 388
Surfactants, 167, 331
Surgical casts, 148
Suspension, 176
Symbols, 20, 73
Syndets, 331
Synthetic organic chemicals, 155
Systeme Internationale, 2

T waves, 471
T_3, 508
T_4, 508
Tachycardia, 291, 470, 490
Tagged atoms, 49
Tannic acid, 363
Tartar emetic, 259
Tartaric acid, 259
Tay Sachs disease, 339, 538, 541
Technetium, 47, 53, 54, 65
Teeth, 56
Teflon, 230
Temperature, 98, 102, 121, 143, 159, 470, 512
  effects of, 95, 371
  optimum, 372
  scales, 8
Tertiary alcohols, 245, 250

Tertiary amines, 262, 263, 264
Tertiary butyl alcohol, 245
Tertiary structure of protein, 357, 373
Testosterone, 279, 342, 517, 522
Tetany 452, 472, 510
Tetrachloromethane, 228
Tetracycline, 381, 537
Tetradecapeptide, 519
Tetraethyl lead, 236
Tetrahedron, 217
Tetrahydrofolic acid, 496
Tetramethyl ammonium iodide, 264
Tetroses, 299, 304
Thallium, 55
Theobromine, 287
Theophylline, 287, 528, 529
Thermal pollution, 155
Thiamine, 264, 286, 292, 377, 479, 491, 499, 528
Thiamine hydrochloride, 264
Thiamine pyrophosphate, 490
Thiazides, 445
Thiazole, 286
Thin-layer chromatography, 366
Thiocyanate, 386
Thioesters, 262
Thiols, 246
Thoracic duct, 392
Three-dimensional arrangement, 217
Threonine, 352, 353, 432, 535
Threose, 304
Thrill, 289
Thrombin, 317, 459, 460
Thrombocytes, 449
Thromboplastin, 360, 459
Thromboxanes, 339, 340, 360
Thrombus, 460
Thymine, 287, 528, 529, 530, 531, 532
Thyrocalcitonin, 508
Thyroglobin, 348, 508, 510
Thyroid
  carcinoma, 508
  condition, 53, 208
  glands, 467
  hormones, 22, 190, 508, 510
  scans, 54, 65
Thyroid-stimulating hormone, 510, 516, 518
Thyroidectomies, 510
Thyrotropic hormone, 514, 516
Thyrotropic-releasing factor, 516, 518
Thyrotropic-releasing hormones, 518
Thyrotropic-stimulating hormones, 518
Thyrotropin, 360
Thyroxine, 508, 509, 510, 516
Tin, 22
Tincture, 159, 242
Titration, 198
TNT, 273
Tobacco mosaic virus, 348

Tobacco smoke, 112
Tocopherols, 244, 486
Tolbutamide, 506
Tollen's reagent, 253, 310
Toluene, 273, 278, 279
Torr, 104
Toxic adenoma, 510
Toxic amines, 393, 431
Toxins, 361
TPP, 490
Trace elements, 22
Tranquilizers, 472
trans structures, 480, 482
Transaminases, 427
Transamination, 427, 429
Transcellular fluid, 467
Transfer RNA, 532, 533
Transferases, 379
Transferrin, 449, 458, 474
Transfusions, 173, 450
Transition elements, 39
Transketolase, 490
Transplantation, 450
Transport potein, 361
trans-retinal, 380
TRF, 516, 517
TRH, 518, 519
Tricylglycerols, 326, 416, 455
Triatomic molecules, 127
Tricarboxylic acid, 258
Trichloracetic acid, 195
Trichloromethane, 228
Triglygerides, 326, 327, 341, 392, 416, 421
Triiodothyronine, 508
Trimethylamine, 263, 264
Trinitrotoluene, 273
Triolein, 329
Triosis, 299, 304
Tripalmitin, 328
Tripeptides, 354, 355, 518
Triplet code, 535
Trisodium phosphate, 153
Tristearin, 325, 328, 329, 348
Trypsin, 370, 372, 375, 377, 379, 382, 383, 391, 392
Trypsinogen, 387, 391
Tryptophan, 350, 353, 363, 364, 393, 427, 432, 492, 493, 507, 535
TSH, 360, 510, 514, 515, 516, 517, 518, 519
TSP, 153
Tuberculosis, 452, 512
Tumors, 58, 60
Tums, 194
Tylenol, 280
Tyndall effect, 178
Typhoid fever, 155
Tyramine, 431
Tyrosinase, 540
Tyrosine, 352, 363, 364, 366, 431, 432, 439, 535, 540

Ubiquinine, 278
UDP, 399, 400, 401
UDPG, 399, 400, 401
UDPG pyrophosphorylase, 399, 400, 401
Ultrasonography, 59
Ultraviolet rays, 113, 363, 483, 484
Units, 2, 47
Unsaturated fatty acids, 323, 417, 418, 486
Unsaturated hydrocarbons, 234
Unsaturated solutions, 162
Unsaturation, 325, 327
"Uppers," 290
Uracil, 287, 399, 528, 532, 533, 535
Urates, 440, 441
Urea, 214, 266, 377, 426, 428, 429, 430, 433, 437, 438, 439, 440, 443, 445, 449, 452, 512
Urea clearance test, 445
Urea cycle, 389, 428, 429
Urea nitrogen, 452
Urease, 377
Uric acid, 126, 433, 439, 440, 441, 442, 449, 452, 474, 512, 516, 528, 529
Uricase, 474
Uridine diphosphate glucose, 399
Uridine triphosphate, 399
Uridyltransferase, 540
Urinary obstruction, 452
Urinary preservative, 273
Urine, 8, 201, 254, 315, 362, 363, 393, 397, 431, 433, 437, 467, 493, 505, 510, 512, 514, 521, 522, 540
Urobilin, 388, 431, 433, 436, 437, 438, 439, 442
Urobilinogen, 388, 431, 433, 439, 442
Urochrome, 388
UTP, 399, 400, 401

Vaccines, 541
Vaccuble, 378
Valence electrons, 39, 72, 73
Valine, 350, 353, 432, 535, 538
Vanadium, 22
Vanillin, 278
van't Hoff, 302
Vapor pressure, 145
Vasoconstrictor, 380
Vasopressin, 438, 517, 522
Vegetable oils, 324
Venoms, 361
Venous blood, 109
Ventilation lung scan, 55
Ventricular fibrillation, 514
Vinegar, 258
Vinyl chloride, 233, 237
Vinyl group, 231

Virucide, 128
Viruses, 64, 433, 531
Viscose, 317
Viscosity, 168, 353, 451
Vision, 465
Visual purple, 482
Vitamins, 283, 292, 375, 376, 377, 386, 442, 449, 474, 479, 503
  A, 244, 302, 328, 480, 486, 487, 510
  B_1, 264, 266, 286, 489, 528
  B_2, 490
  B_6, 286, 377, 427, 474, 493
  B_{12}, 55, 286, 287, 377, 387, 418, 453, 475, 489, 496
  C, 499
  D, 275, 328, 341, 421, 443, 472, 480, 511, 522
  E, 128, 244, 377, 486
  K, 377, 393, 460, 487
VLDL, 360, 455
Vomiting, 65, 209, 289, 309, 439, 450, 452, 465, 467, 470, 471, 473, 486

Warts, 195, 279
Washing soda, 148, 153
Wasting illness, 426
Water, 55, 141, 160, 168, 379, 386, 387, 392, 404, 408, 409, 427, 428, 432, 436, 437, 438, 449, 451, 462, 468, 470, 479, 511, 513, 517, 518
  balance, 449, 456, 466, 518
  constants based on, 143
  of crystallization, 147
  deionized, 154
  distilled, 150, 173
  distribution, 467, 511
  hardness, 330
  of hydration, 147
  impurities of, 152
  ionization of, 199
  pollution, 155, 163
  properties, 141, 147, 149
  purification, 128, 150, 171
  reactions, 147
  retention, 380
  softeners, 153
  structure, 143
  treatment, 134
  vapor pressure, 146
Water-soluble vitamins, 479, 489
Watson, J. D., 526
Watson-Crick DNA model, 529
Waxes, 325, 332
Weight, 2
Weight-volume method, 162
Welding, 236
White blood cells, 63, 448, 449
Whole body scans, 55

Wilson's disease, 382, 383, 458, 474, 540
Wintergreen, 280
Wöhler, Frederick, 214
Wood alcohol, 241, 242

X rays, 45, 48, 55, 65, 207, 208, 363
X-ray scanner, 57
X-ray therapy, 56
Xanthoproteic test, 363

Xenon, 55
Xerophthalmia, 481
Xeroradiography, 58
Xylene, 274
Xylose, 306, 359

Yeast, 310, 314

Zein, 427
Zeolite, 153, 182

Zephiran chloride, 264
Zinc, 22, 372, 391, 474, 482, 494, 505
Zinc stearate, 330
Zinc undecylenate, 330
Zirconium chlorohydrate, 475
Zone electrophoresis, 366
Zwitterions, 352
Zymogens, 383, 387, 391